The Cell Biology of Schistosomes

Implications for Diagnostics and Vaccines

This monograph is dedicated to the postgrads, postdocs, final year project students and visiting researchers from six continents who explored the fascinating world of flukes at York. A special mention for the three individuals who successively maintained the schistosome life cycle for 45 years, without whose endeavours the research would not have been possible. My personal thanks go to Barnesy, Pat and Gill who, down the years, converted my creative ideas into effective experiments.

The Cell Biology of Schistosomes

Implications for Diagnostics and Vaccines

R. Alan Wilson

Department of Biology and
York Biomedical Research Institute
University of York
York
YO10 5NG
UK

CABI

CABI is a trading name of CAB International

CABI
Nosworthy Way
Wallingford
Oxfordshire OX10 8DE
UK

Tel: +44 (0)1491 832111
E-mail: info@cabi.org
Website: www.cabi.org

CABI
200 Portland Street
Boston
MA 02114
USA

Tel: +1 (617)682-9015
E-mail: cabi-nao@cabi.org

A catalogue record for this book is available from the British Library, London, UK.

ISBN-13: 9781800625143 (hardback)
9781800625150 (ePDF)
9781800625167 (ePub)

DOI: 10.1079/9781800625167.0000

Commissioning Editor: Jamie Lee
Editorial Assistant: Theresa Regueira
Production Editor: Helen Elliott

Typeset by Straive, Pondicherry, India
Printed and bound in the UK by CPI Group (UK) Ltd, Croydon CR4 0YY

Contents

Supplementary Content

Acknowledgements

I would like to thank the following for their special contributions to the preparation of this monograph: my former colleague in the York Biology Department, Dr Patricia Coulson, for reading and commenting on all the chapters; Dr Paul McVeigh, School of Biological Sciences, Queen's University, Belfast, for providing a critique of Chapter 5 (The Nervous System); and Dr Govert van Dam, Leiden University Medical Centre, Leiden, for reading Chapter 12 (Diagnostics) and providing his unpublished data for Fig. 12.4.

Prelude: What Are Schistosomes?

The schistosomes that form the subject of this monograph are, in their adult stage, macroscopic threadlike worms parasitic in the bloodstream of mammals. The species of *Schistosoma* infecting humans are located in the vessels of the hepatic portal system between the walls of the intestine and the liver, or in the vesical plexus of the bladder wall. This means that schistosomiasis, the disease they cause, is referred to as intestinal or urogenital. It is also colloquially known as 'bilharzia' after Theodor Bilharz who first described it in Egypt. The World Health Organization (WHO) currently lists the occurrence of human infection as follows: *S. japonicum* in China, Indonesia and The Philippines; *S. mekongi* in Laos and Cambodia; *S. mansoni* in the whole of Africa, parts of the Middle East, the Caribbean, Brazil, Venezuela and Suriname; *S. intercalatum* and *S. guineensis* in Central Africa; and *S. haematobium* (urogenital) in the whole of Africa, parts of the Middle East and most recently in Corsica.

Several schistosomes are also of considerable veterinary importance as parasites of domestic livestock. In Africa these include *S. bovis* in cattle, and *S. curassoni* and *S. mattheei* in sheep and goats. In India and parts of Southeast Asia they include *S. nasale*, *S. indicum* and *S. spindale* in cattle, sheep and goats.

An important feature of schistosomes is that unlike viruses, bacteria or protozoan infectious agents, they do not multiply in the mammalian host. Their impact on the infected human is roughly proportional to the population of worms each accumulates. The major source of morbidity is the eggs which females deposit in the veins of the intestine or bladder wall. When mature, these actively recruit the immune response to aid their escape to the exterior. Some do not make it, triggering the fibrotic pathology that is the hallmark of schistosomiasis. In the average situation in an area endemic for schistosomiasis, most infected people have few worms, but a few people have many. The diagnosis of low-level infections remains a serious problem; the cryptic nature means some individuals can become seriously ill, with irreversible pathology, before infection is detected.

All schistosomes have in common the need for a freshwater gastropod snail as an obligate intermediate host and it is the distribution of the snail that limits disease prevalence. The gastropod hosts of *S. japonicum* are species of *Oncomelania* in a subclass, the Caenogastropoda, related to marine winkles, which can close their shells using a horny operculum. *S. mekongi* uses another caenogastropod, *Neotricula*. Hosts of the remaining human schistosomes are species of the genera *Bulinus* and *Biomphalaria*, members of the family Planorbidae, in the clade Panpulmonata, a distinct group of gastropods. Some biologists suggest that this is part of the evidence that *S. japonicum* is basal in the evolution of the genus. It is certainly the exception in being zoonotic in a wide range of hosts from five orders of the Mammalia.

Schistosomes are members of the class Trematoda (flukes) in the phylum Platyhelminthes (flatworms). From the cell biology viewpoint, they are triploblastic (exoderm, mesoderm and endoderm) with a solid body plan, lacking body cavities; this has manifold implications for their physiology. Taxonomically, they are placed in the Lophotrochozoa, one of two main branches of the Protostomia alongside the Ecdysozoa (nematodes and insects), and distinct from the Deuterostomia (chordates, including their definitive hosts the mammals). Editors of journals sometimes ask why in molecular studies they have not been compared with the "model worm" *Caenorhabditis*, a nematode. In fact, their nearest relatives in the lophotrochzoan clade are the phyla Mollusca and Annelida and attempts to compare schistosome genomes with those of multiple parasitic nematodes actually emphasize the differences between them.

The genus *Schistosoma* contains over 20 species with a complex taxonomy and evolution within the wider Schistosomatidae family, comprising approximately 100 species, also found in waterbirds (e.g. *Trichobilharzia*, etc). Their hosts are warm-blooded and unlike most trematodes they have separate sexes. Other blood flukes of the family Spirorchiidae parasitize marine or freshwater turtles, while those of the Aporocotylidae parasitize marine or freshwater fish. It is unclear if these families are representatives of an evolutionary line, especially as the fish and turtle flukes are hermaphrodite.

There is no fossil record and insufficient molecular data at present, so we can only speculate on the origin of trematodes in general and schistosomes in particular. Free-living flatworms probably originated in the Cambrian radiation while their intermediate host the gastropod molluscs are recorded from the end of the Precambrian (539 million years ago). The Devonian period (419–359 million years ago) is frequently called the age of the fishes. That leaves a long period when flatworms and gastropods coexisted before the first fish appeared. Given the absolute requirement for gastropods in the trematode life cycle it seems a reasonable supposition that flatworms first parasitized snails, potentially with free-living sexually reproducing adults. With the appearance of fish, the adults were added into the life cycle as the vehicle for the sexual reproduction – most trematodes inhabit the alimentary tract, immunologically a relatively safe place. The move into the bloodstream is a much bigger step, because it implies the ability to cope with the emerging vertebrate immune system. If the parasitization of fishes occurred in Devonian times, it would mean that the ancestors of schistosomes subsequently evolved alongside the vertebrate immune system right up to the present day. It would also explain why they can survive and thrive in such a supposedly hostile place as the bloodstream. They had to keep one step ahead of immune system evolution. Perhaps the Tree of Life sequencing projects will provide information to underpin these speculations.

The purpose of this monograph is to examine the cell biology of these remarkable parasites to understand their adaptations. We need also to remember that they can cause debilitating even lethal disease in their human host. Hopefully we can use that knowledge to defeat them.

1

Intramolluscan Development

1.1 Overview

Schistosomes are dependent on several genera and species of aquatic gastropod molluscs (snails) for a complex asexual multiplication process in their two-host life cycle, involving three distinct generations (Fig. 1.1).

- Generation 1: the infective miracidium larva directly penetrates the epithelium of the snail head/foot and transforms into a mother sporocyst near the entry point.
- Generation 2: the morphologically distinct daughter sporocyst develops within the mother sporocyst before emerging to undertake a migration to viscera within the spire of the shell.
- Generation 3: the cercaria larva develops within the body of the daughter sporocyst, before emerging to travel via the snail haemocoel to the mantle cavity where it exits into freshwater. The continuity of the germ line through the three generations is maintained by a cohort of germinal cells. Such cells are already present in the miracidial body, generated during embryogenesis in the egg. After transformation in the snail, they begin to divide and some progeny go on to form the somatic tissues of the daughter sporocyst while others remain undifferentiated. This process is repeated in the daughter sporocyst where the germinal cell progeny form the cercarial body or remain undifferentiated, eventually to become the precursor cells of the adult worm gonads. The asexual replication of consecutive generations in the snail creates a multiplier effect whereby a single miracidium may result in a patent infection releasing up to 3000 cercariae per day. The cercaria infects a human host by direct skin penetration, undergoing another transformation into the schistosomulum larva.

Chapter 1 covers the complex life cycle changes that underlie the progression through the three distinct generations from miracidium to cercaria, within the molluscan host.

1.2 The Miracidium

When considering the miracidium larva, we need to appreciate that it is not just a transmission stage. Its primary biological function may be to locate and penetrate the snail host, but it is also primed with all the material it needs to transform into the next stage in the cycle, the mother sporocyst. It acquired this during development of the egg within the tissues of the mammalian host (see Chapter 11), and after snail entry there is simply no time to synthesize materials required for that transformation. The non-feeding miracidium also lacks the machinery to import the

DOI: 10.1079/9781800625167.0001

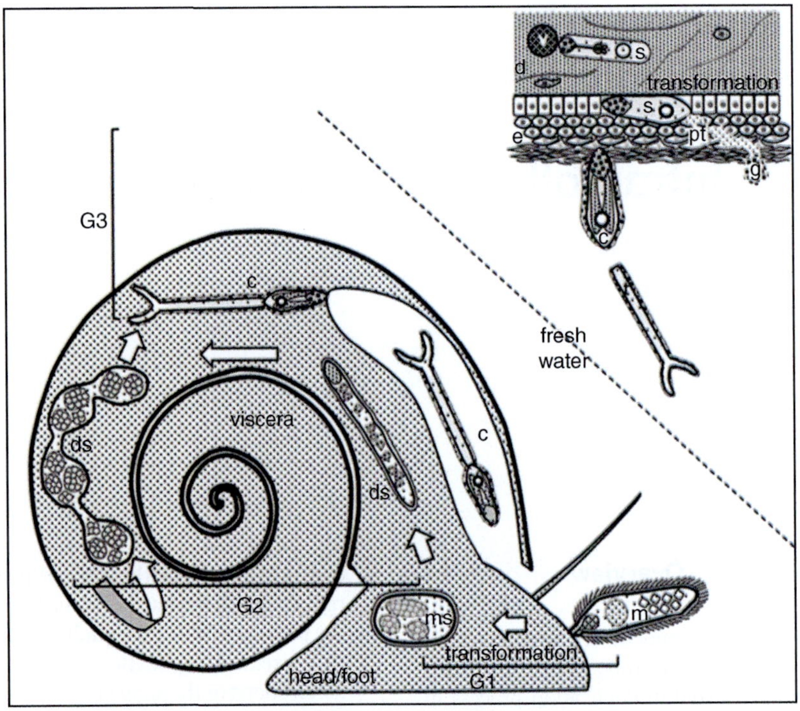

Fig. 1.1. Schematic illustration of the three life cycle generations (G1–G3) associated with the gastropod snail host (not to scale). c, cercaria; d, dermis; ds, daughter sporocyst; e, epidermis; g, glycocalyx; m, miracidium; ms, mother sporocyst; pt, penetration tunnel; s, schistosomulum; t, tail; v, venule. (From Parker-Manuel and Wilson, 2022.)

nutrients for protein synthesis and cell division. It hatches from the egg after entering fresh water in faeces or urine, when the abrupt decrease in osmotic pressure results in a lateral rupture of the shell (there is no operculum) and forceful expulsion of the larva. Apart from a short anterior region, termed an apical papilla or terebratorium, the living miracidium is covered with ciliated plates that provide the motive force for extremely rapid propulsion through freshwater (Fig. 1.2.1). It has a streamlined body form (180 μm long by 40 μm at its widest point) that is seldom captured intact by chemical fixatives and presents a remarkable example of miniaturization. We are reliant of a single transmission electron microscopy (TEM) study to provide an outline of the tissue layout in its compact body (Fig. 1.2.2) (Pan, 1980). Given the recent single-cell sequencing study that has highlighted tissue complexity (Attenborough *et al.*, 2024) there is certainly scope for a new appraisal of miracidial ultrastructure. Knowledge prior to single-cell sequencing is summarized first.

1.2.1 The body wall: propulsion, glycogen, energy metabolism and survival

The pyriform shape of the miracidium is determined by a body wall comprising a meshwork of outer circular and inner longitudinal muscle fibres. Phalloidin staining revealed 12 longitudinal fibres running from the base of the apical papilla to the extreme posterior, tapered at both ends to accommodate body shape (Fig. 1.3.1) (Bahia *et al.*, 2006). In contrast, there are approximately 60 much smaller circular fibres forming closely packed bands around the body (the relationship of these circular fibres to their cell bodies is presently unclear). The two sets of fibres are connected by inter-fibre desmosomes (Meuleman *et al.*, 1978) to form a meshwork that acts on the enclosed interstitial and intracellular fluids as a hydrostatic skeleton. The interplay of the two sets of fibres is under nervous system control, which regulates changes in body shape during swimming and snail penetration. This regulation of shape, rather than locomotion,

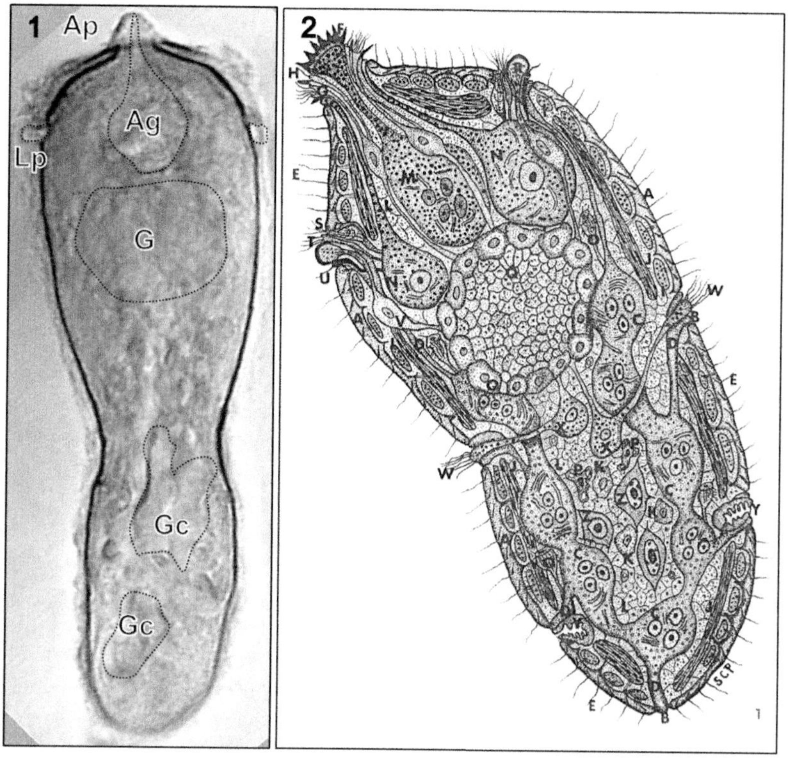

Fig. 1.2. Morphology of the miracidium. **1**) A differential interference contrast image of an *S. mansoni* miracidium that captures the body form of the live organism with apical papilla (Ap), apical gland (Ag), central ganglion (G), lateral papilla (Lp) and large germ cells (Gc). **2**) A simplified schematic of the different tissues, based on TEM: A, epidermal plate; B, epidermal ridge; C, ridge cyton; D, cytoplasmic bridge; E, cilium and rootlet; F, apical papilla; G, multiciliated, deep-pit sensory papilla; H, uniciliated sensory papilla; I, outer circular muscle fibre; J, inner longitudinal muscle fibre; K, interstitial cyton; L, processes of interstitial cells; M, apical gland and secretory duct: N, lateral gland and secretory duct; O, flame cell with excretory tubule; P, cyton of common excretory tubule: Q, neural mass with peripheral ganglia; R, lateral papilla; S, multiciliated saccular sensory organelle; T, multiciliated shallow-pit sensory papilla; U, uniciliated sensory papilla; V, perikaryon of the neuron to lateral papilla; W, multiciliated sensory papilla; X, perikaryon of the multiciliated sensory papilla; Y, excretory vesicle; Z, germ cell. (**1** from Bahia *et al.*, 2006; **2** from Pan, 1980.) Figures used with permission from **1**) Cambridge University Press and **2**) Elsevier.

is the essential property of the very thin body wall muscle fibres.

Groups of ridge cells lie immediately beneath the muscle layer, sending cytoplasmic projections to form a regular pattern of narrow ridges (Fig. 1.3.2) (Meuleman *et al.*, 1978). The ridge cells are biosynthetically active with numerous mitochondria and rough endoplasmic reticulum, but obvious secretory vesicles have not been described. They already contain the material that will form the extruded tegument when the miracidium transforms into the mother sporocyst, but lack the aggregations of small dense vesicles found in the analogous cells of the *Fasciola* miracidium (Wilson, 1971).

The ridge extensions provide the attachment sites for four tiers of densely ciliated epithelial plates, six, eight/nine, four and three cells per tier, respectively (Fig. 1.3.3) (Eklu-Natey *et al.*, 1985). Plates in the first and last tiers are triangular to accommodate the body tapers, the second and third are oblong. They are ~1 μm thick, with 7–10 μm long cilia spaced uniformly apart in all directions. Each cilium is anchored in the cytoplasm by a 1.1 μm forward pointing rootlet, a testament to the motive force generated for

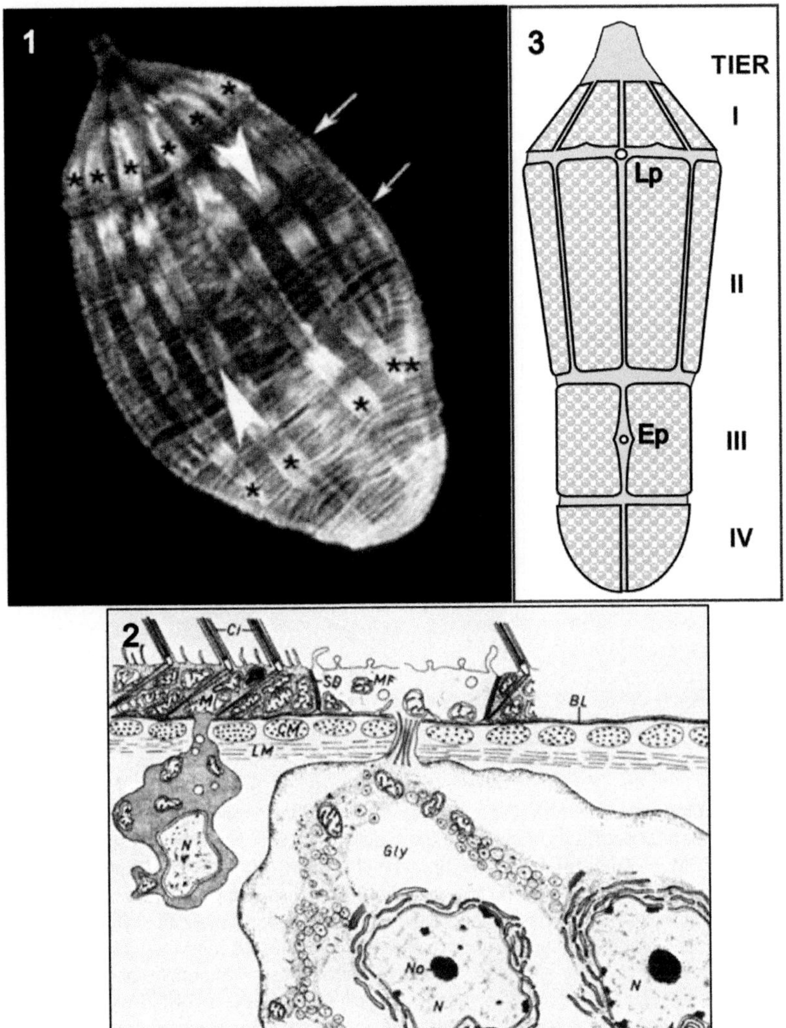

Fig. 1.3. Structure of the body wall. **1**) Z-projection of a differential interference contrast image of miracidial body with circular (arrows) and longitudinal muscle fibres (arrowheads). Accumulations of actin filaments (asterisk). **2**) Diagram summarizing the cellular relationships in the body wall. Ci, cilia; Mi, mitochondria; BL, basal layer; SD, septate desmosome; CM, circular muscle; LM, longitudinal muscle; N, nucleus; No, nucleolus; Gly, glycogen. **3**) Schematic lateral view of the epidermal plate layout with cilia 'shaved off' reveals extent of intercellular ridges (grey), with location of lateral papilla (Lp) and excretory pore (Ep). (**1** from Bahia *et al.*, 2006; **2** from Meuleman *et al.*, 1978.) Figures used with permission from **1**) Cambridge University Press and **2**) Springer Nature. **3**) Figure author's own.

swimming. The cytoplasm below the rootlets is closely packed with mitochondria, an indicator of the high energy demands of cilia-driven locomotion. It is an open question whether the plates are anucleate (Pan, 1980) or are attached to inconspicuous cell bodies below the muscle layer by thin cytoplasmic connections (Fig. 1.3.2) (Meuleman *et al.*, 1978). The beating of the cilia on the separate plates is highly synchronized but it is unclear whether this is achieved by nervous control or some other mechanism (Marinković *et al.*, 2020).

The principal energy reserve of the miracidium is glycogen, laid down during egg development in the host intestinal or bladder tissues (see Chapter 11). It is broken down by cyanide- and oligomycin-sensitive aerobic respiration, implicating the Krebs cycle coupled to the respiratory chain and oxidative phosphorylation. Neither triglycerides nor fatty acids make a contribution (Tielens *et al.*, 1991). Analysis of swimming speed at hourly intervals after hatching has revealed that reserves are adequate for 5 h, before the rates gradually decline (see Section 1.2.7); the impact of this decline on snail infectivity does not appear to have been characterized (cf. the cercaria). The glycogen reserves are held in interstitial/parenchyma cells, estimated to number 20 (Pan, 1980), which fill internal spaces and extend numerous long processes around other cells.

1.2.2 Tissue disaggregation for single-cell sequencing

The most remarkable increment in knowledge of the miracidium has come from the production of a single-cell atlas of the *Schistosoma mansoni* miracidium by enzymatic dissociation of the tissues to obtain a cell suspension (sorted or unsorted) for single-cell RNA sequencing (RNA-Seq) (Attenborough *et al.*, 2024). Counting of nuclei in a confocal Z-stack of whole miracidia gave an estimate of approximately 365 cells. A total of over 20,000 cells provided high-quality transcript data for gene expression analysis. At least 19 transcriptionally distinct clusters were identified, each with putative marker genes allowing discrimination of functions such as propulsion, host location and penetration. The miracidial cells could be split, 7% stem to 93% somatic, with the somatic cells distributed between 57% neural, 19% muscle, 13% epidermal/tegument, 2% parenchymal and 2% protonephridial populations (Fig. 1.4). The miracidium must be one of the 'brainiest' animals in existence.

Single-cell sequencing revealed two transcriptionally distinct muscle clusters, corresponding to the circular and longitudinal fibres (Attenborough *et al.*, 2024). The two have many muscle markers in common, including myosin heavy chain MYH^{+}, but can be distinguished by the expression of specific markers, using *in situ* hybridization. Cluster 1, identified by *wnt11-1* (Smp_156540) expression, highlights 28 circular muscle nuclei, located in two distinct bilaterally symmetrical lines that run from anterior to posterior (Fig. 1.5.1). The density of circular fibres revealed by phalloidin (Fig. 1.5.2) suggests that each circular cell contains multiple copies. Cluster 2, identified by *myoD* (Smp_267400) and Ca^{2+}-activated K^{+} channel (Smp_156150) expression, highlights 32 longitudinal muscle nuclei spaced regularly between the lines of the circular muscle nuclei (Fig. 1.5.2). Given that there are only 12 longitudinal fibres, the presence of 32 nuclei suggests that they could be syncytial. Nevertheless, in both instances, the cell bodies must project inwards beyond the contractile region sufficiently to be detached intact by the tissue disaggregation procedure. A third group of 12 muscle cell bodies, identified by *notum* (Smp_015820) expression, cluster on one side near the apical papilla; they may be the equivalent of the more extensive apical papilla musculature seen in, for example, the miracidium of *Fasciola* (Wilson, 1969).

Although the ridge cells were described as a syncytium (Pan, 1980), they could also be isolated by disaggregation, and were termed tegument cells (Fig. 1.5.3) (Attenborough *et al.*, 2024). Intriguingly they totalled 46, all expressing the adult tegument marker micro-exon gene *meg6* (Smp_163710), which encodes a protein of unknown function. *In situ* hybridization reveals *meg6* expression below the body wall muscles throughout, but strongest in the posterior half, clearly demarcating the ridge extensions (Fig. 1.5.5 and 1.5.6). The inverse expression of *meg6* and Smp_096390 (encoding a calcium-binding protein marker) emphasizes the demarcation between intercellular ridges and ciliated plates (Fig. 1.5.7 and 1.5.8). The plates have been described as the only truly 'miracidium-specific' cell, not found in any other life cycle stage (Attenborough *et al.*, 2024), but their derivation in the larval embryo awaits description.

Single-cell sequencing identified a small group of around nine cells (Fig. 1.5.4), expressing Smp_318890, a marker for parenchymal cells (Attenborough *et al.*, 2024). Two of these cells are located anterior to the brain and five to seven in the posterior body (Fig. 1.5.4). The parenchymal cells split into two subclusters, as in other life cycle stages (see Wendt *et al.*, 2020), but *in situ* hybridization did not distinguish between them in the miracidium. Despite the discrepancy in

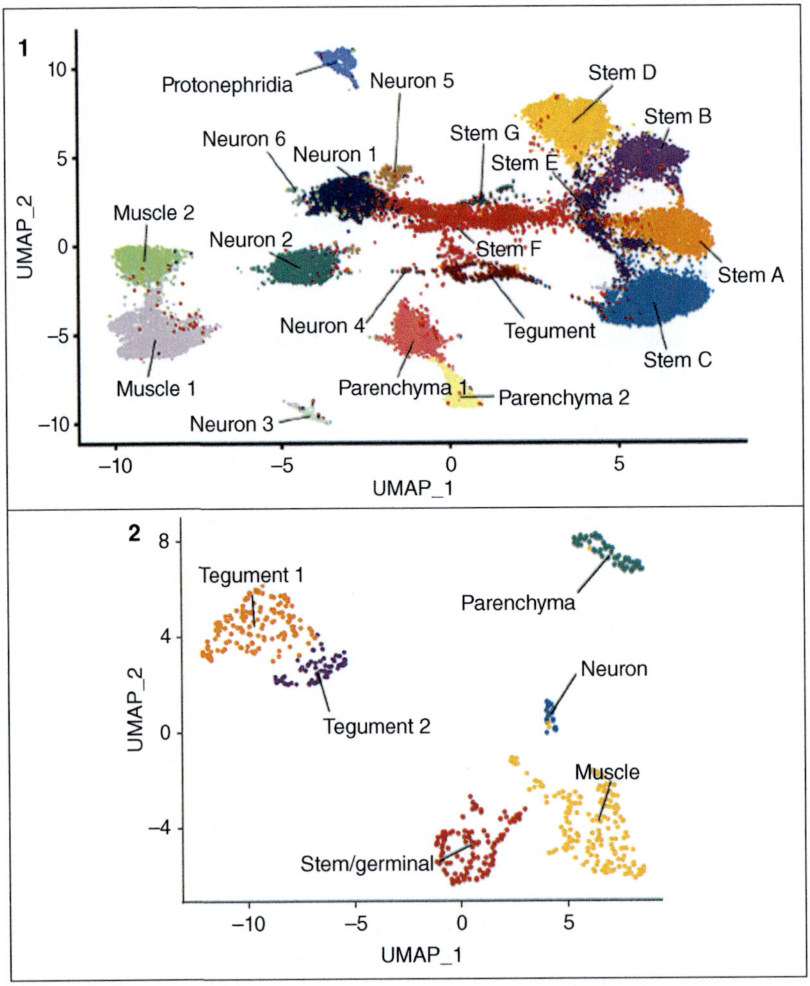

Fig. 1.4. Identification of transcriptionally distinct tissue types in the miracidium and mother sporocyst by single-cell sequencing. **1**) Isolation Uniform Manifold Approximation and Projection (UMAP) representation of 20,478 miracidium single cells. The cell clusters are distinguished by colour and label. **2**) UMAP representation of 601 single cells from mother sporocysts cultured for 5 days. (**1** from Attenborough *et al.*, 2024; **2** from Diaz Soria *et al.*, 2024.) Figures used under license CC-BY-4.0.

number, it is highly likely that the interstitial cells (Pan, 1980) and the parenchymal cells (Attenborough *et al.*, 2024) are identical.

1.2.3 The apical papilla and penetration glands

The most complex surface feature of the miracidium is the 5 μm wide, 4 μm long apical papilla (terebratorium) projecting beyond the ciliated plates at the extreme anterior, covered with a thin cytoplasmic surface extended into a complex pattern of 1 μm folds (Fig. 1.6.1) (Pan, 1980). Phalloidin staining indicated very little actin, with an absence of both retractor and circular fibres, quite unlike the highly muscularized apical papilla of *Fasciola* (Wilson, 1969). Indeed, the apical papilla has more the appearance of a biological gimlet, richly endowed with sensory papillae and gland ducts (Fig. 1.6.1). Much of the anterior quarter of the miracidial body is occupied by three large gland cells, a single apical or penetration gland in the centre, with a lateral

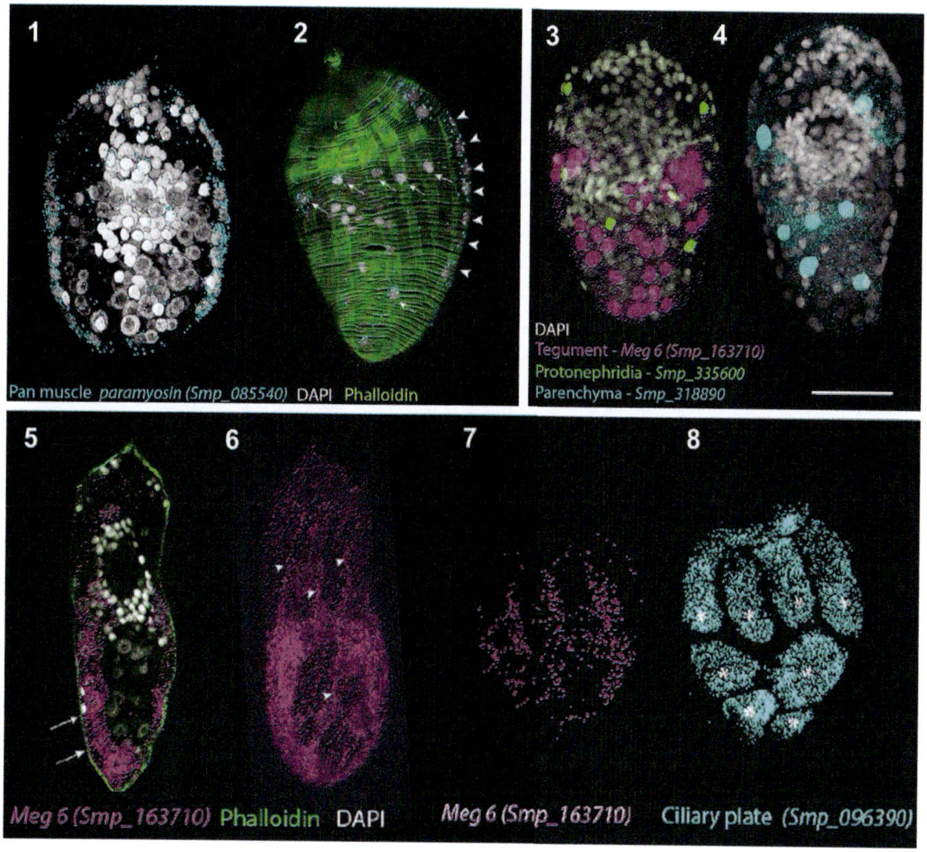

Fig. 1.5. Patterns of miracidial gene expression. **1**) Location of the pan-muscle marker *prm* (paramyosin) in muscle cell bodies revealed by *in situ* hybridization. **2**) *prm* expression counterstained with phalloidin for muscle actin. The nuclei of the circular fibres form two distinct bilaterally symmetrical lines from anterior to posterior pole (arrowhead), those of the longitudinal fibres are regularly spaced around the body (arrows). **3** and **4**) Gene expression analysed by maximum intensity projection with segmentation identifies tegument cells (*meg6*), protonephridia (Smp_335600) and parenchyma (Smp_318890). **5** and **6**) The extent of tegument cell bodies, revealed by *meg6* expression beneath the very thin body wall muscles (green). Arrows in **5** indicate the position of epidermal ridges between ciliated plates. Arrowheads in **6** indicate positions of epidermal ridges. **7** and **8**) The inverse distribution tegument cells (*meg6*) and ciliated cells (Smp_096390). (From Attenborough *et al.*, 2024.) Figure used under license CC-BY-4.0.

gland either side (Fig. 1.2.2). The vesicle contents of the two types differ in appearance, size and presumably in composition (Fig. 1.6.1); peanut agglutinin lectin preferentially stains the lateral glands only implying different glycan residues from the apical gland (Collins *et al.*, 2011). Given their putative function, we can speculate that one or both glands must contain powerful hydrolases, but information is limited. The single-cell sequencing approach failed to capture these large cells so 37 manually isolated glands were selected for sequencing (Attenborough *et al.*, 2024). Most notable among transcripts identified were genes encoding five venom-allergen-like (VAL) proteins and an α-galactosidase/α-*N*-acetylgalactosaminidase (Table 1.1).

Both proteomic and conventional transcriptomic studies on intact larvae or their secretions have also contributed information about miracidial biology. A total of six glycan hydrolases has been identified (Table 1.1) (Wu *et al.*, 2009; Mathieson and Wilson, 2010; Wang *et al.*, 2016; Mameda, 2017) and were among the most strongly upregulated transcripts in

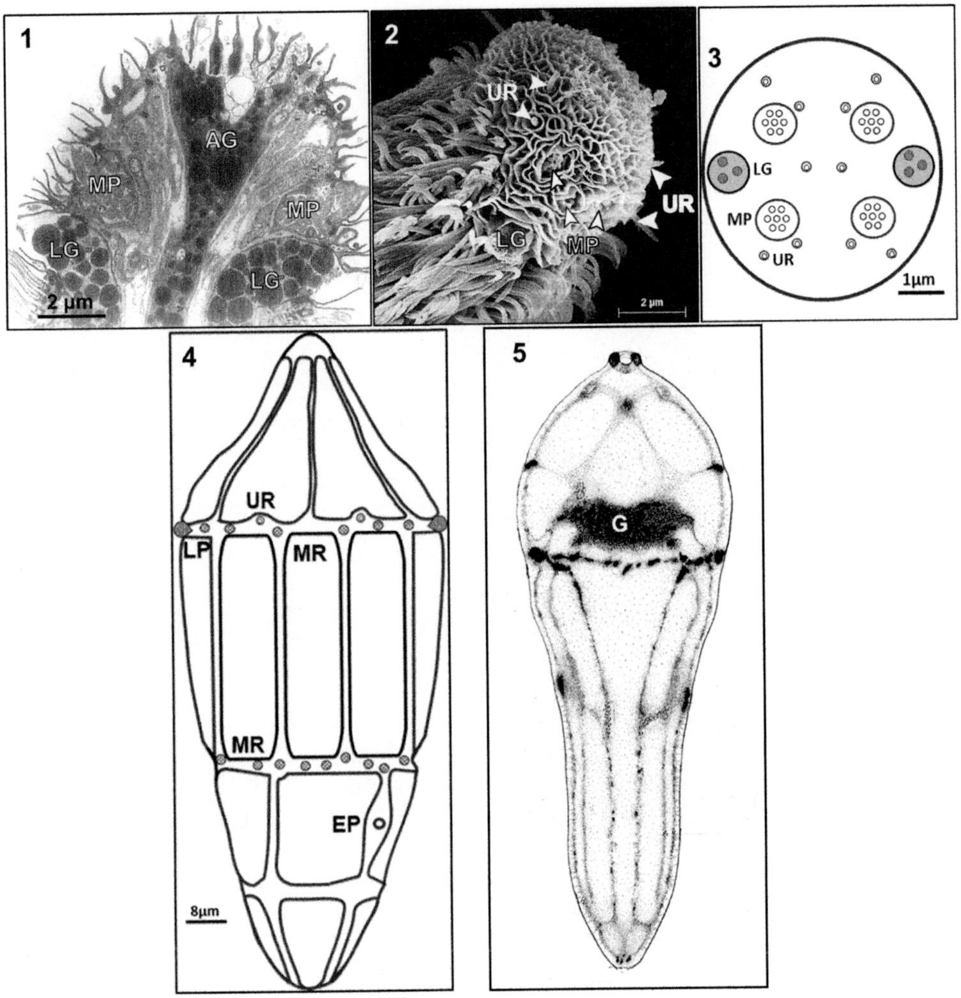

Fig. 1.6. Overview of the apical papilla, nervous system and sensory nerve endings. **1**) Longitudinal TEM section down the apical papilla showing the ducts of the lateral (LG) and apical (AG) glands. Two multiciliate pits (MP) are clearly visible and the thin surface tegument is highly folded. **2**) SEM of the apical papilla of *S. mansoni* in side view showing uniciliate receptors (UR), multicilate pits (MP) and the orifice of a lateral gland duct (LG). **3**) Map of the apical papilla of *S. japonicum* viewed end-on showing the position of lateral gland duct (LG) openings, uniciliate receptors (UR) and multiciliate pits (MP). **4**) Location of superficial sensory endings projecting through the inter-epithelial ridges. MR, multiciliate receptor; LP, lateral papilla; EP excretory pore. **5**) Outline of the miracidial nervous system stained for acetylcholine esterase. Three pairs of longitudinal nerve trunks run from the central ganglion (G) just beneath the body wall. (**1** from Pan, 1980; **2** reproduced with permission from Dr Pierre Poteaux; **3** and **4** redrawn from Eklu-Natey *et al.*, 1985; **5** from Bruckner and Voge, 1974, with permission from *The Journal of Parasitology*, KGL Publishing Services.) Figure 1 with permission from Elsevier.

mature eggs (Lu *et al.*, 2021). In contrast to this implied large capacity for dealing with the snail mucus layer, few proteases have been confidently identified to date (Table 1.1) (Wang *et al.*, 2016; Mameda, 2017; Lu *et al.*, 2021). Proteolytic activity has been detected in the culture medium during the first 24 h of miracidium/sporocyst transformation *in vitro* (Yoshino *et al.*, 1993) but

Table 1.1. Proteins identified in the miracidium; potential constituents of the apical and lateral gland cells.

		References
Glycanases		
α-*N*-acetylgalactosaminidase	Smp_179250, Smp_170830 (now Smp_334700), Smp_186710	1, 2, 3
(α-galactosidase)	Smp_247750, Smp_247760, Smp_179260	4, 5
Selected proteases		
Leishmanolysin (metalloprotease)	Smp_167070, Smp_171350, Smp_167110, Smp_167120	3
Cathepsin D	Smp_013040	
Lysosomal Pro-X carboxypeptidase	Smp_090800, Smp_076610, Smp_002600	
Dipeptidyl peptidase	Smp_019101, Smp_127840	
Calpain A	Smp_089460	
Venom-allergen-like proteins		
VAL-2, -5, -9, -15	Smp_002630, Smp_120670, Smp_176180, Smp_070250	3, 6
VAL-23, -26, -27	Smp_160250, Smp_154260, Smp_154290	3
VAL-14, -28	Smp_078490, Smp_176160	4
Tissue remodelling pathways		
Proteasome subunits		
29 components		3
Ubiquitination pathway		
23 components		3

References: 1, Wu *et al.*, 2009; 2, Mathieson and Wilson, 2010; 3, Mameda, 2017; 4, Wang *et al.*, 2016; 5, Lu *et al.*, 2021; 6, Attenborough *et al.*, 2024. Table author's own.

the suggestion that this might be a cysteine endopeptidase seems misplaced. The pH of snail haemolymph is moderately alkaline (pH ~8.0) and this is the environment into which the miracidium must penetrate. The acid dissociation constant of cysteine endopeptidases is between pH 4 and 6 (Hofer *et al.*, 2020). Serine proteases with an optimum pH of 7–8 are more likely candidates (cf. the cercarial elastases; Chapter 2). Four metalloprotease invadolysins were detected in the miracidial proteome, along with three carboxypeptidases, two dipeptidyl peptidases, cathepsin D and a calpain (Table 1.1) (Mameda, 2017). An enigmatic feature of potential gland secretions is the occurrence of up to nine VAL proteins (or transcripts) (Table 1.1). Most of these VALs are unique to the miracidium/mother sporocyst stage and we can speculate that they play a role in modifying the host environment to favour parasite establishment after penetration.

1.2.4 Protonephridia

For general details of protonephridial structure and function, see Chapter 6. The miracidium contains a dual system comprising a pair of flame cells on each side, one positioned anterior to the central ganglion, the other in the posterior. Each is connected by tubules to lateral excretory pores situated in the ridge between the third and fourth epidermal cells (Fig. 1.3.3) (Eklu-Natey *et al.*, 1985). The platyhelminth 'flame cell' is actually a composite structure of a cap cell and a tubule cell (see Chapter 6) (Wilson and Webster, 1974), with a tubule outgrowth all the way to the excretory vesicle. Single-cell sequencing has identified a marker Smp_335600 that is expressed in the cap cell (Fig. 1.5.3) (but not the barrel) and in the tubules down towards the two excretory pores (Attenborough *et al.*, 2024). Its detection by *in situ* hybridization in six cells suggests that in addition to the four cap cells there must be only two tubule cells in the miracidial system. Each excretory vesicle is a separate cell connected by desmosomes to the tubule and ridge, and its luminal surface is extended into microvilli, suggesting an absorptive function. The flame cells can be visualized by phalloidin staining of actin in the barrel wall and anti-tubulin staining of the flagellar tuft (see Chapter 6). It is surprising that such a tiny larva needs a system to filter fluid from interstitial spaces, suggesting that it possesses barriers that limit simple diffusion of metabolic waste products into the aquatic environment. Potentially this could be the glycocalyx of the epithelial plates.

1.2.5 Nervous system and sensory endings

Arguably, the most remarkable feature of the infective miracidium larva is the number, distribution and diversity of sensory nerve endings (Pan, 1980). The structural features are summarized first before the data from single-cell sequencing. Scanning electron microscopy (SEM) has revealed the pattern of folds on the apical papilla as a rosette or honeycomb, depending on the species (Fig. 1.6.2) (Eklu-Natey *et al.*, 1985; Poteaux *et al.*, 2023). Mapping of sensory endings revealed between 10 and 14 simple uniciliate endings in a symmetrical mirror pattern on the apical papilla, together with two pairs of multiciliate pits (Fig. 1.6.3). A further six uniciliate receptors are situated in the anterior ring between epithelial tiers I and II, at the mid-posterior cell margin (Fig. 1.6.4). Between 10 and 15 endings (depending on species) with multiple projecting cilia are arranged symmetrically around the body in the ridge of cytoplasm between tiers I and II, and a second circle of 18 is located between tiers II and III (except in *Schistosoma japonicum*) (Fig. 1.6.4). Such sensory endings with projecting, apparently stiff non-motile cilia have not been described for other life cycle stages. A pair of non-ciliated endings, termed lateral papillae, are located on the mid-lateral ridge between tiers I and II, rather like shoulder pads (Fig. 1.6.4); they are recorded as being fragile and easily disrupted by sonication.

The complexity of the miracidial peripheral nervous system was first established by whole-mount staining, using the enzyme acetylcholine esterase as a marker (Fig. 1.6.5) (Bruckner and Voge, 1974). A large ganglion is centrally located in the second quarter of the body, comprising a neuropile of axons and dendrites, surrounded by a tight ball of many small neuron nuclei. Six peripheral longitudinal fibres provided the connection between the ganglion and the body wall muscle meshwork. Numerous sensory fibres also ran towards the body surface terminating in ciliated sensory endings. Some ultrastructural details of these endings are available for *S. mansoni* by TEM (Pan, 1980). The uniciliate receptors are firmly anchored into the surface cytoplasm of the apical papilla by a circular septate desmosome, and the projecting cilium is partially protected by the surrounding fold of cytoplasm (Fig. 1.7.1). The cytoplasm of the terminal bulb is packed with 0.15 μm dense vesicles. The multiciliate pits connect to the exterior via a small pore, with 10–15 stubby cilia projecting into the lumen, and a cytoplasm containing 0.1 μm clear vesicles (Fig. 1.7.2). The bulbous lateral papillae contain a dense aggregation of similar vesicles, but the whole structure is covered with a thin layer of cytoplasm (Fig. 1.7.3). The multiciliate endings that project from the surface are attached by a circular desmosome to the intercellular ridge cytoplasm, which projects as a short curtain around the base (Fig. 1.7.4). The cytoplasm is also packed with the ~0.18 μm dense vesicles (Fig. 1.7.5).

Use of *cpx* (complexin; Smp_050220) expression to interrogate single-cell sequencing data identified at least 209 out of the total 365 cells as neurons (Fig. 1.8.1) (Attenborough *et al.*, 2024). These neuron cells have been subdivided in five clusters. A sixth cluster that additionally expresses *p25 alpha* (Smp_097490), a marker of ciliated neurons, is currently attributed to the ciliated epithelial plates (Attenborough *et al.*, 2024). A total of 129 *cpx*$^+$ cells formed the nuclear rind surrounding the neuropile and the remaining 80 were more peripheral, either anterior or posterior to the central ganglion (Fig. 1.8.1 and 1.8.2). Detailed *in silico* expression analysis of cluster 1 and *in situ* hybridization patterns for markers of clusters 2–4 has revealed very complex neural diversity, potentially related to function (Fig. 1.8.3). Neuron cluster 1 could be further subdivided by patterns of neuropeptide expression (e.g. *PWamide, neuropeptide F, neuropeptide Y*; see Chapter 5), while one subcluster expressed two opsin genes (Smp_180350 and Smp_332250). Clusters 2 and 3 were associated with the neuropile (Fig. 1.8.3). Cluster 2 also expressed two further rhabdomeric opsins and a neuropeptide precursor, NPP-43, while cluster 3 expressed a second neuropeptide precursor (NPP-26). The cell bodies of clusters 4 and 5 are situated peripheral to the brain. *In situ* expression of the top marker gene for cluster 4

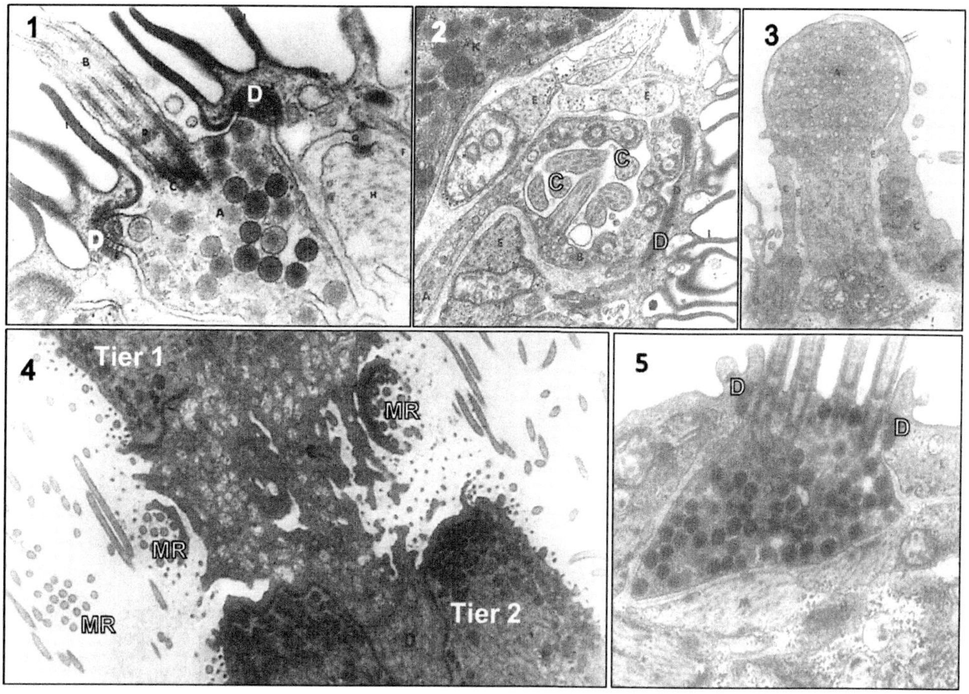

Fig. 1.7. TEM of the sensory nerve endings. **1**) A uniciliate receptor on the apical papilla, firmly attached to the surface cytoplasm by a circular desmosome (D) and surrounded by a projecting curtain. **2**) Insunk multiciliate pit with around 12 cilia (C) projecting into the luminal space, based on the profiles of axonemes and basal bodies. **3**) Bulbous lateral papilla filled with small vesicles and completely covered by a thin layer of tegument. **4**) Surface slice of the miracidium at the junction between tier I and tier II showing three multiciliate receptors (MR) in transverse section bearing 12–15 cilia, two of them with a partial protecting curtain. **5**) Multiciliate receptor in transverse section with cilia projecting above the low surrounding curtain, held in position by a desmosome. (From Pan, 1980.) Figures used with permission from Elsevier.

(Smp_319480, an analogue of human mTORC1) revealed around 26 positive cells; four at the anterior end, with projections leading to the body wall in the first tier of ciliary plates, and around 22 lying lateral and directly posterior to the brain. These 22 cells formed four clusters of around three to seven cells with projections leading into the brain at one pole and extending to the body wall at the other, terminating between the second and third tiers of ciliary plates. This is where around 23 multiciliated nerve endings are located (Fig. 1.6.4) forming a girdle around the larva between the second and third tiers of ciliary plates; Smp_319480 transcripts were expressed at the base of these cilia. Cluster 5, demarcated by Smp_343710 expression, comprises 10–20 cells whose nuclei sit outside of, and anterior to the brain, in and around the paired lateral glands and their secretory ducts. Their location suggests that they are associated with the multiple nerve endings of the apical papilla (Fig. 1.6.2). The lateral papillae are also part of cluster 5 (Fig. 1.7.3).

What can we infer about the function of the different type of nerve ending and can we relate them to the sensory modalities of the miracidium? TEM reveals detailed cell structure but also adds more receptor types not detectable on the surface by SEM. Each terminal nerve bulb bearing cilia invariably has a cytoplasm rich in tiny vesicles. The fact that the vesicle types vary in appearance between endings argues for differences in both composition and function. The uniciliate endings, with or without a protective collar, are common to all life cycle stages and numerous locations; the simplest interpretation is that they are touch/contact receptors. There are two types of multiciliate sensory ending in the schistosome

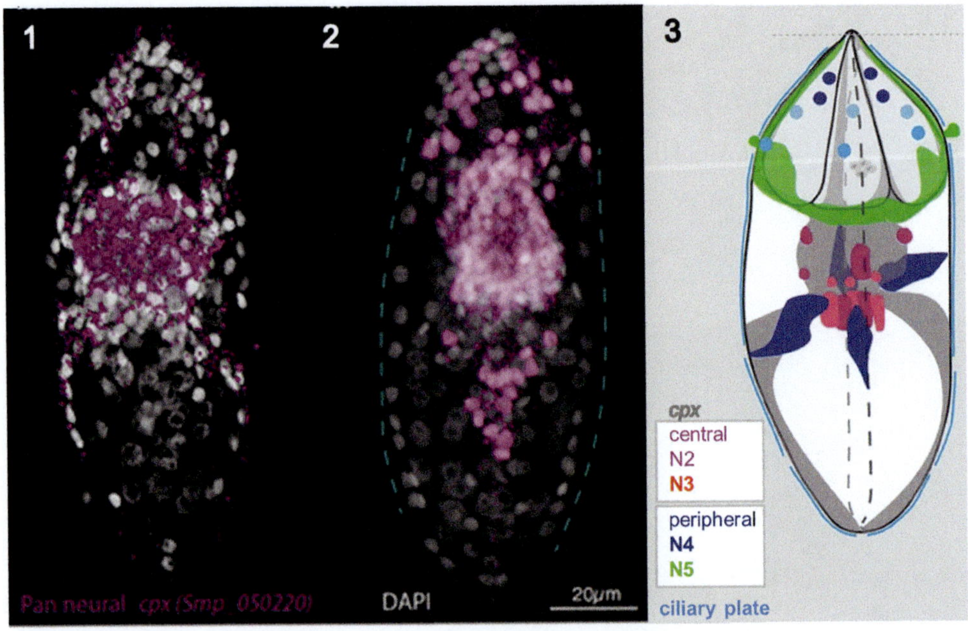

Fig. 1.8. Distribution of miracidial neuron cell bodies identified by the gene encoding complexin (*cpx*). **1**) *In situ* hybridization reveals expression in the central ganglion, in projections running forward to the apical papilla and in two posterior clusters. **2**) Maximum intensity projection with segmentation of *cpx* expression identifies their concentration around the neuropile and in groupings both anterior and posterior to it, most likely associated with ciliated sensory endings. **3**) Summary schematic of the *in situ* expression of marker genes for the different neural cell clusters. (From Attenborough *et al.*, 2024.) Figure used under license CC-BY-4.0.

miracidium. The first, a multiciliated open pit is, by analogy with other invertebrates, believed to function as a chemoreceptor. The second type, with multiple potentially stiff projecting cilia may be unique to schistosomes and is more likely a special type of mechanoreceptor. A fourth type with internal ciliated endings is more enigmatic. Stubby cilia, lacking the central pair of microtubules, project at different angles into a central space, their tips terminating in whorls of membranes. The precise location in *Schistosoma* is unclear but in *Fasciola* a pair of similar club-like structures, with cilia also lacking central microtubules, is located just below the body surface near the lateral papillae (Wilson, 1970). In *Fasciola*, the orientation of 'cilia' in various planes was taken as evidence that it could be stimulated from different directions, potentially detecting changes in the orientation of the miracidium with respect to gravity. The position of the pair on either side at the maximum distance from the mid-line reinforces this idea. The absence of photoreceptors akin to the pigmented eye spots of the *Fasciola* miracidium is notable, but the lack of melanin granules might simply make them difficult to locate by TEM. In fact, a rhodopsin Smp_180350 was found in a proteomic analysis of the miracidial membranes (Mameda, 2017) and also in the transcriptome of mature eggs (Lu *et al.*, 2021). Assigning function to G-protein-coupled receptors (GPCRs) is notoriously difficult but UniProt entry A0A3Q0KTX7 classifies this one as retinal-binding opsin photoreceptor. Thus, it appears on the basis of both protein composition and gene expression, that the miracidium possesses the molecular apparatus to transduce light but the precise cellular location of the receptor(s) remains to be demonstrated.

How do we interpret these sensory structures in the context of host location and penetration? In the absence of electrophysiological recordings, tentative speculations must be made by analogy with other invertebrate sensory endings. The simple uniciliate receptors are likely mechanoreceptors, widespread through the other life cycle stages; the curtain when present around the cilium is a way of filtering out low intensity stimuli. The multiciliate pockets open to the environment are chemoreceptors, capable of detecting host-derived chemical signals. In contrast multiciliate endings with stiff projecting cilia are mechanoreceptors; their position in two rings around the shoulders and mid-body region suggests they are intended to detect a pressure force applied evenly round the body. The obvious source of such a stimulus is the tissues of the snail skin as the parasite enters. If this assumption is correct, then it will be applied twice as the parasite gets deeper into the host.

1.2.6 Germinal cells

The first cell count based on TEM indicated around 20 germinal cells in the posterior third of miracidial body (Pan, 1980). They are large and undifferentiated, with a high nucleus to cytoplasm ratio, polyribosomes, cisternae of endoplasmic reticulum, Golgi bodies and numerous mitochondria This is very much the appearance of cells 'ready to go' when they receive the appropriate stimulus. The fate of germinal cells is covered in Section 1.3.3, but single-cell sequencing of the miracidium has revealed their complexity. Using *ago2-1* gene expression as the marker, 20–29 germinal cells were identified (median 23) (Attenborough *et al.*, 2024). They could be further split into Delta/Phi and Kappa cells on the basis of relevant markers (Fig. 1.9). This means that the dichotomy of germinal cells is already established at the miracidial stage, before cell division could be demonstrated, so must occur during embryogenesis in the egg.

1.2.7 Host location

The first task facing a miracidium, when it is expelled from the egg, is to locate its snail host and it immediately swims away. The swimming behaviour of miracidia has been characterized by recording and successive frame analysis (Carter, 1978; Dixon, 1984). In the unstimulated dispersal phase the direction of travel is in a straight line with only small angular deviations (Fig. 1.10.1 and Video 1.1). The miracidium does not rotate on its long axis as it swims so clearly is aware of the force of gravity; this tallies with the potential function of 'club-like' nerve endings as gravity receptors. Snails are proverbially slow with intermittent movement, and occasional shorts bursts of 1–2 mm/s. At 25°C, a miracidium swims at 2.2 mm/s and can maintain this speed for 5 h, before the rate tails off as energy reserves decline (Dixon, 1984); this gives it an effective dispersal radius of 36 m. The quest for a snail host has the characteristics of an 'active searching strategy', in contrast to the 'sit and wait' strategy employed by the cercaria (see Chapter 2).

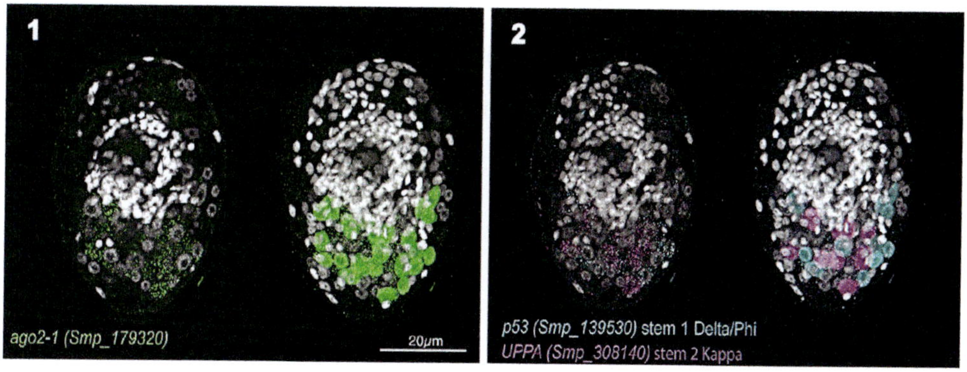

Fig. 1.9. Stem cells/germinal cells revealed by simultaneous multiplexed *in situ* hybridization of three stem cell markers in an individual miracidium. **1**) All cells expressing *ago2-1* (Smp_179320) lie in the posterior half of the body. A maximum intensity projection with segmentation highlights the location of 23 *ago2-1*$^+$ cells. **2**) The *ago2.1*$^+$ cells split into two distinct groups, Delta/Phi and Kappa, based on reciprocal expression of *p53* (Smp_139530) and uridine phosphorylase A (*UPPA*; Smp_308140), respectively. This larva has 15 Delta/Phi and nine Kappa cells. (From Attenborough *et al.*, 2024.)

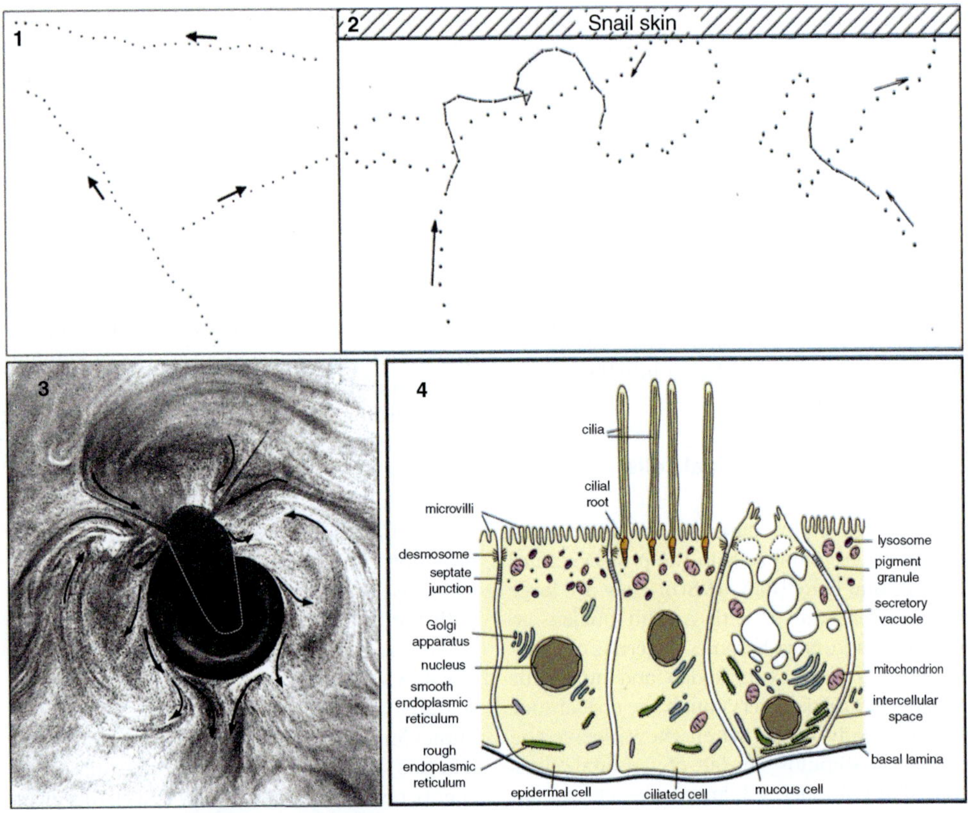

Fig. 1.10. Host location of *B. glabrata* by the miracidium of *S. mansoni.* **1**) Analysis of the swimming path of unstimulated miracidia taken from successive images. The interval between points is 0.091 s, mean speed is 2.2 mm/s and angle of right or left deviation is 8.2°. **2**) Swimming path in the vicinity of a snail. There are frequent changes of direction and turns in three dimensions which makes the larvae appear slightly slower, but the angle of turn is increased to 31°. **3**) Water currents around the snail. The area in front of the head is relatively still and water is drawn by ciliary tracts down the tentacles, across and down the head/foot, setting up mixing vortices on each side that make steep chemical gradients unlikely. **4**) Diagram of snail skin showing three basic types of epithelial cells, epidermal, ciliated and mucus-secreting, found in the molluscan epidermis. (**1–3** reproduced with permission from Carter, 1978; **4** from Ponder *et al.*, 2019.) Figure used with permission from Taylor & Francis Group LLC.

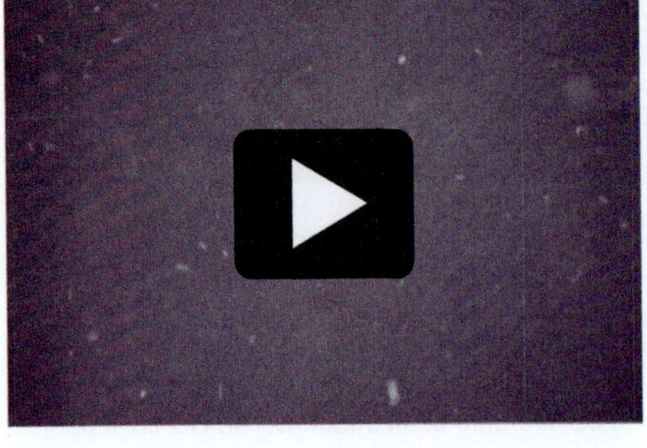

Video 1.1. The random swimming path of miracidia in the horizontal plane, uniformly illuminated from above. Coordinated beating of the epithelial ciliated plates drives a miracidium forward in a virtually straight line. Video courtesy of Dr N.P. Carter.

Changes in behaviour were detected when a miracidium came within 5 mm of a snail, but there is a pronounced variability in response, with >25% showing no change in the linear pattern. However, the majority show a marked increase in turning, right or left (Fig. 1.10.2 and Video 1.2). Miracidia lack an ability to detect the direction of the host snail and navigate towards it, even at very short distances, implying no taxis occurs. (The increased rate of turning, proportional to stimulus intensity, is termed a klinokinesis.) It has been assumed that the behavioural change involves detection of snail chemical products. However, the proximity of proposed receptor pits on the apical papilla makes it unlikely they could be used by the miracidium to navigate up a gradient. A response to the water currents swirling round the head/foot and tentacles has not apparently been considered. However, a complex pattern of such currents is generated around the snail by its epithelial cilia. These can be visualized using colloidal graphite particles (Fig. 1.10.3) (Carter, 1978), and it is entirely possible that they also influence miracidial behaviour.

Attempts to model the impact of increased turning behaviour on location of the snail target produced conflicting results. Laboratory experiments with stimulus boundaries revealed that miracidia respond more quickly to a sudden decrease in the concentration of a chemical stimulus by turning more. This should tend to keep them in or close to the zone of stimulation around the snail (Dixon, 1984). Paradoxically, computer models suggests that an increased rate of turning with successively higher levels of stimulation actually reduces the efficiency of target location because the miracidium ends up chasing its own tail. The better strategy is to have frequent reversals in direction of turn to increase the probability of contact with the snail skin.

The nature of the chemical stimulus released at the snail surface remains uncertain, with a long list of small metabolites and macromolecules proposed as attractants (Jamieson and Haas, 2017). On a personal note, in the York laboratory, steam distillation methods of the perfume industry were applied to *Biomphalaria*-conditioned water and a fraction smelling like a fruity ester was recovered, which had a dramatic effect on miracidial turning behaviour. Unfortunately, the mass spectrometric methods available failed to identify the active compound. Remarkably little research has been performed on the chemical nature of snail pheromones. Gastropods use chemical cues for homing to specific resting positions and for mate location. Predatory snails use them to locate other snails and eat them. Both volatile compounds and proteins isolated from trail mucus may act as cues to drive trail-following (Ng *et al.*, 2013). A protein pheromone, temptin, was identified as an attractant for *Biomphalaria glabrata*, by analogy with the protein pheromone complex of the marine sea snail *Aplysia* (Pila *et al.*, 2017). A recent study of the terrestrial snail *Cornu aspersum* (*Helix aspersa*) identified several proteins and nine volatile components of the secreted mucus trail (Ballard *et al.*, 2021), including one complex ester (2-methyl-1-(1,1-dimethylethyl)-2-methyl-3-propandiyl ester). It seems that identifying snail pheromones may be a fruitful approach to discover the schistosome miracidial attractant(s). In this context, the sequencing of the *B. glabrata* genome (Adema *et al.*, 2017) identified 241 GPCR genes, that are potential chemosensors. Furthermore, expression of one such gene was confirmed in the snail tentacles. The authors concluded that using chemical

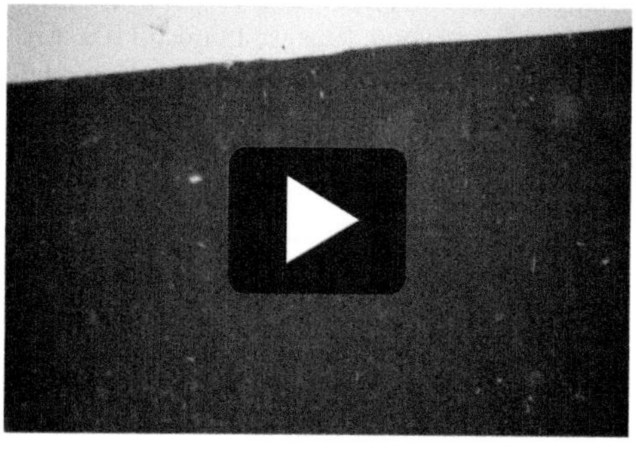

Video 1.2. The swimming path of miracidia within 5 mm of the snail skin of the head/foot region, at the top of the screen. There are frequent changes in direction, which occur in three dimensions, and may be the indirect result of differential changes in body wall muscle contraction, altering larval shape.

communication to interact with other members of your species may also provide host location signals for schistosome miracidia.

1.3 The Mother Sporocyst

1.3.1 The snail surface barrier facing the miracidium

The epidermis of the head/foot in aquatic snails like *Biomphalaria* is covered by a one cell thick epithelium comprising a mixture of three cell types: (i) standard columnar epithelial cells bearing 2 μm long microvilli, (ii) cells of similar appearance but bearing cilia and (iii) mucus-secreting goblet cells responsible for the 10–20 μm thick layer of mucus that covers the whole surface (Fig. 1.10.4) (Ponder *et al.*, 2019). The integrity of the epithelium is maintained by typical septate junctions and desmosomes at the external margin, and the layer never becomes waterproofed by the production of a cuticle (cf. arthropods) or an impervious layer of dead cells (cf. mammals). This barrier, markedly different from human skin encountered by the cercaria, must have implications for the penetration apparatus. The snail head/foot is very plastic, and this is reflected in wide estimates for epithelial thickness of between 9 and 45 μm, depending on the degree of contraction (Zylstra, 1972). The ciliated cells are grouped, the better to generate the previously mentioned water currents around the snail. The *O*-glycan composition of the surface mucus, the first contact layer for the miracidium, has been characterized in *Biomphalaria* (Stepan *et al.*, 2012). In snails generally, there is little variety in the *O*-glycosylation of proteins. A short trisaccharide is linked to a protein serine or threonine OH residue by *N*-acetylgalactosamine, and the only further modification is a methylation of the other hexose constituents. The miracidium, having located this mucus and cell layer, forms a strong attachment and rapidly penetrates it.

1.3.2 Penetration

The initial stages of penetration are hard to capture because, until the process is well under way, attempts to fix the miracidium *in situ* result in it falling off. A miracidium stimulated to attach to an artificial surface slowly rotates on its apical papilla, making it clear that the convolutions on the papilla surface (Fig. 1.6.1 and 1.6.2) interact and mesh with the microvillar extensions of a similar scale on the snail epithelium. Once a firm contact is established the miracidium begins to contract its body, coincident with the start of secretion by the apical and accessory glands. This is a holocrine process in which the entire contents of the gland, cytoplasm as well as vesicles, is voided to the exterior. The identification of several α-*N*-acetylgalactosaminidases in the miracidial proteome (Table 1.1) indicates a capacity to cause a rapid release of the *O*-glycans in the surface coating mucus layer (Stepan *et al.*, 2012). Similarly, the variety of proteases (including multiple metalloproteases) identified may be involved in punching a tight hole in the epithelial layer. Images of penetrating miracidia (Fig. 1.11.1) reveal that only a narrow lesion is created through which the miracidium squeezes, not a broader destruction of the epithelium. The potential release of the several VALs into the penetration hole at this point is intriguing and unexplored. Again, it seems plausible that during this process, the ‘shoulder pads’ are disrupted, potentially releasing neurotransmitters or neuropeptides into the penetration hole to affect the cellular barrier or underlying connective tissue.

1.3.3 Metamorphosis

Mother sporocyst development is hard to follow *in vivo* in the snail host because the transforming larvae remain near the site of penetration and are difficult to extract. However, *in vitro* cultivation methods have been developed, the most successful of which involve sterile co-culture with a *B. glabrata* embryonic (Bge) cell line, all the way to daughter sporocyst production (Yoshino and Laursen, 1995). This culture system was used to analyse the release of proteins during and after *in vitro* transformation, complicated by the presence of the Bge cells and the shed epithelial plates (Lodes and Yoshino, 1989). It was before the advent of proteomic technology that would permit precise identification of products, coupled with immunocytochemistry to localize them, and would be worth revisiting.

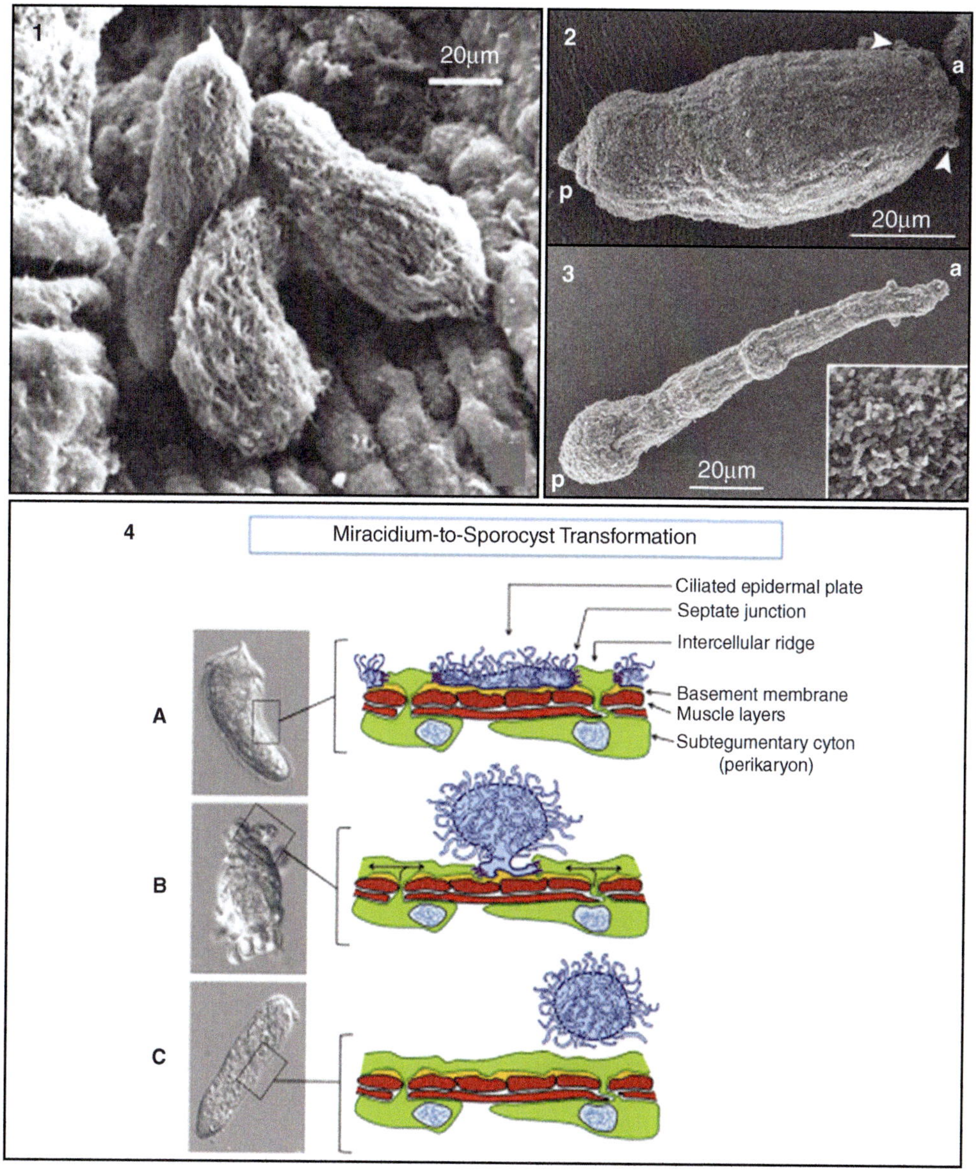

Fig. 1.11. The mother sporocyst of *S. mansoni*. **1**) Three miracidia attached to the snail head/foot adjacent to a tentacle. This shows their dimensions, relative to the snail skin cells between which they penetrate. **2**) A newly transformed mother sporocyst at 6 h in culture. Epithelial plates and apical papilla have been lost, and most sensory structures are no longer visible, but the lateral papillae remain (arrowheads). a, anterior; p posterior. **3**) Mother sporocyst after 97 h in culture. Elongation has occurred and there is a bulbous apex anterior to the lateral papillae. Inset: the body surface is covered in microvilli, presumably to aid nutrient uptake. **4**) Schematic of changes in the body surface during miracidium–mother sporocyst transformation in culture. A: miracidial surface; B: changes during cell shedding; C: newly formed mother sporocyst surface. The time base for A, B and C is 0, 6 and 24 h, respectively. (**1** from Koie and Frandsen, 1976; **2** and **3** reproduced with permission from Dr Pierre Poteaux (Poteaux *et al.*, 2023); **4** from Yoshino *et al.*, 2017.) Figures used with permission from **1**) Springer Nature and **4**) Taylor & Francis Group LLC.

There are detailed structural accounts of the drastic changes in morphology that accompany the metamorphosis of the miracidium into the mother sporocyst, within the snail host (Meuleman *et al.*, 1978; Pan, 1996). One marked difference from the *Fasciola* miracidium is that the ciliated epithelia are not shed as the schistosome miracidium penetrates the snail epithelium but are carried inside and shed later. It takes less than 15 min after attachment for a miracidium to pass completely through the epithelium to the space beneath, with intact plates and beating cilia. By 30 min the plates are detaching and disintegrating. In contrast, the cytoplasmic ridges and their associated ridge cells become very active, extending laterally beneath the detaching plates, with contents below the muscles passing up into the ridges. These fuse together to form the tegument of the mother sporocyst, neatly summarized in Fig. 1.11.4 (Yoshino *et al.*, 2017). Snail amoebocytes arrive in the area to undertake the clearance of the epithelial plate debris by phagocytosis. It has been suggested that the nascent mother sporocyst may be vulnerable at this point because regions not covered by the expanding ridges, such as the basal lamina and muscles, are directly exposed to the host haemolymph (Pan, 1996). In consequence they may be open attack by host amoebocytes or other cells (possibly fibroblasts) with numerous collagenous fibres invested on their surface. Some larvae may be completely surrounded by amoebocytes and fibroblasts, rapidly degenerating thereafter.

From 1 h after entry, the thickness of the mother sporocyst tegument increases and mitochondria appear. The associated cell bodies beneath the muscles become very active, with rough endoplasmic reticulum, Golgi bodies, vesicles and mitochondria evident. Around 2 h, the apical papilla is retracted into the sporocyst body, with shedding of the remnants of the first-tier epithelial plates (Pan, 1996). The passage of vesicles via the cytoplasmic connections to contribute to tegument surface development was confirmed by immunocytochemistry (Dunn and Yoshino, 1988). It was also suggested that other vesicles discharged their contents into the haemolymph, potentially to inhibit amoebocyte attachment (Pan, 1996). At this point, when both the gland secretory phase and the sensing of host-supplied cues are redundant, the tegument closes over the anterior. There is a profound reorganization of the nervous system, with loss of the complex array of redundant sensory endings; by 48 h many tissues are in a degenerative state. This is a highly regulated process, as indicated by the abundance of proteasome components, and the associated ubiquitin system that targets proteins for destruction, in the miracidial proteome (Table 1.1) (Mameda, 2017). It is a testable hypothesis that they are not randomly distributed in the miracidial body but concentrated in those cells destined for destruction. Autophagy may also be responsible for tissue remodelling and it is pertinent that numerous components of the autophagy process were identified in the schistosome transcriptome (Verjovski-Almeida *et al.*, 2003) but there has been little subsequent research interest. By 72 h, metamorphosis is complete and the mother sporocyst is essentially a sessile sac. It comprises the tegument, with dense microvillar extensions and cell bodies beneath sparse body wall muscles, the protonephridia, and the undifferentiated germ cells, which are starting to divide (see Section 1.2.6). A recent SEM study, based on mass *in vitro* culture, revealed that the mother sporocyst develops a specific body form after all ciliated plates have been shed (Poteaux *et al.*, 2023). The two lateral papillae remain as pronounced bulges, with unknown content (Fig. 1.11.2). One or two multiciliate nerve receptors lie near the bulges but uniciliate sensory endings are not evident. A birth pore allowing exit of daughter sporocysts, not found by TEM, was provisionally identified at the extreme anterior where the apical papilla was previously positioned (Poteaux *et al.*, 2023). The energy reserves of the miracidium are exhausted by 72 h, but the mother sporocyst is now fully adapted to acquire requisite nutrients from the snail host via a microvillar tegument surface (Fig. 1.11.3).

From 2 days, the mother sporocyst begins to elongate to accommodate the increasing number of germinal cells and later the developing daughter sporocysts (Meuleman *et al.*, 1978). The musculature gradually reduces in prominence from 3 days onwards, but it is assumed that some muscle persists for the 5–7 weeks lifespan of the essentially sessile mother sporocyst. The tegument of the developing daughter sporocyst begins as an epithelium but as its nuclei degenerate, the surface syncytium becomes connected to internally situated cell bodies. This developmental sequence is an almost exact forerunner of the way the tegument of the cercaria develops within the daughter sporocyst (see Section 1.4.2).

Germinal cells are ideally suited to single-cell transcriptome analysis because of their large size and limited intercellular attachments (see Section 1.2.6 on the miracidial germ cells). The technique applied to germinal cells isolated from *in vitro* cultured 48 h mother sporocysts, confirmed their heterogeneity (Wang *et al.*, 2018), revealing three major cell classes: k-cells (*klf*$^{+}$*nanos2*$^{+}$), j-cells (*fgfrA,B*$^{+}$) and d-cells (*nanos2*$^{+}$ and *fgfrA,B*$^{+}$). However, despite this, sporocyst stem cells largely shared a common transcriptomic profile. The j-cells (also annotated as lower-case phi, φ) were distributed beneath the body wall and excluded from daughter embryos, d-cells were present in large clusters within embryos and k-cells clustered with d-cells in the embryos. The k-cells were also found in extra-embryonic tissues as singlets or doublets, which histological studies suggest are the source of new developing embryos. A hierarchy of development was suggested with the k-cells at the top (Wang *et al.*, 2018), essentially preserving the germ line integrity through both later asexual and sexual stages of reproduction. In the mother sporocyst, the d-cells generate somatic tissues as the larva grows, and downregulation of the *nanos2* gene results in j-cells which terminally differentiate into structures like the tegument cell bodies. By 2 weeks after snail infection, mother sporocysts contain many daughter sporocysts, ready to exit and begin their migration. At this stage k-cells comprised the vast majority (>85%) of stem cells in these daughters; fewer d-cells were observed, and j-cells were mostly excluded.

Single-cell transcript analysis of the 5-day *in vitro* cultured mother sporocysts (Diaz Soria *et al.*, 2024) has highlighted the level of structural simplification and cell destruction resulting from metamorphosis. This can be appreciated from the mean estimate of 169 nuclei (range 112–254) in the transformed larvae versus 365 in the miracidium (Attenborough *et al.*, 2024). Note also that the estimate was made 2–3 days after cell division was reported to begin, so it is safe to conclude that metamorphosis results in destruction of >50% of miracidial cells. The total number of recovered cells available for single-cell sequencing (601) was divided into only six tissue types, compared with the 19 in the disaggregated miracidium (Fig. 1.4.2) (Attenborough *et al.*, 2024; Diaz Soria *et al.*, 2024). The starkest contrast was the neuronal cell complement, representing 4% of recovered cells versus 57% in the miracidium – this is very much in line with the sessile nature of the mother sporocyst. The tegument (34%), muscle (32%), germinal cells (20%) and parenchyma (11%) made up a greater proportion of the tissue mass than in the miracidium. Morphological studies suggest that the absolute number of germinal cells is increasing, but without labelling studies it is not possible to say if the other tissues are increasing too. Indeed, it has been reported that the musculature of the mother sporocyst degenerates with age because it is not motile (Meuleman *et al.*, 1978).

1.3.4 Snail compatibility

Under the light microscope, snail haemolymph contains three types of haemocyte: hyalinocytes (67%), blast-like cells (21%) and granulocytes (12%) (Pichon *et al.*, 2022), Single-cell RNA-Seq has revealed greater complexity and plasticity within these three large populations, with seven clusters, based on exclusive patterns of gene expression; some of the clusters may represent cell activation pathways. The haemocytes can release constitutive plasma molecules, such as opsonizing lectins, which target invaders. They also produce reactive oxygen compounds and nitric oxide (NO) using the enzymes NADPH oxidase and NO synthase, respectively. The downstream products of these compounds (such as H_2O_2) are then directly involved in killing *S. mansoni* sporocysts. (Bayne *et al.*, 2001).

There is a complex genetic interaction between isolates of schistosomes and snails with resistant/susceptible genotypes. There are no differences in miracidial host recognition and penetration of resistant versus susceptible snails; it is what happens shortly afterwards that determines the success or failure of an infection (Bayne *et al.*, 2001). Resistant snails can recognize invading parasites and mount a defence response, while susceptible snails are unable to defend themselves against infection (Coustau *et al.*, 2015). When schistosomes are recognized by haemocytes in resistant snails, they are encapsulated and then exposed to anti-microbial effectors, including reactive oxygen species, leading to their destruction. Susceptible snails either lack the capacity to recognize and react with the invader, or their effector cells are actively suppressed by the mother sporocyst. It is plausible that the glycans detected on the mother sporocyst surface upon metamorphosis from the miracidium (Dunn and Yoshino, 1988), are a part of the evasion mechanism, mimicking snail glycans to avoid alerting haemocytes. (See also the smokescreen hypothesis, Chapter 7.) The mother sporocyst also produces oxidative scavengers such as Cu,Zn superoxide dismutase (Smp_176200) (Moné *et al.*, 2011) that mop up toxic haemocyte products. It appears that the generation of reactive oxygen species by the snail and reactive oxygen scavengers by the mother sporocyst represent a co-evolutionary arms race in the context of resistant and susceptible snails. This has been cited as an example of the Red Queen Hypothesis of reciprocal evolution for functional traits (Moné *et al.*, 2011). Availability of the *B. glabrata* genome sequence has permitted a deeper analysis of the snail parasite interactions. Snail lines have been selected for resistance, with gene regions such as the Guadaloupe Resistance Complex (GRC) being analysed in detail (Allan *et al.*, 2018). In the case of the GRC region, transfer experiments showed that resistance involved proteins encoded in haemocytes, since cell-free plasma was not effective. The proteins in question had features reminiscent of immune recognition proteins. Genetic analysis will clearly be a fruitful area of future research.

1.4 The Daughter Sporocyst

1.4.1 Migration to the hepatopancreas

Daughter sporocysts emerging from the mother sporocyst in the head/foot region begin their migration to the hepatopancreas via the haemocoel. At 25°C in our hands, useful numbers of larvae can be recovered around day 21 for morphological and *in situ* hybridization studies (Parker-Manuel and Wilson, 2022), but Generation 2 is probably the least well understood in the whole life cycle. Generations 1 and 2, the mother and daughter sporocysts, are frequently telescoped in life cycle diagrams as 'the sporocysts' belying the fact that they are distinct biological entities.

During the vermiform migratory phase, daughter sporocysts have a uniform appearance and size (180 μm long and 26 μm wide) (Fig. 1.12.1). The body wall, comprising the tegument syncytium and circular/longitudinal muscles is only 1.5–2.0 μm thick, with a surface extended into microvilli (presumably to enhance nutrient uptake). A layer of small, 4–5 μm diameter cells lies immediately beneath the body wall (tegument cell bodies, parenchyma?), surrounding a core of larger 8–10 μm undifferentiated cells. These are the germinal cells with large nuclei and a 3 μm diameter nucleolus (Fig. 1.12.1, inset a), which occupy the posterior 75% of the body. The anterior is clearly demarcated (Fig. 1.12.1, inset b) but the line is not phalloidin-positive so not analogous to the head capsule of the cercaria. Two enigmatic structures, reminiscent of the cercarial head gland, are enclosed within the anterior tissue mass, but they need further investigation. Phalloidin staining for actin reveals backward-pointing spines within the tegument syncytium, numerous at the anterior, sparse in the mid-region and absent at the posterior (Fig. 1.12.2), presumably providing purchase during transit to the hepatopancreas. It also reveals at least four flame cells and their associated tubules within the body core. The circular muscle fibres are numerous and tightly packed, the longitudinal fibres thicker but more widely spaced (Fig. 1.12.3). Once established in the hepatopancreas, the daughter sporocyst loses its vermiform appearance, with bulbous regions termed brood chambers becoming apparent, separated by actin-rich isthmuses, where circular muscle fibres are contracted. The surface spines are still evident, most numerous and paired on the anterior bulb. The anterior region remains distinct, and differentiates into a cuff of tissue leading to a birth pore at the extreme anterior, through which each cercaria emerges as it matures (Fournier and Théron, 1985).

1.4.2 Development of the germ balls in the daughter sporocyst

Germ ball development from germinal cells is asynchronous, with successive stages present at any one time. The earliest stage germ ball comprises roughly spherical and loosely aggregated cells, varying in diameter from 2 to 9 μm with

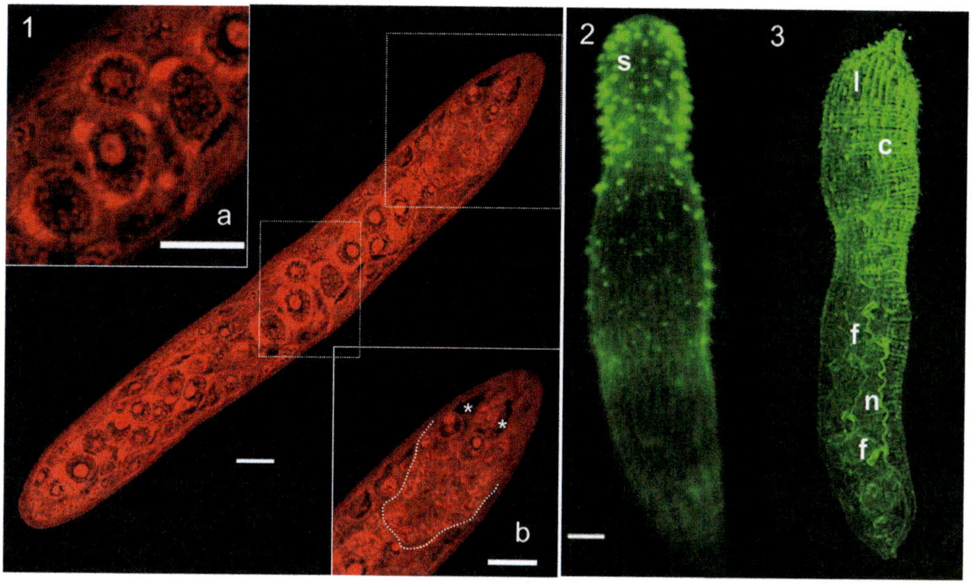

Fig. 1.12. Migratory form of the daughter sporocyst. **1**) The elongate body is packed with large undifferentiated (8–10 μm) germ cells (inset a), each with condensed chromatin, a large nucleolus and intensely stained cytosol. An anterior region (inset b), demarcated from the rest of the body, contains two large cells with lacunae (asterisks) that may be gland cells. **2**) Projection of a confocal Z-stack of a daughter sporocyst stained with phalloidin, showing the numerous projecting spines (s) primarily in the first quadrant. **3**) Projection at a deeper level showing the thin meshwork of longitudinal (l) and circular (c) fibres in the body wall, plus flame cells (f) and nephridial canals (n). Scale bars: 10 μm. (From Parker-Manuel and Wilson, 2022.) Figure used under license CC-BY-4.0.

prominent nucleoli and a bright ring of cytoplasm (Fig. 1.13.1) (Parker-Manuel and Wilson, 2022). As development proceeds, a thin layer of cytoplasm, which will become the tegument, envelops the entire germ ball (Fig. 1.13.2). The internal cells become more closely apposed and appear to be organizing themselves into structures. The thin surface layer becomes more apparent as an epithelium (possibly a syncytium) with visible nuclei (Fig. 1.13.3). Ultimately, bridges of cytoplasm link internal cell bodies with the outer epithelial layer and the nuclei disappear. By the time the germ ball has developed a stubby tail (Fig. 1.13.4), its cells are well organized into future recognizable cercarial tissues. The cells of the first quarter will become the head capsule, those of the second the neural ganglion, visible as an anucleate mass. The third quarter contains the large precursors of acetabular gland cells, with distinct lateral bands of cells on each side, while the fourth quarter contains undifferentiated potential germinal cells. The cells in the emerging tail are neatly arranged in lateral rows that will differentiate into the muscle fibres.

It is at this stage that the muscle cells of the cercarial body wall develop, the circular before the longitudinal, and flame cells can be discerned. The longitudinal fibres are formed from bands of distinct myocytes, arranged in circular tiers around the body. These differentiate after the head capsule muscle boundary has formed. The myofilaments of each longitudinal myocyte appear to be organized into pairs of myofibrils (Fig. 1.13.5). Starting at the two extremes the myocytes appear to extend until they meet and dovetail with those of the preceding and succeeding tiers. It is unclear whether the resulting longitudinal muscle fibre is a syncytium of around seven or eight myocytes, or individual cells are simply tightly adherent.

The pattern of gene expression in developing germ balls has been explored using a comprehensive microarray platform for cDNA hybridization without PCR amplification (Parker-Manuel

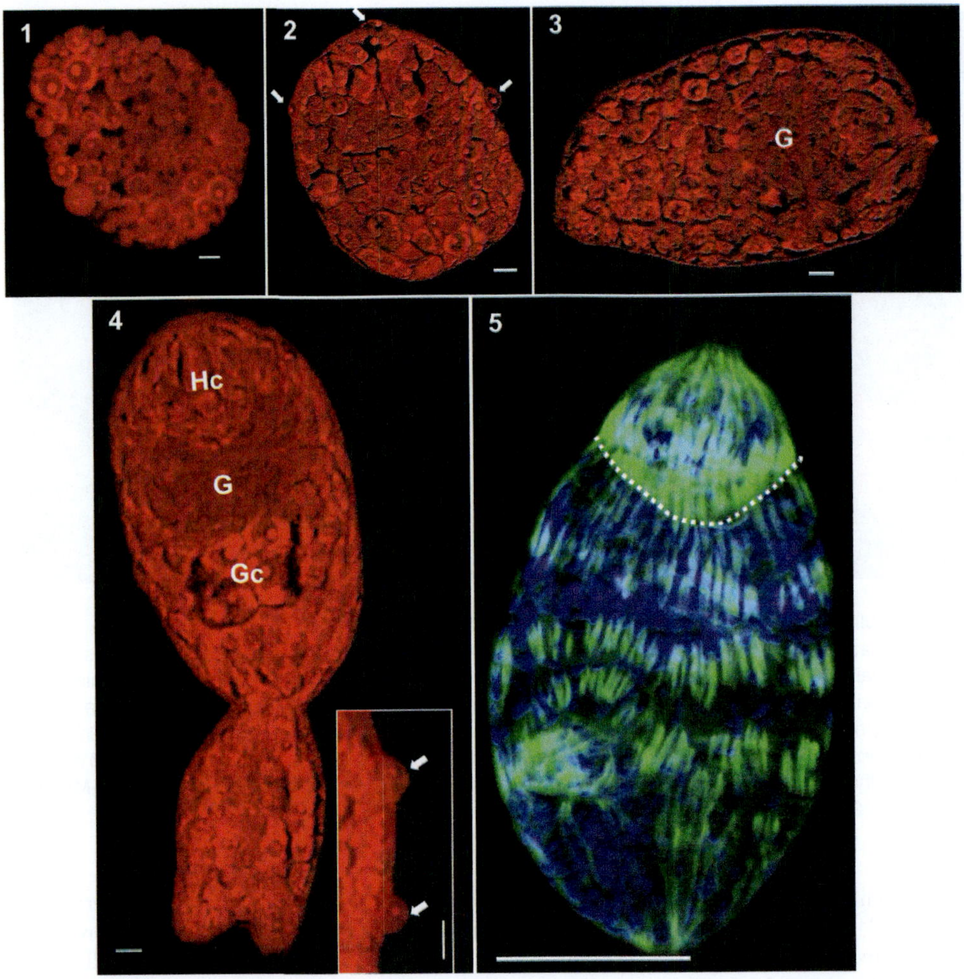

Fig. 1.13. Development of germ balls within the daughter sporocyst. **1**) Early germ ball comprising more than 100 loosely packed spherical cells. **2**) At the next stage, the germ ball is enveloped by a thin epithelial layer with nuclei (arrowed). **3**) It then elongates, and cells begin organizing into tissues, the ganglia (G) appearing first. **4**) A stubby tail sprouts from the posterior, as the head capsule (Hc), neural ganglia (G) and acetabular gland cells (Gc) differentiate. Epithelial nuclei are still visible at the surface (inset) but are soon lost as the surface layer connects to internal cell bodies. **5**) The muscle layers develop, circular fibres first (not shown), the head capsule boundary (dashed line) and distinct longitudinal myocytes in bands around the body. Each appears to contain two myofilaments, and they can be seen aligning to form the longitudinal fibres (actin stained green with phalloidin and nuclei blue with DAPI). Scale bars: **1–4**, 5 μm; **5**, 50 μm. (From Parker-Manuel and Wilson, 2022.)

et al., 2011). The germ balls were obtained by microdissection of snails 22–26 days post-infection (to exclude mature cercariae) and compared with those of the cercaria and day 2 schistosomulum. Genes were categorized using the Gene Ontology (GO) resource to aid interpretation of biological processes. These data confirm that the germ balls are the most and cercariae the least mitotically active of the three stages. All of the 48 genes upregulated in the 'DNA replication' category were most enriched in the germ balls, as were 27 of the 31 genes enriched in the 'translation' category. The extent of biosynthetic activity in germ balls was confirmed by their transcription of 14 out of the 21 upregulated 'glycosyl transferases'. Among specific tissue markers, four early neural patterning genes were upregulated, coincident with the appearance of the central ganglia and nervous system at the 'stubby tailed' stage. A total of 27 serine proteases were differentially transcribed, including 11 elastase genes that were 10–65-fold more highly expressed in the germ balls, along with 22 out of 35 differentially expressed metalloproteases; the five most highly upregulated (13–28-fold) were invadolysins. Again, this is evidence for synthesis of acetabular gland constituents at the stubby tail stage, early in cercarial development. Also of note were six VAL-encoded proteins genes (VAL-4, -24, -19, -20, -18 and -25), most highly transcribed in the germ ball. Intriguingly, none of these overlaps with the approximately nine VALs identified in the miracidium (see Section 1.2.3). Finally, three micro-exon gene (MEG) transcripts MEG-7, -10 and -18 were enriched. These are outliers from the main MEG grouping in adult worms. MEG-7 and -18 have not been identified in other stages but MEG-10 is expressed in the back end of adult males.

The expression sites of selected genes were confirmed by *in situ* hybridization (Parker-Manuel and Wilson, 2022). Elastase 1a (*ce1a*) is expressed in all stages, except the small spherical germ balls, and is most intense at the stubby tail stage (Fig. 1.14.1–1.14.3). As the tail enlarges, expression declines until in the most mature larvae it is present only as a central band, in the anterior cytoplasm of the pre-acetabular glands (Fig. 1.14.4). The reason is that the protein synthetic machinery is progressively displaced to one pole of each gland cell by the accumulating secretion bodies. This is equally evident with both Sm*pepm8* (invadolysin) (Fig. 1.14.5) and *val10* genes, where expression occurs at a later stage and mRNA is confined to a transverse band (Fig. 1.14.6). Conversely, invadolysin protein accumulates in the fundus of each gland cell and reaches up the ducts to the head capsule (Fig. 1.14.8). An independent study also using *in situ* hybridization, showed that VAL-4 and -24 had the same expression pattern as VAL-10 (Fernandes *et al.*, 2017). As an aside, the expression of a supposed secreted immunomodulator, Sm16, was also investigated (Parker-Manuel and Wilson, 2022). Expression of *sm16* mRNA was not limited to any particular tissue and was first transcribed in early germ balls. At the 'stubby tailed' stage it was distributed throughout the body and nascent tail (Fig. 1.14.7). Conversely, the tissue patches that lacked staining corresponded to the location of the acetabular gland cell fundi and ducts. The evidence points to Sm16 not being a secreted protein.

The first phase of development in each germ ball is dominated by cell division followed by protein/glycan synthesis and finally a period of maturation into the cercaria before emergence from the snail. It takes ~28 days at 26°C for the first cercariae to emerge after exposure to miracidia (Fried *et al.*, 2001). If the first daughter sporocysts leave the mother sporocyst after 11 days, then the minimum time for cercarial development is 17 days. From snail labelling studies we know that incorporation of amino acids into proteins is maximal between 9 and 5 days before emergence (Wilson and Coulson, 1986). We can therefore estimate the duration of the cell division phase as 7 days, protein synthesis as 5 days, and the maturation process as 5 days. There is negligible amino acid incorporation into the cercaria in the final 3 days before emergence, so it is likely they have left the daughter sporocyst and are migrating through the haemocoel to the exit points. Mature cercariae require a photo stimulus to trigger emergence – under natural circumstances most likely daybreak. They emerge into freshwater primarily through the mantle collar (57%) and to a lesser extent the pseudobranch (31%) and head/foot (13%) (Tucker *et al.*, 2014). It has been assumed that enzymatic secretions are involved in breaching the tissues, but tail-first and mass escapes have also been observed. The appearance of snail haemoglobin in the water is often a corollary of mass shedding. Once in freshwater the cercaria is free to progress to the next stage of the life cycle.

1.5 Summary

- The miracidium stage, which infects the snail host, is covered by ciliated epithelial plates that provide the propulsive force for dispersal after hatching from the egg. In contrast, the role of the slight body wall muscles is largely the maintenance of body shape. Its lifespan and infectivity depend on stored

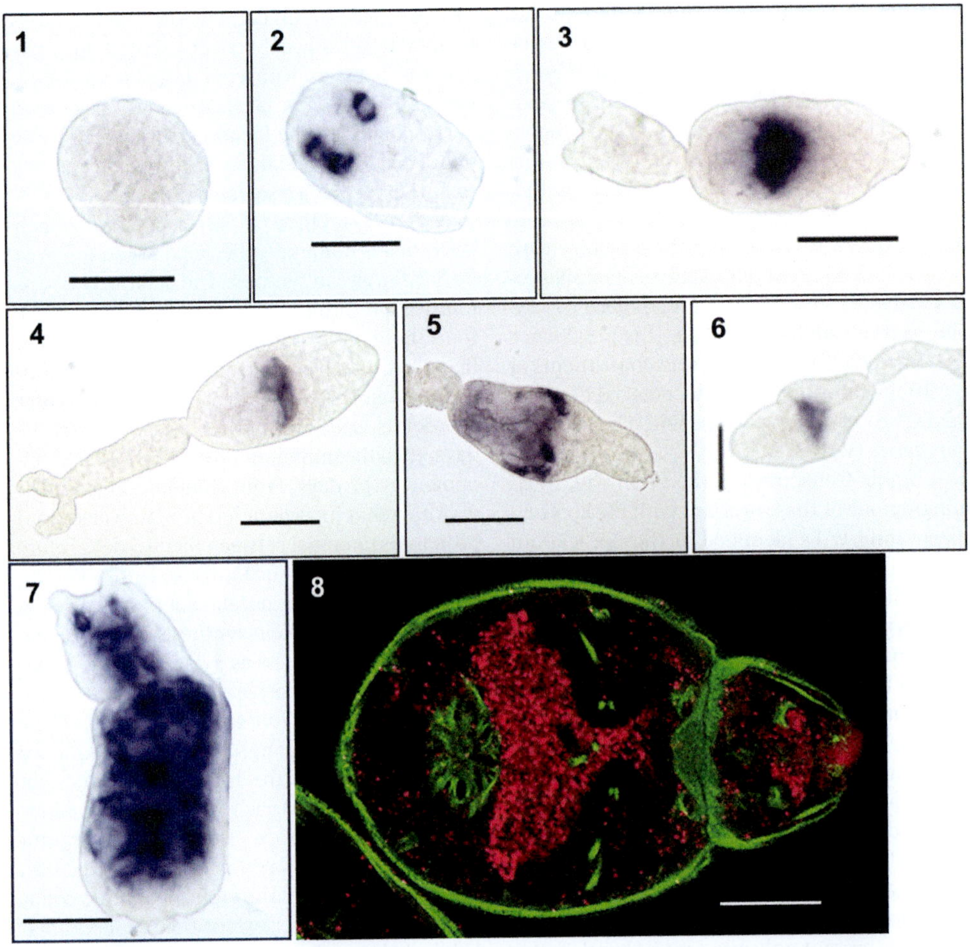

Fig. 1.14. Gene/protein expression in developing germ balls of the daughter sporocyst. **1–4**) The pattern of expression of cercarial elastase gene *ce1a* from **1**) early germ ball (negative) through **2**) elongating germ ball with intense expression in precursor cells of acetabular glands to **3**) the pre-acetabular gland cell bodies full of mRNA, at the stubby tail stage. Finally, in **4**) gene expression is confined to the leading edge of the gland as accumulating protein products compress the biosynthetic area. **5**) Expression of the metalloprotease gene Sm*pepm8* around the leading edge of the gland cells. **6**) Weaker expression of *val-10* in the same location. **7**) The gene encoding *sm16* is expressed in virtually all cells of the body and tail, at the stubby tail stage. **8**) Immunocytochemistry for SmPepM8 (invadolysin) protein stained with rat anti-invadolysin protein (purple) reveals it is present in discrete 'particles' of the gland cell bodies and ducts. Muscle actin (green) was detected by phalloidin 488. Scale bars: **1–7** = 20 μm; **8** = 50 μm. (From Parker-Manuel and Wilson, 2022.)

glycogen reserves which are expended at a constant rate by aerobic respiration during the active quest for a snail host.

- It is a marvel of miniaturization capable of a myriad of diverse functions all packed into its approximately 365 cells. Tissue disaggregation and single-cell sequencing has provided a wealth of information on patterns of gene expression in assembled cell clusters. Unfortunately, there is a gulf between the expression data and the original ultrastructural descriptions that needs to be bridged by new high-resolution serial TEM to clarify such questions as the identity of photoreceptors. A TEM study of the embryonic miracidium would also aid interpretation of epithelial and parenchymal origins.

- The central ganglion is a large mass of neurons around a neuropile which, together with peripheral sensory neurons, comprises 57% of the total cell complement. Unfortunately, it is difficult to relate the functions of the multiple types of sensory ending to the processes of host location and snail penetration. Snail chemicals are a key in these processes, with the recent suggestion that snail pheromones may be a crucial specific element in the miracidium/snail interaction.
- The miracidium possesses a central apical and two lateral accessory glands involved in penetration, but their secretions are not yet well characterized. The obstacle to infection presented by the snail host is a coat of mucus overlying a single layer of epithelial cells. Current information points to both proteases and polysaccharidases as important constituents. The barrier is rapidly breached once a stable interlocking contact is made between host cell microvilli and matching apical papilla projections.
- There are morphological descriptions of the profound metamorphosis of the miracidium into the mother sporocyst beneath the snail epithelium. However, no single-cell sequencing has been applied before 48 h for germs cells or 5 days for the mother sporocyst. A massive structural simplification occurs but nothing is known about underlying gene expression patterns or whether cytological processes like autophagy accompany the morphological changes.
- The cytology of the second life cycle generation, the daughter sporocyst, is also enigmatic. There is limited structural information on the early migratory stage that leaves the head/foot and ascends into the viscera, or how this is actively achieved. Once there, the contained germ balls rapidly grow into the infective cercarial stage. Both morphological and gene expression patterns have been described for this phase, which takes a minimum of 17 days before protein synthesis tails off. In the ensuing days the cercaria exits the daughter sporocyst, and then the snail, to begin its brief non-feeding life in fresh water.

References

Adema, C.M., Hillier, L.W., Jones, C.S., Loker, E.S., Knight, M. *et al.* (2017) Whole genome analysis of a schistosomiasis-transmitting freshwater snail. *Nature Communications* 8, 15451. DOI: 10.1038/ncomms15451

Allan, E.R.O., Gourbal, B., Dores, C.B., Portet, A., Bayne, C.J. *et al.* (2018) Clearance of schistosome parasites by resistant genotypes at a single genomic region in *Biomphalaria glabrata* snails involves cellular components of the hemolymph. *International Journal for Parasitology* 48(5), 387–393. DOI: 10.1016/j.ijpara.2017.08.008

Attenborough, T., Rawlinson, K.A., Diaz Soria, C.L., Ambridge, K., Sankaranarayanan, G. *et al.* (2024) A single-cell atlas of the miracidium larva of *Schistosoma mansoni* reveals cell types, developmental pathways, and tissue architecture. *eLife* 13, RP95628. DOI: 10.7554/eLife.95628

Bahia, D., Avelar, L.G.A., Vigorosi, F., Cioli, D., Oliveira, G.C. *et al.* (2006) The distribution of motor proteins in the muscles and flame cells of the *Schistosoma mansoni* miracidium and primary sporocyst. *Parasitology* 133(3), 321–329. DOI: 10.1017/S0031182006000400

Ballard, K.R., Klein, A.H., Hayes, R.A., Wang, T. and Cummins, S.F. (2021) The protein and volatile components of trail mucus in the common garden snail, *Cornu aspersum*. *PLoS ONE* 16(5), e0251565. DOI: 10.1371/journal.pone.0251565

Bayne, C.J., Hahn, U.K. and Bender, R.C. (2001) Mechanisms of molluscan host resistance and of parasite strategies for survival. *Parasitology* 123(Suppl.), S159–S167. DOI: 10.1017/s0031182001008137

Bruckner, D.A. and Voge, M. (1974) The nervous system of larval *Schistosoma mansoni* as revealed by acetylcholinesterase staining. *The Journal of Parasitology* 60(3), 437–446. DOI: 10.2307/3278359

Carter, N.P. (1978) The host-location mechanisms of the miracidium and cercaria of *Schistosoma mansoni*. PhD thesis, University of York, York, UK. Available at: https://etheses.whiterose.ac.uk/id/eprint/36331

Collins, J.J., King, R.S., Cogswell, A., Williams, D.L. and Newmark, P.A. (2011) An atlas for *Schistosoma mansoni* organs and life-cycle stages using cell type-specific markers and confocal microscopy. *PLoS Neglected Tropical Diseases* 5(3), e1009. DOI: 10.1371/journal.pntd.0001009

Coustau, C., Gourbal, B., Duval, D., Yoshino, T.P., Adema, C.M. *et al.* (2015) Advances in gastropod immunity from the study of the interaction between the snail *Biomphalaria glabrata* and its parasites: a review of research progress over the last decade. *Fish & Shellfish Immunology* 46(1), 5–16. DOI: 10.1016/j.fsi.2015.01.036

Diaz Soria, C.L., Attenborough, T., Lu, Z., Fontenla, S., Graham, J. *et al.* (2024) Single-cell transcriptomics of the human parasite *Schistosoma mansoni* first intra-molluscan stage reveals tentative tegumental and stem-cell regulators. *Scientific Reports* 14(1), 5974. DOI: 10.1038/s41598-024-55790-3

Dixon, M.D. (1984) Strategies of host location employed by larval trematodes. PhD thesis, University of York, York, UK. Available at: https://etheses.whiterose.ac.uk/id/eprint/10916

Dunn, T.S. and Yoshino, T.P. (1988) *Schistosoma mansoni*: origin and expression of a tegumental surface antigen on the miracidium and primary sporocyst. *Experimental Parasitology* 67(2), 167–181. DOI: 10.1016/0014-4894(88)90064-1

Eklu-Natey, D.T., Wüest, J., Swiderski, Z., Striebel, H.P. and Huggel, H. (1985) Comparative scanning electron microscope (SEM) study of miracidia of four human schistosome species. *International Journal for Parasitology* 15(1), 33–42. DOI: 10.1016/0020-7519(85)90098-0

Fernandes, R.S., Barbosa, T.C., Barbosa, M.M.F., Miyasato, P.A., Nakano, E. *et al.* (2017) Stage and tissue expression patterns of *Schistosoma mansoni* venom allergen-like proteins SmVAL 4, 13, 16 and 24. *Parasites & Vectors* 10(1), 223. DOI: 10.1186/s13071-017-2144-2

Fournier, A. and Théron, A. (1985) Morpho-anatomic and functional sectorization of *Schistosoma mansoni* daughter sporocysts. *Zeitschrift für Parasitenkunde* 71(3), 325–336. DOI: 10.1007/BF00928335

Fried, B., Muller, E.E., Broadway, A. and Sherma, J. (2001) Effects of diet on the development of *Schistosoma mansoni* in *Biomphalaria glabrata* and on the neutral lipid content of the digestive gland-gonad complex of the snail. *The Journal of Parasitology* 87(1), 223–225. DOI: 10.1645/0022-3395(2001)087[0122:EODOTD]2.0.CO;2

Hofer, F., Kraml, J., Kahler, U., Kamenik, A.S. and Liedl, K.R. (2020) Catalytic site pK_a values of aspartic, cysteine, and serine proteases: constant pH MD simulations. *Journal of Chemical Information and Modeling* 60, 3030–3042. DOI: 10.1021/acs.jcim.0c00190

Jamieson, B.G.M. and Haas, W. (2017) Miracidium of *Schistosoma*. In: Jamieson, B.G.M. (ed.) *Schistosoma, Biology, Pathology, Control*. CRC Press, Boca Raton, FL, chapter 6. DOI: 10.1201/9781315368900

Koie, M. and Frandsen, F. (1976) Stereoscan observations of the miracidium and early sporocyst of *Schistosoma mansoni*. *Zeitschrift für Parasitenkunde* 50(3), 335–344. DOI: 10.1007/BF02462978

Lodes, M.J. and Yoshino, T.P. (1989) Characterization of excretory-secretory proteins synthesized *in vitro* by *Schistosoma mansoni* primary sporocysts. *The Journal of Parasitology* 75(6), 853–862. DOI: 10.2307/3282863

Lu, Z., Sankaranarayanan, G., Rawlinson, K.A., Offord, V., Brindley, P.J. *et al.* (2021) The transcriptome of *Schistosoma mansoni* developing eggs reveals key mediators in pathogenesis and life cycle propagation. *Frontiers in Tropical Diseases* 2, 713123. DOI: 10.3389/fitd.2021.713123

Mameda, M.S.L. (2017) Complexidade do proteoma de *Schistosoma mansoni* na miniatura da fase larval miracídio [Complexity of the proteome of *Schistosoma mansoni* in miniature of the miracidial larval phase]. Master's thesis, Universidade Federal de Ouro Preto, Ouro Preto, Brazil. https://repositorio.ufop.br/items/7c9a0bcc-7630-4f9a-a2a7-c4583967b3e7

Marinković, M., Berger, J. and Jékely, G. (2020) Neuronal coordination of motile cilia in locomotion and feeding. *Philosophical Transactions of the Royal Society of London. Series B, Biological Sciences* 375(1792), 20190165. DOI: 10.1098/rstb.2019.0165

Mathieson, W. and Wilson, R.A. (2010) A comparative proteomic study of the undeveloped and developed *Schistosoma mansoni* egg and its contents: the miracidium, hatch fluid and secretions. *International Journal for Parasitology* 40(5), 617–628. DOI: 10.1016/j.ijpara.2009.10.014

Meuleman, E.A., Lyaruu, D.M., Khan, M.A., Holzmann, P.J. and Sminia, T. (1978) Ultrastructural changes in the body wall of *Schistosoma mansoni* during the transformation of the miracidium into the mother sporocyst in the snail host *Biomphalaria pfeifferi*. *Zeitschrift für Parasitenkunde* 56(3), 227–242. DOI: 10.1007/BF00931716

Moné, Y., Ribou, A.-C., Cosseau, C., Duval, D., Théron, A. *et al.* (2011) An example of molecular co-evolution: reactive oxygen species (ROS) and ROS scavenger levels in *Schistosoma mansoni/Biomphalaria glabrata* interactions. *International Journal for Parasitology* 41(7), 721–730. DOI: 10.1016/j.ijpara.2011.01.007

Ng, T.P.T., Saltin, S.H., Davies, M.S., Johannesson, K., Stafford, R. *et al.* (2013) Snails and their trails: the multiple functions of trail-following in gastropods. *Biological Reviews of the Cambridge Philosophical Society* 88(3), 683–700. DOI: 10.1111/brv.12023

Pan, S.C. (1980) The fine structure of the miracidium of *Schistosoma mansoni*. *Journal of Invertebrate Pathology* 36(3), 307–372. DOI: 10.1016/0022-2011(80)90040-3

Pan, S.C. (1996) *Schistosoma mansoni*: the ultrastructure of larval morphogenesis in *Biomphalaria glabrata* and of associated host–parasite interactions. *Japanese Journal of Medical Science & Biology* 49(4), 129–149. DOI: 10.7883/yoken1952.49.129

Parker-Manuel, S.J. and Wilson, R.A. (2022) An atlas of the germ ball–cercaria–schistosomulum transition in *Schistosoma mansoni*, using confocal microscopy and *in situ* hybridisation. *Current Research in Parasitology & Vector-Borne Diseases* 2, 100087. DOI: 10.1016/j.crpvbd.2022.100087

Parker-Manuel, S.J., Ivens, A.C., Dillon, G.P. and Wilson, R.A. (2011) Gene expression patterns in larval *Schistosoma mansoni* associated with infection of the mammalian host. *PLoS Neglected Tropical Diseases* 5(8), e1274. DOI: 10.1371/journal.pntd.0001274

Pichon, R., Pinaud, S., Vignal, E., Chaparro, C., Pratlong, M. *et al.* (2022) Single cell RNA sequencing reveals hemocyte heterogeneity in *Biomphalaria glabrata*: plasticity over diversity. *Frontiers in Immunology* 13, 956871. DOI: 10.3389/fimmu.2022.956871

Pila, E.A., Peck, S.J. and Hanington, P.C. (2017) The protein pheromone temptin is an attractant of the gastropod *Biomphalaria glabrata*. *Journal of Comparative Physiology. A, Neuroethology, Sensory, Neural, and Behavioral Physiology* 203(10), 855–866. DOI: 10.1007/s00359-017-1198-0

Ponder, W.F., Lindberg, D.R. and Ponder, J.M. (2019) Shell, body, and muscles. In: Ponder, W.F., Lindberg, D.R. and Ponder, J.M. (eds) *Biology and Evolution of the Mollusca. Volume 1*. CRC Press Boca Raton, FL, chapter 3. DOI: 10.1201/9781351115667

Poteaux, P., Gourbal, B. and Duval, D. (2023) Time series analysis of tegument ultrastructure of *in vitro* transformed miracidium to mother sporocyst of the human parasite *Schistosoma mansoni*. *Acta Tropica* 240, 106840. DOI: 10.1016/j.actatropica.2023.106840

Stepan, H., Pabst, M., Altmann, F., Geyer, H., Geyer, R. *et al.* (2012) *O*-glycosylation of snails. *Glycoconjugate Journal* 29(4), 189–198. DOI: 10.1007/s10719-012-9391-4

Tielens, A.G., Van de Pas, F.A., Van den Heuvel, J.M. and Van den Bergh, S.G. (1991) The aerobic energy metabolism of *Schistosoma mansoni* miracidia. *Molecular and Biochemical Parasitology* 46(1), 181–184. DOI: 10.1016/0166-6851(91)90211-n

Tucker, M.S., Lewis, F.A., Driver, J.D. and Granath, W.O., Jr (2014) Determination and quantification of *Schistosoma mansoni* cercarial emergence from *Biomphalaria glabrata* snails. *The Journal of Parasitology* 100(6), 778–783. DOI: 10.1645/14-531.1

Verjovski-Almeida, S., DeMarco, R., Martins, E.A.L., Guimarães, P.E.M., Ojopi, E.P.B. *et al.* (2003) Transcriptome analysis of the acoelomate human parasite *Schistosoma mansoni*. *Nature Genetics* 35(2), 148–157. DOI: 10.1038/ng1237

Wang, B., Lee, J., Li, P., Saberi, A., Yang, H. *et al.* (2018) Stem cell heterogeneity drives the parasitic life cycle of *Schistosoma mansoni*. *eLife* 7. DOI: 10.7554/eLife.35449

Wang, T., Zhao, M., Rotgans, B.A., Strong, A., Liang, D. *et al.* (2016) Proteomic analysis of the *Schistosoma mansoni* miracidium. *PLoS ONE* 11(1), e0147247. DOI: 10.1371/journal.pone.0147247

Wendt, G., Zhao, L., Chen, R., Liu, C., O'Donoghue, A.J. *et al.* (2020) A single-cell RNA-seq atlas of *Schistosoma mansoni* identifies a key regulator of blood feeding. *Science* 369(6511), 1644–1649. DOI: 10.1126/science.abb7709

Wilson, R.A. (1969) Fine structure and organization of the musculature in the miracidium of *Fasciola hepatica*. *The Journal of Parasitology* 55(6), 1153–1161.

Wilson, R.A. (1970) Fine structure of the nervous system and specialized nerve endings in the miracidium of *Fasciola hepatica*. *Parasitology* 60(3), 399–410. DOI: 10.1017/s0031182000078197

Wilson, R.A. (1971) Gland cells and secretions in the miracidium of *Fasciola hepatica*. *Parasitology* 63(2), 225–231. DOI: 10.1017/s0031182000079543

Wilson, R.A. and Coulson, P.S. (1986) *Schistosoma mansoni*: dynamics of migration through the vascular system of the mouse. *Parasitology* 92, 83–100. DOI: 10.1017/s0031182000063472

Wilson, R.A. and Webster, L.A. (1974) Protonephridia. *Biological Reviews of the Cambridge Philosophical Society* 49(2), 127–160. DOI: 10.1111/j.1469-185x.1974.tb01572.x

Wu, X.-J., Sabat, G., Brown, J.F., Zhang, M., Taft, A. *et al.* (2009) Proteomic analysis of *Schistosoma mansoni* proteins released during *in vitro* miracidium-to-sporocyst transformation. *Molecular and Biochemical Parasitology* 164(1), 32–44. DOI: 10.1016/j.molbiopara.2008.11.005

Yoshino, T.P. and Laursen, J.R. (1995) Production of *Schistosoma mansoni* daughter sporocysts from mother sporocysts maintained in synxenic culture with *Biomphalaria glabrata* embryonic (Bge) cells. *The Journal of Parasitology* 81(5), 714–722.

Yoshino, T.P., Lodes, M.J., Rege, A.A. and Chappell, C.L. (1993) Proteinase activity in miracidia, transformation excretory-secretory products, and primary sporocysts of *Schistosoma mansoni*. *The Journal of Parasitology* 79(1), 23–31. DOI: 10.2307/3283272

Yoshino, T.P., Gourbaland, B. and Théron, A. (2017) Schistosoma sporocysts. In: Jamieson, B.G.M. (ed.) *Schistosoma, Biology, Pathology, Control*. CRC Press, Boca Raton, FL, chapter 7. DOI: 10.1201/9781315368900

Zylstra, U. (1972) Histochemistry and ultrastructure of the epidermis and the subepidermal gland cells of the freshwater snails *Lymnaea stagnalis* and *Biomphalaria pfeifferi*. *Zeitschrift für Zellforschung und Mikroskopische Anatomie* 130(1), 93–134. DOI: 10.1007/BF00306996

2

The Cercaria and the Mammalian Infection Process

2.1 Overview

In some respects the cercaria, the second aquatic transmission stage, could not be more different from the first, the miracidium. Where the miracidium is lightly muscularized, with a flexible body propelled rapidly by cilia, the cercaria is much more heavily muscularized and propelled by tail lashing movements. Hidden in this disparity is a profound truth about the evolutionary origins of the digenetic trematodes, if we could only crack the code. The cercaria is the first phenotype in the third generation of the life cycle that will undergo morphological, developmental and physiological changes, which ultimately culminate after about 5 weeks in an adult male or female worm. This chapter follows the same plan as Chapter 1, first dealing with the cellular morphology of the cercaria, before covering its brief non-feeding life in freshwater and the way it locates the mammalian host. Then follows the manner of skin penetration and ensuing metamorphosis into the schistosomulum, before the next phase of the cycle begins – migration to the hepatic portal system (Chapter 3).

2.2 The Cercaria

The mature cercaria is much larger than the miracidium, comprising in excess of 1000 cells, estimated from counting of nuclei. It is ~0.5 mm long, in a ratio of one-third body to two-thirds tail. Its normal orientation is to hang tail-up, head-down in the water, implying a greater density for the head (Fig. 2.1.1). The layout of tissues and organs is illustrated diagrammatically in Fig. 2.1.2 (Bogitsh *et al.*, 2019). Both body and tail have a complex musculature, and the body surface is covered in spines. The tail terminates in two furcae, each held at ~90° to its axis in the resting (sinking) position. The large sucker (acetabulum) is located on the mid-ventral surface, while the anterior of the body forms a discrete head capsule (also referred to as an anterior organ, and incorrectly as an oral sucker). Acetabular (penetration) glands are the principal internal feature of the body, while a head gland occupies the internal core of the head capsule. Together these glands take up far more of the internal space than those of the miracidium, potentially related to their respective targets. The mouth is subterminal on the ventral surface of the head capsule and connects via a long oesophagus to a rudimentary caecum in the centre of the body. A neural ganglion lies dorsally, astride the oesophagus, from which arises a system of peripheral nerves, and a rich variety of sensory endings. A protonephridial system runs through the body and tail, and an aggregation of germinal cells lies centrally, posterior to the acetabulum between the posterior gland cell fundi.

DOI: 10.1079/9781800625167.0002

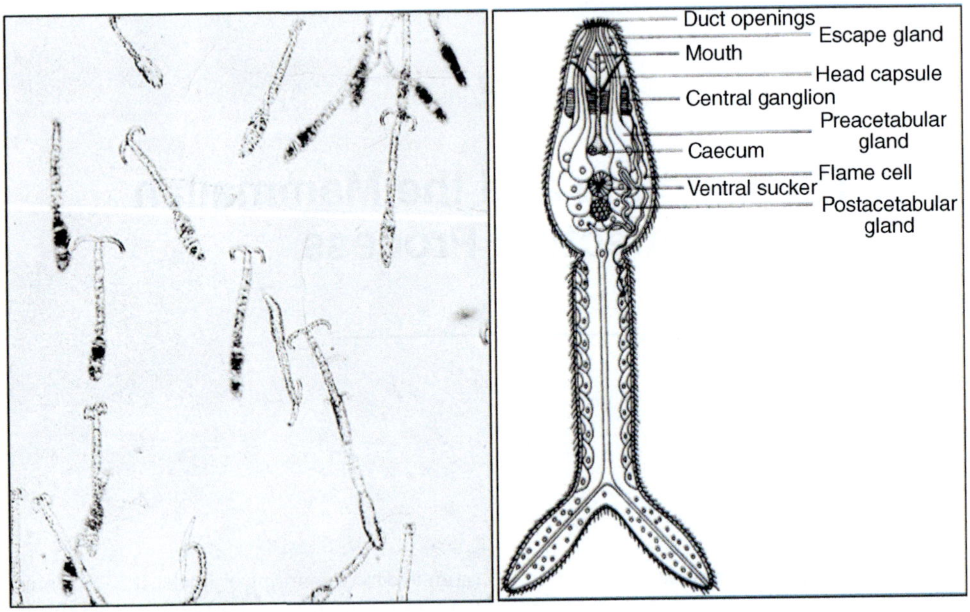

Fig. 2.1. Morphology of the cercaria. **1**) The normal orientation of an unstimulated cercarial population, hanging tail-up, head-down below the water surface, with the position maintained by alternating short bursts of upward swimming and long periods of sinking. **2**) Diagram of a cercaria in ventral view with major tissues labelled. The existence of escape glands is unconfirmed. (**2** from Bogitsh *et al.*, 2019.) **1**) Figure author's own. **2**) Figure used with permission from Elsevier.

2.2.1 Tegument and muscles

The syncytial tegument that covers the entire body of the mature cercaria is quite thin (~0.5 μm), with a dense granular cytoplasm containing a few small mitochondria and two types of inclusion (Fig. 2.2.1) (Morris, 1971; Hockley, 1972). The numerous backward-pointing spines are enclosed entirely within the cytoplasm and composed predominantly of actin. It is important, in view of what follows, to emphasize that the outer and basal tegument surfaces are delimited by conventional membranes, originally described as trilaminate because of their 'black–white–black' appearance in the electron microscope (Hockley, 1972). The base of the tegument rests on an extracellular fibrous lamella, while its outer surface is coated with a filamentous glycocalyx 1 μm thick (Fig. 2.2.2). Physiologically this glycan layer, a heterogeneous population of multi-fucosylated complex oligosaccharides (Khoo *et al.*, 1995), provides osmotic protection in freshwater. We can surmise this because when the glycocalyx is shed during skin penetration, the larva acquires osmotic sensitivity. The tegument is connected at intervals by microtubule-lined processes to cell bodies situated beneath the body wall muscles. These contain the endoplasmic reticulum, Golgi bodies and preformed inclusions that will be deployed during metamorphosis into the schistosomulum. If anything, the tegument overlying the tail is even thinner, plausibly because it is rendered obsolete at infection (Morris, 1971).

A detailed appraisal of muscle physiology is covered in Chapter 4, with only the layout and role of the cercarial muscles considered here. The way the circular and longitudinal fibres develop was covered in Section 1.4.2. There may be as many as 200 outer circular fibres positioned immediately below the tegument (Fig. 2.3.1) (Parker-Manuel and Wilson, 2022). Beneath them lie the much larger longitudinal fibres, which run the whole length of the body, branching and anastomosing as they do so. They are at their broadest in the mid-body region, tapering over the head capsule and extreme posterior to accommodate the rotund body termini. It is

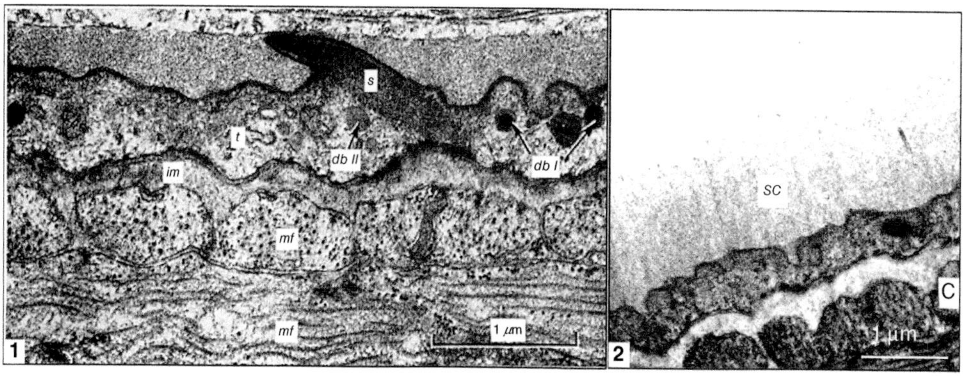

Fig. 2.2. The cercarial body wall. **1**) The syncytial tegument (t) contains spines (s) and two types of dense inclusions (db). It lies on a thick layer of interstitial material (im) beneath which there is a tight meshwork of outer circular and inner longitudinal muscle fibres (mf). **2**) The surface coat (sc) consists of long oligosaccharide chains anchored to the outer plasma membrane. (From Hockley, 1972.) Figures used with permission from Cambridge University Press.

difficult to estimate their number because of the branching, but there are probably around 30 fibres. The overall thinness (~0.1 µm) of this body wall muscle layer needs to be emphasized (Fig. 2.3.2), with frequent inter-fibre connections via dense bodies, so that the muscles act as a single unit to compress the cells and fluids of the body core that comprise the hydrostatic skeleton. Fine muscle fibres associated with the alimentary tract can also be visualized, predominantly in multiple rings around the oesophagus, plus a few longitudinal fibres along the length of the nascent organ (Fig. 2.3.2, inset). The short bifurcated caecal lobes are also enveloped by a coat of tiny fibres.

Arguably, it is the muscle systems additional to those of the body wall that play the most important role in cercarial biology. Principal of these are the ventral sucker and head capsule (anterior organ). The ventral sucker is roughly spherical in shape, packed with muscle fibres, and enclosed by a fibrous capsular matrix to create a virtually autonomous organ, only perforated by motor and sensory neurons. However, the sucker is anchored firmly to the dorsal body wall by a series of dorsoventral muscle fibres (Nuttman, 1975). The muscles of the sucker are arranged as an outer complement of circular fibres, forming the flexible 'lips' below which lie blocks of thicker radially arranged fibres connecting the central cavity surface with the outer capsule wall (Fig. 2.3.3) (Nuttman, 1975). The central cavity is lined by a thin layer of tegument bearing impressive backward-pointing spines to provide purchase, plus an array of four mechanoreceptor endings (see Section 2.2.4), clearly intended to supply the central ganglion with tactile information (Short and Cartrett, 1973). The head capsule is similarly demarcated from the rest of the body by a fibrous diaphragm through which pass the gland ducts, alimentary tract and neurons. A series of radial (circular) fibres runs around the anterior surface of the diaphragm, while a set of longitudinal retractor fibres interdigitate with those of the body wall at the posterior of the head capsule but detach part way forward to insert at the extreme anterior of the capsule (Fig. 2.3.4) (Nuttman, 1975). Collectively the muscles of the head capsule allow it to operate independently, exerting pressure on its contents, largely the acetabular gland ducts and head gland (see Section 2.2.2). These contractions of the head capsule muscles can be envisaged as exerting a squeezing effect on the gland structures, like a tube of toothpaste, forcing the contents out.

The tail and furcae comprise the third element of cercarial locomotory system. A layer of subtegumentary muscle is present along the entire length of the tail stem, with closely spaced outer circular and inner longitudinal fibres. The contractile regions of the circular fibres in transverse section are consistently smaller than those of the body. The major structural difference lies in the six separate blocks of longitudinal muscle lying immediately beneath the circular muscle

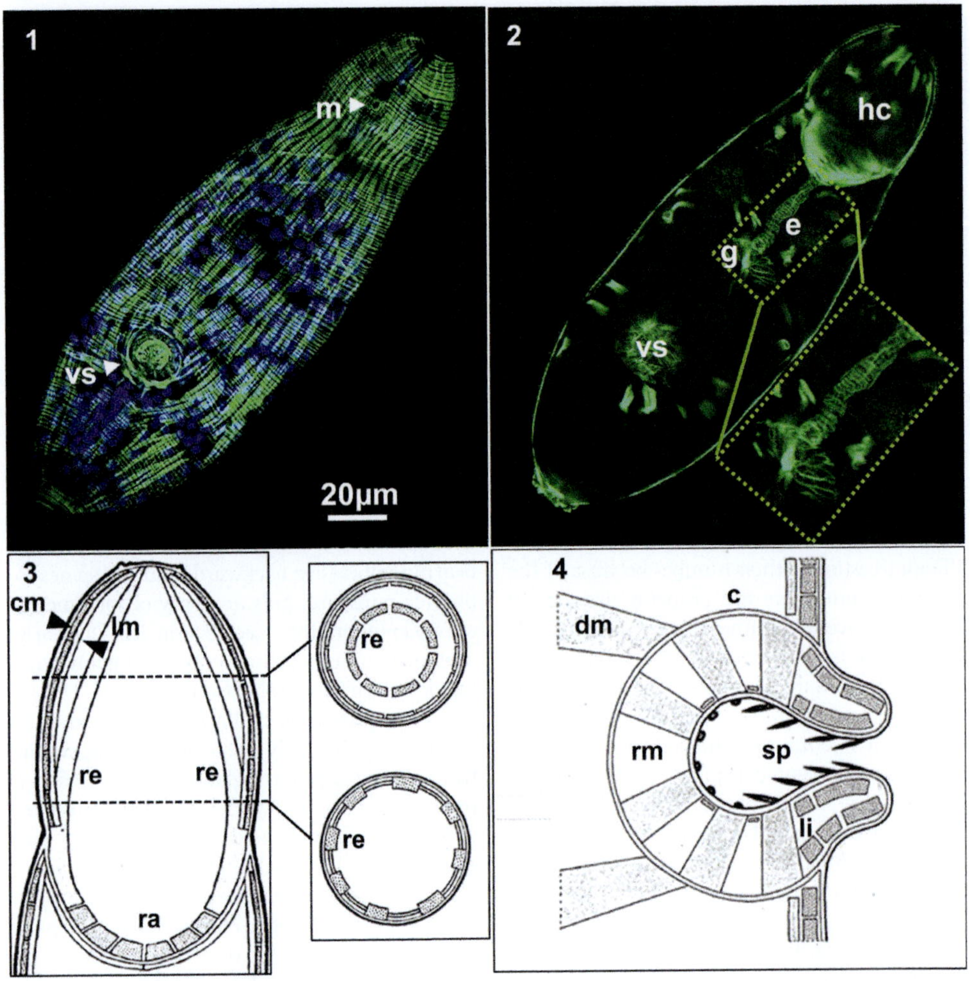

Fig. 2.3. Layout of the cercarial body musculature. **1**) Three-dimensional projection of a confocal Z-stack showing circular and longitudinal muscle actin of the body wall stained by AF488 phalloidin (green). The separate muscles of the ventral sucker (vs), and the subterminal mouth (m) are also visible. **2**) Single slice through the central body showing the thin body wall muscles, the head capsule (hc), oesophagus (e) and gut (g) (see inset). **3**) Schematic of the head capsule muscles. Additional to the circular (cm) and longitudinal (lm) muscles of the wall, eight thicker retractor fibres (re) insert on the extreme anterior at one end and interdigitate with the body wall at the other. A series of radial fibres (ra) form the base of the capsule. Transverse sections through the head capsule illustrate muscle arrangements. **4**) The ventral sucker, enclosed within a fibrous capsule (c) and attached by muscles (dm) to the dorsal body wall. The sucker bulb comprises radially arranged muscle fibres (rm) while rings of circular fibres form the lips (li). The sucker cavity is lined with prominent tegument spines (sp). (**1** and **2** from Parker-Manuel and Wilson, 2022; **3–5** from Nuttman, 1975.) **1** and **2**) Figures used under license CC-BY-4.0. **3** and **4**) Figures used with permission from Dr Chris Nuttman.

layer (Fig. 2.4.1). These longitudinal fibres are not contiguous with the longitudinal fibres of the body but insert within the terminal cylinder of the body fibres around the bladder. This explains why the tail 'snaps off' during skin penetration. The mid-dorsal and mid-ventral caudal blocks are relatively small, with a conventional structure comprising two closely adjacent fibres, circular in cross-section anteriorly but flattened dorsoventrally towards the distal end of the tail. The remaining four blocks consist of up to five fibres at any one point, each of which lies at an angle of ~10–12° to the longitudinal axis (Fig. 2.4.2). Viewed under a light microscope, this arrangement appears as a herringbone pattern, crossed by transverse lines with a periodicity of 1 μm. The anterior extremity of each fibre is located laterally with its posterior inserted close to the mid-line, and each appears U-shaped in cross-section when it is adjacent to another fibre. The fine structure of the striations, the associated dense bodies and the sarcoplasmic reticulum is covered in Chapter 4. Suffice it to say here that the thin actin filaments are inserted on the dense bodies and the thick myosin filaments are always shorter than the 1 μm repeating striations. This is the equivalent of one sarcomere in vertebrate striated muscle. The furcae have their own system of outer circular and inner non-striated longitudinal muscle fibres. How these connect to the tail is unclear, but the important feature is that the furcae are motile, and can flex laterally through a 90° arc, presumably under nervous system control. This flexing property affects the direction of swimming, head-first or tail-first (see Section 2.3.1).

2.2.2 Gland cells

Each of the four pre- and six post-acetabular glands are single cells that ultimately grow to an enormous volume and dimensions (Fig. 2.5.1). They comprise a body or fundus, complete with nucleus and protein/glycan synthetic machinery, leading to a long duct that opens at the extreme anterior of the head capsule (Fig. 2.5.2) (Collins *et al.*, 2011). Use of labelled ^{35}S-methionine as a marker for protein synthesis in the developing cercaria has revealed that the tail accounts for 32% of total protein. The acetabular glands secrete ~25% of labelled body protein in the first 3 h of transformation, a good indication of their sheer size (Harrop and Wilson, 1993). Enzymes and venom-allergen-like (VAL) proteins are synthesized in and secreted from the pre-acetabular glands but the precise composition of the posterior glands is less well characterized. The 'best guess' is that the secretions are sticky mucins that aid the cercaria in its attachment to the substratum; the larva leaves deposits behind when it crawls over a surface (Stirewalt, 1959). Both pre- and post-acetabular glands bind the plant lectin, peanut agglutinin, whereas the *Pisum sativum* agglutinin labels only the posterior glands,

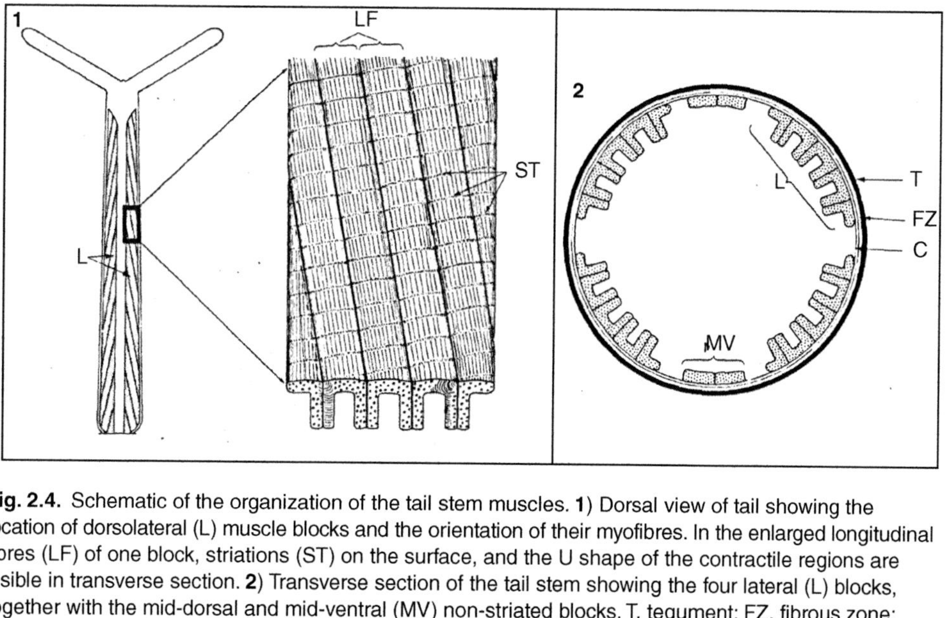

Fig. 2.4. Schematic of the organization of the tail stem muscles. **1**) Dorsal view of tail showing the location of dorsolateral (L) muscle blocks and the orientation of their myofibres. In the enlarged longitudinal fibres (LF) of one block, striations (ST) on the surface, and the U shape of the contractile regions are visible in transverse section. **2**) Transverse section of the tail stem showing the four lateral (L) blocks, together with the mid-dorsal and mid-ventral (MV) non-striated blocks. T, tegument; FZ, fibrous zone; C, thin circular muscle layer. The sarcoplasmic regions of longitudinal myofibres are omitted. (From Nuttman, 1975.) Figure used with permission from Dr Chris Nuttman.

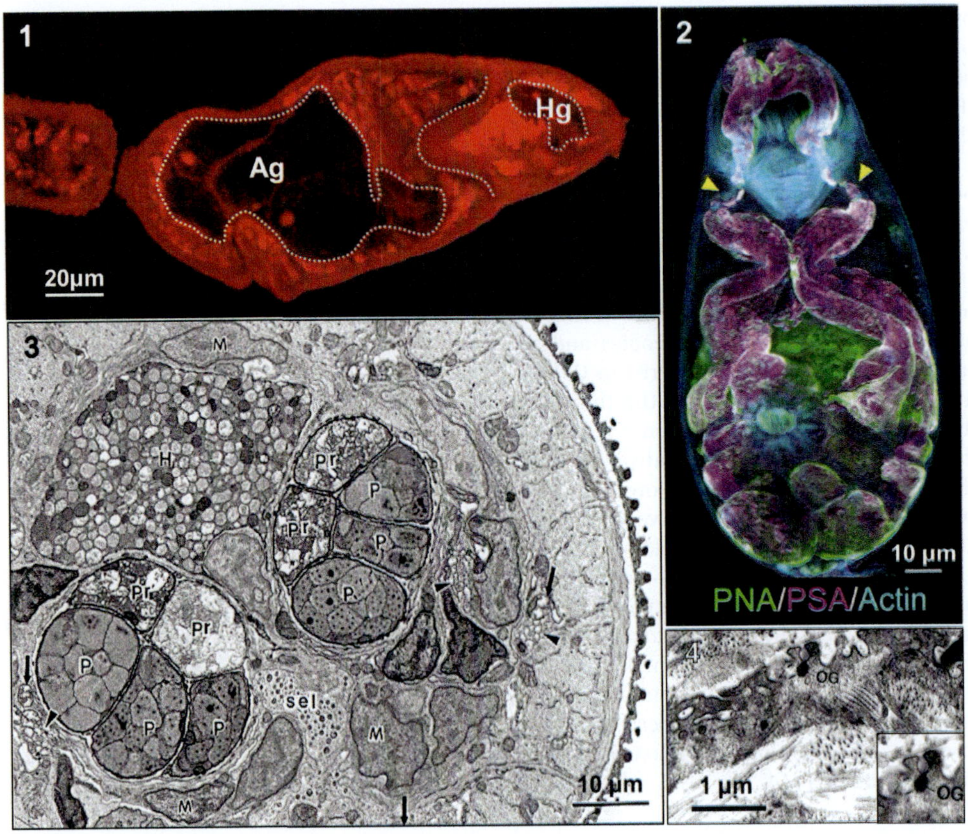

Fig. 2.5. The cercarial glands. **1**) Longitudinal confocal slice through a cercaria showing the body volume occupied by the acetabular glands (Ag) and the head gland (Hg) within the head capsule. **2**) Confocal projection of lectin staining to highlight pre-acetabular and post-acetabular gland cells and ducts, with muscles picked out by actin staining. Arrowheads indicate muscles around the ducts. **3**) TEM taken transversely across the head capsule to highlight the different appearance of pre- (Pr), post- (P) acetabular and head (H) gland contents. **4**) TEM of the tegument at the anterior showing the merocrine secretion of head gland vesicles by fusion with the surface plasma membrane (**1** from Parker-Manuel and Wilson, 2022; **2** from Collins *et al.*, 2011; **3** from Dorsey *et al.*, 2002; **4** from Crabtree and Wilson, 1985.) **1** and **2**) Figures used under license CC-BY-4.0. Figures used with permission from **3**) Elsevier and **4**) Cambridge University Press.

implying differences in glycan composition (Fig. 2.5.2) (Collins *et al.*, 2011). Certainly, at the ultrastructural level, the ovoid membrane-packaged secretions of the two glands (0.5 × 0.7 µm) differ in appearance (Fig. 2.5.3) (Dorsey *et al.*, 2002).

A third gland, the head gland, is located dorsally within the head capsule (Fig. 2.5.1). It has variously been described as having between one and four nuclei, so may be a syncytium (Dorsey, 1974). Its structure is quite different to that of the acetabular glands, and the cytoplasm is packed with small (~0.2 µm diameter) electron-dense, membrane-bound vesicles (Fig. 2.5.3). The gland is connected to the tegument cytoplasm at the extreme anterior of the head capsule via multiple microtubule-lined projections, in the manner of a tegument cell body (Fig. 2.5.4). The vesicle cargo is released by conventional merocrine secretion, in which the vesicle membrane fuses with the plasma membrane, so that the gland cytoplasm remains intact (Fig. 2.5.4). Unlike the acetabular glands, the head capsule and the gland it contains persist for some days after infection. Judging from the way numbers of vesicles in the head gland decline over time (Crabtree and Wilson, 1985), the period of secretion is prolonged and the secretions are potentially involved in several processes. In function it clearly differs from the destructive one-shot holocrine process employed for the acetabular glands during epidermal entry.

2.2.3 Protonephridia

The protonephridial system of the cercaria consists of 10 flame cells, eight bilaterally distributed along the body and a pair lying within the base of the tail (Fig. 2.6.1) (Collins *et al.*, 2011). Two body pairs are positioned between the ventral sucker and the head capsule, and two pairs posterior to it. As described in Chapter 6, each flame cell is a composite structure comprising a cap cell and a tubule cell. Further tubule cells convey the filtrate towards the bladder; their number has not been defined and their intracellular tubules follow a very convoluted path that is hard to map (Fig. 2.6.2). The tubules on each side unite to create two larger ducts at the level of the ventral sucker (Fig. 2.6.3). The walls of these ducts are thicker and the cytoplasm highly vesiculated, perhaps indicative of secretory activity. These wider ducts pass posteriorly to join a thin-walled bladder, situated just above the body/tail junction. Fortuitously, investigations of protein kinase A signalling in the cercariae highlight the activity of this enzyme on the walls of the nephridial tubules (Hirst *et al.*, 2016). From the bladder two tubules emerge and unite to pass down the centre of the tail (Fig. 2.6.4). They bifurcate before reaching the furcae, running to a vesicle in each, before terminating at a pore at the tip (Fig. 2.6.5). The collecting tubules leading to the bladder are also stained (Fig. 2.6.6). Why does the cercaria need a nephridial system when no cercarial tissue is more than 25 μm from an external surface so products of metabolism such as lactic acid should readily diffuse out? It is plausible that the osmotic barrier required by life in freshwater makes the cercarial surface too impermeable for adequate diffusion of metabolites, and the protonephridia provide an alternative route. Another possibility is that the cercaria needs to conserve inorganic salts during its free life in freshwater, as it has no way of replenishing them. Inspection of the protein kinase A interactome (Hirst *et al.*, 2016) did identify a Ca^{2+}-activated K^+ channel (Smp_166910).

2.2.4 Nervous system and sensory endings

The cercaria has an extensive central and peripheral nervous system. Staining for the nerve marker synapsin reveals a bilobed central ganglion astride the oesophagus (Fig. 2.7.1) (Collins *et al.*, 2011). In transverse section, the ganglion occupies all of the cercarial body within the body wall, apart from the bundle of gland cell ducts (Fig. 2.7.4) (Cousin and Dorsey, 1991). As in the miracidium, there is a rind of nerve cell bodies (perikarya) with their axons and dendrites forming a tangled knot in the central neuropile. From the ganglion, longitudinal nerves run to the posterior, uniting before the junction with the tail and then running along its length as a single commissure before bifurcating into each furca (Fig. 2.7.1). En route there is significant innervation of the acetabulum, and the muscles of the body wall and tail. There is a similar intensity of innervation of the head capsule muscles, with neurons investing the numerous sensory endings of the apical area.

A second and peripheral nerve net can be visualized by staining for the marker SmKK7 (Parker-Manuel and Wilson, 2022). The KK7 protein was first found in cercarial secretions and identified (incorrectly) as a K^+ channel blocker (Curwen *et al.*, 2006) but fortuitously serves as a marker for the nerve net (Chapter 5). *In situ* hybridization on cercariae revealed that the transcript was expressed in six cells in the body and two distally in the tail (Fig. 2.7.2). The protein product was localized, using specific antibodies, to the six cell bodies and a diffuse nerve net beneath the body wall. The anterior cell pair lies within the head capsule, the second is situated in the centre of the body, and the third towards the posterior. Overall, the peripheral nerve network comprises six ventral and six dorsal strands (Fig. 2.7.3) positioned along the body between the anterior and posterior, with some lateral connections (see Chapter 5 for the adult worm). There are also KK7-positive 'knobs' at the very anterior of the cercaria, external to the phalloidin-stained muscles, which equate to the bulbous sensory endings of the apical area (see below).

The variety of exposed and internal sensory nerve endings identified by light and electron microscopy has much in common with those of

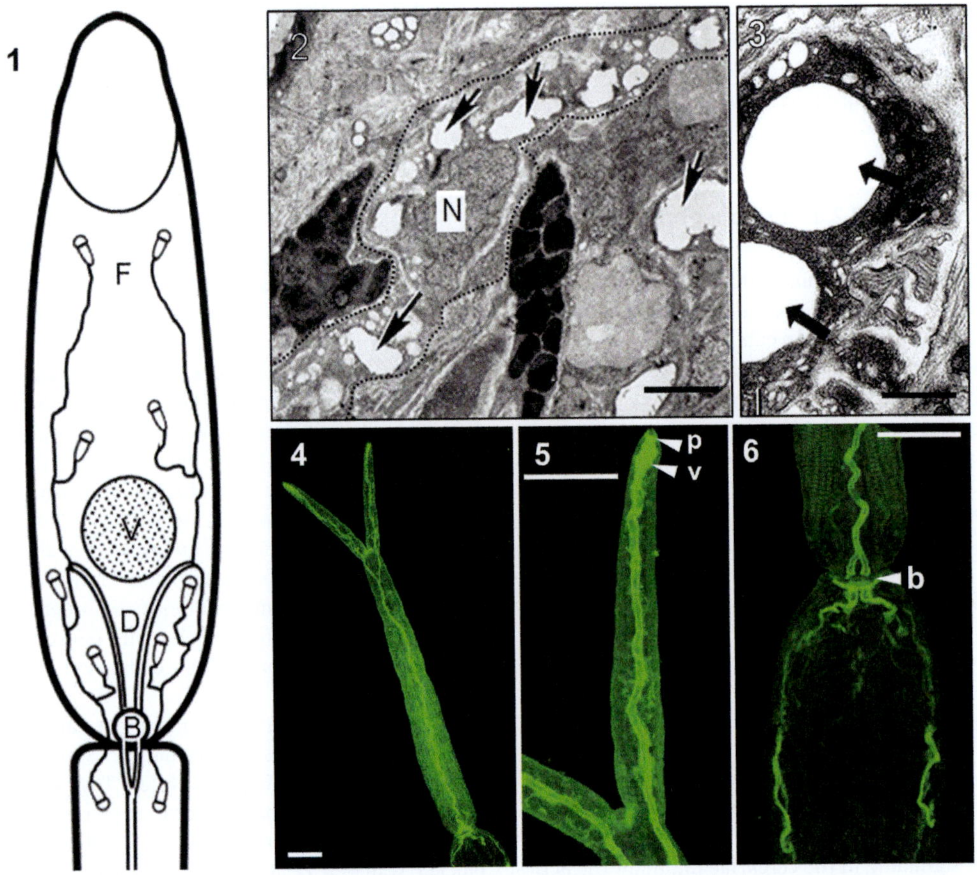

Fig. 2.6. The protonephridial system. **1**) Schematic of the layout in the head and tail (truncated). Four pairs of flame cells (F) in the body and one in the tail are connected via fine tubules to thicker walled collecting ducts (D) which convey fluid to a bladder (B). V, ventral sucker. **2**) TEM of a tubule cell with nucleus (N) showing the tortuous path of the tubules (arrowed) through the cytoplasm. **3**) TEM of the pair of collecting ducts in transverse section (arrowed), with highly vesiculated cytoplasm. **4–6**) Confocal images of a cercaria stained to detect activated protein kinase A (green). **4**) Activity in the tail is present along the narrow tubule that runs from the bladder down the centre, bifurcating to pass along the furcae. **5**) An excretory pore (p) is situated at the tip of each furca, preceded by a bulbous vesicle (v). **6**) The bladder region (b) showing the two collecting ducts entering and two thinner ducts exiting before fusing to form the tail tubule. Scale bars: **2** and **3**, 0.5 μm; **4–6**, 20 μm. (**2** and **3** from Dorsey *et al.*, 2002; **4–6** from Hirst *et al.*, 2016.) **1**) Figure author's own. **2** and **3**) Figure used with permission from Elsevier. **4–6**) Figures courtesy of Professor Anthony J. Walker.

the miracidium. However, their distribution appears rather different, and this is likely related to the behaviour patterns involved in location of, and penetration through the mammalian host skin. The front face of the head capsule, where the five pairs of acetabular gland ducts empty to the exterior, has been mapped by scanning electron microscopy (SEM) (Parker-Manuel and Wilson, 2022). It bears two symmetrical arcs of five sensory endings, each comprising two with short cilia, one with a long cilium and two with short fat cilia (Fig. 2.8.1 and 2.8.2). The pattern of such single ciliated receptors scattered over the surface of the body and tail is diagnostic of different *Schistosoma* species and was used in 'chaetotaxy' before the advent of molecular techniques. A total of 76 papillae was counted on the cercarial body of *Schistosoma mansoni*,

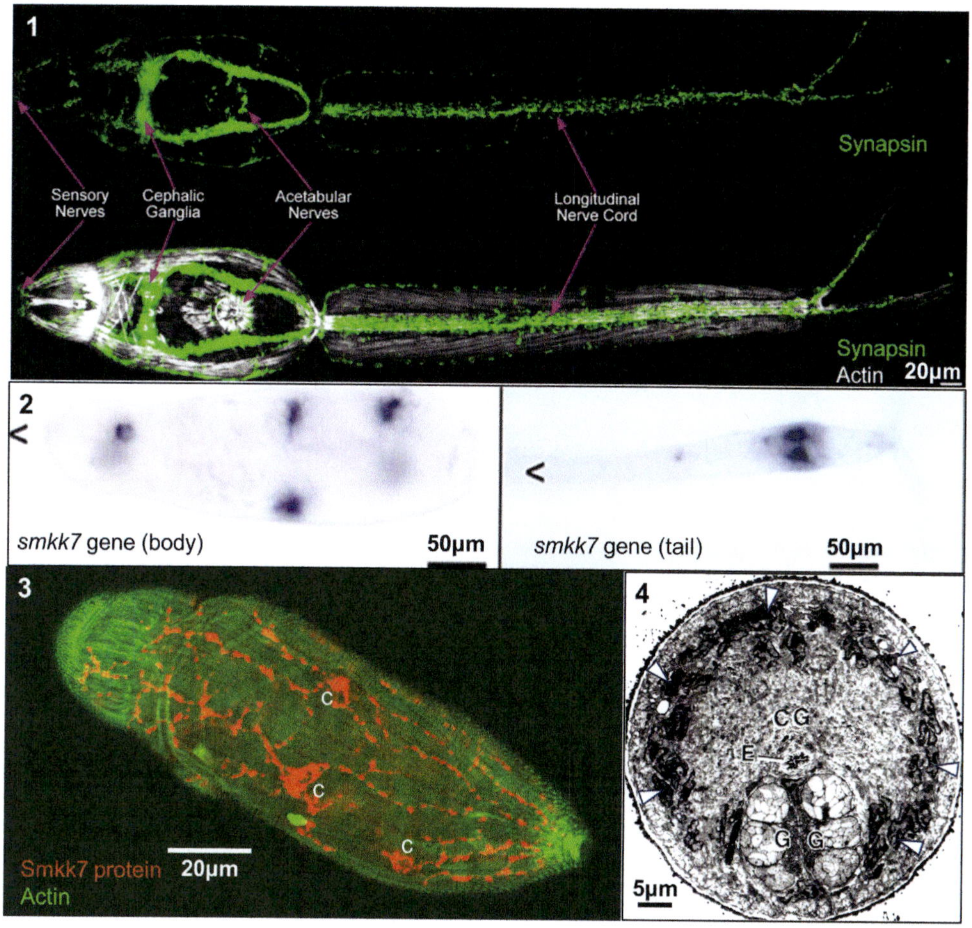

Fig. 2.7. The cercarial nervous system. **1**) Staining with an anti-synapsin antibody labels the cephalic ganglia and many peripheral neural structures, +/– phalloidin staining for muscle actin. **2**) Detection of Sm*kk7* gene expression by *in situ* hybridization reveals six cells in the body and two distally in the tail. **3**) Staining of SmKK7 protein with specific antibody shows its site of synthesis in cell bodies (c) and its distribution along nerves of the peripheral network but not the ganglion. **4**) TEM of the central ganglion (CG) astride the oesophagus (E) showing the rind of perikarya (arrowed) and the neuropile occupy all the space apart from the gland cell ducts (G). (**1** from Collins *et al.*, 2011; **2** and **3** from Parker-Manuel and Wilson, 2022; **4** from Cousin and Dorsey, 1991.) **1**) Figure used under license CC-BY-2.5. **2** and **3**) Figures used under license CC-BY-4.0. **4**) Figure used with permission from Springer Nature.

plus 50 on the tail (Fig. 2.9.1) (Short and Cartrett, 1973; Nuttman, 1975). The uniciliate endings clearly supply the cercaria with abundant positional data when it contacts a substratum, and they include a group of papillae within the bulb of the ventral sucker. It is plausible that the sensory papillae on the furcae inform the cercaria of its arrival at the water surface, to terminate the swimming activity (see below).

At the ultrastructural level, the presumed mechanoreceptors fall into two groups (Fig. 2.9.2) (Nuttman, 1975). The simplest is a nerve bulb anchored in the tegument by a circular septate desmosome, from which projects a single cilium (Fig. 2.9.3), in a few instances up to 10 µm long. A second type is a simple nerve bulb with a short projecting cilium, surrounded by a collar of tegument cytoplasm (Fig. 2.9.4) which

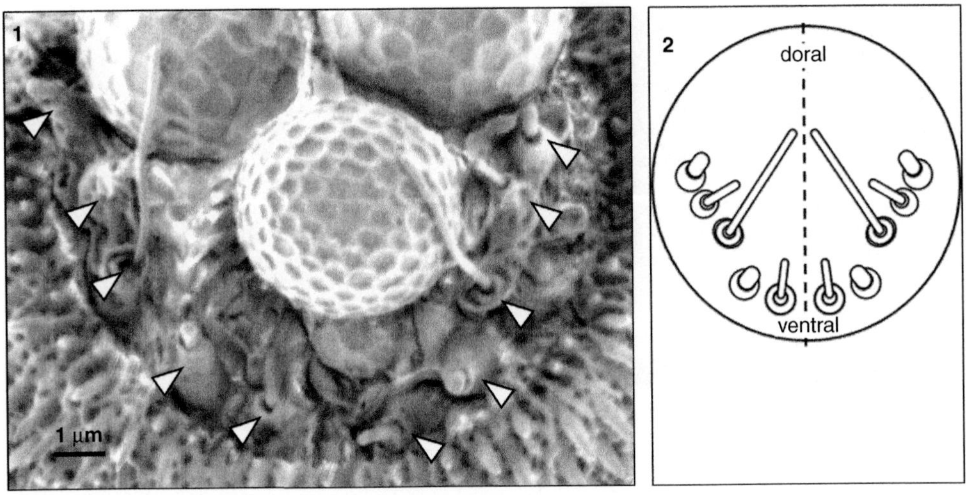

Fig. 2.8. Cercarial mechanoreceptor endings. **1**) SEM image of the front face of the head capsule showing three types of ciliate ending. The geodesic domes are droplets of extruded viscous gland cell secretions. **2**) Schematic of the same area showing the three types of sensory ending with projecting cilia: short fat sheathed, short thin unsheathed, and long thin. These represent the first point of contact between the cercaria and skin that will trigger attachment and penetration behaviour. (**1** and **2** from Parker-Manuel and Wilson, 2022 from an image courtesy of Professor James McKerrow and Dr Stephanie Hopkins, UCSF, San Francisco, CA, USA.)

presumably acts to dampen down the mechanical signal. In cross-section the cilia have the classical 9 + 2 arrangement of microtubules in epithelial plates and flame cells but there is no evidence that they are motile (Nuttman, 1975). More likely they serve a signal transducing function. The nerve bulb of these ciliated nerve endings contains numerous large membrane-bound vesicles extending down the exon. One potential constituent of unknown function is the SmKK7 protein, mentioned above.

A third and enigmatic structure, termed a laminate receptor (Nuttman, 1975), is positioned at the front lateral edge of the head capsule (Fig. 2.9.5). A pair of these nerve endings is entirely enclosed beneath the body wall, and similar in structure and appearance to the proposed 'balance receptor' of the miracidium. The nerve bulb consists of a thin-walled sac into four to six laminated membrane whorls project. These may be degenerate cilia, each with the remnants of a basal body. Given the location of the lamellate receptors, it was suggested that they function as 'squeeze receptors' (Nuttman, 1975), so that when a cercaria is probing under the plates of the stratum corneum during skin penetration, the receptors would be stimulated. It is also worth recording that the laminate structures have been suggested as photoreceptors (Short and Gagné, 1975), but see below. A fourth receptor type comprises multiciliated pits open to the exterior (cf. the miracidium), which are the best candidates for chemoreceptors (Fig. 2.9.6). Transmission electron microscopy (TEM) investigations have identified such pits distributed ventrally posterior to the sucker, approximately dorsal to the sucker, along the line of the lateral nerve cords, and most numerous around the head capsule (Nuttman, 1975), but a map is not available. Each pit is attached to the overlying tegument by a circular desmosome, leaving a pore 0.2 μm in diameter, open to the exterior. Five to six cilia, at least 1.0 μm long, project into the lumen of the pit which also contains numerous small (~50 nm) dense vesicles of unknown content, origin and function. Ciliary basal bodies lie within the cytoplasm of the pit wall, and numerous clear spherical vesicles are present, as in other sensory endings. If these pits are capable of detecting host skin chemicals, then their widespread distribution may result in a complex pattern of behaviour, depending on which pits are stimulated.

Finally, that leaves the conundrum of a photoreceptor. The schistosome cercaria is clearly

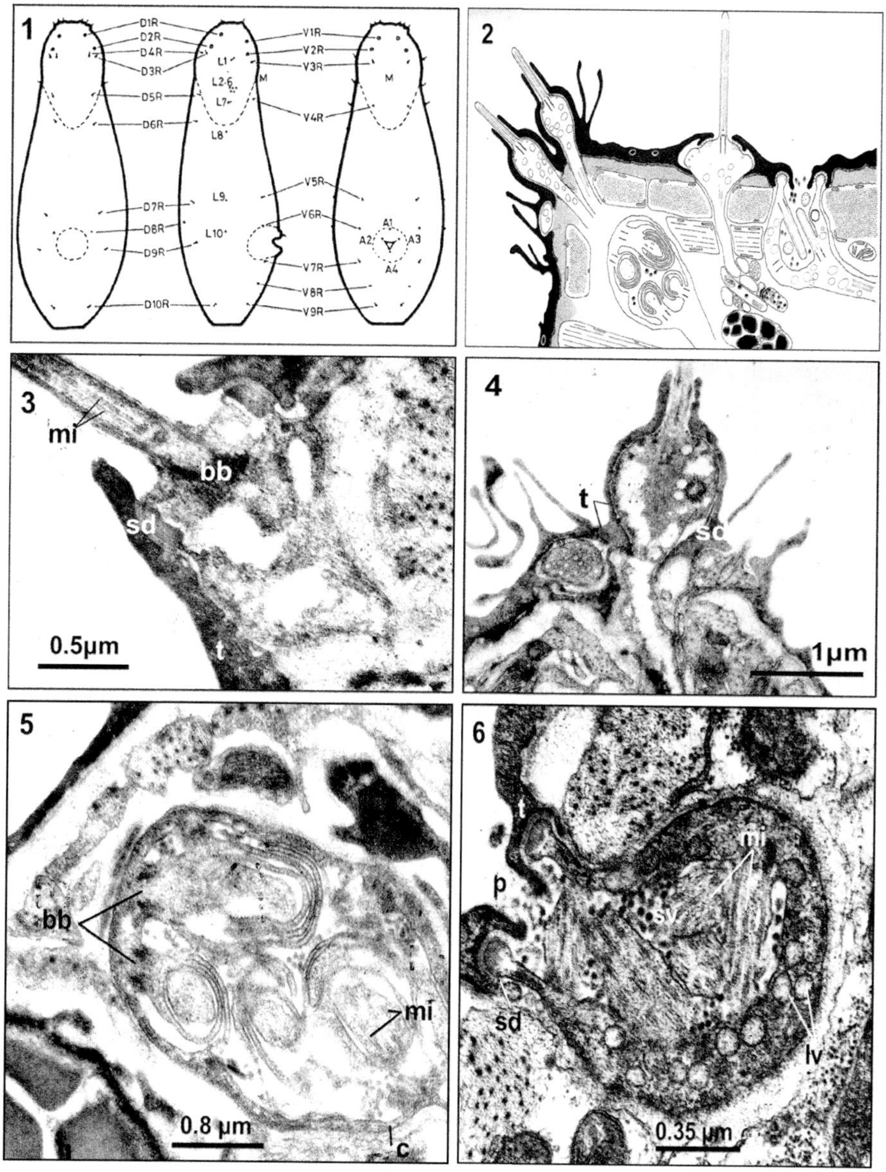

Fig. 2.9. Sensory nerve endings of the cercaria. **1**) Map of the projecting single cilia mechanoreceptor endings on the cercarial body from dorsal, lateral and ventral views. **2**) Schematic of the four main classes of sensory ending at the anterior of the head capsule. **3**) Single cilium (of varying length) with basal (bb) body, projecting from a nerve bulb held in the tegument (t) by a circular septate desmosome (sd). **4**) Single ciliated nerve bulb surrounded by a circlet of tegument cytoplasm, presumed to dampen tactile stimulation. **5**) Lamellate body with whorls of membrane projecting from the bounding capsule (c) into the central cavity, each anchored by a much-reduced basal body and microtubules (mi). **6**) Multiciliated pit anchored into the tegument by a septate desmosome, open to the exterior by a narrow pore (p). Numerous small dense vesicles (sv) are present in the cavity. Abundant larger vesicles are present in the cytoplasm, and the short cilia are anchored by a reduced basal body. (From Nuttman, 1975.) Figures used with permission from Dr Chris Nuttman.

able to respond to light, but how is it detected? For a possible explanation we have to turn to bird schistosomes, in different genera from *Schistosoma* spp., but still within the Schistosomatidae. Cercariae of *Trichobilharzia* spp., parasites of ducks, have two very prominent eyespots partially surrounded by a cup of pigment granules to provide directionality (Fig. 2.10.1) (Neuhaus, 1952). These eyespots are situated dorsally, posterior to and directly connected to the neural ganglion. The eyespots in *T. ocellata* are even more sophisticated, with a transparent lens, potentially to focus the light on to a series of membranous structures (Fig. 2.10.2 and 2.10.3) (van der Roemer and Haas, 1984). These membranes are typical of other simple eyes that carry rhodopsin, the light transducing chemical. It would be worth investigating by TEM or *in situ* hybridization whether unpigmented receptors reside in the same location in *Schistosoma* spp.

2.2.5 Gene expression in cercariae

In the comparison of patterns of gene expression between the germ ball, cercaria and day 3 schistosomulum, the cercaria was the least biosynthetically active stage (Parker-Manuel *et al.*, 2011). This is not surprising as it has no access to external sources of materials and must rely on what has been accumulated within its snail host. Nevertheless, some genes were more highly expressed at the cercarial stage reflecting the switch to aerobic processes. These included: acyl CoA dehydrogenase required for the cycle of fatty acid oxidation, 13 members of the citric acid cycle (e.g. isocitrate dehydrogenase) and members of the electron transport chain (e.g. cytochrome *c* reductase). Surprisingly in this context, the phosphorylase enzymes involved in glycogen mobilization were not upregulated. The extensive and specialized musculature of the cercaria (see Section 2.2.1) is matched by the differential expression of a small group of 20 genes encoding 'actin binding' proteins. Two groups of genes encoding alimentary tract proteins were already active in the cercaria but more strongly expressed at day 3. They comprised 20 enzymes and saposins from the gastrodermis, and eight micro-exon genes (MEGs) from the oesophageal glands. This cercarial expression of alimentary tract genes may indicate an earlier onset of tissue function than anticipated. Five genes encoding members of the VAL family of proteins VAL-1, -2, -16, -17 and -21, were most highly transcribed in the cercaria. Apart from VAL-2, these were distinct from the nine VAL genes/proteins identified in the miracidium (see Table 1.1). Nevertheless, expression of these VAL genes indicates the potential of their protein products to modify host processes during skin penetration (see below).

On the assumption that the cercaria was about to experience 'stress' during the infection process, the expression pattern in the stress-related gene category was investigated. Three out of 29 genes were upregulated: universal stress protein, glutathione peroxidase and a multidrug resistance pump (MDR; Smp_151290). A small heat shock protein, Smp40, was also upregulated 18-fold. It is notable that this same chaperone

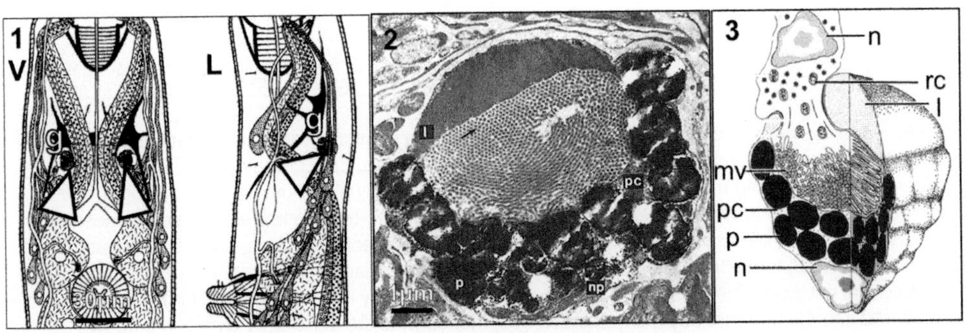

Fig. 2.10. The cercarial photoreceptor of bird schistosomes, *Trichobilharzia* spp. **1**) Schematic of eyespot location (arrowed) in *T. szidati*, posterior to the ganglion (g) in ventral view (V), and close to the dorsal surface in lateral view (L). **2**) TEM of the pigment cup (pc), lens (l) and microvilli (mv) of *T. ocellata*. **3**) Schematic of the way in which the retinular cell (rc) terminating in photoreceptor microvilli, the pigment cup cell with pigment granules (p) and the lens are assembled to create the directional light detector. (**1** from Neuhaus, 1953; **2** and **3** from van der Roemer and Haas, 1984.) Figures used with permission from Springer Nature.

comprises 15% of the soluble miracidial proteome (see Chapter 11, Section 11.3.2) (Mathieson and Wilson, 2010), and may protect proteins from irreversible aggregation upon stress-induced denaturation, in an energy independent manner. Given the extent of the remodelling starting immediately after infection, the upregulation of genes encoding proteins involved in apoptosis, autophagy or intracellular protein degradation by the proteasome pathway might be anticipated (again cf. the miracidium). Surprisingly, these were not evident, potentially indicating gene expression and protein synthesis had occurred earlier in the developing germ ball. The limitation of characterizing gene expression patterns in a dynamic transition, such as an infection process, is that we cannot know if they reflect current protein levels or those yet to come in the immediate future as the transition proceeds. At the time of writing there does not appear to be a detailed analysis of the whole cercarial proteome that might provide information on putative constituents of remodelling processes that occur immediately after skin penetration.

2.3 Life in Freshwater

2.3.1 Swimming

The strategy used by the cercaria when it emerges from the snail is quite different to that followed by the miracidium. It is best viewed as a 'sit and wait' behaviour, conserving energy for as long as possible until the final host passes by. On receipt of appropriate stimuli its behaviour changes dramatically, presumably to increase the probability of host contact. If that is not achieved, the behaviour reverts to 'sit and wait'. Movement is achieved by very rapid threshing of the tail that needs high speed image capture to record (Graefe *et al.*, 1967). The tail can oscillate at 22 Hz, due to the specialized structure of the longitudinal muscles, contracting alternately on its right and left sides. This equates to a maximum speed of 1.4 mm per second equivalent to three body lengths. (Note that the miracidium propelled by cilia actually moves faster, swimming continuously at 1.2 mm/s.) The contractions of the tail muscles are possibly unique among platyhelminths, faster than the tail beats of an amphibian tadpole or fish larva, but slower than hummingbird or insect flight. The direction of propulsion is determined by the position of the tail furcae. Held at an angle of 90°, the furcae have been likened to oar blades when the tail is active, and the cercaria swims tail-first. Conversely, when the furcae are closely apposed they function like an elastic tail fin and the cercaria swims head-first. Moreover, the cercaria can alternate these furcal positions instantaneously when stimulated, achieving frequent reversals of direction. A detailed physical analysis of this elastohydrodynamic 'T swimmer gait' has been reported (Krishnamurthy *et al.*, 2017). After escape from the snail a cercaria rapidly rises to the water surface by active swimming, and then sinks slowly, head-first (Video 2.1). Once established this alternating swim/sink behaviour just below the surface persists for hours, essentially maintaining the cercaria in one place, apart from the vagaries of water currents (see Section 2.3.3). After a time, a gradual increase in the sink period results in a cercaria transitioning to the bottom of the cell.

2.3.2 Energetics and survival

Snails incubated in water containing ^{14}C-glucose will take it up and it is incorporated both into the

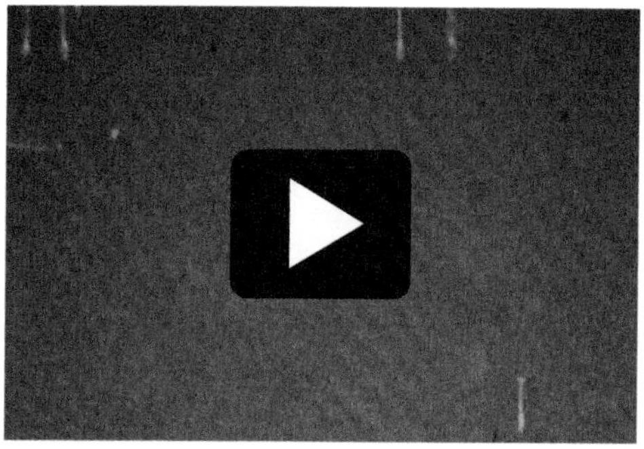

Video 2.1. Cercariae recorded at the surface (top) of the glass cell shortly after shedding from the snail host into pond water. They hang tail uppermost and display alternate brief periods of upward swimming with slow sinking. Arrival at the meniscus terminates the swim period. (Note that the minute objects swimming randomly through are protozoa in the pond water.) Video courtesy of Dr N.P. Carter.

tissues of the hepatopancreas and developing cercaria, which later emerge with a cargo of labelled glycogen (Bruce *et al.*, 1969). Cercaria can also be labelled by a brief incubation in water containing high specific activity ^{14}C-glucose (with the caveat that this is an artificial situation). During the ensuing 18 h of free life the labelled glycogen is consumed and the ^{14}C label appears in CO_2 (79%), pyruvate (12%) and lactate (9%) (Van Oordt *et al.*, 1989). This indicates that the cercaria has an aerobic energy metabolism centred on the Krebs cycle, with no evidence for other constituents such as lipids as an energy source (Bruce *et al.*, 1969). This makes the glycogen content accumulated by the developing cercaria an important determinant of its lifespan and infectivity. Measured by a specific enzymatic method in small samples of newly emerged cercariae, it was found to vary between 4.78 and 14.15 ng per cercaria (mean 9.4 ng), the range presumably reflecting the nutritional status of the snail host (Lawson and Wilson, 1980). The survival curves of cercariae, maintained at different temperatures, were measured in an ecologically realistic window between 15°C and 35°C. They had a reverse sigmoid form (Fig. 2.11.1 at 25°C) indicating that there was a time lag before death became appreciable and as might be anticipated, the higher the temperature the shorter the half-life ($t_{1/2}$) of the population (Fig. 2.11.2). This relationship with ambient water temperature has implications for transmission.

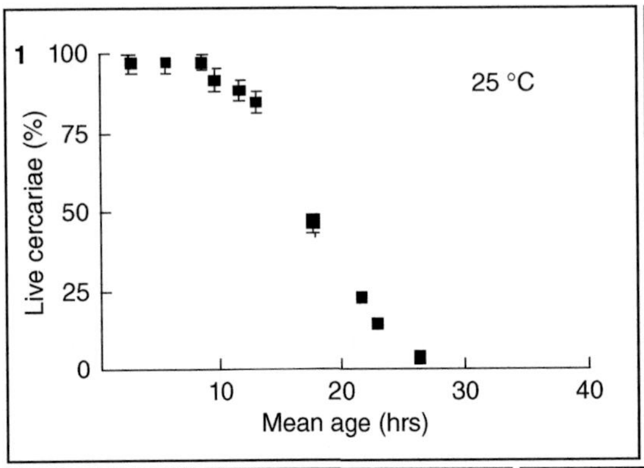

2

Temp	Survival
°C	t½(h)
35	10.7
30	17.9
25	23.1
20	31.5
15	53.3

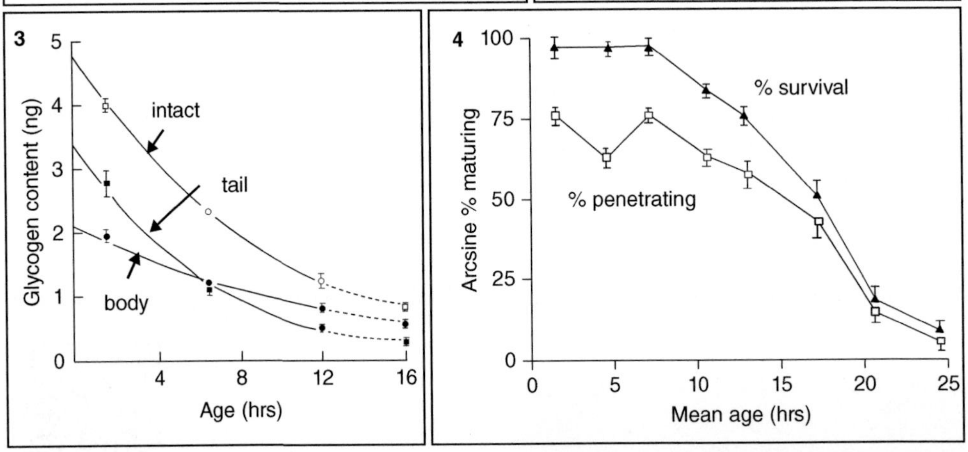

Fig. 2.11. The energetics and survival of cercariae with time after shedding. **1**) Survival curve of cercariae at 25°C. There is a latent period before any death is observed. **2**) The $t_{1/2}$ of survival at a range of temperatures, calculated by probit transformation of % survival. **3**) The mean glycogen content per cercaria, measured in intact parasites, and separated bodies and tails. The solid line represents the best fit exponential model of the form $G_t = G_0 \exp^{(gt)}$. **4**) The relationship between survival, ability to penetrate and % maturation in mice. (**1–3** from Lawson and Wilson, 1980; **4** from Lawson and Wilson, 1983.) Figures used with permission from Cambridge University Press.

The glycogen content of whole cercariae and separated bodies and tails was measured during ageing at 27°C, over the first 9–12 h to avoid complications due to mortality (Fig. 2.11.3) (Lawson and Wilson, 1980). At the outset, the tails contained ~55% of the glycogen. Total glycogen declined in a negative exponential manner, but faster in the tail than body so that the level of glycogen in the tail rapidly fell below that of the body as ageing proceeded.

The ability of cercariae to penetrate the skin and establish an infection has been a major source of controversy that has taken decades to disentangle (see Chapter 3). Nevertheless, standardized exposures of, for example, mice can be performed to chart the fate of the skin penetrants. Setting aside controversies about what happens in the skin and simply looking at the number of parasites maturing at 5 weeks, it is possible to obtain information on the decline in cercarial infectivity with time (Fig. 2.11.4) (Lawson and Wilson, 1983). For ~8 h, the ability of cercariae to penetrate and mature is unaffected, but thereafter there is a gradual decline as they age and consume their glycogen reserves. Measuring the utilization of glycogen reserves during penetration through an excised skin membrane revealed that the process consumed 24% of the body glycogen; incubation for a further period in culture medium consumed another 11%. Thus, it is feasible that a cercaria with only a feeble swim response, may still have sufficient body reserves to penetrate skin and undergo transformation.

2.3.3 Host location

A potential mammalian (or avian) schistosome host entering water may bring shadows, water turbulence, a temperature gradient and numerous skin chemicals into the orbit of a cercaria. The influence of temperature on host location was discounted because the differential between human skin in water at 28°C was only 0.5°C after 1 min of immersion, so it is very unlikely that this stimulus could be remotely sensed (Nuttman, 1975). A response to a shadow stimulus of 3–4 s was readily demonstrable (Fig. 2.12.3 and Video 2.2) (Carter, 1978), markedly increasing the percentage activity of the population at the top of the cell and persisting up to 30 s. The ability of cercariae to respond to water turbulence was tested by the simple expedient of filling the test cell with cercariae and waiting 15 s for mixing to subside before recording activity. There was a great increase in the duration of the swimming period directly after the cell was filled, before it slowly returned to basal levels, but the duration of the sinking period was unaffected. The result was an increase in the overall activity but not in the speed, direction and angularity of the swimming. It appears that both shadows and turbulence activate the swimming phase but impart no information about directionality of the stimulus.

That brings us to the question of skin chemicals as a stimulus. Which are important and how do they aid host location? It was well known that human skin lipids smeared on to glass slides would stimulate cercarial attachment (Stirewalt and Walters, 1973) but could these same lipids alter cercarial behaviour at a distance? Cercarial swimming behaviour was recorded in the presence of an aqueous swab of human forearm skin, and in proximity to an anaesthetised mouse tail (Fig. 2.12.2 and Videos 2.3 and 2.4) (Carter, 1978). The duration of the swim period was dramatically increased by the presence of skin surface chemicals and the stimulus of rapid mixing enhanced the response. Initially, all the cercariae were swimming, and although this activity slowly subsided, 5 min after filling the cell, 35.6% of the cercariae were still actively swimming. The important feature of this activity is that both close to a mouse tail and in human skin wash, the cercariae swam in all directions. Many also showed reversals in the mode of swimming, i.e. the normal tail-first swimming briefly became head-first. A few cercariae were also observed to attach briefly to the glass walls of the test cell. The cercariae do not show a directed response to host chemicals (i.e. not a taxis), rather it is a chemoklinokinesis (Haeberlein and Haas, 2008). It makes no difference whether the skin surface chemicals were diffuse (from a skin swab) or in the form of a possible gradient from a mouse tail (Carter, 1978). Precisely how the change in behaviour induced by host skin chemicals increases the chance of a cercaria contacting its host is unclear. Computer simulations did not resolve the question, but an active cercaria will have a better chance of hitting the host than an inactive one. It is worth noting that if host contact is not made and the stimulus is removed,

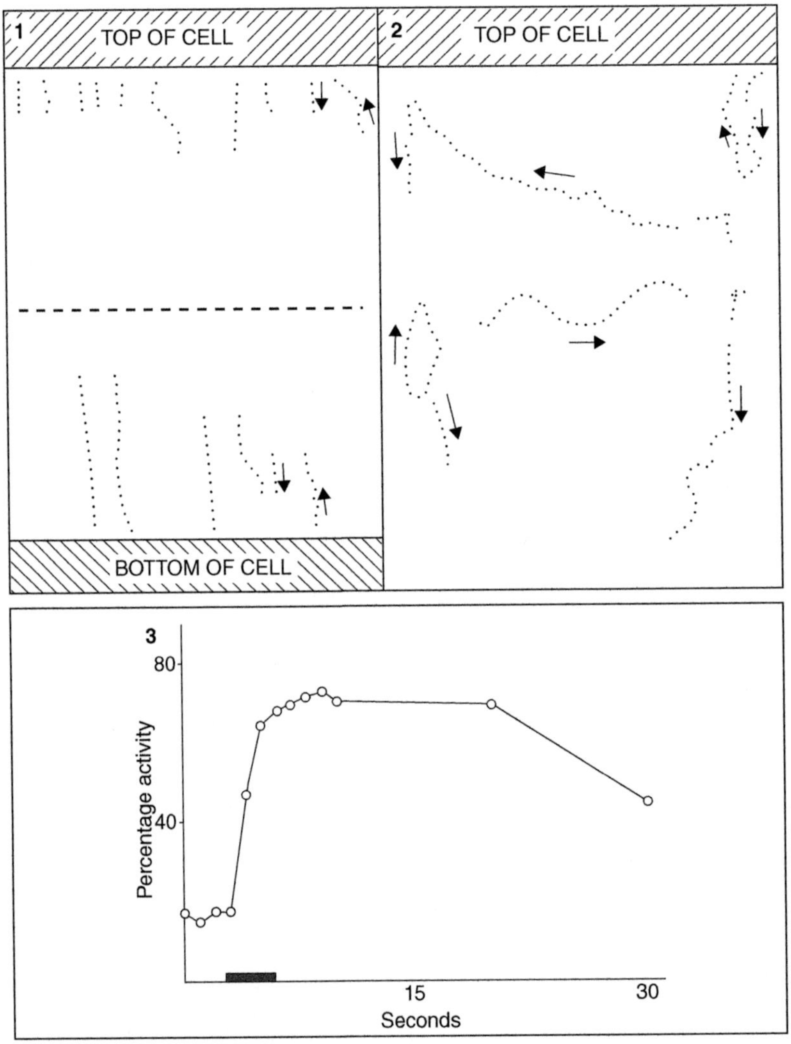

Fig. 2.12. Behaviour of cercariae during location of the host. **1**) Tracks of cercariae alternately swimming and sinking at the top and at the bottom of a test cell. The time intervals are 0.185 s for swimming and 0.926 s for sinking tracks. **2**) Sample tracks of cercariae swimming in skin-conditioned water directly after the cell was filled. **3**) The percentage activity of 1-h-old cercariae at the top of a test cell after application of a shadow stimulus. (From Carter, 1978.) Figures used with permission from Dr N.P. Carter.

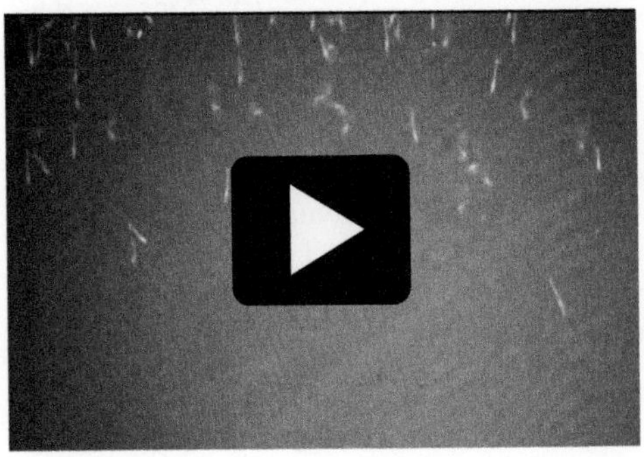

Video 2.2. A dense population of cercariae suspended at the top of the cell, showing the sinking swimming pattern. Activity is abruptly triggered by the application of an external shadow stimulus, but then rapidly subsides to the background rhythm. Video courtesy of Dr N.P. Carter.

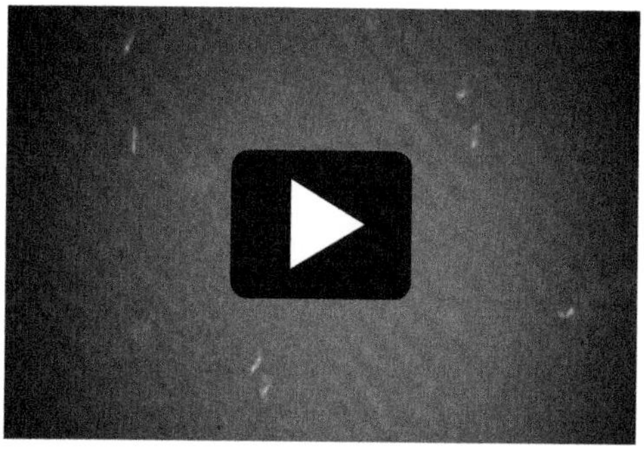

Video 2.3. Cercariae added to human skin-conditioned water before pipetting into the recording cell. The cercariae swim continuously in all directions, with occasional reversal, and this behaviour persists for some time. Video courtesy of Dr N.P. Carter.

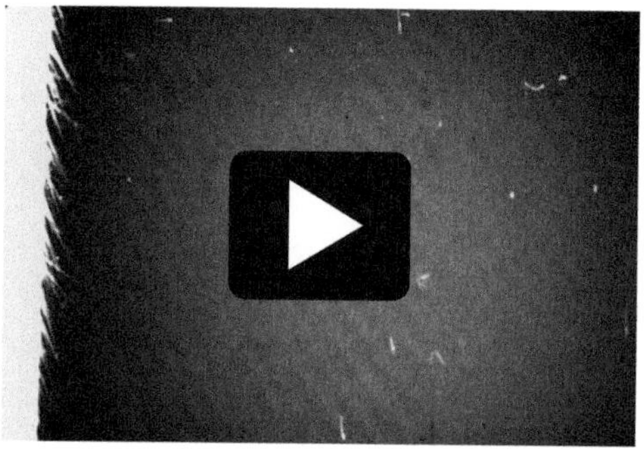

Video 2.4. A record of cercariae swimming in the vicinity of an anaesthetised mouse tail (left edge). There is no directed movement towards the tail but rather, an increase in swimming activity. Some cercariae are stimulated to attach to the glass surface of the cell, especially in the vicinity of the tail where skin chemical concentration will be highest. Video courtesy of Dr N.P. Carter.

the cercarial behaviour returns to the unstimulated state to conserve energy and await another attempt.

The chemicals present on human skin have been characterized, and constituents assayed for their effect on cercarial behaviour, to identify the active agents (Haeberlein and Haas, 2008). Initial fractionation involved separation of an aqueous extract into hydrophilic and lipophilic components; both increased the frequency with which cercariae changed their direction of swimming – the 'shift rate'. Among skin surface lipids, only fatty acids had a significant effect on the shift rate, down to a 0.1 μM threshold. Specifically, these were saturated C_{10} to C_{14} aliphatic chain, and an unsaturated C_{18} series, their stimulant activity increasing with the number of *cis*-double bonds (this grouping hints at solubility in water as the important parameter). Small molecular compounds (<3 kDa) in the hydrophilic fraction also stimulated the chemokinetic response, with activity restricted to the basic amino acids. L-Arginine at concentrations as low as 100 nM was the exclusive stimulant in the mixture and a weaker chemokinetic response to a tetrapeptide with terminal L-arginine was also observed. The existence of two distinct chemo-stimulants implies the presence of different chemoreceptor specificities. The presence of multiple receptor pits on the body and apical area of the cercaria could accommodate this (see Section 2.2.4).

2.4 The Skin Barrier

Mammalian (and avian) skin presents a much greater obstacle for the infective cercaria than the single layer of snail epidermis did for the miracidium. This explains why proportionally much more of the cercarial body is occupied by gland cells. The layout of skin is a cellular epidermis overlying a thicker and largely extracellular dermis that rests on a subcutaneous layer, rich in adipose tissue (Fig. 2.13.1). Skin thickness varies according to location on the body, but for the purposes of cercarial infection that of arms or legs has an overall thickness of ~1 mm, one-tenth of which is epidermis. This outer layer is primarily a stratified squamous epithelium of keratinocytes, plus minor cell types, resting on a basal lamina, incorrectly referred to as a membrane. The basal lamina comprises a mixture of collagens, laminin, perlecan and entactin, secreted by cells of the stratum basale, bound together in a highly

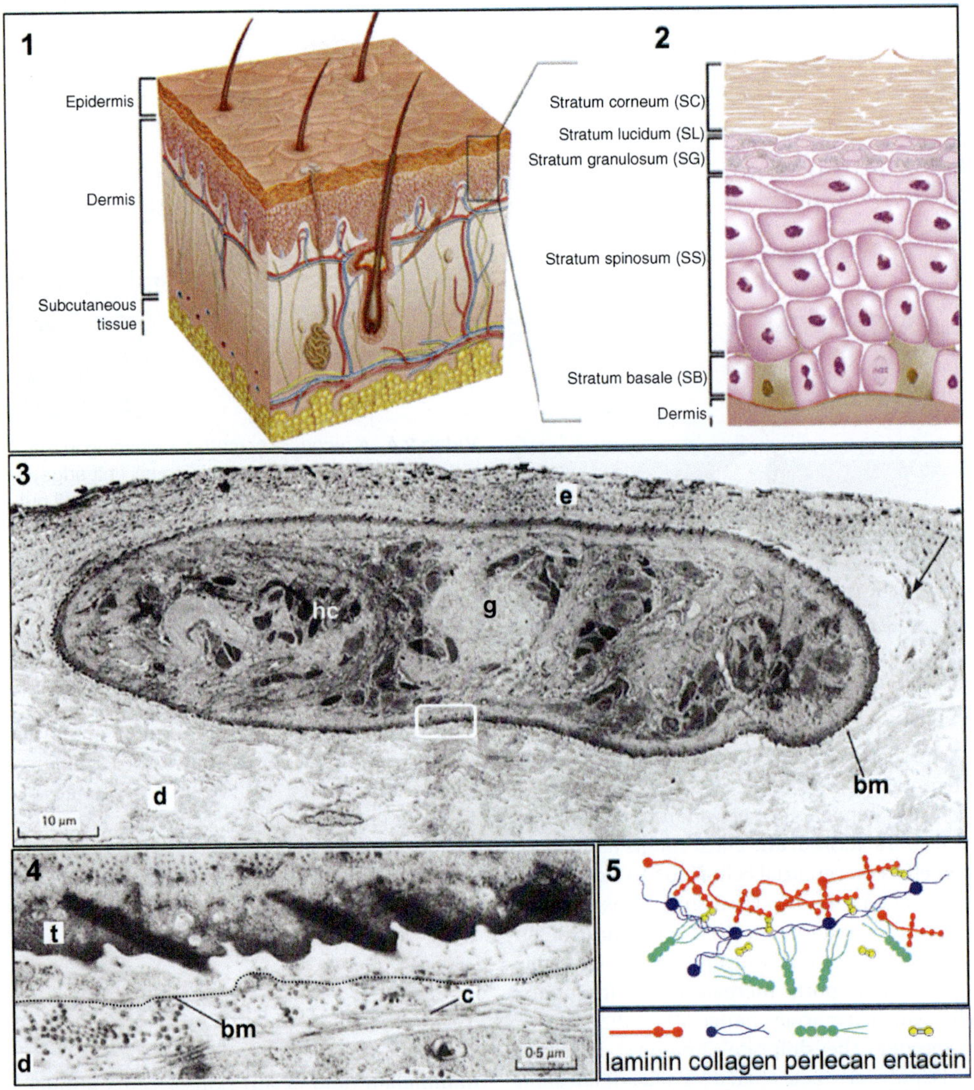

Fig. 2.13. Cercarial penetration into the skin. **1**) Diagram of the human skin barrier showing the epidermis and underlying dermis, with hair follicles and sebaceous glands, sweat glands and blood supply. **2**) The epidermis enlarged to show the four cell layers. **3**) The body of a cercaria 30 min after exposure to hamster cheek pouch skin, lying in a penetration tunnel (arrowed) at the base of the epidermis (e) external to the basement membrane (bm). The head capsule (hc) and ganglion (g) are visible, but most acetabular gland material has been used (d) dermis. **4**) Enlarged area in **3**, the cercarial tegument (t) and spines with tissue debris. The basement membrane is intact and collagen fibres (c) make up the dermal matrix below it. **5**) The molecular composition of the basal lamella. (**1** and **2** from Dijkhoff *et al.*, 2020; **3** and **4** from Crabtree and Wilson, 1985; **5** courtesy of Professor Michelle Peckham, University of Leeds, Leeds, UK) **1** and **2**) Figures used under license CC-BY-4.0. **3** and **4**) Figures used with permission from Cambridge University Press.

cross-linked extracellular matrix (https://www.histology.leeds.ac.uk/tissue_types/connective/con_basal_lam.php). It appears to delay progress of the invading larva into the dermis.

The epidermis can be divided histologically into four layers (Fig. 2.13.2) but importantly, the keratinocytes are continually generated by mitosis of stem cells at the base and gradually differentiate as they move up towards the surface. This involves the synthesis of multiple types of keratin, and other markers. Ultimately, the cells lose their nuclei and organelles to become corneocytes, which make up the stratum corneum. Adjacent corneocytes are bound together by intercellular adhesive proteins and become embedded in a matrix of specialized lipids, including ceramides, cholesterol and free fatty acids, mostly originating in lamellar bodies deeper in the epidermis. These hydrophobic components fuse together to form multiple bilayers of lipids between corneocytes to act as the principal barrier to the transcutaneous movement of water and electrolytes. The corneocytes are eventually shed by desquamation. The penetrating cercaria appears to make very short work of this epidermal layer.

The dermis consists of connective tissue, a conglomeration of fibres and extracellular matrix in which a number of cell types are located. Hair follicles, sebaceous glands and sweat glands are also embedded in the matrix, and it is supplied with blood vessels, lymphatics and nerves (Fig. 2.13.1). Scattered fibroblasts are the principal cell type responsible for production of collagen, elastin and the hyaluronan, proteoglycans and glycoproteins of the matrix. Macrophages and mast cells, elements of the immune system, are also residents of the dermis. It is important to note that the sebaceous glands and hair follicles, although situated deep in the dermis, are still surrounded by an extension of the epidermal basal lamella so penetrant larvae entering those locations are not yet in the dermis proper.

2.4.1 Penetration

When a cercaria does make contact with the skin surface, the response is very rapid. The concentration of lipids is undoubtedly much higher than in the surrounding water, triggering attachment via the ventral sucker. This is followed by a sequence of behavioural responses, described as phases of invasion (Haeberlein and Haas, 2008). Enduring contact with the skin is followed by creeping activity using alternating attachment of apical organ and ventral sucker. The apical organ passes under exposed corneal squamae, and secretion of acetabular gland contents begins. Intravital labelling of the cercaria with the fluorescent tracer CFDA-SE (carboxyfluorescein succinimidyl ester) has permitted cercarial penetration of mouse skin to be analysed (Paveley *et al.*, 2009). In this study, the initial stage forcing under the stratum corneum took about 20 min, during which time the lashing tail broke off and was left behind. A squeezing phase followed during which the glycocalyx was shed, and the larva began to move more rapidly through the living cellular layers, creating a penetration tunnel up to 250 μm long. The cercarial head comes to rest lying parallel to the basal lamella (Fig. 2.13.3 and 2.13.4) (Crabtree and Wilson, 1985).

2.4.2 Cercarial secretions

It is possible to trigger the cercaria to secrete the contents of its acetabular glands *in vitro* and these were among the first preparations to be subjected to proteomic analysis (Knudsen *et al.*, 2005; Curwen *et al.*, 2006). Prior to that, conventional biochemical separation and molecular biology techniques had been used to isolate a group of serine proteases from *S. mansoni* cercariae, which were named elastases (Salter *et al.*, 2002). This nomenclature became another point of controversy because elastins are constituents of the dermis, only encountered by *S. mansoni* after the glands have been cleared (Curwen and Wilson, 2003). Two of the five genes identified in *S. mansoni* accounted for >90% of the protease activity, and closely related orthologues were present in *Schistosoma haematobium*. There are multiple variants of the *in vitro* methods used to stimulate secretion and transformation. These have included incubating cercariae in water in a petri dish coated in human skin lipid – this results in cytolysis as osmoprotection is lost. Forcing cercariae through a hypodermic needle to break off the tails also results in shear damage to the larval surface and leakage of internal proteins. The author's preferred method involves a brief vortexing to detach the tails, followed by immediate transfer to RPMI-1640 culture medium for 3 h, at 37°C (Ramalho-Pinto *et al.*, 1974). The viability of larvae generated in this way has been tested by *in vitro* culture for 7–12 days before transfer to the superior mesenteric vein of mice. The subsequent recoveries of adult worms 5 weeks later ranged from 70% to 87% (Harrop and Wilson, 1993). This approach provides a metric against which to assess induced larval necrosis.

The proteins released by 3 h in culture included the previously mentioned 'elastases' but additionally a metalloproteinase 'invadolysin' and a dipeptidyl peptidase (Table 2.1) (Curwen *et al.*, 2006). The three previously mentioned VAL proteins (VAL-4, -10 and -18; Section 2.2.5) were identified along with Sm16, and SmKK7 covered in Section 2.2.4. Given that secretion from the acetabular glands is holocrine, cytosolic and cytoskeletal proteins were also identified, particularly glycolytic enzymes. The analysis of potential penetration enzymes has been extended to other schistosome species as the sensitivity of mass spectrometric techniques improved. Initial studies on *Schistosoma japonicum* failed to find any serine proteases, but a cathepsin B (cysteine protease) was abundant (Dvorák *et al.*, 2008). This led to the hypothesis that cysteine proteases were the archetypal penetration enzymes, with the serine proteases arising later in schistosome evolution. With time, the situation has become more complex and nuanced. The use of laser capture microdissection on the acetabular glands of the bird schistosome *Trichobilharzia szidati* has provided a very different angle (Vondráček *et al.*, 2022). It proved possible to isolate the post-acetabular and pre-acetabular glands (circum-acetabular in *T. szidati*) for separate analysis, by intravital staining of the calcium present at high levels in the circum-acetabular glands. Assuming this method is valid, resulting in very limited mixing of the two gland constituents, then the surprise was that both types contained proteases. Indeed, peptidases of five catalytic types accounted for around 8% and 6% of reliably identified proteins in the post- and circum-acetabular glands, respectively. These included invadolysin (cf. Curwen *et al.*, 2006), nardilysin (M16 family protease), cathepsins B2 and L3, and elastase 2b. The presence of the elastase appears to invalidate the hypothesis about the late evolution of the serine proteases. Protease inhibitors cystatin and serpin were identified – are these present to regulate protease activation or are their intended targets host proteases from, for example, macrophages encountered during epidermal penetration? VAL-4, -10 and -18 were also found in the circum-acetabular glands (cf. Curwen *et al.*, 2006).

2.4.3 Metamorphosis

Information on this important transition is fragmentary, but it is possible to build up an impression of the process. The first irreversible event is loss of the osmo-protective glycocalyx as the cercaria passes through the stratum corneum, but the process is only completed when parasite growth is initiated in the hepatic portal system a week later. By 2–3 h after the start of penetration,

Table 2.1. Proteins in cercarial secretions identified by proteomics of two-dimensional gel separations.

Protein identity	Smp v4	Smp v10	Spot volume %	Function
Cercarial elastase 1a, 1b	119130	9 current identifiers	34.4	Serine protease
Cercarial elastase 2a	112090	5 current identifiers		Serine protease
Invadolysin	090100	090100	12.8	Metalloprotease
VAL-4	002070	002070	1.91	Immunomodulation
VAL-18	001890	001890	0.61	Immunomodulation
VAL-10	002060	002060	0.44	Immunomodulation
Sm16	113780	331920	3.38	? In all tissues
SmDPPIV	057530	057530	<0.5	Dipeptidylpeptidase
SmKK7	194830	194830	0.56	Nervous system
SmSerpin	003300	003300	4.9	Protease inhibitor

References: Curwen *et al.*, 2006. Table author's own.

the cercarial body (in *S. mansoni* at least) is lying in its penetration tunnel parallel to the epidermal basal lamella and metamorphosis is under way (Crabtree and Wilson, 1985). The morphological changes that accompany infection were characterized 50 years ago in an ultrastructural study, partly using parasites *in situ* in the skin and partly after *in vitro* transformation (Hockley and McLaren, 1973). The incorporation of an extra uranyl acetate fixation step during specimen preparation was a technical breakthrough that stabilized surface membrane structures. At 30 min, numerous ovoid vesicles (100–150 nm diameter) were present in the subtegumental cells and connections to tegument (Fig. 2.14.1). These contained whorls of membranous material around a denser core. By 60 min these vesicles were contributing to the tegument surface by membrane fusion, with their membranous contents spreading to give the surface a multilaminate appearance. As this process proceeded, the cercarial tegument membrane bilayer was displaced into microvillus-like projections (1500 nm long by 50 nm wide) covered with a thin filamentous coat; their fate was to be shed externally (Fig. 2.14.2 and 2.14.3) (Hockley and McLaren, 1973).

In the original study the new surface was described as heptalaminate, comprising two closely applied trilaminate membranes and the space between (Hockley and McLaren, 1973). This terminology needs to be seen in the context of the debate about membrane structure at the time, from the 1960s, when the concept of the

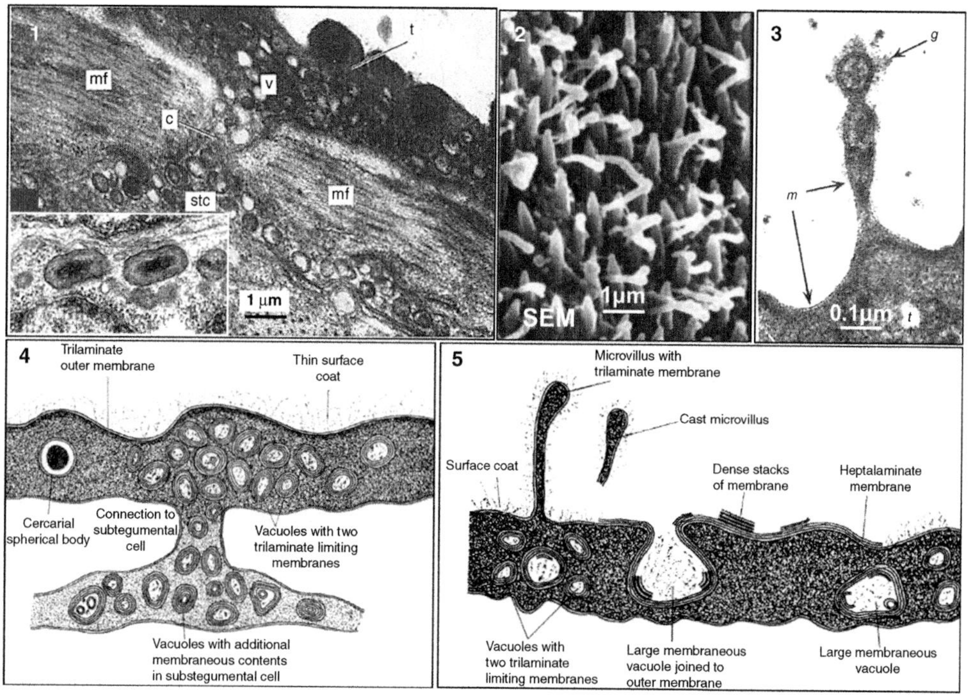

Fig. 2.14. Changes in the outer membrane of the tegument during transformation from cercaria to schistosomulum. **1**) A tegument cell body (stc) in the cercaria separated by muscle fibres (mf) but connected (c) to the tegument (t); numerous vesicles are present (v). The inset shows these contain membranous whorls around a dense core. **2**) SEM of the surface taken 30 min after *in vitro* transformation. Short microvilli are evident between the tegument spines. **3**) TEM at the same time showing that the microvillus has the normal trilaminate surface continuous with the tegument surface. **4**) Schematic of the relationship between the subtegumental cell and the cercarial tegument. **5**) Schematic of membraneous vesicles fusing with the surface to deliver their laminate cargo while at the same time replacing the cercarial tegument by shedding of microvilli and surface coat. (**1**, **4** and **5** from Hockley and McLaren, 1973; **2** and **3** from McLaren and Hockley, 1976; inset **1** from Dorsey *et al.*, 2002.) **1–5**) Figures used with permission from Cambridge University Press.

lipid bilayer unit membrane was introduced (Robertson, 1967) to the fluid mosaic model of cell membrane structure put forward in 1972 (Singer and Nicolson, 1972). The surface of the intra-mammalian schistosome after transformation is here interpreted as two bilayers originating as the vesicle membrane and its lamellar contents (see Chapter 7 on the tegument). For the parasite, this shedding of on old surface and its replacement with a new one ought to be a moment of extreme hazard. *In vitro* this is the case, but *in vivo* an attack on larvae newly penetrated into the skin has not been documented (see Chapter 9).

The sequence of membrane events during transformation to the schistosomulum was confirmed using the surface glucose transporter (SGTP-4) of adult worms as a marker for the process (Skelly and Shoemaker, 2001). At 0 h most cercarial bodies exhibit little or no visible staining for SGTP-4. After 60 min incubation in RPMI medium, the parasite surface stains in a regular but patchy manner as vesicles deliver their contents (Fig. 2.15.1 and 2.15.2); by 3 h the surface SGTP-4 pattern has become more uniform (Fig. 2.15.3). From then onwards, the larva can acquire glucose (and potentially other nutrients) across its new double bilayer surface (see Chapter 7).

Replacement of the tegument surface is only the first event in body remodelling that follows infection. Over the next 48–72 h, before the schistosomulum begins to migrate out of the skin, other changes occur. Experiments using ^{14}C-glucose revealed that at 3 h after penetration, energy metabolism was in transition but still sensitive to cyanide (i.e. still reliant on cytochrome *c* oxidase) (Thompson *et al.*, 1984). However, by 24 h CO_2 production was reduced by 77% while lactate had increased by 84%, almost identical with the levels in adult worms. Over this same period the remnants of the spent acetabular glands disappear. This coincides with the appearance by 24 h of acidic organelles inside the schistosomulum body, which take up the lysosome indicator LysoTracker Red (Al-Adhami *et al.*, 2005). The suggestion is that metamorphosis requires induction of the autophagy pathway to scavenge redundant tissues, and this deserves further scrutiny. The head gland is not subject to such a clearance mechanism at this stage. Given the extent of this remodelling, we might anticipate the upregulation of genes encoding proteins involved in apoptosis, autophagy

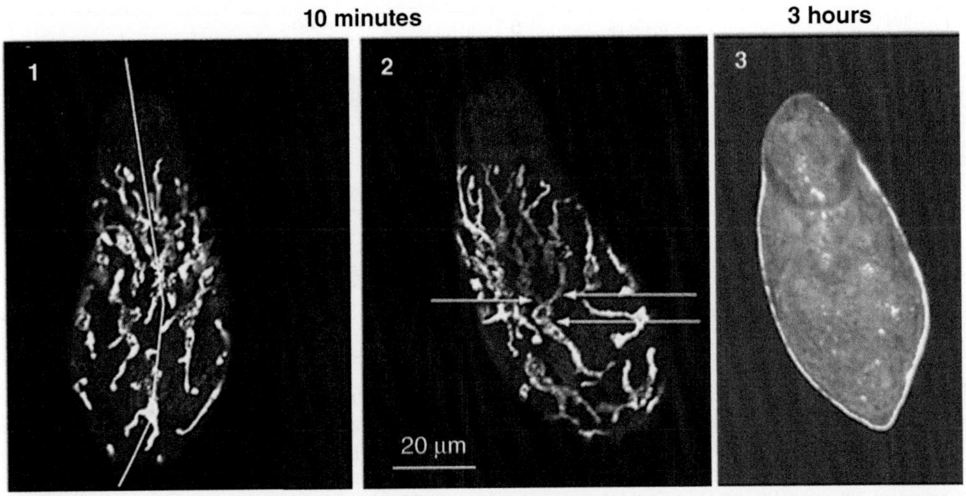

Fig. 2.15. Formation of the schistosomulum tegument by eruption over the surface of membrane vesicles from underlying cell bodies. **1**) The detection of the surface glucose transporter SGTP-4 by confocal microscopy. The bilateral symmetry of the cyton network is indicated by the white line. **2**) Its interconnected nature is indicated by the arrows. **3**) Optical section through a schistosomulum after 3 h reveals that the new surface is complete. (**1** and **2** from Skelly and Shoemaker, 2001.) Figures used with permission from Cambridge University Press.

or intracellular protein degradation by the proteasome pathway. However, expression of genes in these pathways was not evident in the day 3 schistosomulum (Parker-Manuel *et al.*, 2011). It is more plausible that the necessary components for tissue remodelling were pre-synthesized during cercarial development; a future proteomic analysis would illuminate this point.

2.4.4 Gene expression and protein synthesis: when does the alimentary tract become active?

In vivo, the migrating schistosomulum shows no evidence of mitosis before it reaches the hepatic portal system, and nor does it increase in mass (Lawson and Wilson, 1980). It does however undergo marked morphological changes that adapt it for intravascular migration (see Chapter 3). This must involve protein synthesis, and potentially new patterns of gene expression. In fact, this turns out to be a difficult question to address because all studies have relied on the maintenance of schistosomula in M169 medium with high nutrient levels (Basch, 1981). Such *in vitro* schistosomula in Basch medium are the equivalent of schistosomula newly arrived in the portal system at 7–10 days, not *in vivo* day 2–3 skin schistosomula. This conclusion is reinforced by the observation that when skin-transformed schistosomula were assayed for proliferation, by incorporation of the thymidine analogue 5-ethynyl-2′-deoxyuridine (EdU) into dividing cells (Wang *et al.*, 2018), five EdU^+ cells were observed around the penetration glands, between 22 and 36 h. Over the next 12 h they completed mitosis, with the appearance of five EdU^+ doublets; thereafter the number of EdU^+ nuclei steadily increased. By 1 week, two clusters of around two to three EdU^+ cells appeared in the germinal cell region posterior to the ventral sucker. How this relates to *in vivo* events is difficult to interpret and it must be assumed that these mitoses would normally be triggered after arrival in the portal vein.

With these caveats in mind about whether schistosomula cultured for 2–3 days represent newly arrived liver worms, it is worth summarizing observations made on gene expression. After the relative transcriptional desert of the cercaria, the day 3 schistosomulum showed upregulation of some gene categories related to its future development (Parker-Manuel *et al.*, 2011). The switch to anaerobic metabolism was accompanied by a 14-fold increase in lactate dehydrogenase transcripts. Upregulation of genes for a multidrug resistance protein, a superoxide dismutase and a thioredoxin peroxidase suggests a potential role in defence against oxidative attack from phagocytes. Alimentary tract genes upregulated included 10 of the 12 saposins, together with five cathepsins and an asparaginyl endopeptidase. Oesophageal gland MEG proteins MEG-4.1, -8.1, -8.2, -9, -12, -14, -15, -16 and -17 were also highly transcribed at day 3. Although ingestion of erythrocytes does not begin until the portal system is reached, this early transcription suggests that the alimentary tract may already be active at day 3 in skin schistosomula. Most genes encoding tegument proteins were upregulated in the day 3 schistosomulum, including five CD59-like analogues; their proteins are now in search of a function (Farias *et al.*, 2013). Additional to the glucose transporter SGTP-4, an aquaporin, an ectonucleotide pyrophosphatase and two amino acid transporters were upregulated. The activity of these alimentary tract and tegument surface genes attests to the skin schistosomulum readying itself for a life in the bloodstream, with the tegument changes essential for nutrient uptake. It thus appears possible that the alimentary tract is functional before the schistosomulum begins feeding on erythrocytes in the portal system and this has implications for vaccine targets (Chapter 9).

Single-cell RNA sequencing has been applied to 2-day-old schistosomula of *S. mansoni*, to produce a comprehensive cell type atlas of the early intra-mammalian stage (Diaz Soria *et al.*, 2020). Thirteen transcriptionally distinct populations were identified, comprising three muscle-like, two tegument, two parenchyma, one stem cell, four nervous system and one oesophageal gland (Fig. 2.16.1 and 2.16.2). The head gland, the protonephridial system and the nascent gut were not found. How the three muscle populations relate to intravascular migration or the vast expansion of the musculature in the hepatic portal growth phase is not presently clear. Cells of the tegument 1 population expressed a previously characterized Annexin B2 (Smp_077720) (Tararam *et al.*, 2010) (Fig. 2.17.1). Intriguingly,

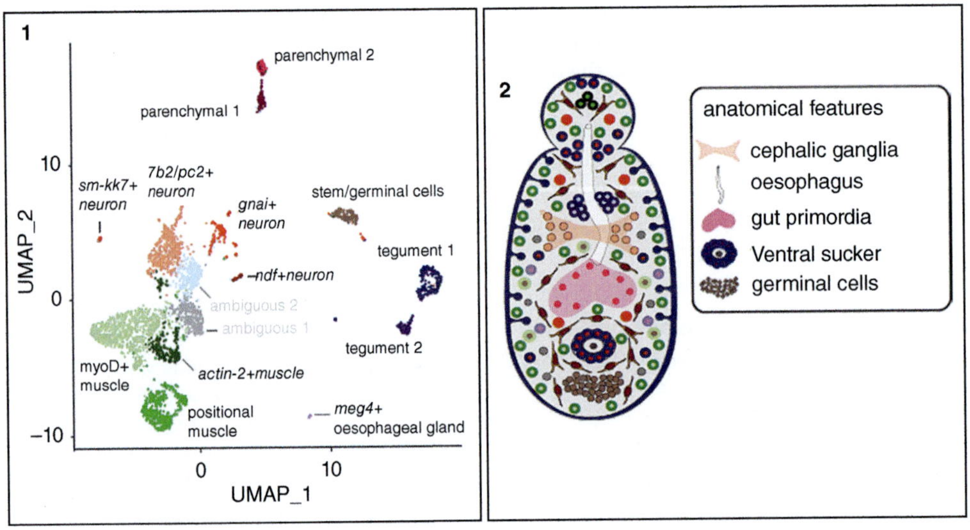

Fig. 2.16. Patterns of gene expression in day 2 *in vitro* cultured schistosomula. **1**) Uniform Manifold Approximation and Projection (UMAP) representation of single cells in 13 cell clusters. **2**) Schematic of cell and tissue locations in the day 2 schistosomulum. (From Diaz Soria *et al.*, 2020.) Figures used under license CC-BY-4.0.

the tegument 1 population also expressed one of the *meg3* family members (Smp_138070), in cells between the ventral sucker and the head capsule (Fig. 2.17.2). The expression of *meg4.1* (now Smp_307220) was demonstrated by *in situ* hybridization in the oesophageal gland cluster (Fig. 2.17.3), which also expressed *meg8.2*, *meg9*, *meg11*, *meg15* and *meg32.1* genes. Use of *in situ* hybridization confirmed the expression of *cathepsin B* in the nascent gut alongside lysosomal marker *lap* (leucine amino peptidase) with a broader tissue pattern (Fig. 2.17.4 and 2.17.5).

These studies of gene expression reveal a parasite larva getting ready for growth to the adult stage. However, it is emphasized that at the skin/lung stage *in vivo*, development must be paused while the schistosomulum makes the transit from the skin infection site to the distant location in the portal tract. How this pause is controlled remains to be established.

2.5 Summary

- The cercarial stage which infects the vertebrate host has marked contrasts with the miracidium. Propulsion is provided by the flexing of a muscular tail endowed with a special type of myocyte capable of rapid contraction/relaxation cycles. The body, which will ultimately grow to become the adult worm, has a muscular head capsule, ventral sucker and internal fibres, additional to the body wall. The largest discrepancy is the presence of gland cells comprising ~30% of body volume, which provide the secretions for skin penetration (acetabular glands) and onward migration (head gland).
- Single-cell sequencing has not been reported but analysis of cercarial gene expression patterns has revealed it is much less active than preceding germ balls or succeeding day 3 schistosomula. Little protein synthesis is also evident, so our understanding relies on ultrastructure and confocal microscopes atlases of specific transcripts and proteins.
- The central ganglion astride the oesophagus occupies less volume that in the miracidium but has a similar structural complexity. It connects via nerve cords to the musculature, and to multiple types of sensory ending, predominantly located at the extreme anterior; a peripheral nerve net has also been described. Bird schistosome cercariae possess defined photoreceptors and their existence

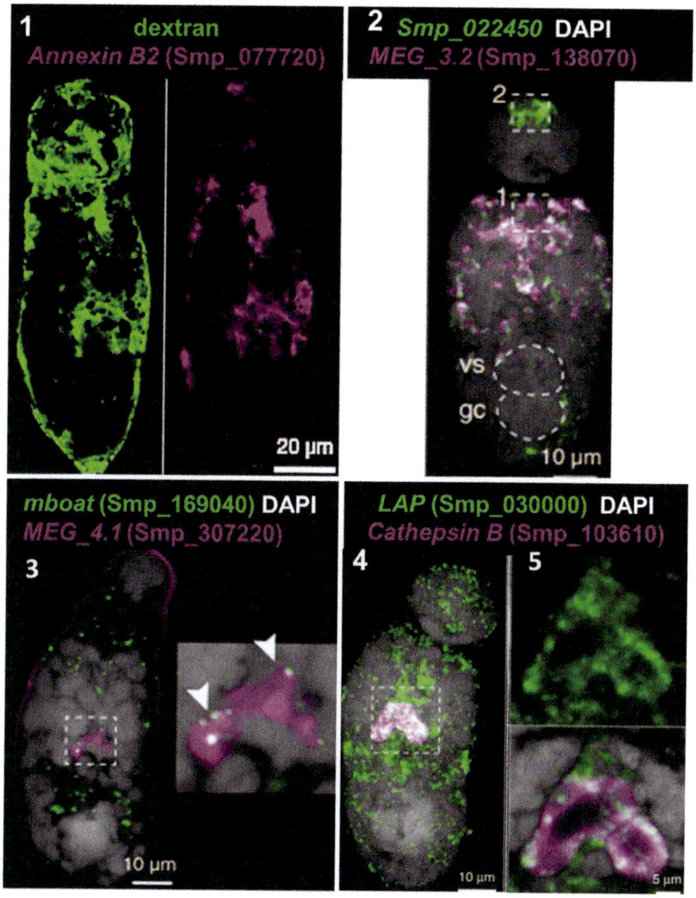

Fig. 2.17. Patterns of gene expression in day 2 *in vitro* cultured schistosomula by *in situ* hybridization. **1**) Tegument location by glycan infiltration, and cell bodies by *annexin B2* expression. **2**) *meg3.2*, strongly expressed in the mid-body region (tegument cell bodies) and weakly in the head gland alongside Smp_022450. **3**) The oesophageal gland identified by *meg4.1* expression. **4** and **5**) *cathepsin B* expression in the nascent gastrodermis and leucine amino peptidase (*lap*) throughout the body parenchyma as well as the nascent gastrodermis. (Diaz Soria *et al.*, 2020.)

in mammalian schistosomes is inferred from a demonstrable response to light. Chemoreceptor pits open to the exterior mediate detection of human skin chemicals, potentially of several modalities; their G-protein-coupled receptors await identification. The existence of a gravity receptor has also been inferred.

- The behaviour and energetics of the non-feeding cercaria, which adopts 'a sit and wait strategy', is another contrast with the miracidium. The aerobic expenditure of glycogen reserves is conserved by alternating brief bursts of upward swimming generated by tail flexing, and longer periods of downward quiescent sinking using tail furcae like a parachute. How is this rhythmicity controlled? The swimming pattern alters markedly with the transient appearance of a host in the vicinity, with reversals of direction and longer swim periods. Responses to shadows, water turbulence and skin products have all been described.
- Skin penetration is initiated after a stable attachment of the cercarial body and insertion of the apical organ beneath the flakes on stratum corneum. It is facilitated by expulsion of proteases and other proteins from the acetabular glands, identified by

proteomic analysis of secretions *in vitro*. The tail and protective glycocalyx surface are shed in the process of creating a penetration tunnel.

- The epidermal barrier confronting the penetrant is much thicker and keratinized than that posed by the snail epithelium, which accounts for the larger gland volume and longer time taken to penetrate. By ~30 min the *S. mansoni* cercaria comes to rest external to the extracellular basal lamella of the epidermis. The situation in other species needs clarification.
- The process of metamorphosis into the schistosomulum then begins, with the entire cercarial tegument surface being replaced by preformed vesicular secretions exported from underlying tegument cell bodies. As in the miracidium, there is a period of profound tissue reorganization about which little is known, apart from a suggestion of enhanced lysosomal activity and autophagy; it is a major outstanding question. By 24 h the skin schistosomulum is ready to begin its protracted journey to the hepatic portal system.

References

Al-Adhami, B.H., Noble, C., Sharaf, O., Thornhill, J., Doenhoff, M.J. *et al.* (2005) The role of acidic organelles in the development of schistosomula of *Schistosoma mansoni* and their response to signalling molecules. *Parasitology* 130(3), 309–322. DOI: 10.1017/s0031182004006511

Basch, P.F. (1981) Cultivation of *Schistosoma mansoni in vitro*. II. production of infertile eggs by worm pairs cultured from cercariae. *The Journal of Parasitology* 67(2), 186–190. DOI: 10.2307/3280633

Bogitsh, B.J., Carter, C.E. and Oeltmann, T.N. (2019) *Blood flukes*. In: Bogitsh, B.J., Carter, C.E. and Oeltmann, T.N. (eds) *Human Parasitology*, 5th edn. Academic Press, London, pp. 193–209. DOI: 10.1016/B978-0-12-813712-3.00011-4

Bruce, J.I., Weiss, E., Stirewalt, M.A. and Lincicome, D.R. (1969) *Schistosoma mansoni*: glycogen content and utilization of glucose, pyruvate, glutamate, and citric acid cycle intermediates by cercariae and schistosomules. *Experimental Parasitology* 26(1), 29–40. DOI: 10.1016/0014-4894(69)90092-7

Carter, N.P. (1978) The host-location mechanisms of the miracidium and cercaria of *Schistosoma mansoni*. PhD thesis, University of York, York, UK. Available at: https://etheses.whiterose.ac.uk/id/eprint/36331

Collins, J.J., King, R.S., Cogswell, A., Williams, D.L. and Newmark, P.A. (2011) An atlas for *Schistosoma mansoni* organs and life-cycle stages using cell type-specific markers and confocal microscopy. *PLoS Neglected Tropical Diseases* 5(3), e1009. DOI: 10.1371/journal.pntd.0001009

Cousin, C.E. and Dorsey, C.H. (1991) Nervous system of *Schistosoma mansoni* cercaria: organization and fine structure. *Parasitology Research* 77(2), 132–141. DOI: 10.1007/BF00935427

Crabtree, J.E. and Wilson, R.A. (1985) *Schistosoma mansoni*: an ultrastructural examination of skin migration in the hamster cheek pouch. *Parasitology* 91(1), 111–120. DOI: 10.1017/s0031182000056559

Curwen, R.S. and Wilson, R.A. (2003) Invasion of skin by schistosome cercariae: some neglected facts. *Trends in Parasitology* 19(2), 63–66. DOI: 10.1016/s1471-4922(02)00019-3

Curwen, R.S., Ashton, P.D., Sundaralingam, S. and Wilson, R.A. (2006) Identification of novel proteases and immunomodulators in the secretions of schistosome cercariae that facilitate host entry. *Molecular & Cellular Proteomics* 5(5), 835–844. DOI: 10.1074/mcp.M500313-MCP200

Diaz Soria, C.L., Lee, J., Chong, T., Coghlan, A., Tracey, A. *et al.* (2020) Single-cell atlas of the first intra-mammalian developmental stage of the human parasite *Schistosoma mansoni*. *Nature Communications* 11(1), 6411. DOI: 10.1038/s41467-020-20092-5

Dijkhoff, I.M., Drasler, B., Karakocak, B.B., Petri-Fink, A., Valacchi, G. *et al.* (2020) Impact of airborne particulate matter on skin: a systematic review from epidemiology to *in vitro* studies. *Particle and Fibre Toxicology* 17(1), 35. DOI: 10.1186/s12989-020-00366-y

Dorsey, C.H. (1974) *Schistosoma mansoni*: ultrastructure of cercarial escape glands. *Experimental Parasitology* 36(3), 386–396. DOI: 10.1016/0014-4894(74)90078-2

Dorsey, C.H., Cousin, C.E., Lewis, F.A. and Stirewalt, M.A. (2002) Ultrastructure of the *Schistosoma mansoni* cercaria. *Micron* 33(3), 279–323. DOI: 10.1016/s0968-4328(01)00019-1

Dvorák, J., Mashiyama, S.T., Braschi, S., Sajid, M., Knudsen, G.M. *et al.* (2008) Differential use of protease families for invasion by schistosome cercariae. *Biochimie* 90(2), 345–358. DOI: 10.1016/j.biochi.2007.08.013

Farias, L.P., Krautz-Peterson, G., Tararam, C.A., Araujo-Montoya, B.O., Fraga, T.R. *et al.* (2013) On the three-finger protein domain fold and CD59-like proteins in *Schistosoma mansoni*. *PLoS Neglected Tropical Diseases* 7(10), e2482. DOI: 10.1371/journal.pntd.0002482

Graefe, G., Hohorst, W. and Dräger, H. (1967) Forked tail of the cercaria of *Schistosoma mansoni* – a rowing device. *Nature* 215(5097), 207–208. DOI: 10.1038/215207a0

Haeberlein, S. and Haas, W. (2008) Chemical attractants of human skin for swimming *Schistosoma mansoni* cercariae. *Parasitology Research* 102(4), 657–662. DOI: 10.1007/s00436-007-0807-1

Harrop, R. and Wilson, R.A. (1993) Protein synthesis and release by cultured schistosomula of *Schistosoma mansoni*. *Parasitology* 107(3), 265–274. DOI: 10.1017/s0031182000079245

Hirst, N.L., Lawton, S.P. and Walker, A.J. (2016) Protein kinase a signalling in *Schistosoma mansoni* cercariae and schistosomules. *International Journal for Parasitology* 46(7), 425–437. DOI: 10.1016/j.ijpara.2015.12.001

Hockley, D.J. (1972) *Schistosoma mansoni*: the development of the cercarial tegument. *Parasitology* 64(2), 245–252. DOI: 10.1017/s003118200002967x

Hockley, D.J. and McLaren, D.J. (1973) *Schistosoma mansoni*: changes in the outer membrane of the tegument during development from cercaria to adult worm. *International Journal for Parasitology* 3(1), 13–25. DOI: 10.1016/0020-7519(73)90004-0

Khoo, K.H., Sarda, S., Xu, X., Caulfield, J.P., McNeil, M.R. *et al.* (1995) A unique multifucosylated –3GalNAcβ1→4GlcNAcβ1→3Gal alpha 1– motif constitutes the repeating unit of the complex *O*-glycans derived from the cercarial glycocalyx of *Schistosoma mansoni*. *The Journal of Biological Chemistry* 270(29), 17114–17123. DOI: 10.1074/jbc.270.29.17114

Knudsen, G.M., Medzihradszky, K.F., Lim, K.-C., Hansell, E. and McKerrow, J.H. (2005) Proteomic analysis of *Schistosoma mansoni* cercarial secretions. *Molecular & Cellular Proteomics* 4(12), 1862–1875. DOI: 10.1074/mcp.M500097-MCP200

Krishnamurthy, D., Katsikis, G., Bhargava, A. and Prakash, M. (2017) *Schistosoma mansoni* cercariae swim efficiently by exploiting an elastohydrodynamic coupling. *Nature Physics* 13(3), 266–271. DOI: 10.1038/nphys3924

Lawson, J.R. and Wilson, R.A. (1980) Metabolic changes associated with the migration of the schistosomulum of *Schistosoma mansoni* in the mammal host. *Parasitology* 81(2), 325–336. DOI: 10.1017/s0031182000056067

Lawson, J.R. and Wilson, R.A. (1983) The relationship between the age of *Schistosoma mansoni* cercariae and their ability to penetrate and infect the mammalian host. *Parasitology* 87(3), 481–492. DOI: 10.1017/s0031182000083001

Mathieson, W. and Wilson, R.A. (2010) A comparative proteomic study of the undeveloped and developed *Schistosoma mansoni* egg and its contents: the miracidium, hatch fluid and secretions. *International Journal for Parasitology* 40(5), 617–628. DOI: 10.1016/j.ijpara.2009.10.014

McLaren, D.J. and Hockley, D.J. (1976) *Schistosoma mansoni*: the occurrence of microvilli on the surface of the tegument during transformation from cercaria to schistosomulum. *Parasitology* 73(2), 169–187. DOI: 10.1017/s0031182000046850

Morris, G.P. (1971) The fine structure of the tegument and associated structures of the cercaria of *Schistosoma mansoni*. *Zeitschrift für Parasitenkunde* 36(1), 15–31. DOI: 10.1007/BF00328972

Neuhaus, W. (1952) Biology and development of *Trichobilharzia szidati* n. sp. (Trematoda, Schistosmatidae), a parasite causing dermatitis in man. *Zeitschrift für Parasitenkunde* 15(3), 203–266. DOI: 10.1007/BF00260453

Nuttman, C.J. (1975) The structure and behaviour of the cercaria of *Schistosoma mansoni*. PhD thesis, University of York, York, UK. Available at: https://etheses.whiterose.ac.uk/id/eprint/14197

Parker-Manuel, S.J. and Wilson, R.A. (2022) An atlas of the germ ball–cercaria–schistosomulum transition in *Schistosoma mansoni*, using confocal microscopy and *in situ* hybridisation. *Current Research in Parasitology & Vector-Borne Diseases* 2, 100087. DOI: 10.1016/j.crpvbd.2022.100087

Parker-Manuel, S.J., Ivens, A.C., Dillon, G.P. and Wilson, R.A. (2011) Gene expression patterns in larval *Schistosoma mansoni* associated with infection of the mammalian host. *PLoS Neglected Tropical Diseases* 5(8), e1274. DOI: 10.1371/journal.pntd.0001274

Paveley, R.A., Aynsley, S.A., Cook, P.C., Turner, J.D. and Mountford, A.P. (2009) Fluorescent imaging of antigen released by a skin-invading helminth reveals differential uptake and activation profiles by antigen presenting cells. *PLoS Neglected Tropical Diseases* 3(10), e528. DOI: 10.1371/journal.pntd.0000528

Ramalho-Pinto, F.J., Gazzinelli, G., Howells, R.E., Mota-Santos, T.A., Figueiredo, E.A. *et al.* (1974) *Schistosoma mansoni*: defined system for stepwise transformation of cercaria to schistosomule *in vitro*. *Experimental Parasitology* 36(3), 360–372. DOI: 10.1016/0014-4894(74)90076-9

Robertson, J.D. (1967) Origin of the unit membrane concept. *Protoplasma* 63(1), 218–245. DOI: 10.1007/BF01248039

Salter, J.P., Choe, Y., Albrecht, H., Franklin, C., Lim, K.-C. *et al.* (2002) Cercarial elastase is encoded by a functionally conserved gene family across multiple species of schistosomes. *The Journal of Biological Chemistry* 277(27), 24618–24624. DOI: 10.1074/jbc.M202364200

Short, R.B. and Cartrett, M.L. (1973) Argentophilic 'papillae' of *Schistosoma mansoni* cercariae. *The Journal of Parasitology* 59(6), 1041–1059. DOI: 10.2307/3278640

Short, R.B. and Gagné, H.T. (1975) Fine structure of possible photoreceptor in cercariae of *Schistosoma mansoni*. *The Journal of Parasitology* 61(1), 69–74. DOI: 10.2307/3279110

Singer, S.J. and Nicolson, G.L. (1972) The fluid mosaic model of the structure of cell membranes. *Science* 175(4023), 720–731. DOI: 10.1126/science.175.4023.720

Skelly, P.J. and Shoemaker, C.B. (2001) The *Schistosoma mansoni* host-interactive tegument forms from vesicle eruptions of a cyton network. *Parasitology* 122(1), 67–73. DOI: 10.1017/s0031182000007071

Stirewalt, M.A. (1959) Isolation and characterization of deposits of secretion from the acetabular gland complex of cercariae of *Schistosoma mansoni*. *Experimental Parasitology* 8(3), 199–214. DOI: 10.1016/0014-4894(59)90020-7

Stirewalt, M.A. and Walters, M. (1973) *Schistosoma mansoni*: histochemical analysis of the postacetabular gland secretion of cercariae. *Experimental Parasitology* 33(1), 56–72. DOI: 10.1016/0014-4894(73)90009-x

Tararam, C.A., Farias, L.P., Wilson, R.A. and Leite, L.C. de C. (2010) *Schistosoma mansoni* annexin 2: molecular characterization and immunolocalization. *Experimental Parasitology* 126(2), 146–155. DOI: 10.1016/j.exppara.2010.04.008

Thompson, D.P., Morrison, D.D., Pax, R.A. and Bennett, J.L. (1984) Changes in glucose metabolism and cyanide sensitivity in *Schistosoma mansoni* during development. *Molecular and Biochemical Parasitology* 13(1), 39–51. DOI: 10.1016/0166-6851(84)90100-2

Van Oordt, B.E., Tielens, A.G. and Van den Bergh, S.G. (1989) Aerobic to anaerobic transition in the carbohydrate metabolism of *Schistosoma mansoni* cercariae during transformation *in vitro*. *Parasitology* 98(3), 409–415. DOI: 10.1017/s0031182000061497

Vondráček, O., Mikeš, L., Talacko, P., Leontovyč, R., Bulantová, J. *et al.* (2022) Differential proteomic analysis of laser-microdissected penetration glands of avian schistosome cercariae with a focus on proteins involved in host invasion. *International Journal for Parasitology* 52(6), 343–358. DOI: 10.1016/j.ijpara.2021.12.003

van der Roemer, A. and Haas, W. (1984) Fine structure of a lens-covered photoreceptor in the cercaria of *Trichobilharzia* ocellata. *Zeitschrift für Parasitenkunde/Parasitology Research* 70(3), 391–394. DOI: 10.1007/BF00927826

Wang, B., Lee, J., Li, P., Saberi, A., Yang, H. *et al.* (2018) Stem cell heterogeneity drives the parasitic life cycle of *Schistosoma mansoni*. *eLife* 7, e35449. DOI: 10.7554/eLife.35449

3

Migration and Maturation

3.1 Overview

If there is one topic in schistosome biology which has been mired in controversy right up to the present, it is the route and quantitative aspects of migration to the site of parasitization. How does the schistosome, having penetrated host skin and undergone metamorphosis there, then reach the portal system and grow to maturity, a process which takes a minimum of 4–5 weeks. Briefly, the uncertainty arose from the difficulty of finding and accurately counting the parasites after they have entered the skin. Over time, numbers decrease at the penetration site, a population is subsequently found in the lungs, and schistosomula gradually accumulate in the portal tract, reaching a plateau after some weeks. Where have they been in the meantime?

3.2 The Skin Phase

3.2.1 Duration of skin transit

At the end of Chapter 2 we left the majority of newly transformed schistosomula sitting external to the basal lamella of the epidermis while the numerous cellular processes of metamorphosis were completed. Independent of the details of their fate, there is one simple technique which objectively establishes the duration of skin migration, namely excision of the infection site at intervals after exposure to cercariae. Parasites that have left before excision have the possibility of maturing, those still *in situ* do not. Adult worm numbers recovered by portal perfusion 40 days later for a *Schistosoma mansoni* experiment are shown in Fig. 3.1 (Miller and Wilson, 1978). A logistic curve fitted to the data can be used to estimate the half-life ($t_{1/2}$) for duration of stay in the skin. The mean ± SD for mouse abdominal skin was 88 ± 23 h and for Syrian hamsters (*Mesocricetus aureus*) was 64.5 ± 9 h. Note that in this experiment 36% of applied cercariae matured in the mouse and 72% in the hamsters. This tells us that a lot of penetrants fail to mature in a naïve host. Given the uncertainty about the rapidity of skin migration in *Schistosoma japonicum* (see below) and potentially in *Schistosoma haematobium*, objective data for these species would be very useful.

3.2.2 The pitfalls of mincing and incubation

Schistosomula can be recovered from the skin and lungs of exposed hosts by a mincing and incubation technique, but not from other tissues in significant numbers. Two factors are crucial to interpretation, namely the incubation conditions and the efficiency of the technique. First,

DOI: 10.1079/9781800625167.0003

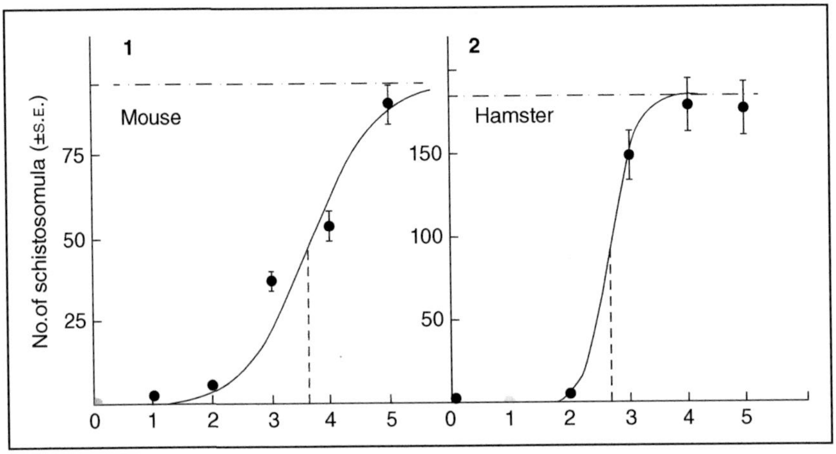

Fig. 3.1. Transit of schistosomula out of the skin infection site in **1**) mice and **2**) hamsters, each exposed to 250 cercariae. The method is based on excision of the skin infection sites at daily intervals followed by recovery of adult worms from the portal tract 40 days later. The vertical dashed lines represent the $t_{1/2}$ of exit. (From Miller and Wilson, 1978.) Figures used with permission from Cambridge University Press.

if appreciable numbers of dead parasites are recovered, are they representative of the whole population, or simply an artefact of the extraction technique? Second, if the efficiency of extraction varies with time, is it possible to create a balance sheet of numbers in skin or lungs? The author's opinion is a firm negative to both questions. The use of Hanks balanced salt solution as an extraction medium (Clegg and Smithers, 1968) is not optimal. Indeed, a comparison of skin extraction using nutrient-rich medium with data from the skin excision technique (Fig. 3.2) (Miller and Wilson, 1978; Wilson, 2009) revealed a broad and variable discrepancy with time, in the apparent numbers of parasites in the skin. In a perplexing twist, the proponents of mincing and incubation stated that while 'it was known that many of the schistosomula seen in our sections of skin were dead, no histological distinction could be made between living and dead parasites' (Clegg and Smithers, 1968). The best advice is to treat any data that claims to make quantitative estimates of parasites from tissue extraction techniques with extreme caution.

3.2.3 How long do the parasites spend in each skin compartment?

Inevitably, this question can only be answered by microscopical examination. Predominantly, this means histopathological and ultrastructural studies of parasites *in situ* in fixed skin. However, there is one living skin preparation that lends itself to direct observation, namely the everted hamster cheek pouch (Wilson and Lawson, 1980). The pouch has a simplified structure without hair follicles, sweat glands or lymphatic drainage, so the venous system is the only route of egress. Maturation after infection via the Syrian hamster cheek pouch was not significantly different from infection via the skin, indicating that the absence of lymphatic drainage does not affect parasite maturation (Miller and Wilson, 1978). Repeated visual observations were made on the same cheek pouches of the Chinese hamster (*Cricetus griseus*), using the pattern of blood vessels as geographical markers. Lateral migration in the penetration tunnels of the epidermis had virtually ceased by 10 h post-exposure. The first schistosomula unequivocally entered the dermis by ~40 h, by which time all traces of acetabular glands had disappeared (Crabtree and Wilson, 1985), with $t_{1/2}$ of stay in the epidermis of ~52.5 h. Once in the dermis, a schistosomulum took about 10 h to locate a dermal venule, and a mean of 8 h to penetrate the vessel wall (Wilson and Lawson, 1980). Most had left the dermis by 60–80 h by penetrating a venule of mean diameter 22.7 μm. Since the diameter of day 2–3 skin schistosomula calculated from scanning electron microscopy (SEM) images is ~16 μm, exit down a venule is not a tight squeeze (Crabtree and Wilson, 1980).

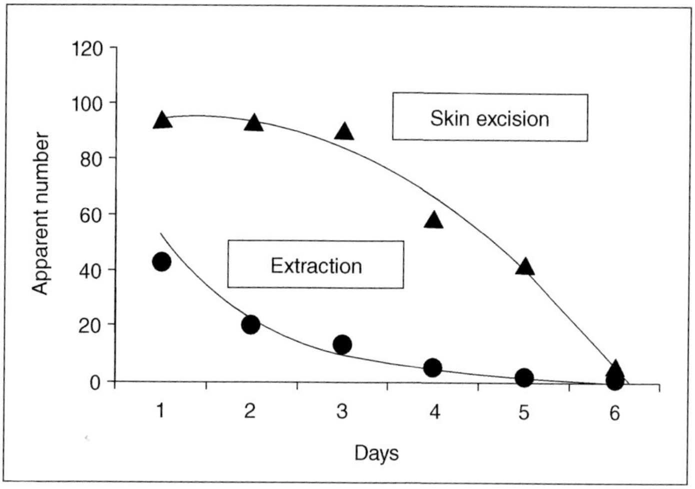

Fig. 3.2. The apparent profiles of schistosomula in the skin of mice with time post-exposure. The values were determined by mincing and incubation to extract parasites versus the numbers present revealed by the skin excision method. (From Wilson, 2009.) Figures used with permission from Cambridge University Press.

Direct histopathological studies on fixed skin add to the *in vivo* observations but are inevitably more subjective. In one such study, mouse abdominal skin exposed to 1000 cercariae (a high density) was excised at 15 min, 1, 2, 3, 4 and 5 days post-exposure (Wheater and Wilson, 1979). Within 15 min, 84% of penetrants were in the epidermis and 16% in the dermis and hypodermis. On day 1, the density had not changed with about half of epidermal schistosomula in penetration tunnels (Fig. 3.3.1) and half in sebaceous glands (Fig. 3.3.2). By day 2, 62% of schistosomula were in the connective tissue of the dermis and hypodermis while 38% remained within sebaceous glands and the epidermis; some schistosomula were observed closely approximated to dermal venules. On day 3, the mean absolute density of schistosomula had decreased to about half, with 90% of those remaining in the connective tissue of the dermis and hypodermis. About 20% were either closely applied to dilated blood vessels or in the process of penetrating (Fig. 3.3.3). On day 4, the mean absolute density of schistosomula had greatly decreased, the dermis was extremely haemorrhagic, but no inflammatory foci were present at either this or earlier stages. In summary, for *S. mansoni* these observations support the skin excision studies, revealing a prolonged residence external to the basement membrane of the epidermis, and notably the lack of evidence for dead schistosomula in the skin of naïve mice. The approximate $t_{1/2}$ of stay in the skin in this histopathology study was about 72 h.

A more recent study of three species using a human skin organ culture system (He *et al.*, 2002) has broadly confirmed the observations for *S. mansoni*. At 8 h after exposure of human skin to cercariae, 94% of schistosomula were present in the epidermis and by 24 h the number had decreased slightly to 89%. By 72 h most observed parasites were close to blood vessels or inside them. It is noteworthy that as this was an isolated skin preparation, the observations suggest that venules are not located on the basis of oxygen tension gradients. The situation for *S. haematobium* schistosomula was very similar with >93% located in the epidermis at 8 h after exposure to infection. They also appeared to enter the dermis in large numbers around 48 h and approach dermal vessels around 72 h after exposure. Surprisingly, the situation for *S. japonicum* was strikingly different, with much faster migration through human skin. At 8 h after exposure to infection 73% of the schistosomula had already entered the dermis and this rose to >90% at 24 h. Individual parasites were observed inside dermal blood vessels as early as 2 h post-exposure. The extent to which this is a product of the *in vitro* preparation, or a true reflection of *in vivo* events is unclear. It is not explicitly stated but this is believed to be a Chinese strain

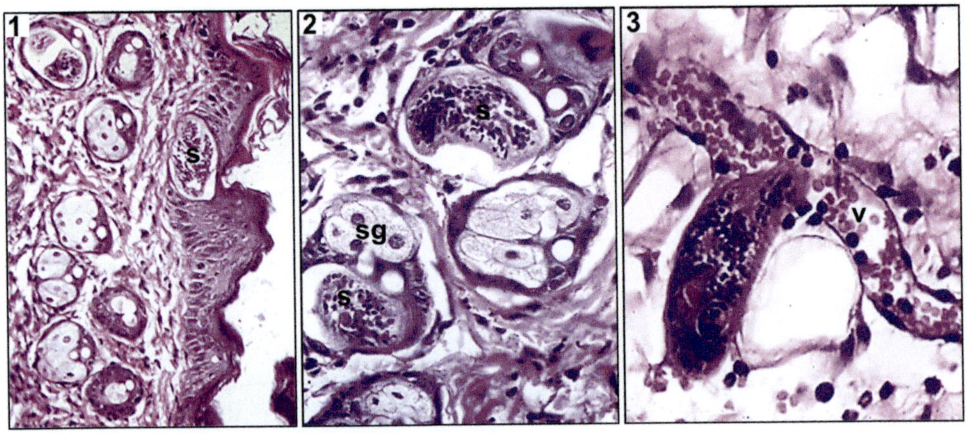

Fig. 3.3. Transit through skin compartment. **1**) Schistosomulum (s) in a mouse epidermal penetration tunnel at 24 h. **2**) Two schistosomula (s) in sebaceous gland (sg) ducts at 24 h, still external to the epidermal basal lamella. **3**) A schistosomulum in the process of penetrating a dermal venule (v) at 72 h. (From Wheater and Wilson, 1979.) Figures used with permission from Cambridge University Press.

of the parasite. Note that parasite tracking of the Philippine strain of *S. japonicum* recorded a slower migration of schistosomula out of the skin (Laxer and Tuazon, 1992) (see Section 3.3.4).

3.2.4 The mechanics of skin migration

How does the fully transformed schistosomulum breach the basal lamella of the epidermis, traverse the dermis, locate a venule and penetrate its wall to exit the skin in the direction of blood flow? Focusing on *S. mansoni*, it seems clear that the acetabular glands have been completely resorbed before transit from epidermis to dermis occurs. The head gland is the obvious source of lytic enzymes but information about the composition of its secretions is limited (see Section 3.3.2 on lung schistosomula secretions). There are no ultrastructural images of head gland secretions being applied to the epidermal basal lamella but another possibility arises. We now know that the alimentary tract is transcriptionally active, starting in the cercaria and increasing in the day 2/3 schistosomulum (Parker-Manuel *et al.*, 2011), and the gut caecum can ingest marker dyes (Fig. 3.4.1). Since the mouth is subterminal, it is ideally placed to release proteolytic secretions from the tract to dissolve the fibrous proteins of the basal lamella. A corollary to the resorption of the acetabular glands is that the so-called cercarial elastases are not available to react with the elastase and collagen fibres of the dermal matrix. Movement of the schistosomulum through the dermis is quite rapid and may be related to the presence of body spines. These can provide traction through the dermal ground substance, although their size is diminishing (Fig. 3.4.2) and there is little evidence for inflammation impeding progress in a naïve animal.

It must be a matter of conjecture how the schistosomulum locates a venule. SEM images show that the array of sensory papillae is no longer present on the apical area, but the projected chemosensory pits may still be intact. A chemical cue would appear ideal, but its nature is unknown. Transmission electron microscopy (TEM) images have revealed schistosomula probing a vessel wall from the outside with the apical area (Fig. 3.5.1). Cytological evidence for a lytic process was provided by fusion of head gland vesicles with the surface (Chapter 2, Fig. 2.5.4), ultimately making a breach in the vessel wall, complete with a fibrin clot (Fig. 3.5.2). A more detailed understanding requires information on the head gland secretions. Once in the vessel lumen, the schistosomulum rapidly leaves, carried passively in the direction of the blood flow to the vena cava, then via the right atrium and ventricle of the heart to arrive in the lungs via the pulmonary arterioles.

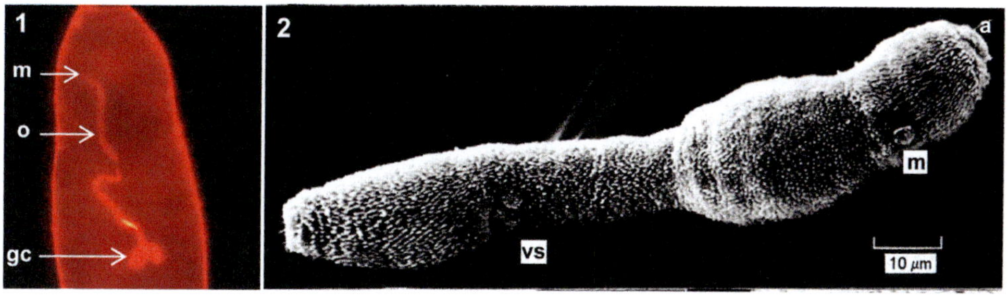

Fig. 3.4. Transit through the skin. **1**) Skin schistosomulum incubated with membrane impermeant lucifer yellow takes up the dye into the oesophagus (o) and gut caecum (gc) via the mouth (m). **2**) Day 2 skin schistosomulum viewed from a lateroventral aspect. vs, ventral sucker; m, mouth. Elongation of the body has commenced and there is a slight reduction in the size of the spines in the mid-body region. The apical area (a) is modified leaving a raised spineless knob. (**1** courtesy of Professor J. Kusel, Glasgow University, Glasgow, UK; **2** from Crabtree and Wilson, 1980.) Figure used with permission from Cambridge University Press.

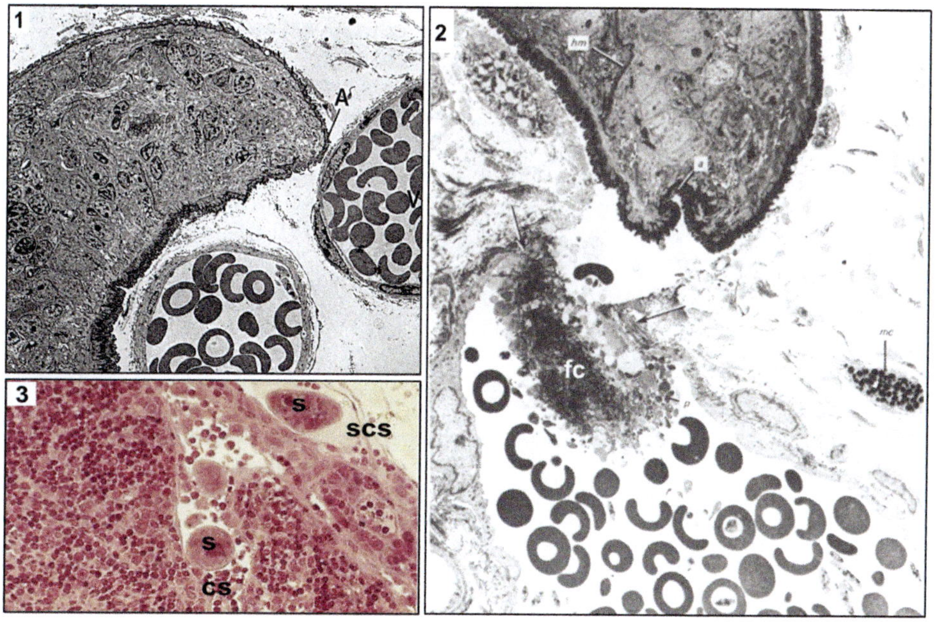

Fig. 3.5. Exit from the skin. **1**) A 68-h schistosomulum probing a venule wall with its apical area (A). **2**) A 72-h schistosomulum further into the process. The venule wall has been breached (arrows) by the head gland secretions and a fibrin clot (fc) has formed in the vessel lumen. **3**) A skin-draining node showing the alternative route of exit via the lymphatics. A schistosomulum (s) is located in the subcapsular sinus (scs) while a second has already entered a cortical sinus (cs). (**1** and **2** from Crabtree and Wilson, 1985.) **1** and **2**) Figures used with permission from Cambridge University Press. **3**) Figure author's own.

In the murine host, ~16% of schistosomula exit the skin via lymphatic vessels to lodge in lymph nodes draining the exposure site (Mountford *et al.*, 1988). By histopathology, schistosomula were observed within all the lymphatic channels including the afferent lymphatics and the hilar efferent lymphatics (Fig. 3.5.3) (Wheater and Wilson, 1979). Schistosomula have been recovered from the axillary lymph nodes of mice, hamsters and rats, amounting at peak to ~4% of those parasites that will mature. If such schistosomula recovered from mice are injected into the tail vein of uninfected mouse hosts, they have the same chance of maturing as comparable skin schistosomula (Miller and Wilson, 1978) so apparently are not harmed by their lymph node transit. Passage through lymph nodes may be relevant in the radiation-attenuated (RA) vaccine model of immunity (see Chapter 9).

3.3 The Intravascular Phase

3.3.1 Elusive migrating parasites

It is relatively easy to extract schistosomula from lung tissues by mincing and incubation, from which a profile of numbers recovered with time can be constructed. The technique has the same shortcomings as those already outlined for parasite extraction from the skin (see Section 3.2.2). Similarly, the arrival of schistosomula in the portal tract can also be estimated by vascular perfusion, with care needed in the early days not to miss the small newly arrived worms. The data derived from such experiments in mice and hamsters plotted in Fig. 3.6 are intended to make three points. First, after an early lung peak around day 6 in both species the numbers undergo a gradual decline out to day 20–22, after which further parasites cannot be recovered. Second, the number of parasites arriving in the portal system does not match the decline in the lungs. This is very noticeable in the hamster, where there is a decided dearth of larvae for a period of ~10 days. Third, accumulation of schistosomula in the mouse portal system is essentially over by day 21, when all those that will mature have arrived. In contrast, schistosomula continue to arrive in the hamster portal tract up to day 40. This discrepancy between hosts is undoubtedly related to their respective levels of parasite maturation (~30% versus 70%).

The gap between the 'disappearance' of schistosomula from the lungs and their accumulation in the portal tract inevitably led to speculation about their migration route from the lungs to the portal system. An early suggestion was that they traversed the pulmonary capillaries and travelled via the left side of the heart to reach the systemic circulation (Faust *et al.*, 1934; Yolles *et al.*, 1949). Some would be distributed to the splanchnic circulation leading to the portal system, the rest to other organs, through which they would pass to return to the lungs. Strongly against this hypothesis was the fact that few if any schistosomula could be recovered from systemic organs. In direct contrast was the suggestion that schistosomula travelled from the lungs to the liver by direct migration through the tissues. This requires that they exit the pulmonary tissues to the pleural cavity and traverse the diaphragm, bringing them into direct contact with the liver capsule. By penetrating through the capsule and liver tissues schistosomula would eventually reach the hepatic portal vessels (Wilks, 1967; Pereira *et al.*, 1972; Bruce *et al.*, 1974). Large numbers of schistosomula were reported in washes of the pleural cavity in one of these studies (Wilks, 1967). Notwithstanding, no schistosomula were found in the

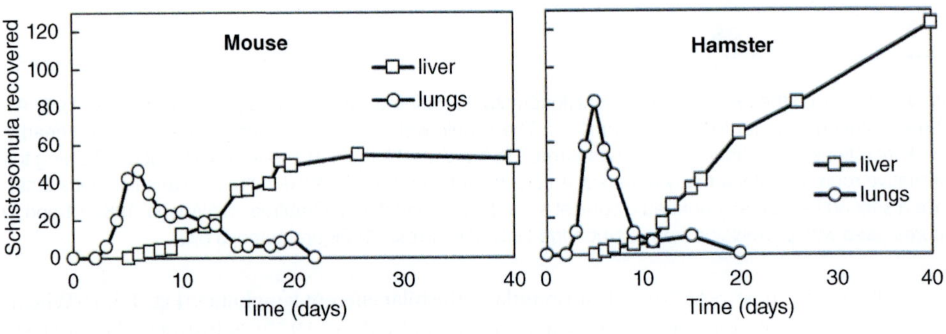

Fig. 3.6. The missing parasites. **1**) Profile of schistosomula recovered from mouse lungs by mincing and incubation of tissue compared the number of schistosomula recovered by perfusion of the portal system. **2**) A similar data-set obtained from the Syrian hamster. (Adapted from Miller and Wilson, 1980.) Figure used with permission from Cambridge University Press.

pleural cavity of both mice and hamsters in the study shown in Fig. 3.6 (Miller and Wilson, 1980). The third route of migration from the lungs to liver is mentioned for completeness. It was suggested from work on *Schistosoma mattheei* in sheep, based on parasite recovery from sections of the clamped blood vessels (Kruger *et al.*, 1969). The proposal was that when schistosomula reached the lungs, they reversed direction and migrated against the bloodstream via the pulmonary artery, right ventricle and atrium, posterior vena cava and hepatic vein into the liver. If this might seem implausible, just consider that we do not know how the migrating schistosomula of *Schistosoma nasale* reach and mature in the blood vessels of the nasal mucosa in the bovine host.

3.3.2 The morphology and biochemistry of intravascular parasites

In spite of the difficulty of locating schistosomula in systemic organs, several factors pointed to migration by an intravascular route. Among them was the observation that schistosomula, recovered *ex vivo* during migration, underwent remarkable changes in morphology not so apparent in cultured worms (Fig. 3.7) (Wilson *et al.*, 1978). Between days 3 and 6 after infection, schistosomula become capable of extending and contracting their bodies between a minimum length of 100–150 and up to >400 μm. This elongation reaches a maximum in day 8 schistosomula, which can constrict regions of the body to <10 μm diameter. The obvious explanation for this process of extension in the lungs is that it facilitates migration through vascular beds. On arrival in the hepatic portal system around day 8, schistosomula undergo a transition taking about 2 days from the elongate, migratory to a short liver form. Thus, migration has not been accompanied by an increase in worm mass since the liver schistosomula are now indistinguishable in size from day 0–3 skin worms, just no longer capable of negotiating hepatic sinusoids or capillaries. How is this elongation achieved?

One notable feature of the cercarial body wall, revealed by TEM studies, is the thick layer of interstitial material situated between the tegument and underlying muscle layers of (Fig. 3.8.1) (Hockley, 1972). Thinning of the layer begins in the skin schistosomulum and is further reduced in the day 4 schistosomulum (Crabtree and Wilson, 1986b). By day 7 it has disappeared altogether in the elongated migrating schistosomulum (Fig. 3.8.2). In many invertebrates this extracellular matrix comprises highly conserved laminin, collagen IV and fibronectin, and its gradual disappearance implies controlled proteolysis. Such processes are normally effected by matrix metalloproteases but a search of the differentially

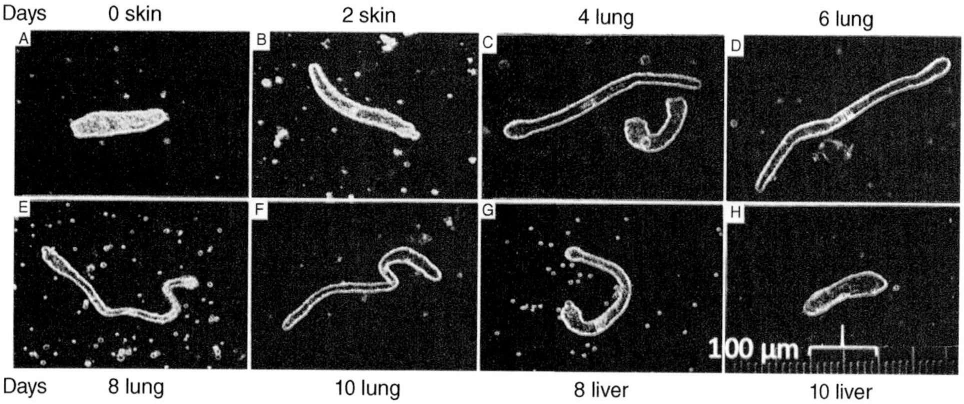

Fig. 3.7. The morphology of *ex vivo* schistosomula filmed at 37°C. Each image is a single film frame. The larval body increases in length and becomes narrower in lung worms, reaching maximum length by day 8. On arrival in the portal distributaries of the liver, the larvae contract back to a size indistinguishable from those in the skin. (From Wilson, *et al.*, 1978.) Figure used with permission from Cambridge University Press.

expressed transcripts from day 6 lung schistosomula (Wangwiwatsin *et al.*, 2020) failed to find any, so the dissolution of the layer must remain a mystery. Its absence allows the circular and longitudinal muscles, acting on the body core, to modify body shape, but there is a corollary. The surface area of the schistosomulum increases by >50% between day 3 and day 8 to accommodate the elongated body (Crabtree and Wilson, 1980). Another change is the disassembly of the tegumental spines, already evident at day 2, so that by day 4 they remain only at the extreme anterior and posterior.

The advantages of these morphological changes are that they will facilitate passage along the lumina of capillaries (Fig. 3.9.1) (Crabtree and Wilson, 1980). The anterior spines provide purchase on the walls of the blood vessel while the body is contracted up, the posterior spines while the body is extended forward along

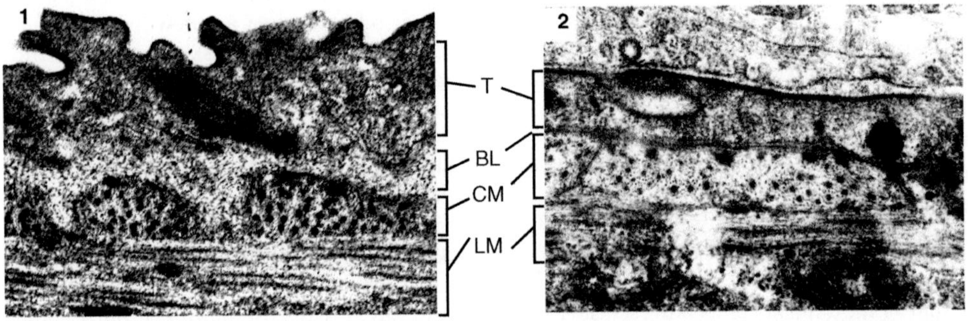

Fig. 3.8. Modifications in the parasite body wall that make intravascular migration possible. Longitudinal sections through the body wall of **1**) a day 2 skin schistosomulum (left) and **2**) a day 7 lung schistosomulum in a capillary (right). By day 7 the tegument (T) is much thinner with a smooth surface minus spines. The fibrous subtegumental basal layer (BL) has completely disappeared. The circular muscle (CM) fibres are flattened but the number of thick filaments has not changed. The longitudinal muscle (LM) fibres are much thinner to accommodate the increase in length, with fewer thick filaments visible. The result is a body that can oscillate in length between ~130 and ~400 μm. Figure author's own.

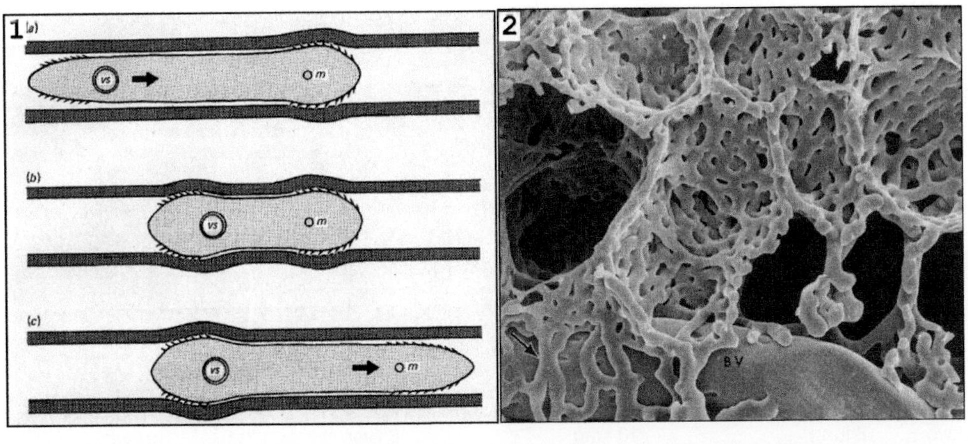

Fig. 3.9. Migration through capillary beds. **1**) Diagram showing the envisaged integration of morphology and contractile rhythm to drive progression along the capillary lumen. m, mouth; vs, ventral sucker. **2**) SEM of a latex cast of the pulmonary microcirculation showing the labyrinthine layout of vessels around each alveolus that a schistosomulum must negotiate. (**1** from Crabtree and Wilson, 1980; **2** from Guntheroth *et al.*, 1982.) Figure used with permission from **1**) Cambridge University Press and **2**) American Physiological Society.

the vessel lumen. This neatly explains the rhythmical extensions and contractions of *ex vivo* lung schistosomula. The absence of spines over the mid-body region will minimize friction between the worm surface and the capillary endothelium. It is worth drawing attention to the particular layout of the pulmonary capillaries at this point, where they form a labyrinth of routes over the surfaces of alveoli (Fig. 3.9.2) (Guntheroth *et al.*, 1982). When schistosomula eventually reach the portal system, the flexible organization of musculature goes into reverse with a reappearance of the basal lamella, increased complexity of the tegument with reassembly of the spines and the formation of an oral sucker around the mouth by day 14 (Crabtree and Wilson, 1980).

From the early 1980s onwards there was significant interest in lung schistosomula as targets of protective immunity elicited by the RA cercarial vaccine in the mouse model (Coulson, 1997) (see Chapter 9). In consequence, attempts were made to characterize their secretory and surface-exposed proteins that might serve as antigens in the live worm. Initially, culturing schistosomula to the lung stage required complex media, unsuited to identification of the minute amounts of released material. To an extent this could be circumvented by culture in complex media with added ^{35}S-methionine, followed by electrophoretic separation of released products and autoradiography to pinpoint labelled proteins in the medium (Harrop and Wilson, 1993). These studies revealed that migrating schistosomula had active biosynthetic capacity, rising from a very low level at 24 h to a peak at day 8, before declining sharply (Fig. 3.10.1). They were poised to start growth but lacked the signal. Autoradiography revealed one major secreted product of 20 kDa and two minor ones of 45 and 61 kDa (Fig. 3.10.2). It was another 17 years before the ~20 kDa band was identified by proteomics as a cluster of micro-exon gene (MEG)-3 family isoforms (Fig. 3.10.3) (DeMarco *et al.*, 2010). This family was identified by *in situ* hybridization as expressed in the head gland and tegument cell bodies of day 7 lung worms. Paradoxically, the MEG-3 isoforms were also identified in egg secretions, alongside numerous MEG-2 isoforms (see Chapter 11 on the egg). Most recently two MEG-2 transcripts were also identified in day 6 lung worms (Wangwiwatsin *et al.*, 2020). Thus, it appears that two intravascular stages, the lung schistosomulum and the mature egg, are secreting the same MEG proteins and it is tempting to conclude that they must interact with the surrounding vascular endothelium. Alternatively, as a result of transcytosis across the endothelium, the MEGs might also interact with components of the interstitial space to facilitate intravascular migration. This is a topic worth future investigation.

3.3.3 Autoradiographic tracking of labelled parasites

What was needed to solve the 'elusive parasite' conundrum was a way of finding the tiny migrating larvae in the mass of host tissues. The tracking technique had its origins in work showing that ^{75}Se-labelled methionine was taken up by *Biomphalaria* snails from pond water, and subsequently incorporated by developing schistosome sporocysts, which produced labelled cercariae (Christensen, 1977). The ^{75}Se isotope emits energetic γ-rays which are not blocked by animal tissues and can be detected in a γ-counter or by autoradiography of tissues. The first study showed, both by estimating the counts in whole tails, and by autoradiography of flattened tail skin, that the number of parasites declined from 48 h in a sigmoid curve, with a $t_{1/2}$ of 91 and 101 h in replicate experiments (Georgi, 1982). This was in good agreement with the 88 h determined from excision of abdominal skin (Miller and Wilson, 1978). The technique was quickly extended to lung tissues, gently compressed on to cardboard before autoradiography, and applied to longitudinal studies of migration (Dean *et al.*, 1984). One of the first observations was that >90% of cercarial penetrants could be located as late as day 7 when 86% of them were in the lungs (bad news for proponents of early death in the skin) (Mangold and Dean, 1983). The technique was sufficiently sensitive to produce a profile of lung schistosomula numbers up to 14 days post-exposure (Georgi *et al.*, 1983).

With small additions to the technique, such as use of intensifying screens and film exposure at −80°C, the sensitivity of detection was increased out to day 35. The challenge was to create a two-dimensional version of the mouse host, suitable for exposure to X-ray film. The entire mouse pelt was laid out on card, organ

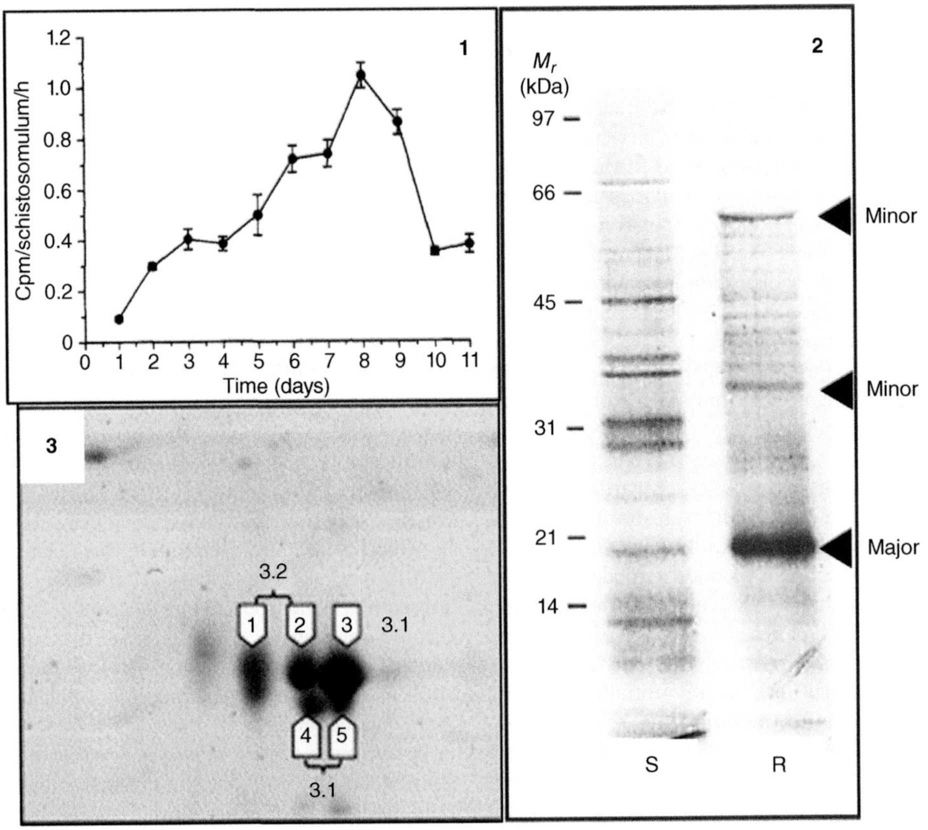

Fig. 3.10. The biosynthetic capacity of migrating schistosomula. **1**) Protein synthetic capacity on consecutive days determined by a 24-h pulse of ^{35}S-methionine. **2**) Electrophoretic separation of the soluble body fraction and proteins secreted into the medium, detected by autoradiography. One major and two minor secreted bands were detected. **3**) Proteomic analysis of the major band after two-dimensional separation identified it as a mixture of MEG-3 isoforms. (**1** and **2** from Harrop and Wilson, 1993; **3** from DeMarco *et al.*, 2010.) **1** and **2**) Figures used with permission from Cambridge University Press. **3**) Figure used under license CC-BY-4.0.

compression was standardized with a steel roller, and the muscles were squeezed from the eviscerated and de-brained carcase with a hydraulic press (Wilson *et al.*, 1986). Each parasite, represented as a spot on the film, could be counted to construct an accurate balance sheet of numbers with time post-infection. From this, the pattern of migration and site(s) of attrition could be deduced.

There was a rapid decline in the numbers of parasites in the skin of mice from day 4 onwards and their commensurate appearance in the lungs (a small proportion of parasites lingered in the skin out to day 35) (Fig. 3.11.1). Numbers peaked in the lungs at day 8 (Fig. 3.11.2) before undergoing a gradual decline out to day 35. Parasites were first detected in systemic organs (e.g. carcase, kidney, brain) from day 4 with a peak of 24% of the day 0 total at day 12 (Fig. 3.11.3). Their distribution was in good agreement with data for the fractional distribution of cardiac output in the mouse, but even at peak the total systemic population was only half that of the lung population. Parasites were detected in the organs of the splanchnic circulation (spleen, alimentary tract) from day 10, but only in small numbers (4% of the day 0 total at day 14), in spite of receiving ~31% of cardiac output (see next paragraph) (Wilson and Coulson, 1986). The first parasites were detected in the liver at day 10 (Fig. 3.11.4), rapidly accumulating in the ensuing days and

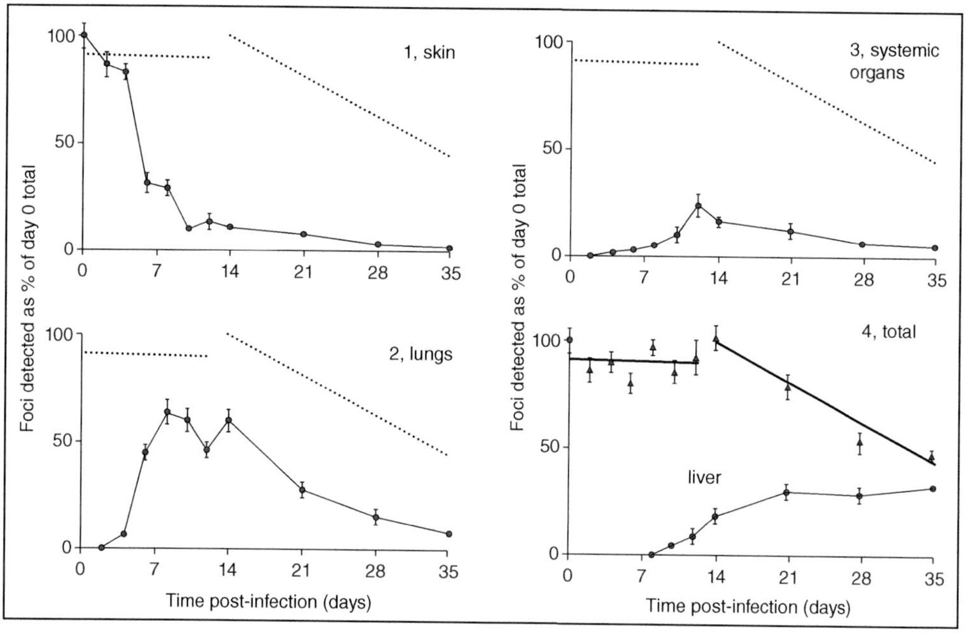

Fig. 3.11. Parasite tracking of all mouse tissues permits creation of a balance sheet of numbers out to 35 days. The dotted lines in each plot are the total in panel **4**, for reference. **1**) Numbers in tail skin. **2**) Profile of numbers in the lungs with a peak at day 8. **3**) Numbers in non-splanchnic systemic organs reach a peak at day 12. **4**) Parasites accumulating in the liver reach a plateau at day 21. The total number detectable does not begin to decline until after 14 days, in a linear manner. (From Wilson *et al.*, 1986.) Figure used with permission from Cambridge University Press.

reaching a plateau at day 21. The percentage maturation in this experiment was 33.4% of the initial burden so clearly a large number of parasites had perished during migration. No significant loss of parasites occurred before day 12, after which there was a gradual virtually linear decline from day 14 until day 35 (Fig. 3.11.4). This means that at day 21, although the portal population was complete, 50% of the day 0 total was still present in other locations, declining to 16% at day 35. Were these parasites alive or dead?

Subsequent experiments on the persistence of dead parasites appear to confirm their likely viability. Heat-killed schistosomula, injected intravenously to the lungs, had disintegrated beyond recognition by 40 h, albeit in previously vaccinated mice (Kassim *et al.*, 1992). Additionally, the rapid clearance of injected dead schistosomula in naïve mice was confirmed by measuring the autoradiographic spot intensity; this declined with a $t_{1/2}$ of 34 h (Dean and Mangold, 1992). These observations strongly suggest that parasites detected in locations other than the liver, when the portal population is complete, are most likely still alive but trapped. They are relevant to assessment of immune elimination mechanisms after vaccination experiments (see Chapter 9). The autoradiographic technique also made it possible to measure the kinetics of migration by administering a pulse of labelled *ex vivo* day 7 lung schistosomula to different locations in mice, and then tracking their movements (Fig. 3.12) (Wilson and Coulson, 1986).

When schistosomula were introduced directly to the pulmonary vessels via a femoral vein injection, 99% were detected in the lungs minutes later (Fig. 3.13.1). There was a linear decline in numbers out to 70 h, and a regression against time gave a $t_{1/2}$ value of 55 h for the population. However, by then it will contain individuals that had passed through a systemic capillary bed and returned to the lungs, so the first transit is probably ~30–35 h. When schistosomula were delivered via the left ventricle to all systemic organs, the total dose was detected in the ratio 0.63:0.37, systemic to splanchnic beds

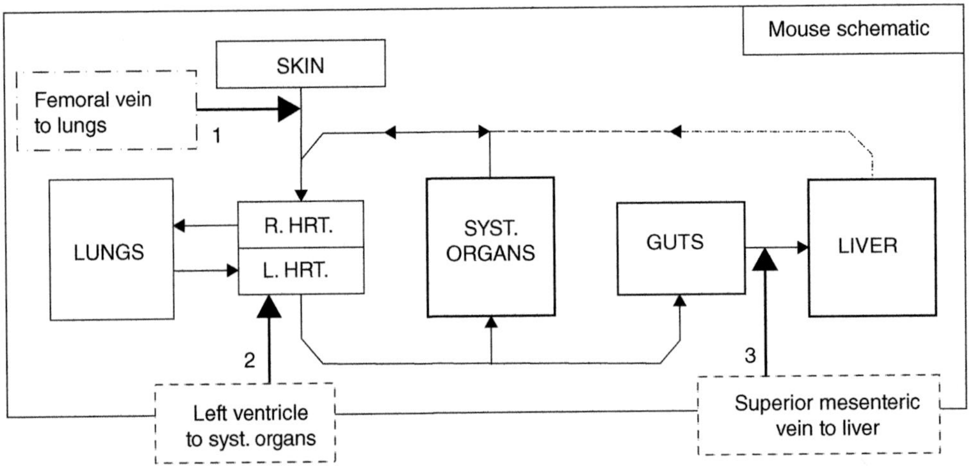

Fig. 3.12. Schematic of mouse circulation to show delivery points of radiolabelled day 7 *ex vivo* lung schistosomula. **1**) The femoral vein via the right side of the heart to the pulmonary arterioles. **2**) The left ventricle to all systemic organs including guts. **3**) The superior mesenteric vein to the hepatic portal distributaries of the liver only. (Modified from Wilson and Coulson, 1986.) Figures used with permission from Cambridge University Press.

(Fig. 3.13.2 and 3.13.3). The decline in numbers in both the systemic and splanchnic beds followed a negative exponential form. Regression of the early values, linearized by a ln transformation, permitted the mean transit time through systemic and splanchnic capillary beds to be determined (Wilson and Coulson, 1986). The estimates of 16 and 6.5 h, respectively, confirmed that the lung capillaries really were a greater obstacle to transit. The rapid decline in both systemic and splanchnic vascular beds was matched by an almost equal and opposite rise in the respective downstream organs. If proof was still needed to convince doubters about intravascular migration, this was it. After left ventricle injection and passage through systemic organs, the number arriving in the lungs peaked at 25 h, and then began to decline as schistosomula continued their migration. Those schistosomula delivered to the intestines and spleen had the fastest transit time through the capillary beds to accumulate in the liver but with an unanticipated complication.

When schistosomula were delivered to the superior mesenteric vein, the vast majority were detectable in the liver immediately afterwards. Surprisingly, the number had declined to 71% at 24 h when 13–15% were detected in the lungs, revealing that the hepatic sinusoids were not a completely efficient filter (P of trapping = 0.79–0.86). It is plausible that some then continued their migration, potentially entering the portal system for a second time. Based on these injection experiments, it appears that two to three circuits of the systemic and pulmonary vasculature of a mouse, each taking >50 h, would be sufficient to deliver the entire portal population via the splanchnic circulation. However, the extended period of accumulation in the hamster portal vein (Fig. 3.6) and higher percentage maturation in that host (Crabtree and Wilson, 1986a), suggests that schistosomula may make further circuits of the vasculature up to 40 days post-infection, before reaching their goal.

The 'elusive parasite' question (see Section 3.3.1) was answered by the quantitative data provided by parasite tracking. At the day 12 peak, 24% of schistosomula were present in systemic organs versus 50% in the lungs. Compare these numbers with the wet weight of the lungs (~0.2 g) versus 20 g for other body tissues in a 25 g mouse, a ratio of 1:200. Migrating schistosomula are concentrated in the lungs but dispersed throughout all the other body tissues so the probability of finding a schistosomulum in, for example, a kidney is only 0.005 that in the lungs. Add in the fact that the lungs are very elastic so more likely to expel loosely trapped parasites and it is clear to see why they are so hard to extract from systemic tissues.

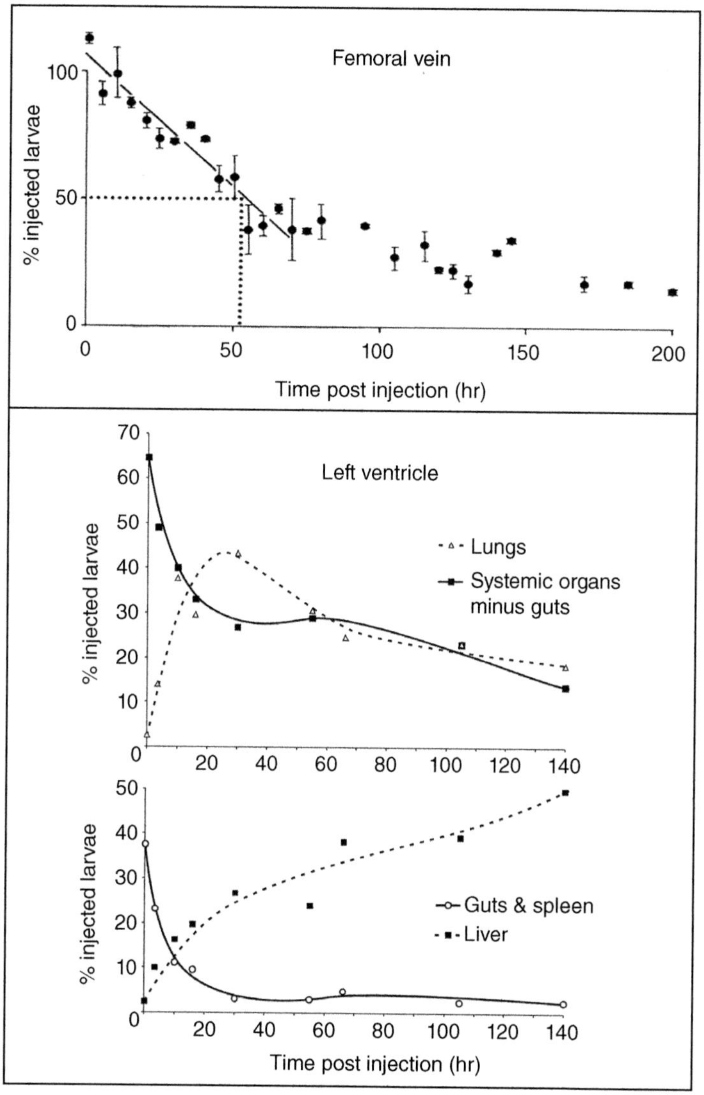

Fig. 3.13. Kinetics of migration through vascular beds. **1**) Profile in the lungs after femoral vein injection. The dotted line is the apparent $t_{1/2}$ based on linear regression of numbers against time. **2**) After left ventricle injection the larvae are delivered in the ratio 0.63:0.37 between systemic organs (upper half) and the guts and spleen (lower half). Numbers in both rapidly decline in a negative exponential manner. Not shown is the data from superior mesenteric vein injection where the vast majority are trapped in the portal system. (From Wilson and Coulson, 1986.) Figures used with permission from Cambridge University Press.

Both the balance sheet and schistosomula injection experiments revealed that the lungs of mice presented a particular obstacle to migration. In a histopathology study of mouse lungs (Mastin *et al.*, 1983), it was observed that from day 11 onwards an increasing proportion of parasites had left the blood vessels and were in the alveoli. Subsequently this was confirmed in an ultrastructural study (Fig. 3.14.1) (Crabtree and Wilson, 1986b) and provides a plausible explanation of why more than half of penetrant cercariae fail to mature in the mouse. During passage through the labyrinth of alveolar capillaries, they rupture the vessels and enter the alveoli

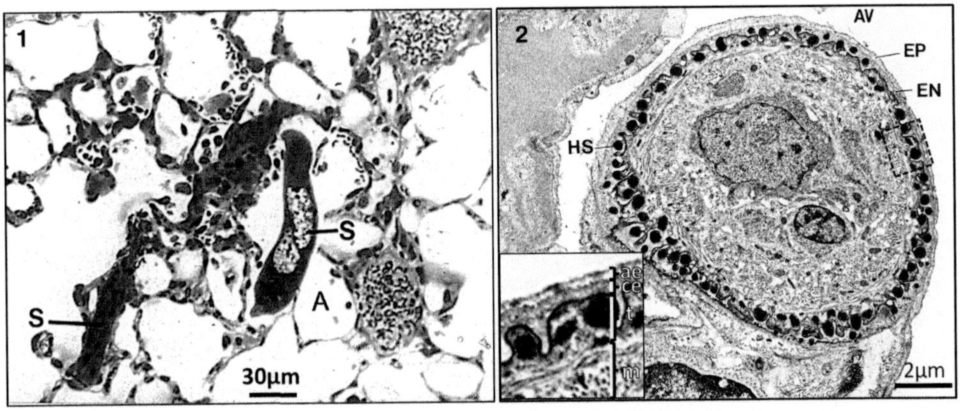

Fig. 3.14. Schistosomula in the mouse lung. **1**) An elongate day 11 schistosomulum (S), partly intravascular and partly alveolar. A small leucocytic infiltrate is present around the site of emergence but adjacent alveoli are clear. **2**) Day 7 schistosomulum in a pulmonary capillary. The head spines (HS) indent into the vascular endothelium (EN). The combined width of vascular endothelium and alveolar epithelium (EP) is <0.3 µm. AV, alveolus. The inset shows at greater magnification the scale of the schistosomulum body wall muscles (m) and overlying tegument (t) compared to the very thin capillary endothelium (ce) and overlying alveolar epithelium (ae). (**1** and **2** from Crabtree and Wilson, 1986a and b, respectively.) **1**) Figure used with permission from Cambridge University Press. **2**) Figure used with permission from John Wiley & Sons.

from which they have a limited capacity to re-enter tissues. The combined thickness of the pulmonary capillary endothelium and alveolar epithelium in the mouse is ~0.3 µm (Fig. 3.14.2). The exertions involved in passage along the lumen in many cases clearly leads to rupture. Indeed, this fragility has been linked to the limited success of penetrant cercariae (~32%) reaching maturity in the mouse (Wilson *et al.*, 2016). The larger Syrian hamster is better and a primate like the baboon best of all for % cercarial maturation, quite feasibly because they have more robust pulmonary capillaries. It is unfortunate that no tracking studies were carried out with Syrian hamsters that would have tested the capillary fragility hypothesis. Extrapolating to the human host, given their size, it is plausible that like primates they too have a high level of maturation of cercarial skin penetrants. The controlled human cercarial challenge experiments may provide information on this question.

3.3.4 Migration in *S. haematobium* and *S. japonicum*

A tracking experiment which compared *S. haematobium* with *S. mansoni* in the skin, lungs and liver of the laboratory mouse found a slower migration out the skin for *S. haematobium* giving rise to a later lung peak at day 8 (Georgi *et al.*, 1986). Parasites persisted in the lungs in some numbers out to day 22, and it was apparent that relatively few reached and matured in the liver. The average maturation of penetrant *S. haematobium* cercariae was recorded as only 17% in 15 separate experiments with two isolates (Agnew *et al.*, 1988). In the York group, three experiments with cohorts of 20 BALB/c mice exposed to 300 cercariae resulted in recovery of ~10% as adult worms by portal perfusion at 16 weeks, with a ratio of three males to two females (Dr P. Coulson, unpublished data). Even in the Syrian hamster, which is favoured for life cycle maintenance, there is slow migration and a very variable recovery of adult worms (mean 14% at 18 weeks) (Le *et al.*, 2015). Faecal eggs were not detected until between 57 and 130 days after exposure. It is not possible to infer from the above observations the true situation for *S. haematobium*. They could simply reflect the lack of a suitable laboratory model host, especially when it comes to migration of paired worms from the portal system to the vesicle plexus of the bladder wall.

Based on histopathology, *S. japonicum* parasites apparently migrate extremely rapidly through the skin, being reported in dermal blood vessels as soon as 2 h after penetration (see Section

3.3.2) (He *et al.*, 2002). However, a parasite tracking study performed with the Philippine strain (Laxer and Tuazon, 1992) does not support this very rapid skin exit (Fig. 3.15). Numbers detected in the skin started to fall by 24 h and had declined to ~17% by 72 h. The first parasites were found in the lungs at 48 h rising to a peak at 72 h, followed by a gradual decline. Parasites were detected in systemic locations such as the brain and kidney, as well as the spleen and intestines, and first appeared in the liver on day 3 reaching a plateau of 40% of the initial cercarial dose as early as day 6. These rates of migration, appreciably faster than for *S. mansoni*, were confirmed by unpublished data from a second tracking study using a Chinese strain of *S. japonicum* (Dr P. Coulson, unpublished data). Mice received a mean dose of 32 cercariae on the abdominal skin. By day 4, 16% remained in the skin, 59% were located in the lungs, 23% in systemic organs (especially the kidneys and carcase) and 11% in the intestines and liver. By day 8, 76% of the remaining parasites were located in the intestines and liver versus 34% in all other locations. This represented 94% of the adult worm population at day 28, confirming that the portal population was virtually complete by day 8, when arrival of *S. mansoni* schistosomula was only just beginning. An additional factor unique to *S. japonicum* was the reported occurrence of numerous petechial haemorrhages in mouse lungs (Moloney and Webbe, 1983); these were not observed during the lung migration of four other schistosome species (Rheinberg *et al.*, 1998). It thus appears that *S. japonicum* schistosomula have more of a bulldozer capacity than those of other species, potentially related to their basal evolutionary position in the genus and wide host range. This rapid migration may be relevant to vaccine development (see Chapter 9).

3.4 Initiation of Growth in the Portal Tract

3.4.1 The hepatic portal switch

As we have already seen from observation of *ex vivo* schistosomula (Fig. 3.7), it takes ~2 days for the elongate migrating form to convert to a short hepatic portal worm. The nutrient levels in portal blood or culture medium are important (high glucose levels of Earle's balanced or amino acid levels contributed by lactalbumin hydrolysate) but not sufficient in themselves; a supply of erythrocytes must be provided. The start of erythrocyte ingestion is accompanied by quite dramatic changes in physiology and metabolism, the precise triggers for which are unknown (Lawson and Wilson, 1980). Wet weight, oxygen consumption and lactic

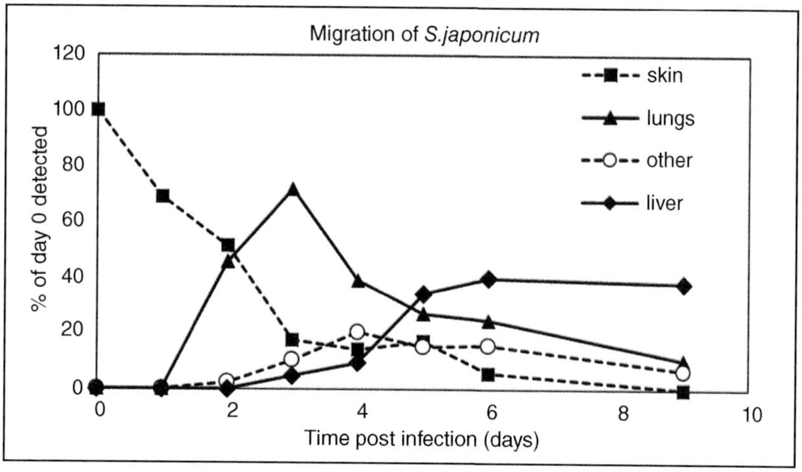

Fig. 3.15. Migration profile for radiolabelled *S. japonicum* larvae. Note that in this study, day 1 appears to be time 0, so day 2 is 24 h post-exposure, day 3 is 48 h and so on. The 'other' category of systemic organs does not include the carcase. (Replotted from data in Laxer and Tuazon, 1992.) Figure used with permission Oxford University Press.

dehydrogenase activity all increased exponentially following arrival of schistosomula in the hepatic portal system, while a rapid increase in nitrogen content indicated the onset of protein synthesis. Little is known about the genes which are activated at the crucial point but the comparison of day 6 and day 13 transcriptomes (Wangwiwatsin *et al.*, 2020) did record a number of developmental genes (*prospero homeo box*, *achae*, *hand1*, *frizzled* and *krueppel*) among the 75 most differentially upregulated at the later time. Unfortunately, the study characterizing stem cells throughout the life cycle (Wang *et al.*, 2018) sampled juvenile worms at day 21 so missed this critical juncture after erythrocyte ingestion around day 10. The ensuing development changes are a feature of schistosome biology worth more detailed scrutiny.

3.4.2 Growth, pairing and migration to the site of egg laying

Around day 30–35 post-infection the adults of *S. mansoni* and *S. japonicum* mate and begin their journey to the sites of oviposition. The factors which control pairing and the maturation of the gonads in males and females are covered in Chapter 10 on reproduction. If there is an excess of one sex, the worms remain in the intrahepatic portal vessels until the relevant partner appears. This might be some time, during which the males are virtually fully grown, whereas a female needs physiological input from a male to undergo full maturation, a rapid process once pairing has occurred. The highly muscularized male then transports the female in his ventral gynaecophoric canal up a vessel in the portal drainage to reach the tissues. Based on sites of egg deposition this can be any organ from the stomach wall or spleen to the rectum (Fig. 3.16). The preferred routes and locations are illustrated and a detailed evaluation provided of the evidence collected over decades, much of it from human autopsy studies (Nation *et al.*, 2020). Two points to note are that mouse intestines are thin walled so the large size of a schistosome pair means it cannot reach far into the mucosa, compared with human or larger mammalian hosts. Second, the worm pairs are not static but constantly move up a vessel, where the female presses forward from the male to lay a string of eggs, before retracting and moving up an adjacent portal venule. It is entirely possible that the female is able to release vasodilator secretions to assist its move forward up mucosal or submucosal vessels.

The situation with *S. haematobium* was highlighted in Section 3.3.4. In infected humans, adult pairs travel from the liver up the inferior vena cava to the rectal veins and through the rectal venous plexus to the vesical plexus of the bladder wall (Fig. 3.16). Eggs are laid in the human bladder wall and can escape to the bladder lumen to be voided in urine. However, once in the venous circulation of the lower abdomen *S. haematobium* pairs can also migrate in human females to the wall of the cervix, vagina, uterus, fallopian tubes and ovaries. In human males they can reach the epididymis, prostate, seminal vesicles, vas deferens, and testes (Nation *et al.*, 2020). In what are essentially dead-end locations, the eggs they lay will not continue transmission. However, they do cause female or male urogenital schistosomiasis, respectively, pathological conditions whose importance has only recently been appreciated (Chapter 10).

3.5 Summary

- Penetrating *S. mansoni* cercariae spend several days in the skin, the first 48 h in an epidermal location transforming into schistosomula. How the barrier of the epidermal basement membrane is breached remains unclear. Transit through the dermal matrix is rapid but the cue(s) for venule location are unknown. Secretions from the apical area breach a venule wall, the larva enters and is carried away in blood flow. More information about head gland secretions would be helpful.
- The advent of autoradiographic tracking techniques has clarified the route and timing of migration. For the three primary human species it is safe to conclude that migration to the hepatic portal system is intravascular, in the direction of blood flow, with one to several circuits of the vasculature. For schistosomes of veterinary importance, and those of birds, there is insufficient information to reach any conclusion.

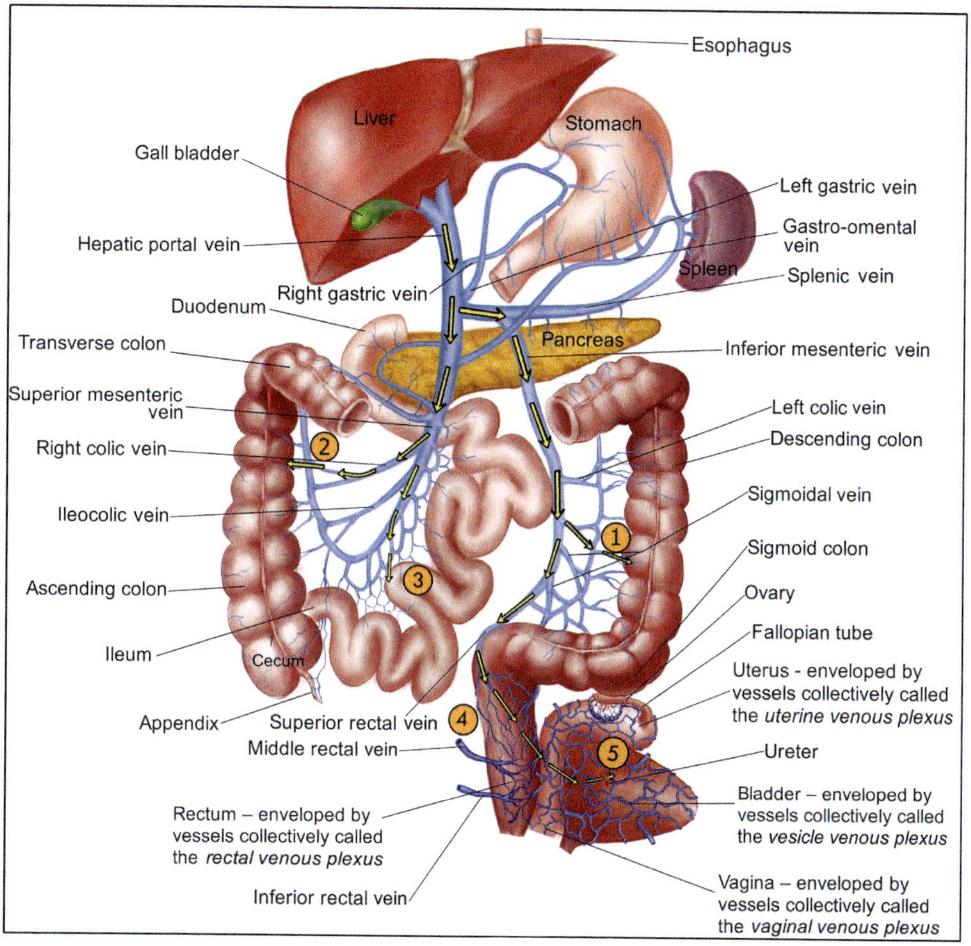

Fig. 3.16. Migration to the site of egg laying. Pathways are: **1**, the splenic vein, then inferior mesenteric vein to the descending colon; **2**, the superior mesenteric vein to right colic vein and the ascending colon; **3**, the superior mesenteric vein, then the jejunal and ileal veins to the small intestine; **4**, the inferior mesenteric vein and the superior rectal vein to the rectum; **5**, beyond the vasculature of the rectum via the rectal venous plexus through the uterine and vaginal venous plexuses in a human female. Pathways **1–4** are followed by *S. japonicum* and *S. mansoni*. Pathway **5** is *S. haematobium* only. (Reproduced from Nation *et al.*, 2020.)

- Elongation of the schistosomulum body in the lungs is facilitated by dissolution of the subtegumental fibrous layer. Reorganization of the tegument spines then permits transit through the pulmonary, and systemic capillary beds, with varying rates of migration, those of the lungs presenting a particular obstacle.
- The fragility of the alveolar/endothelial wall is the principal hazard for a migrating larva, with many deflected into the alveoli in mice, which for *S. mansoni* is a dead end. Migrating larvae of *S. japonicum* may have a greater capacity to re-enter tissues to continue their journey.
- The studies of gene expression in larvae of migrating age have used media that effectively convert them into newly arrived liver worms. This means that mechanisms suspending cell division and differentiation, while migration is in progress, are not understood. Equally, the cues that terminate migration in the portal vessels of the liver, triggering erythrocyte ingestion, have not yet been established.

References

Agnew, A.M., Lucas, S.B. and Doenhoff, M.J. (1988) The host–parasite relationship of *Schistosoma haematobium* in CBA mice. *Parasitology* 97(3), 403–424. DOI: 10.1017/s0031182000058820

Bruce, J.I., Pezzlo, F., Yajima, Y. and McCarty, J.E. (1974) *Schistosoma mansoni*: pulmonary phase of schistosomule migration studied by electron microscopy. *Experimental Parasitology* 35(1), 150–160. DOI: 10.1016/0014-4894(74)90018-6

Christensen, N.O. (1977) A method for the *in vivo* labelling of *Schistosoma mansoni* and *S. intercalatum* cercariae with radioselenium. *Zeitschrift für Parasitenkunde* 54(3), 275–288. DOI: 10.1007/BF00390119

Clegg, J.A. and Smithers, S.R. (1968) Death of schistosome cercariae during penetration of the skin. II. Penetration of mammalian skin by *Schistosoma mansoni*. *Parasitology* 58(1), 111–128. DOI: 10.1017/S0031182000073479

Coulson, P.S. (1997) The radiation-attenuated vaccine against schistosomes in animal models: paradigm for a human vaccine? *Advances in Parasitology* 39, 271–336. DOI: 10.1016/s0065-308x(08)60048-2

Crabtree, J.E. and Wilson, R.A. (1980) *Schistosoma mansoni*: a scanning electron microscope study of the developing schistosomulum. *Parasitology* 81(3), 553–564. DOI: 10.1017/s003118200006193x

Crabtree, J.E. and Wilson, R.A. (1985) *Schistosoma mansoni*: an ultrastructural examination of skin migration in the hamster cheek pouch. *Parasitology* 91(1), 111–120. DOI: 10.1017/s0031182000056559

Crabtree, J.E. and Wilson, R.A. (1986a) The role of pulmonary cellular reactions in the resistance of vaccinated mice to *Schistosoma mansoni*. *Parasite Immunology* 8(3), 265–285. DOI: 10.1111/j.1365-3024.1986.tb01038.x

Crabtree, J.E. and Wilson, R.A. (1986b) *Schistosoma mansoni*: an ultrastructural examination of pulmonary migration. *Parasitology* 92(2), 343–354. DOI: 10.1017/S0031182000064118

Dean, D.A. and Mangold, B.L. (1992) Evidence that both normal and immune elimination of *Schistosoma mansoni* take place at the lung stage of migration prior to parasite death. *The American Journal of Tropical Medicine and Hygiene* 47(2), 238–248. DOI: 10.4269/ajtmh.1992.47.238

Dean, D.A., Mangold, B.L., Georgi, J.R. and Jacobson, R.H. (1984) Comparison of *Schistosoma mansoni* migration patterns in normal and irradiated cercaria-immunized mice by means of autoradiographic analysis. Evidence that worm elimination occurs after the skin phase in immunized mice. *The American Journal of Tropical Medicine and Hygiene* 33(1), 89–96. DOI: 10.4269/ajtmh.1984.33.89

DeMarco, R., Mathieson, W., Manuel, S.J., Dillon, G.P., Curwen, R.S. *et al.* (2010) Protein variation in blood-dwelling schistosome worms generated by differential splicing of micro-exon gene transcripts. *Genome Research* 20(8), 1112–1121. DOI: 10.1101/gr.100099.109

Faust, E.C., Jones, C.A. and Hoffman, W.A. (1934) Studies on *Schistosomiasis mansoni* in Puerto Rico. III. Biological studies. 2. The mammalian phase of the life cycle. *Puerto Rico Journal of Public Health and Tropical Medicine* 10, 133–196.

Georgi, J.R. (1982) *Schistosoma mansoni*: quantification of skin penetration and early migration by differential external radioassay and autoradiography. *Parasitology* 84, 263–281. DOI: 10.1017/s0031182000044826

Georgi, J.R., Dean, D.A. and Mangold, B.L. (1983) *Schistosoma mansoni*: temporal distribution of radioselenium-labelled schistosomula in lungs of mice during the first two weeks of infection. *Parasitology* 86(1), 31–36. DOI: 10.1017/s0031182000057140

Georgi, J.R., Wade, S.E. and Dean, D.A. (1986) Attrition and temporal distribution of *Schistosoma mansoni* and *S. haematobium* schistosomula in laboratory mice. *Parasitology* 93(1), 55–70. DOI: 10.1017/s0031182000049829

Guntheroth, W.G., Luchtel, D.L. and Kawabori, I. (1982) Pulmonary microcirculation: tubules rather than sheet and post. *Journal of Applied Physiology* 53(2), 510–515. DOI: 10.1152/jappl.1982.53.2.510

Harrop, R. and Wilson, R.A. (1993) Protein synthesis and release by cultured schistosomula of *Schistosoma mansoni*. *Parasitology* 107(3), 265–274. DOI: 10.1017/s0031182000079245

He, Y.X., Chen, L. and Ramaswamy, K. (2002) *Schistosoma mansoni*, *S. haematobium*, and *S. japonicum*: early events associated with penetration and migration of schistosomula through human skin. *Experimental Parasitology* 102(2), 99–108. DOI: 10.1016/s0014-4894(03)00024-9

Hockley, D.J. (1972) *Schistosoma mansoni*: the development of the cercarial tegument. *Parasitology* 64(2), 245–252. DOI: 10.1017/s003118200002967x

Kassim, O.O., Dean, D.A., Mangold, B.L. and Von Lichtenberg, F. (1992) Combined microautoradiographic and histopathologic analysis of the fate of challenge *Schistosoma mansoni* schistosomula in mice immunized with irradiated cercariae. *The American Journal of Tropical Medicine and Hygiene* 47(2), 231–237. DOI: 10.4269/ajtmh.1992.47.231

Kruger, S.P., Heitman, L.P., Van Wyk, J.A. and McCully, R.M. (1969) The route of migration *Schistosoma mattheei* from the lungs to the liver in sheep. *Journal of the South African Veterinary Medical Association* 40, 39–43. DOI: 10.10520/AJA00382809_4377

Lawson, J.R. and Wilson, R.A. (1980) Metabolic changes associated with the migration of the schistosomulum of *Schistosoma mansoni* in the mammal host. *Parasitology* 81(2), 325–336. DOI: 10.1017/s0031182000056067

Laxer, M.J. and Tuazon, C.U. (1992) Migration of ^{75}Se-methionine-labeled *Schistosoma japonicum* in normal and immunized mice. *The Journal of Infectious Diseases* 166(5), 1133–1138. DOI: 10.1093/infdis/166.5.1133

Le, T-L.P., Boyett, D.M., Hurley-Novatny, A. and Hsieh, M.H. (2015) Hamster weight patterns predict the intensity and course of *Schistosoma haematobium* infection. *The Journal of Parasitology* 101(5), 542–548. DOI: 10.1645/14-600

Mangold, B.L. and Dean, D.A. (1983) Autoradiographic analysis of *Schistosoma mansoni* migration from skin to lungs in naive mice. Evidence that most attrition occurs after the skin phase. *The American Journal of Tropical Medicine and Hygiene* 32(4), 785–789. DOI: 10.4269/ajtmh.1983.32.785

Mastin, A.J., Bickle, Q.D. and Wilson, R.A. (1983) *Schistosoma mansoni*: migration and attrition of irradiated and challenge schistosomula in the mouse. *Parasitology* 87(1), 87–102. DOI: 10.1017/s0031182000052446

Miller, P. and Wilson, R.A. (1978) Migration of the schistosomula of *Schistosoma mansoni* from skin to lungs. *Parasitology* 77(3), 281–302. DOI: 10.1017/s0031182000050253

Miller, P. and Wilson, R.A. (1980) Migration of the schistosomula of *Schistosoma mansoni* from the lungs to the hepatic portal system. *Parasitology* 80(2), 267–288. DOI: 10.1017/s0031182000000743

Moloney, N.A. and Webbe, G. (1983) The host–parasite relationship of *Schistosoma japonicum* in CBA mice. *Parasitology* 87(2), 327–342. DOI: 10.1017/s0031182000052677

Mountford, A.P., Coulson, P.S. and Wilson, R.A. (1988) Antigen localization and the induction of resistance in mice vaccinated with irradiated cercariae of *Schistosoma mansoni*. *Parasitology* 97(1), 11–25. DOI: 10.1017/s0031182000066701

Nation, C.S., Da'dara, A.A., Marchant, J.K. and Skelly, P.J. (2020) Schistosome migration in the definitive host. *PLoS Neglected Tropical Diseases* 14(4), e0007951. DOI: 10.1371/journal.pntd.0007951

Parker-Manuel, S.J., Ivens, A.C., Dillon, G.P. and Wilson, R.A. (2011) Gene expression patterns in larval *Schistosoma mansoni* associated with infection of the mammalian host. *PLoS Neglected Tropical Diseases* 5(8), e1274. DOI: 10.1371/journal.pntd.0001274

Pereira, L.H., Coelho, P.M., Fonseca, J.J., Bredt, A. and Pellegrino, J. (1972) Migration of *Schistosoma mansoni* larvae in the albino mouse. *Revista do Instituto de Medicina Tropical de Sao Paulo* 14(5), 306–309.

Rheinberg, C.E., Moné, H., Caffrey, C.R., Imbert-Establet, D., Jourdane, J. *et al.* (1998) *Schistosoma haematobium*, *S. intercalatum*, *S. japonicum*, *S. mansoni*, and *S. rodhaini* in mice: relationship between patterns of lung migration by schistosomula and perfusion recovery of adult worms. *Parasitology Research* 84(4), 338–342. DOI: 10.1007/s004360050407

Wang, B., Lee, J., Li, P., Saberi, A., Yang, H. *et al.* (2018) Stem cell heterogeneity drives the parasitic life cycle of *Schistosoma mansoni*. *eLife* 7, e35449. DOI: 10.7554/eLife.35449

Wangwiwatsin, A., Protasio, A.V., Wilson, S., Owusu, C., Holroyd, N.E. *et al.* (2020) Transcriptome of the parasitic flatworm *Schistosoma mansoni* during intra-mammalian development. *PLoS Neglected Tropical Diseases* 14(5), e0007743. DOI: 10.1371/journal.pntd.0007743

Wheater, P.R. and Wilson, R.A. (1979) *Schistosoma mansoni*: a histological study of migration in the laboratory mouse. *Parasitology* 79(1), 49–62. DOI: 10.1017/s0031182000051970

Wilks, N.E. (1967) Lung-to-liver migration of schistosomes in the laboratory mouse. *The American Journal of Tropical Medicine and Hygiene* 16(5), 599–605. DOI: 10.4269/ajtmh.1967.16.599

Wilson, R.A. (2009) The saga of schistosome migration and attrition. *Parasitology* 136(12), 1581–1592. DOI: 10.1017/S0031182009005708

Wilson, R.A. and Coulson, P.S. (1986) *Schistosoma mansoni*: dynamics of migration through the vascular system of the mouse. *Parasitology* 92(1), 83–100. DOI: 10.1017/s0031182000063472

Wilson, R.A. and Lawson, J.R. (1980) An examination of the skin phase of schistosome migration using a hamster cheek pouch preparation. *Parasitology* 80(2), 257–266. DOI: 10.1017/s0031182000000731

Wilson, R.A., Draskau, T., Miller, P. and Lawson, J.R. (1978) *Schistosoma mansoni*: the activity and development of the schistosomulum during migration from the skin to the hepatic portal system. *Parasitology* 77(1), 57–73. DOI: 10.1017/s0031182000048721

Wilson, R.A., Coulson, P.S. and Dixon, B. (1986) Migration of the schistosomula of *Schistosoma mansoni* in mice vaccinated with radiation-attenuated cercariae, and normal mice: an attempt to identify the timing and site of parasite death. *Parasitology* 92(1), 101–116. DOI: 10.1017/s0031182000063484

Wilson, R.A., Li, X.H. and Castro-Borges, W. (2016) Do schistosome vaccine trials in mice have an intrinsic flaw that generates spurious protection data? *Parasites & Vectors* 9, 89. DOI: 10.1186/s13071-016-1369-9

Yolles, T.K., Moore, D.V. and Meleney, H.E. (1949) Post-cercarial development of *Schistosoma mansoni* in the rabbit and hamster after intraperitoneal and percutaneous infection. *The Journal of Parasitology* 35(3), 276–294. DOI: 10.2307/3273303

4

Muscle, Parenchyma and Cell Adhesion

4.1 Overview

In the adult male schistosome, the musculature and parenchymal tissues comprise in excess of 81% of the cellular mass, versus 9.5% for dorsal and ventral tegument syncytium and associated cell bodies and 4% for the gastrodermis (Fig. 4.1) (Wilson and Barnes, 1979). The protonephridia, testes and nervous tissue make up the rest. In the female the situation is very different with the musculature far less prominent, reflecting her position as a passenger of the male and a factory for egg production. The vitellaria occupy much of the interior in the rear two-thirds and the ovary, ootype and uterus are prominent in the front third. This could explain why females are more susceptible to starvation than males (Wilson *et al.*, 2008; Li *et al.*, 2015). They have more demanding metabolic needs, but also less parenchymal tissue to serve as a nutrient buffer. In this chapter, the contrasting role of the muscles and parenchyma in male and female worms are examined.

4.2 Muscle

4.2.1 The muscular system in adult males and females

The muscle layout in adult males and females is readily visualized by the staining of F-actin with fluorescently labelled phalloidin (Fig. 4.2) (Skelly *et al.*, 2014). The body wall of the male ventral surface and the whole of the female immediately beneath the syncytial tegument is broadly similar to that of the cercaria (see Chapter 2 on the cercaria). It consists of a single layer of circular fibres, overlying a single layer of larger longitudinal fibres. In contrast, the male dorsal surface comprises the same circular layer, beneath which lie multiple layers of longitudinal fibres, as many as five centrally but tapering to one or two at the edges of the dorsoventrally flattened male body. A second feature present predominantly only in the male is the numerous dorsal–ventral fibres that give the male its flattened appearance. These are not apparent in the female, which in consequence has an approximately circular profile. (Other muscles, such as those investing the alimentary tract and reproductive organs are visualized by phalloidin staining and are covered in other chapters.)

A more detailed impression of muscle organization can be found in a Z-scan of a FITC-phalloidin-stained female worm (Mair *et al.*, 2000). The very small circular fibres (<1.0 μm diameter) are closely packed around the circumference of the body (Fig. 4.3.1), with no apparent branching; it is possible that each fibre forms a continuous ring. The associated nuclei and cell bodies must lie below the longitudinal muscle layer and it seems plausible, given the frequency of the

DOI: 10.1079/9781800625167.0004

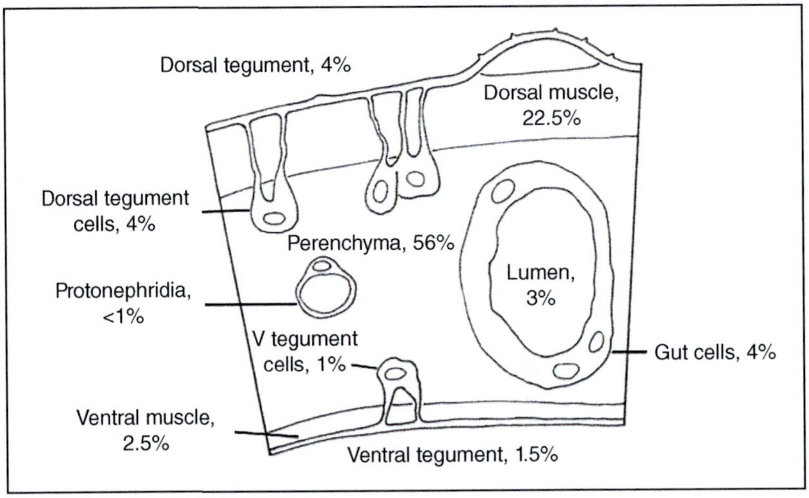

Fig. 4.1. Diagrammatic representation of the relative contributions of the different tissues in a transverse section through mid-body region of an adult male. The dorso-ventral fibres which maintain the flattened body shape are omitted. The parenchyma comprises by far the largest share, followed by the smooth muscles. The largely muscular oral and ventral suckers will increase smooth muscle overall contribution. (From Wilson and Barnes, 1979.) Figure used with permission from Cambridge University Press.

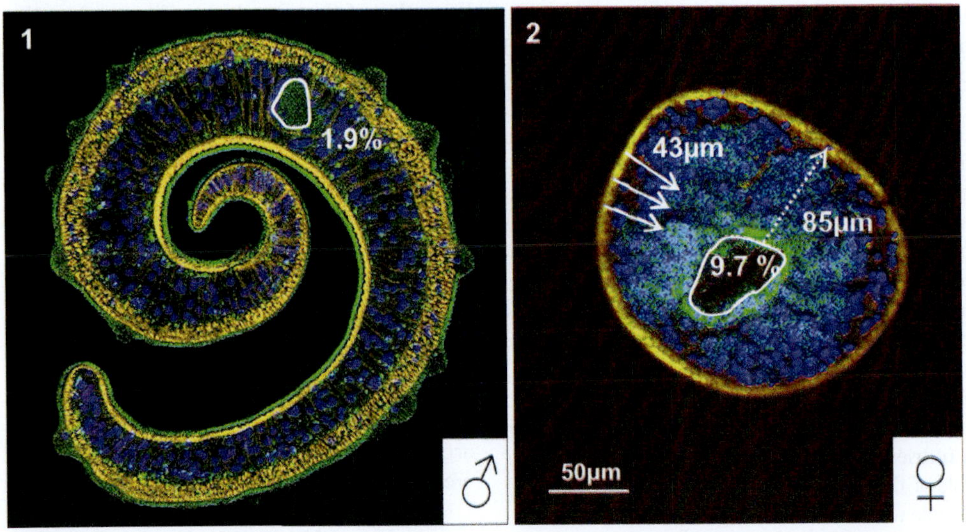

Fig. 4.2. Layout of musculature in adult *S. mansoni* revealed by phalloidin staining of actin (chrome yellow; nuclei blue). **1**) Adult male in transverse section. **2**) Adult female, to scale. The relative proportions of body volume occupied by the gut are shown. Also, the short distances that nutrients must diffuse from gut or tegument in the female. (Modified from Skelly *et al.*, 2014.) Figure used under license CC-BY-4.0.

circular fibres, that several of them are associated with a single nucleated cell body (cf. the cercaria). The longitudinal fibres are larger (at least 2.0 µm wide) and closely packed, with some evidence for branching (Fig. 4.3.2). They show a distinct spindle shape, tapering at the ends, and each is 20–40 µm long. A special feature revealed by the Z-scan is the presence beneath the longitudinal fibres of a further set of diagonal fibres, comparatively few in number and often in

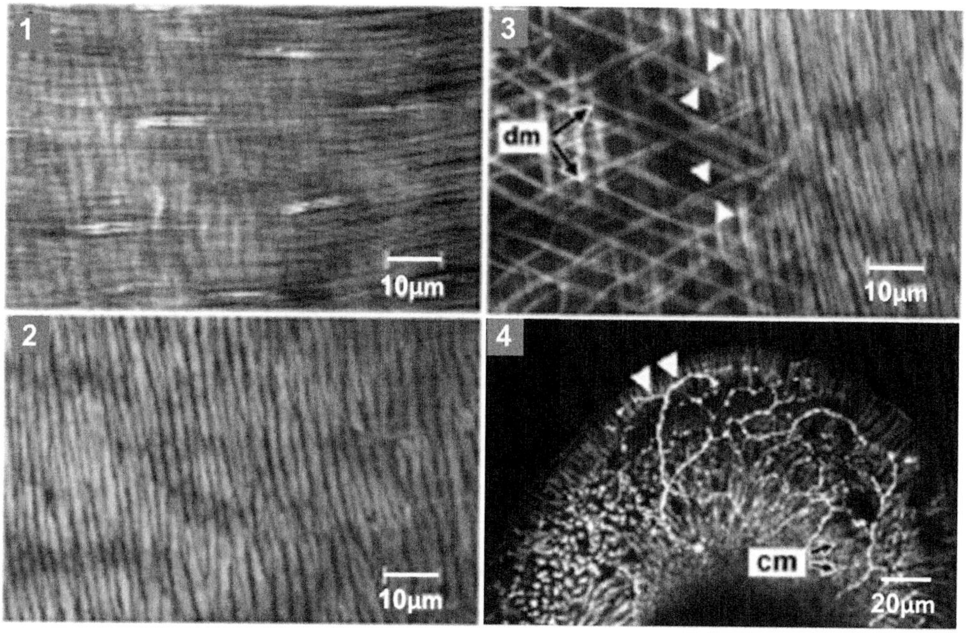

Fig. 4.3. Organization of myocytes in the body wall of female adult *S. mansoni* revealed by a confocal Z-scan from the surface downwards, after staining with FITC-phalloidin. **1**) Superficial closely packed circular fibres with little branching. **2**) Underlying perpendicular, spindle shaped, longitudinal fibres 20–40 μm long, with some branching. **3**) The innermost widely spaced layer of diagonal fibres, often arranged in pairs, forming a diamond pattern (dm). **4**) Serotonergic innervation of the male oral sucker against a background of actin-stained muscle fibres (cm). (From Mair *et al.*, 2000.) Figure used with permission from Cambridge University Press.

pairs (Fig. 4.3.3). Their diamond pattern layout and similar size in the males and females suggests their function, working in opposition, is to limit the possible extensions of the male or female body. It is presently uncertain if diagonal fibres are present beneath the male dorsal surface, given its already complex structure.

4.2.2 Fine structure of muscle fibres

Examination of the body wall muscles by transmission electron microscopy (TEM) revealed the salient features of invertebrate smooth muscle but also others related to the schistosome lifestyle (Silk and Spence, 1969). (Note that muscle cytology has its own special terms: sarcolemma for plasma membrane, sarcoplasmic reticulum for endoplasmic reticulum and sarcoplasm for cytoplasm.) The sarcoplasm contains a loose arrangement of thin actin (5 nm diameter) and thick myosin (20–40 nm diameter) filaments, arranged longitudinally (Fig. 4.4.1). The myosin filaments are shorter than the actin filaments, with tapered ends. The highly organized sarcomeres of striated muscle in higher animals have a 1:2 ratio of thick to thin filaments. In contrast, for smooth muscle the ratio can be as high as 1:15 and this is very evident in transverse sections of fibres (Fig. 4.4.2). At high magnification cross connections can be seen between thick and thin filaments. The thin filaments insert on dense bodies attached to the sarcolemma and additionally positioned at intervals throughout the sarcoplasm (Fig. 4.4.1). These bodies are integral to the transmission of contractile forces to the entire muscle fibre, and beyond to composite structures like the body wall (Fig. 4.4.3) (Sweeney and Hammers, 2018). Deposits of glycogen are scattered among the filaments and dense bodies as a readily available source of energy (Fig. 4.4.1). The sarcoplasmic reticulum, which acts as a calcium store,

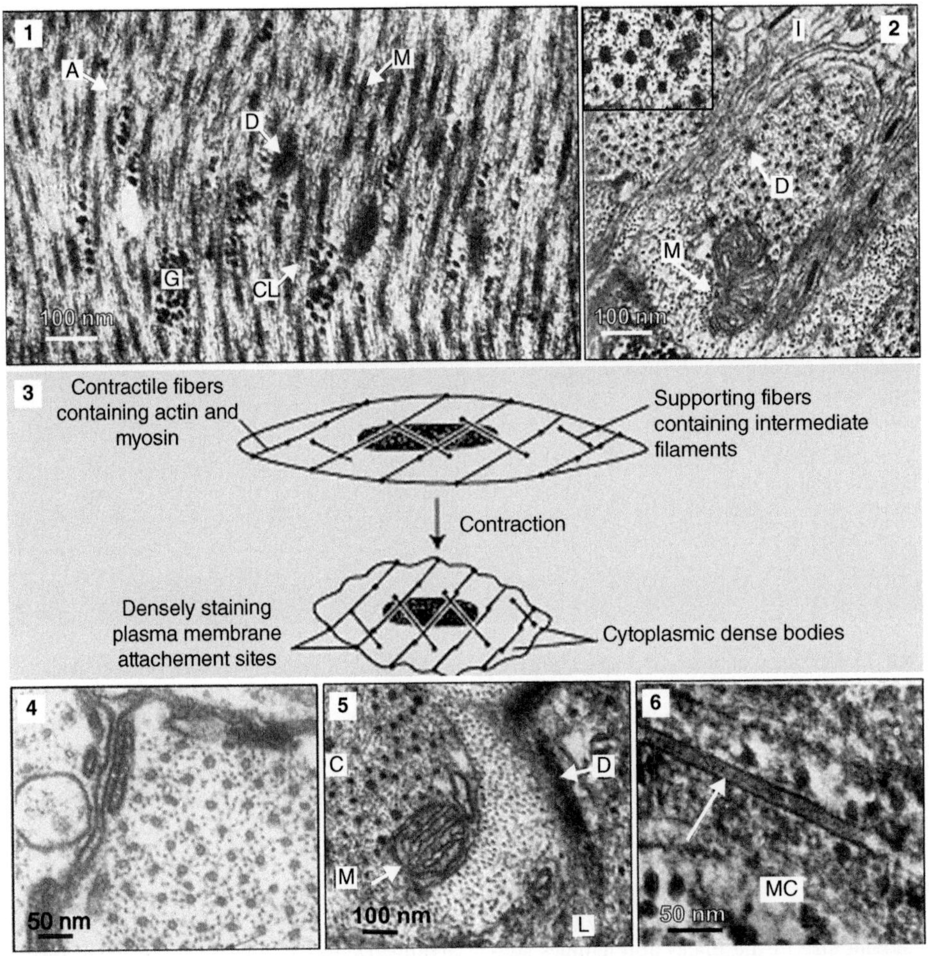

Fig. 4.4. Muscle ultrastructure. **1**) Longitudinal section through a longitudinal fibre showing thin actin (A) and thick myosin (M) filaments, glycogen granules (G) and sarcoplasmic dense bodies (D). Cross-links are present between actin and myosin (CL). **2**) Transverse section through a circular fibre showing sarcolemma dense bodies (D) and small mitochondria (M). Inset: higher magnification of actin and myosin filaments. **3**) Diagram showing how actin/myosin interactions are transmitted to via the muscle cell cytoskeleton during contraction. **4**) High-resolution TEM image of myosin thick filaments showing the hollow core formed by paracrystalline paramyosin. **5**) Fibrillar interstitial material between circular (C) and longitudinal (L) muscle fibres. A dense body (D) is present on the sarcolemma of the longitudinal fibre. M, mitochondria. **6**) A junctional complex (arrowed) between the sarcolemmas of two adjacent myocytes. (**1**, **2**, **5** and **6** from Silk and Spence, 1969; **3** from Sweeney and Hammers, 2018, reprinted courtesy of Cold Spring Harbour Laboratory Press; **4** from Reger, 1976.) Figures used with permission from **3**) Cold Spring Harbour Laboratory Press and **4**) Elsevier. **1**, **2**, **5** and **6**) Permission unavailable.

is located peripherally beneath the sarcolemma (Fig. 4.4.4 and 4.4.5). Small mitochondria are similarly located, but they are less frequent than in the cercarial tail fibres or the miracidial ciliated epithelia. This suggests that the energetics of the body wall is centred on slow sustained contractions not rapid propulsive movements.

At a gross level, the contractile regions containing the actin and myosin are distinct from the cell bodies containing the nucleus and biosynthetic areas, which generally reside centrally on the inner surface and may be fairly easily detached if the results of single-cell sequencing are a guide (Wendt *et al.*, 2020). The body wall muscles are separated from the overlying tegument by a layer of finely fibrillar interstitial connective tissue, and each fibre is surrounded by a thinner layer of the same material (Fig. 4.4.5). TEM of the muscle cell bodies indicates that fibrils are synthesized there and accumulate in distended vacuoles of sarcoplasmic reticulum before being extruded directly across the sarcolemma; the composition of the fibres has not been formally characterized. Tangential sections across the interstitial layer reveal that the fibres are randomly orientated. Note this is the same layer that is 'dissolved' to allow lung worms to extend their length 2–3-fold, so it provides another constraint on adult body shape (see Chapter 3 on migration). The spines of the tegument are firmly attached to its basal membrane and each in turn is anchored to the sarcolemma of an underlying muscle fibre. This means concerted movements of the body wall muscles are efficiently transmitted to the worm surface during intravascular migration. These movements of the body wall muscles are further reinforced by junctional complexes (see Section 4.4) between adjacent muscle fibres, binding the two interacting sarcolemmas over a distance of ~40 nm (Fig. 4.4.6).

It is pertinent to consider what is special about the structure of cercarial tail longitudinal muscle, given its extremely rapid oscillations (see Section 2.3.1). The thin actin and thick myosin filaments occupy the bulk of the sarcoplasm (in a ratio 10:1 or 12:1) (Nuttman, 1975). However, both filaments are ~0.8–1.0 μm long, forming contractile units in the manner of striated muscle sarcomeres. This is unlike the smooth muscles of the body wall, where the filaments are probably several microns long in the longitudinal fibres (Mair *et al.*, 2000). The thin filaments insert on to dense bodies at both ends, with the slightly shorter thick filaments lying between in parallel. The dense bodies are arranged in regular arrays stretching from the outer surface deep into the sarcoplasm (Fig. 4.5.1 and 4.5.2) (Nuttman, 1975). A fenestrated sarcoplasmic reticulum is very extensive, and situated just beneath the sarcolemma, but also penetrating from the inner surface deep into the sarcoplasm, alternating with the dense bodies between the contractile units. This organization presumably ensures that regulators of contraction, e.g. calcium, are conveyed deep into the interior before release into the sarcoplasm. The upshot is an extremely rapid alternating cycle of contraction and relaxation that gives the tail its burst of continuous activity on receipt of stimulation from the passing mammalian host. The spaces between the U-shaped contractile regions of the longitudinal fibres are filled with mitochondria (Fig. 4.5.3), situated centrally to provide an abundant supply of ATP, by metabolism of the glycogen stores via the Krebs cycle and oxidative phosphorylation.

4.2.3 Muscle cell proteins

There appears to have been no dedicated proteomic analysis of isolated smooth muscle cell populations, although such preparations have been used for *in vitro* physiological studies (Blair *et al.*, 1991). To understand the molecular basis of muscle function we therefore need to rely on transcriptome data. By far the most information about muscle cell composition has come from the single-cell RNA sequencing (RNA-Seq) analysis of 43,642 cells from adult *Schistosoma mansoni* (Wendt *et al.*, 2020). The cells clustering into 68 distinct populations, were visualized using a Uniform Manifold Approximation and Projection (UMAP) plot (Fig. 4.6). It is possible to interrogate the data-set by downloading it (https://www.science.org/doi/suppl/10.1126/science.abb7709/suppl_file/abb7709_tables1.xlsx) or investigate it on the SchistoCyte website (https://www.collinslab.org/schistocyte). The study identified eight clusters of muscle cells, based on differential expression of unique markers (Fig. 4.7). Some populations occur diffusely throughout the worm (muscle 1 and muscle 2) whereas others, such as muscle 7 cells, are anatomically restricted around the gut suggesting that they are the enteric muscles. A combination of whole-mount *in situ* hybridization (WISH) and double fluorescence *in situ* hybridization (FISH) revealed that muscle 3 cells are associated with the oesophagus, which morphologically has its own musculature facilitating peristalsis. There is also sexual dimorphism in non-reproductive tissues with three muscle clusters (5, 6, and 8) appearing to be largely restricted to female parasites, with muscle 8 representing muscle cells that surround the ovary. We can only conjecture what these specializations mean for muscle function, but putting that aside, there is a strong commonality of composition between the eight clusters, representing

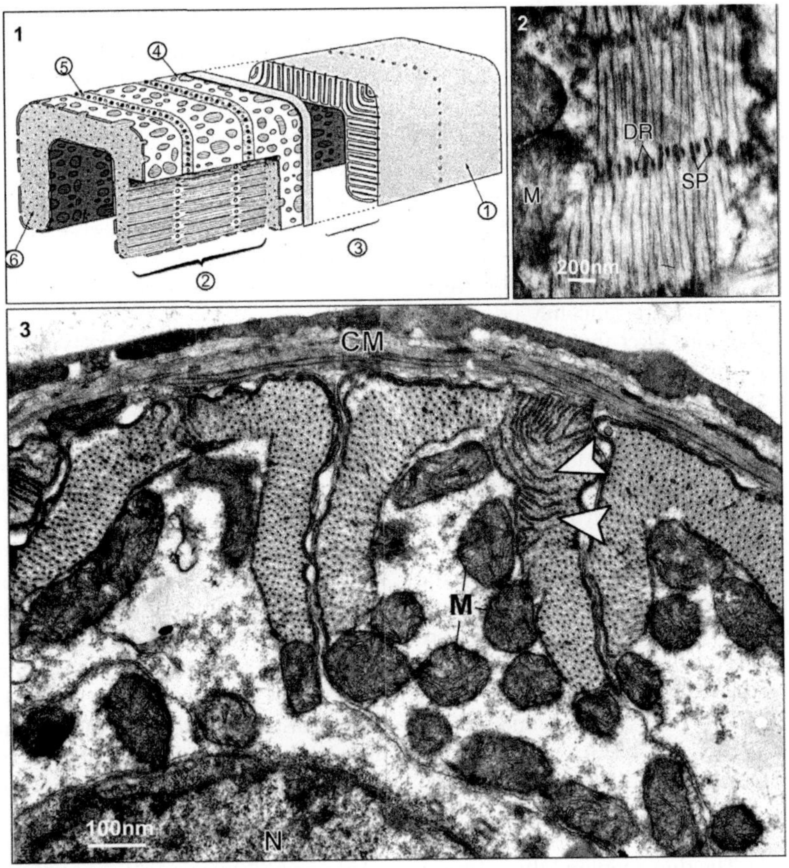

Fig. 4.5. Structure of cercarial tail 'striated' muscle. **1**) Schematic diagram of a single U-shaped longitudinal contractile unit. 1, sarcolemma covers entire fibre; 2, sarcomere in longitudinal section showing striations comprising tubules and dense rods between which run the thick and thin filaments; 3, segment removed to reveal striations in TS; 4, surface view of fenestrated sarcoplasmic reticulum; 5, striations below the sarcolemma; 6, transverse section of fibre showing thick filaments surrounded by numerous thin filaments. **2**) TEM of alternating dense bodies (DR) and sarcoplasmic tubules (SP) that comprise a single striation. M, mitochondria. **3**) Tail in transverse section showing three distinct longitudinal myocytes with U-shaped regions, one with a nucleus (N). Numerous large mitochondria are present, and the alternating sarcoplasmic tubules and dense bodies are visible (arrowed). (From Nuttman, 1975.) Figures used with permission from Dr Chris Nuttman.

the complete molecular assembly participating in contraction. The transcripts include multiple actins, myosin heavy and two light chains, myosin light chain kinase, calponin and calmodulin calcium regulating proteins, G-protein-coupled receptors (GPCRs), etc. We can conclude that the mechanism of smooth muscle contraction is similar to that in other platyhelminths, and the Lophotrochozoa in general.

One unanticipated discovery was the enrichment of 'extracellular matrix structural components' in muscle clusters, suggesting that muscles are the source of extracellular matrix in schistosomes, similar to the situation in planarians (Cote *et al.*, 2019). This neatly confirms the TEM observation more than 50 years ago, of muscle cells secreting fibrillar material across the sarcolemma (see Section 4.2.2) (Silk and Spence, 1969). In muscle cluster 8 located around the ovary, seven of the top 30 most highly expressed genes encode variants of α-collagen. Furthermore, the ovary is known to be

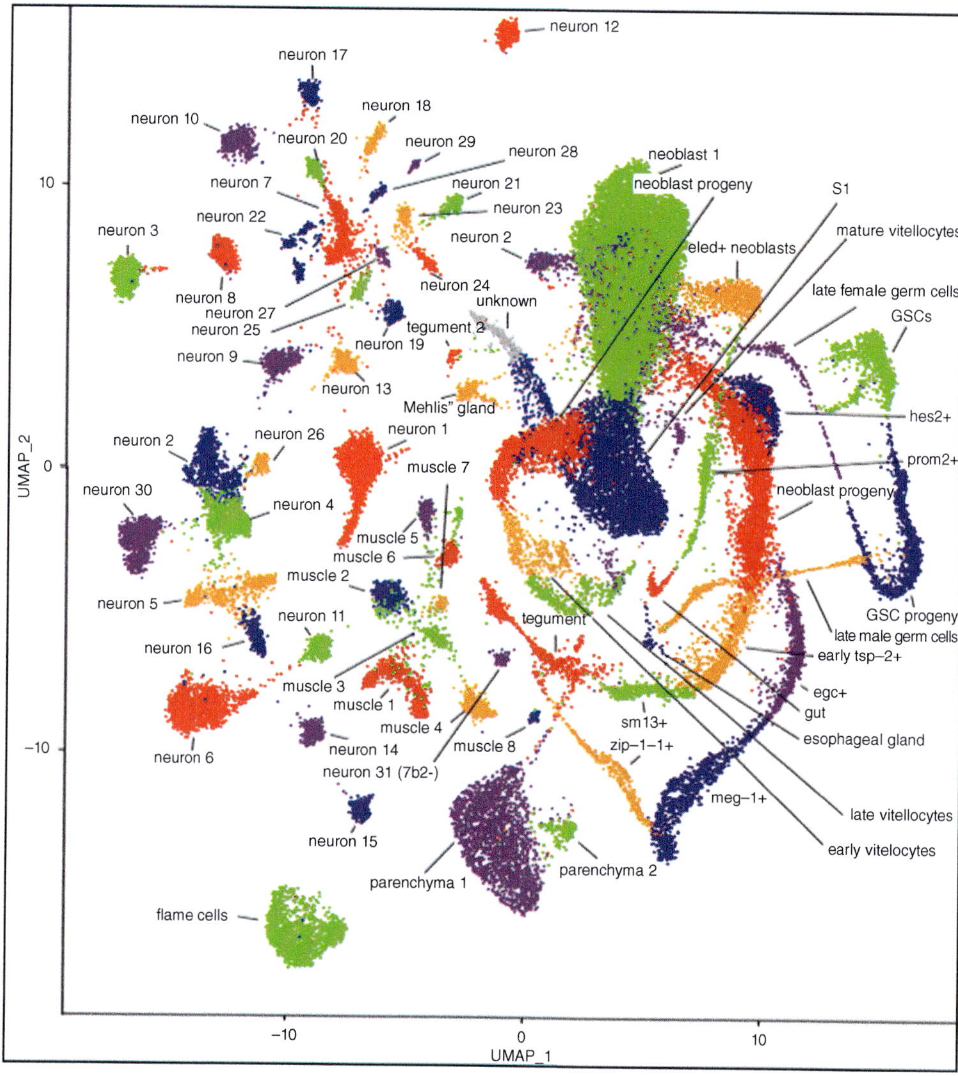

Fig. 4.6. A UMAP plot of the 68 cell clusters and their annotations, resulting from single-cell RNA-Seq analysis cells from adult worms. (An original image kindly provided by Professor J.J. Collins, UTSouthwestern Medical Center, Dallas, TX, USA; published by Wendt *et al.*, 2020.) Figure used with permission from Professor J.J. Collins.

surrounded by a capsule of matrix proteins so tough that the organ can be isolated intact for gene expression studies (Hahnel *et al.*, 2013) (see Chapter 10 on reproduction). Transcripts for two basement membrane-specific heparan sulphate proteoglycan core proteins (Smp_020550 and Smp_310170) and a fibrillin (Smp_001100) are present in the muscle clusters. UniProt indicates that the encoded proteins are expressed in an extracellular surface location making them putative matrix components. However, there appears to be no schistosome equivalent of the fibronectins and elastins that are constituents of vertebrate extracellular matrix. This suggests that collagen fibres are the principal constituents of the fibrils revealed by TEM.

There is one muscle protein, paramyosin, that has been a source of controversy, with reports concluding that it was present in the tegument, for example (Gobert *et al.*, 1997;

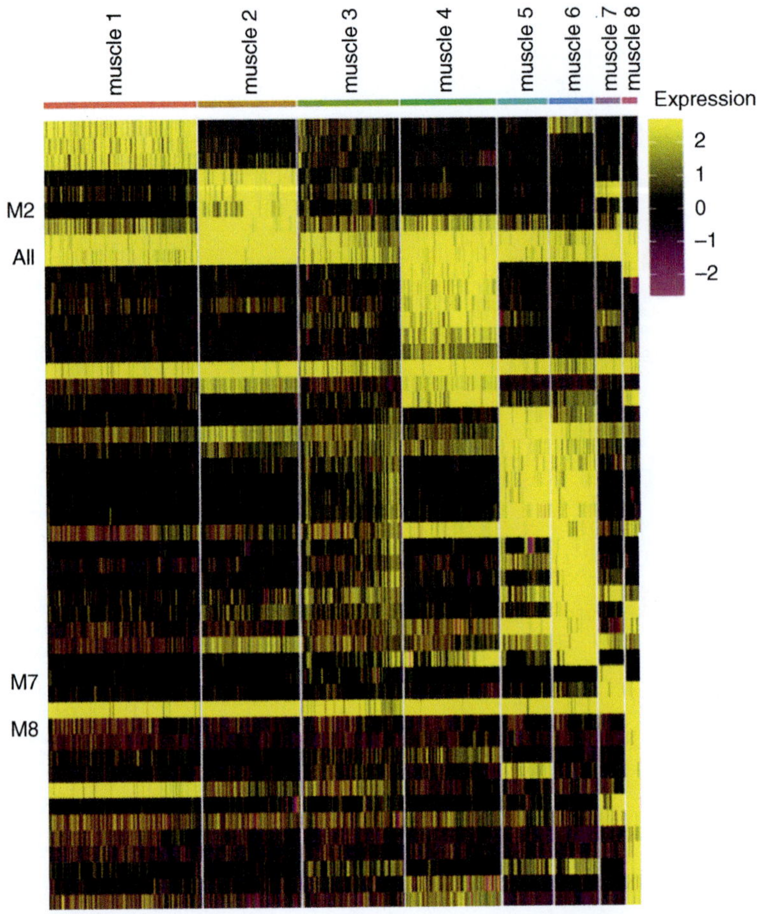

Fig. 4.7. Heatmap of the most uniquely expressed genes from the eight muscle clusters grouped by cluster number. Each row represents a gene and each column represents a cell. Clusters are indicated on the top of the panel. The number of cells sequenced per cluster ranged from 593 (M1) to 58 (M8). Key to listed markers: M2, Smp_068240, zinc finger protein; All, Smp_086330, myophilin; M7, Smp_343800, homeobox protein engrailed-like; M8, Smp_200110, uncharacterized. The power of the approach is that the list of genes expressed in any cluster can be mined to identify those associated with a selected biological function in that cell type. (An original image kindly provided by Professor J.J. Collins, UTSouthwestern Medical Center, Dallas, TX, USA; published by Wendt *et al.*, 2020.) Figure used with permission from Professor J.J. Collins.

Matsumoto *et al.*, 1988). However, this was not a unanimous conclusion (Fig. 4.8.1) (Riengrojpitak, 1987). Most invertebrate thick filaments contain a core of paramyosin, a coiled-coil protein ~124 nm long (Craig and Woodhead, 2006), and there is no reason to suppose that schistosomes would differ in this respect. The paramyosin has a paracrystalline organization, with the myosin heavy chain forming a thin surface layer of loosely attached molecules. The thick paramyosin core may strengthen these large myosin filaments against the high loads they must bear due to their greater length than in a striated sarcomere, and hence the larger number of actin filament interactions they make. It is notable that some high-resolution TEM images show the myosin heavy filament as hollow in transverse section (Fig. 4.4.4) (Reger, 1976). Both Southern blotting (Schmidt *et al.*, 1996) and database searching (WormBase

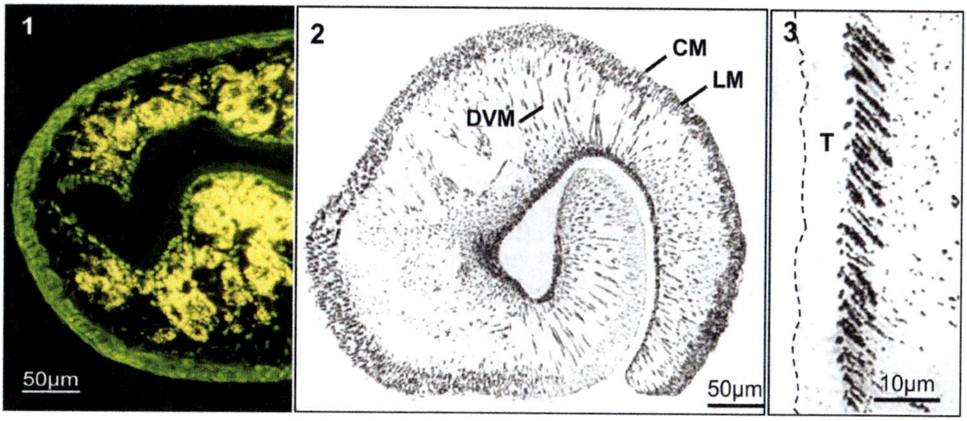

Fig. 4.8. Localization of paramyosin in adult *S. mansoni* worms. **1**) Transverse section of the posterior half of a female stained with mouse monoclonal anti-paramyosin, detected by FITC-labelled goat anti-mouse IgG (green). The outer circular and inner longitudinal fibres of the body wall and the musculature surrounding the gut are positive. (Shell granules in vitelline cells autofluoresce bright yellow.) **2**) Low magnification of adult male transverse section stained with anti-paramyosin antibody and detected by immunogold/silver labelling on thin sections. The circular (CM), longitudinal (LM) and dorsoventral (DVM) fibres are all positive. **3**) High magnification of the adult surface to show that the tegument (T) is negative while the circular, longitudinal and dorsoventral fibres are strongly positive. (**2** and **3** from Schmidt *et al.*, 1996.) **1**) Figure author's own. **2** and **3**) Figures used with permission from Cambridge University Press.

ParaSite, NCBInr) reveals only a single copy gene for paramyosin (Smp_021920; UniProt P06198). A thorough and detailed investigation of the localization of paramyosin (Schmidt *et al.*, 1996) revealed that in cercariae, schistosomula and adults, the circular and longitudinal muscles of the body wall (Fig. 4.8.2), the dorsoventral muscles and those surrounding the gut and oesophagus, as well as the cercarial tail (Fig. 4.8.3), intensely reacted with a specific antibody. Conversely, neither staining of sections nor Western blots of isolated tegument syncytium, indicated the presence of paramyosin there. In addition, it was demonstrated that phosphorylation of the serine and tyrosine residues of paramyosin is likely responsible for the generation of multiple isoforms, with implications for function.

4.2.4 Regulation of motility

The way in which adult schistosomes migrate around the hepatic portal vasculature has recently been visualized in a remarkable study using advanced microscopical techniques (Zhang *et al.*, 2019; Yeh *et al.*, 2024). We need to put this motility in the context of worm biology. After pairing, between days 28 and 35 in the mouse, the male acts as a chauffeur for the female, carrying her up into the finer branches of the mesenteric venules. She then progresses a little further upstream to deposit eggs within the intestinal tissues (see Chapter 11 on the egg). A study of the wandering capacity of a worm revealed that the female laid a cluster of eggs along a venule, before the male withdrew and carried her to a new venule that might be centimetres away, to repeat the process. How is this peregrination achieved?

Traction force microscopy with hydrogel incorporating fluorescent beads as the substrate, was used to measure the forces generated as the worm travels across that surface, by the changes in motion of the beads. When an adult male is not confined, as in the main portal vein, it uses its oral and ventral suckers to maintain position and 'march', either forward or backward. When marching, the region between the oral and ventral suckers alternates between extensions and contractions as each sucker engages and then releases the substrate (Fig. 4.9.1) (Yeh *et al.*, 2024). The traction forces exerted by these suckers are complex; one principal feature is an

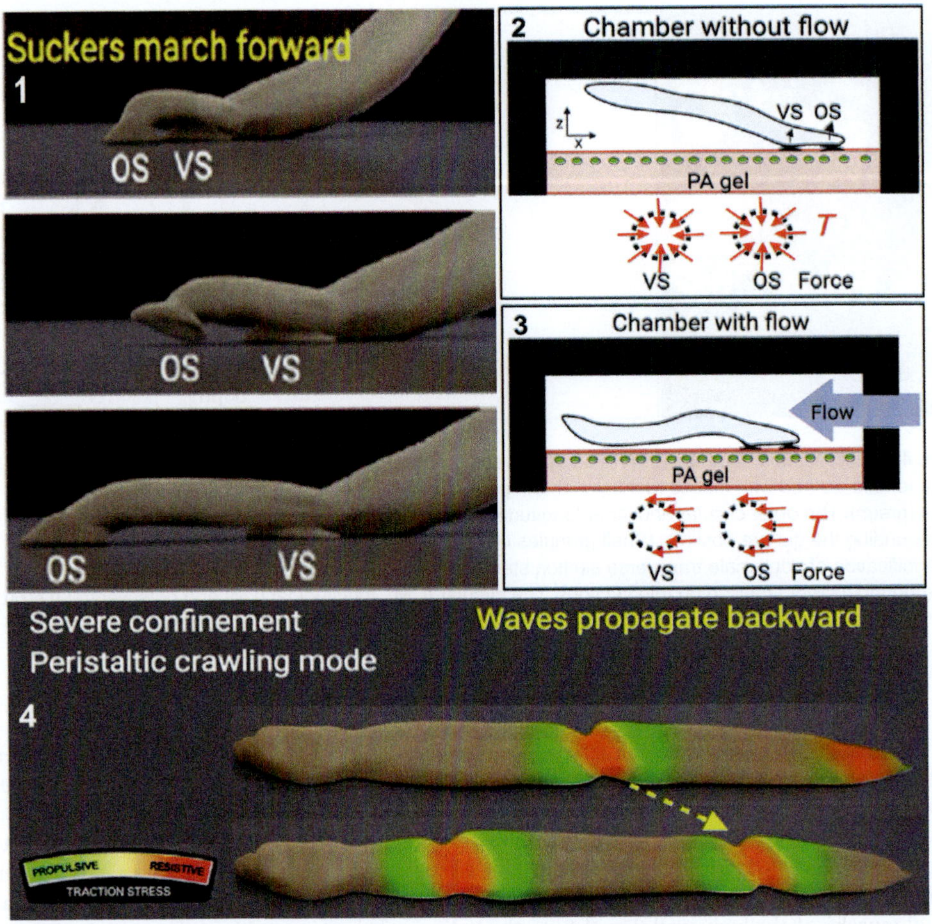

Fig. 4.9. The mechanism of male *S. mansoni* locomotion. **1**) Two-anchor marching mode under unconfined conditions such as those experienced in the lower mesenteric and hepatic portal vein. **2**) Use of a microfluidics device and traction force microscopy to quantify adhesion forces and mechanics of locomotion by *S. mansoni* worms. Under no-flow conditions the worm generates a uniform suction pressure with its oral and ventral suckers to anchor to the substrate as it marches forward. **3**) Under flow conditions, the sucker forces adjust to balance the hemodynamic resistance experienced by the worm. T, traction stress vector; VS, ventral sucker; OS, oral sucker; PA, polyacrylamide gel with fluorescent beads. **4**) Under confined conditions the worm switches to crawling mode, generating peristaltic waves. If these propagate backward, the worm is propelled forward. (From Yeh *et al.*, 2024.) Figure used with permission from Elsevier.

inward contraction that creates a suction pressure inside the sucker to hold fast to the substrate (Fig. 4.9.2). When the worm encounters blood flow, more force is applied to the leading edge of the suckers to counteract its strength (Fig. 4.9.3). One conclusion of the study is that the parasite can both sense and rapidly respond to changes in fluid flow in its environment, working very hard to maintain its position in the blood vessel. When the worms move into the confined space of small venules, the male exhibits a different behaviour. He switches from sucker-based propulsion to the generation of peristaltic waves that originate posterior of the ventral sucker and propagate backward (retrograde) to move the worm forward up the vessel, carrying the female (Fig. 4.9.4). Conversely, anterograde peristalsis allows the male to travel backward down the small venule, into which the pair have crawled, without the need to physically turn his body. Impressively, the male can also coordinate sucker marching with peristaltic crawling, leading to faster migratory speeds, compared to either modality alone. Videos showing antero and retrograde peristalsis are available at figshare: https://doi.org/10.6084/m9.figshare.c.4380302.v1 (Zhang *et al.*, 2019).

This complex coordination of suckers and body wall muscles, within and between worms implies the presence of a complex neural network linking the detection of external sensory stimuli to motor instructions. Here, it is simply worth noting that the spiny bosses covering the male dorsal surface are richly supplied with numerous morphologically identical mechanoreceptor endings (see Section 4.3) that can provide information on the amount of pressure in the confined venule space. The sensory endings on the cercarial ventral sucker have been mapped but no similar ventral sucker map for the adult, or one for the oral sucker, appear to have been made.

4.2.5 Regulation of contraction

The acoelomate structure of the schistosome worm body always presented a problem for experiments on muscle physiology. For decades the only method available to investigate the action of suspected neurotransmitters was the direct application of the agent to the intact worm followed by some optical or direct measurement of its response (Pax and Bennett, 1991). This approach revealed that application of acetylcholine 'paralysed' worms while serotonin (5-hydroxytryptamine) stimulated contraction. A tantalizing glimpse at the complexity of muscular control was provided by an *in vitro* preparation in which uniform 0.3 mm worm 'steaks' were cut from the mid-body of anaesthetised males, then returned to medium at 37°C, and mounted in a motion-recording device before application of physiological agents (Pax *et al.*, 1984). Other studies had implicated acetylcholine, serotonin and dopamine as major neurotransmitters, and this proved to be the case for both circular and longitudinal fibres, but not in an identical way. In brief, dopamine was an effective relaxant of longitudinal muscle but appeared to have a complex effect on the circular muscle. Serotonin induced rhythmic contractile activity in both sets of muscles, while decreasing tone in the circular and increasing it in the longitudinal muscle. The cholinergic agonist carbachol produced flaccid paralysis of both sets of muscles but eserine, an anticholinesterase, produced significant relaxation only in the longitudinal, not in the circular muscle. It is notable that known neurotransmitters in other invertebrate systems (γ-aminobutyric acid (GABA), norepinephrine, epinephrine and octopamine) had no measurable effects on muscle tone or contractile activity in this male body wall muscle preparation.

A second avenue of investigation by the same research group was the development of an isolated muscle cell preparation that permitted electrophysiological recording (Blair *et al.*, 1991). Chopped up male worms incubated for 30 min at 37°C in culture medium, containing papain as the preferred protease, released distinct fibres. The cytoplasmic bridges connecting the muscle cell nuclei to the contractile spindle were severed during the process of dispersion (cf. Wendt *et al.*, 2020) but the fibres were otherwise functional and excluded trypan blue dye. These isolated fibres responded to high K^+ concentrations by alternately relaxing and contracting, an effect that could be blocked by Co^{2+} ions. The study identified a Ca^{2+}-activated K^+ channel in the muscle membrane, similar to ones in other invertebrates, with a 10:1 selectivity for K^+ over Na^+. Subsequent work with isolated muscle cells of different morphologies suggested at least two types of K^+-gated channels (Day *et al.*, 1993). One gene encoding a voltage-gated K^+ channel was subsequently cloned and characterized by molecular biology techniques (Smp_069240) (Kim *et al.*, 1995). The function of such membrane channels is that during action potentials they return the depolarized cell to the resting state.

The isolated muscle cell preparation was also used to investigate directly the role of serotonin in muscle cell contraction (Day *et al.*, 1994). Ca^{2+} in the incubation medium was necessary to elicit contractions in response to the elevated K^+ level. Moreover, there was a dose-dependent relationship over the range 10–300 nM serotonin in the incubation medium, and the muscle response to elevated K^+. Judicious use of a variety of serotonin agonists and antagonists, mostly gleaned from mammalian neurotransmitter receptor studies to substitute for serotonin or to interfere with its action, demonstrated at least one receptor site on muscle cell membranes. Serotonin was a prerequisite for high K^+ depolarization to cause contraction of isolated muscles fibres, those contractions required extracellular Ca^{2+}, and were blocked by the Ca^{2+} channel blocker, nicardipine. Thus, contraction of the schistosome muscle was also dependent on an influx of Ca^{2+} through voltage-gated Ca^{2+} channels. It had originally been proposed that a serotonin receptor coupled to a G-protein membrane receptor functioned by activating intracellular adenylate cyclase to elevate cAMP levels (Kasschau and Mansour, 1982). The observation that a protein kinase A inhibitor (H89) was able to block the contractile response of muscle fibres to the presence of serotonin supported this mode of action in isolated fibres (Day *et al.*, 1994).

The isolated muscle cell preparation was also used to explore another angle on the control of muscle cell contractility (Day *et al.*, 1994). It was apparent from work on other platyhelminths, and also molluscs, that neuropeptides were major components of the nervous system. Furthermore, such short FMRFamide (Phe-Met-Arg-Phe-NH_2)-like peptides were capable of producing potent myoexcitation. Two peptides, from a tapeworm and a turbellarian, caused dose-dependent contractions of isolated fibres from *S. mansoni*. This was the first demonstration of a direct excitatory effect of a putative peptide neurotransmitter on the muscle of a platyhelminth and implied the presence of peptide receptors on the sarcolemma. Work continued, using heterologous peptides, to define the mechanism of fibre stimulation (Novozhilova *et al.*, 2010), revealing that the peptide-induced contractions utilized extracellular Ca^{2+}, while the pharmacological profile implicated voltage-gated Ca^{2+} channels as the entry conduit. By analogy with other species, GPCRs were the likely signal mediators, associated with voltage-gated Ca^{2+} channels, acting via a protein kinase C-dependent pathway. Interrogation of the SchistoCyte database (Wendt *et al.*, 2020) (see below) revealed that all eight muscle clusters in the adult worm expressed a cAMP-dependent protein kinase C catalytic subunit α (Smp_164380), which supports this proposed mode of operation. Four of the muscle clusters also expressed three different FMRFamide receptors, which could imply a differential mode of stimulation. The topic of neuropeptides is covered in Chapter 5.

The publication of the *S. mansoni* transcriptome in 2003 (Verjovski-Almeida *et al.*, 2003) and the full genome in 2009 (Berriman *et al.*, 2009) finally removed a major obstacle to progress in the characterization of genes and proteins involved in muscle function. At the same time, the data tabulations revealed just how extensive were the lists of receptors and ion channels potentially involved in neuromuscular coordination. At least 92 genes encoding putative GPCRs were identified. One group in the α subfamily (30 members) includes amine receptors, and a second in the β subfamily (24 members) includes neuropeptide and hormone receptors. Unfortunately, bioinformatics alone cannot identify putative ligands, which need to be confirmed by functional studies. Each of the three major ligand-gated ion channel families were represented, namely the Cys-loop family, glutamate-activated cation channel and ATP-gated ion channel. Among the 13 Cys-loop members, nine encode nicotinic acetylcholine receptor subunits. The remaining four anion channel subunits were GABA, glycine and glutamate receptors. There were at least 41 members of voltage-gated K^+ channel families. Other K^+ channels include the KQT, large Ca^{2+}-activated, small Ca^{2+}-activated and cyclic nucleotide-gated groups. There were also four α and two β subunits of voltage-gated Ca^{2+} channels.

After 2009, the challenge for researchers was to associate this diversity of components with specific tissues. In this they have been aided by single-cell RNA-Seq from adult worms (Wendt *et al.*, 2020). Focusing in on genes expressed in the muscle clusters, the previously cloned voltage-gated K^+ channel (Smp_069240) (Kim *et al.*, 1995) was expressed in seven out of eight muscle clusters (and several neuron clusters). In contrast, the putative serotonin receptor (Smp_126730) (Patocka *et al.*, 2014) localized only to neurons. Ironically, in view of the finding that isolated muscle fibres did not respond to GABA as an applied stimulus (Pax *et al.*, 1984), seven out of eight muscle clusters expressed a GABA receptor subunit γ-3 (Smp_336620), implying susceptibility to the ligand. Muscle clusters 1 and 8 also expressed dopamine receptors at low transcript levels. Two acetylcholine-gated

Cl^- channels (SmACCs), SmACC-1 (Smp_176310) and SmACC-2 (Smp_306240), have been cloned and characterized (MacDonald *et al.*, 2014). They localized to regions of the peripheral nervous system that innervated the body wall muscles but neither appeared to be expressed directly on the muscle cells. Thus, they are unlikely candidates for the muscle acetylcholine receptor that causes flaccid paralysis. However, muscle clusters 2 and 7 express a different nicotinic acetylcholine receptor (Smp_031680) that may be a better candidate to mediate the effect.

4.3 Parenchyma

4.3.1 Exactly what is the parenchyma?

The parenchyma is probably the least investigated or appreciated tissue of the adult worm body. Basically, any space within the confines of the body wall muscles that is not an organ is filled with a packing tissue, given the name 'parenchyma'. Therein lies the problem – it is defined by what it is not, namely not muscle cells, alimentary tract, protonephridial system, nervous system and reproductive organs. In the male worm, an early TEM report concluded that the contents of the dorsal tubercles were 'herniations of the medullary parenchyma' passing through gaps between the body wall muscles (Smith *et al.*, 1969). The interstitial spaces between adjacent longitudinal and circular fibres are penetrated by the tubular cytoplasmic connections coming from both tegumental cell bodies and parenchymal cells (Fig. 4.10.1), as well as the terminal insertions of the dorsoventral muscles. Within the core of each tubercle the extensions from the parenchyma cells balloon out to fill the space creating its raised appearance (Fig. 4.10.2). Neurons also enter the tubercles terminating in uniciliated sensory endings on the body surface. There is a striking dichotomy between the tubercles, which is relevant to the peristaltic propulsion described in Section 4.2.4 above. They alternate between fully spined and relatively smooth rows across the dorsal surface (Fig. 4.10.3), and it is the smooth tubercles that bear the sensory endings (Fig. 4.10.4). The utility of this arrangement is that the heavily spined tubercles provide traction against the blood vessel surface, while the projecting cilia on the smooth tubercles can signal the intensity of that contact.

A second TEM study treated the parenchyma as synonymous with the cell bodies of muscle fibres (Reissig, 1970) which leaves us in an awkward situation. To get a convincing picture of the ultrastructure of the parenchyma, and the role it might play in worm physiology, we have to turn to a description of the tissue in the liver fluke (*Fasciola hepatica*) (Threadgold and Gallagher, 1966). There, parenchymal cells were polymorphic in shape, sometimes long and slender with pseudopodia-like extensions when lying adjacent to organ systems, embedded in a layer of interstitial material. The cytoplasm contained sparse endoplasmic reticulum proximal to nuclei, mitochondria and various inclusion bodies, but Golgi bodies were not evident. Clearly this was not a cell destined to secrete quantities of proteins into its environs. There was a marked tendency for mitochondria to be concentrated in large numbers in small areas of the cell leaving other regions virtually devoid. Both α- and β-forms of glycogen were present, sometimes in aggregations, together with lipid droplets. This parenchymal cell structure gives the impression of serving as an energy store. In the absence of a circulatory system the authors posited that it could also function as a transport route between other tissues, due to its intimate association with them via the pseudopodial processes.

To what extent can this description be applied to schistosomes? Two studies have suggested that a glutathione *S*-transferase (GST) might be a good parenchyma marker. The first used a polyclonal antibody against protein purified from worms (Holy *et al.*, 1989) so we cannot be certain of the molecular target. The second used polyclonal antibody against a recombinant 28 kDa vaccine candidate (Porchet *et al.*, 1994) (Smp_333010). Interrogation of the data-set from single-cell sequencing (Wendt *et al.*, 2020) reveals that there is a GST exclusively expressed in parenchyma clusters 1 and 2, namely Smp_152710, whereas Smp_333010 is expressed in germ cell and tegument lineages. It seems unlikely that a GST isoform can provide an exclusive parenchymal marker protein, suitable for unequivocal immunolocalization, which would aid characterization of this tissue.

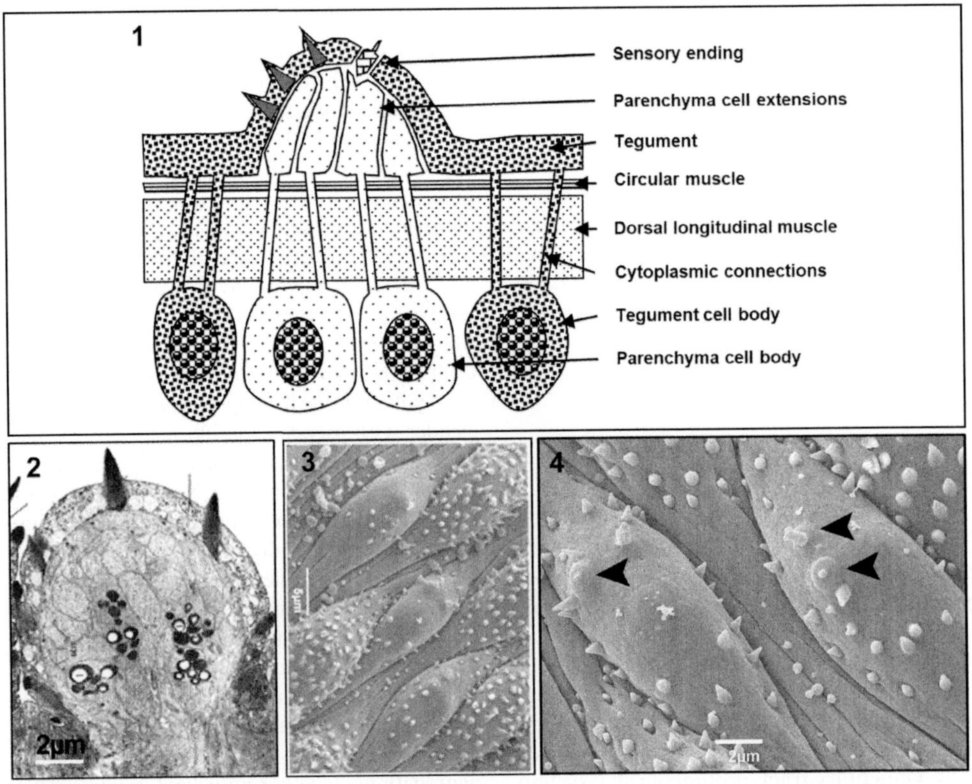

Fig. 4.10. The male dorsal tubercle. **1**) Simplified schematic showing how both tegument cell bodies and parenchymal cell extend cytoplasmic connections through the dorsal longitudinal and circular muscle layers. Those from the parenchymal cells balloon out to form the packing tissue of each dorsal tubercle. **2**) A dorsal tubercle filled with parenchymal cytoplasm and lipid droplets. **3**) Alternating spiny and smooth rings of tubercles across the dorsal male surface. **4**) At higher magnification ciliated sensory endings are visible (arrowed) only on the smooth tubercles. (**2** from Smith *et al.*, 1969; **3** and **4** from Parker-Manuel and Wilson, 2022.) **1**) Figure author's own. **2**) Figure used with permission from *The American Journal of Tropical Medicine and Hygiene*. **3** and **4**) Figures used under license CC-BY-4.0.

4.3.2 Metabolic processes in the parenchyma

Visual inspection of the transverse sections of adult worms (Fig. 4.2) suggests that the male proportionally has far more parenchymal tissue than the female. The abundance of glycogen in parenchyma and muscles provides another way of looking at the properties of these tissues (Bueding and Koletsky, 1950). Direct compositional analysis of worms freshly removed from the portal system gave remarkable values for glycogen as a percentage of dry weight. It was 19.6% ($n = 59$) in males versus only 4.3% ($n = 29$) in females, so the male has 4.5 times the glycogen content of the female, distributed largely between muscle and parenchyma. The male has a greater requirement for ATP production in its role as chauffeur for the female but the total energy requirements of the female for egg production are far greater. The smaller size of the female glycogen 'buffer' may thus contribute to its excess mortality in some vaccine models (see Chapter 9 on vaccines).

The abundance of glycogen underlines its central importance in adult worm metabolism, while *in vitro* investigations showed it is in a dynamic relationship with free glucose availability (Tielens and Van den Bergh, 1987). The enormous capacity of tegument membrane transporters in both males and females to take up glucose from the blood, covered in Chapter 7, posed a question about why there was a need for a large glycogen store (Tielens and Van den Bergh, 1987). This was addressed in a series of *in vitro* experiments which showed that worms rapidly utilized their glycogen reserves when placed in culture medium. Recovery slowly followed, or degradation could be prevented, if the medium was enriched with 100 mM glucose and 1% bovine serum albumin. The existence of glycogen stores strongly suggests that the worms sometimes encounter conditions where the externally available glucose is in limited supply. The authors rejected the idea that this might occur between meals, when the glucose level in the portal tract fluctuates several fold, because even at low molarities glycogen reserves could still be replenished, *in vitro*. They suggested instead that the movement of a worm pair into a small mesenteric vein could have an even more profound effect since the flow of blood through a vein occupied by a worm pair would be severely restricted, leading to consumption of glycogen reserves. Indeed, they tied this into the wanderings of worm pairs around the portal system (see Section 4.2.4 and Chapter 11 on the egg). It is feasible that depletion of glycogen reserves is the trigger for worm reversal to wider vessels where the blood flow can irrigate the tegument surfaces.

A second study (Tielens *et al.*, 1989) added more details, labelling worms by incubation in the presence of 6-^{14}C-glucose, after an initial reduction of their glycogen content. Subsequent breakdown by the parasite revealed that newly synthesized labelled glycogen was degraded only to lactate and carbon dioxide. The former metabolite is by far the larger end-product confirming the adult worm as a homolactate fermenter, with minimal use of the Krebs cycle and oxidative phosphorylation. Glycogen metabolism was regulated by the balance between external glucose concentration and the level of the endogenous glycogen stores. Studies on paired and unpaired worms also showed that no interaction between male and female was necessary for the synthesis of glycogen by females, confounding the view that the male not only transported the female, but also supplied her with glucose (Cornford and Fitzpatrick, 1985). The idea that glycogen stores in the parenchyma tide over the parasite when external glucose supplies are limiting, may be a basic feature of the trematode lifestyle (Halton, 1967). In a comparative study of 15 species, the principal reserves of glycogen were found in the cells of the parenchyma and, to a lesser extent in association with the musculature. Furthermore, from quantitative estimates, those parasites living under conditions of low oxygen tension contained far more glycogen than those inhabiting the more aerobic habitats.

The consensus from biochemical and cytological studies is that adult worms, the males especially, have large glycogen stores that can be mobilized or augmented according to external circumstances. We would therefore expect the transcripts of genes encoding proteins involved in glycogen synthesis and breakdown to be preferentially found in muscle and parenchymal clusters. The publication of a study comparing the total transcriptome of eight life cycle stages, which can be interrogated via the Schisto.xyz website (https://lifecycle.schisto.xyz) allows the overall expression intensity of the genes involved in glycogen metabolism to be scrutinized (Buddenborg *et al.*, 2023). This approach confirms that transcripts are present for all the requisite enzymes of glycogen metabolism in all samples analysed from the eight life cycle stages but can say nothing about tissue site. Focusing on the muscle and parenchyma clusters identified by the single-cell RNA-Seq of adults (Wendt *et al.*, 2020), the same exercise can be performed producing somewhat surprising results (Table 4.1). Transcripts encoding proteins of the glycogen synthesis pathway are well represented while those involved in glycogen breakdown are not, in spite of the biochemical studies indicating that the two pathways are balanced in the adult worm. One reason for the low level of transcripts for glycogenolysis may be that the enzymes involved have a long half-life ($t_{1/2}$), which would be reflected in a low transcript level. This has been demonstrated for glycogen phosphorylase in mouse skeletal muscle, with a $t_{1/2}$ of 11.9 days (Butler *et al.*, 1985).

Schistosomes clearly need lipids and sterols for the production of membranes (Rumjanek and Simpson, 1980) and potential mediators such as lysophosphatidylcholine and prostaglandin D_2 (Bexkens *et al.*, 2019); they are abundant components of the alimentary tract, gastrodermis and by extension, the parenchyma. The weight of evidence, gathered over decades, was that adult schistosomes were homolactic

Table 4.1. Glycogen metabolism.

Enzyme	Adults									
	M1	M2	M3	M4	M5	M6	M7	M8	P1	P2
Hexokinase	✓	✓	✓	✓		✓	✓	✓	✓	✓
Phosphoglucomutase										✓
UTP-glucose-1-phosphate uridylyltransferase	✓	✓	✓	✓	✓	✓	✓	✓		
1,4-α-glucan branching enzyme					✓				✓	✓
Glycogenin Smp_008490	✓			✓	✓		✓	✓		✓
Glycogenin Smp_197950				✓	✓	✓				
Glycogen synthase	✓	✓	✓	✓	✓	✓	✓	✓		
α1,4-glucan phosphorylase	✓	✓	✓	✓	✓	✓	✓	✓	✓	✓
Glycogen debranching enzyme			✓							
Phosphoglucomutase										✓
Glucose-6-phosphatase								✓		

From Wendt *et al.*, 2020, interrogation of muscle (M) and parenchyma (P) clusters. Table author's own.

fermenters strictly dependent on carbohydrates in their energy metabolism. Whether schistosomes could use the pathway of β-oxidation to metabolize lipids as an energy source was questionable. However, the first version of the *S. mansoni* genome published in 2009 (Berriman *et al.*, 2009) stated that the genes necessary for a complete β-oxidation pathway were present, with a caveat that this usually inactive pathway might operate in reverse to perform syntheses. To address this conundrum, a comprehensive study of the lipid metabolism of *S. mansoni* was performed by incubating adults, eggs and miracidia with ^{14}C-labelled fatty acids (Bexkens *et al.*, 2019). None of these stages oxidized the fatty acids, as no $^{14}CO_2$ production could be detected. The authors therefore re-examined the *S. mansoni* genome annotations using the known genes involved in fatty acid oxidation from six eukaryotic model reference species. They found not just that the presumed *S. mansoni* genes for fatty acid oxidation were incorrectly annotated, but that no genes encoding β-oxidation enzymes were present (Bexkens *et al.*, 2019); the same was true for *Schistosoma japonicum* and all other schistosome species. This conclusively demonstrated that *S. mansoni* cannot use the β-oxidation pathway in any life cycle stage. It also provides a cautionary tale to treat gene annotations with care and check them against multiple sources (WormBase ParaSite; UniProt; NCBInr). Even then, rogue annotations may be encountered, not backed by any functional studies.

The absence of β-oxidation does not imply that schistosomes have no use for host lipids (Bexkens *et al.*, 2019). Adult schistosomes can acquire and modify fatty acids from their host for biosynthetic purposes, incorporating them in phospholipids and neutral lipids. Female worms deposit large amounts of these lipids in the eggs they produce, which explains why interference with the lipid metabolism in females will disturb egg formation (see Chapter 11 on the egg).

4.4 Cellular Adhesion

The evolution of intercellular adhesion was a major feature that permitted the development of the complex cellular structures in primitive animals, which led ultimately to the tissues and organs of higher animals (Wilson, 2012). An overview of cellular adhesion structures in schistosomes was first attempted in 2006 based on transcriptome data and version 4 of the genome assembly before later publication (Wilson, 2012). Many of the suggestions were based on speculative annotations, which subsequent research, an updated version of the genome (Protasio *et al.*, 2012), further sequencing deposited on WormBase ParaSite (currently v10), and chromosome assembly (Buddenborg *et al.*, 2021) means that a reappraisal of cell adhesion is desirable (Fig. 4.11). It can also be linked to the single-cell RNA-Seq atlas of adult worms (Wendt *et al.*, 2020) to establish tissue

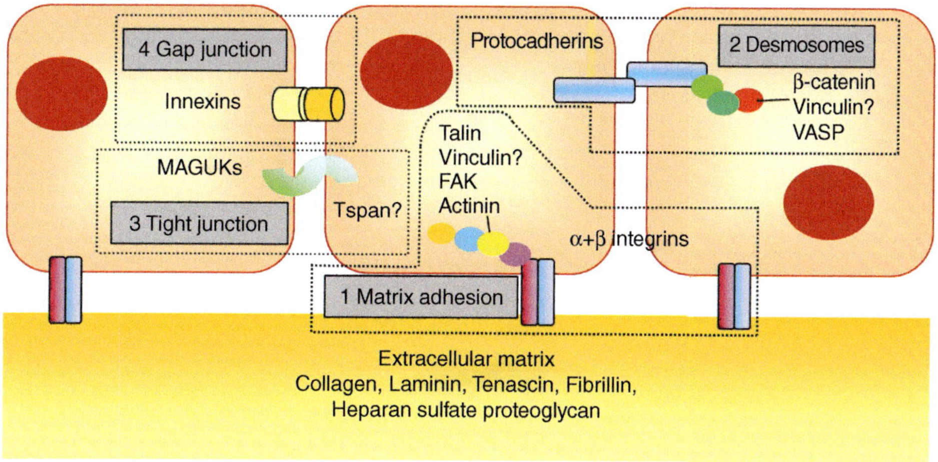

Fig. 4.11. Potential cell adhesion mechanisms. Diagram based on mining of the genome and interrogation of the RNA-Seq single-cell clusters. The four interactions underpinned by adequate transcript expression are: **1**) matrix adhesion by which the cells attach to the extracellular protein matrix; **2**) desmosomes, the most morphologically visible means of cell-to-cell binding; **3**) tight junctions, between closely apposed regions of membrane, which do not reach the complexity of septate junctions; and **4**) gap junctions, important in coordinating activity between cells. MAGUK, membrane-associated guanylate kinases; FAK, focal adhesion kinase; VASP, vasodilator-stimulated phosphoprotein. (From Wilson, 2012, based on original analysis by Dr Gary Dillon.) Figure used with permission from Elsevier.

sites of expression, here confined to the muscles and parenchyma, the subject of Chapter 4.

The components of the schistosome extracellular matrix were covered in Section 4.2.3. Under the heading 'Matrix adhesion' at least four α-integrins and four β-integrins are encoded in the genome, facilitating cell attachment to the matrix as heterodimers (Fig. 4.11.1). Currently, the precise α/β pairings or which matrix components they bind are unknown. Within the cytoplasm, linking the integrins to the cytoskeleton and to signalling pathways, are the proteins actinin, focal adhesion kinase (FAK), vinculin and talin. Interrogation of the adult worm atlas reveals that actinin (Smp_034550) is expressed in all muscle clusters, while FAK (Smp_122680) and talin (Smp_167010 and Smp_343540) transcripts are present in the two parenchyma clusters. (A vinculin transcript is only present in the Mehlis gland.)

Cell-to-cell attachment occurs via desmosomes, morphologically visible in TEM, and involving homodimeric interaction of protocadherins (Fig. 4.11.2). Within the cytoplasm of invertebrate cells these proteins are directly linked to the actin cytoskeleton via β-catenin, vasodilator-stimulated phosphoprotein (VASP) and vinculin; α-catenin binds to β-catenin as part of the interacting chain. In the worm atlas, transcripts for two protocadherins are present (Smp_167470 and Smp_247030), the first in muscle cluster 6 and the second in clusters 2, 3, 4 and 8. Neither α- nor β-catenin transcripts were found in muscle or parenchyma clusters, but less well researched δ-catenin transcripts were present in muscle clusters 2, 4, 5, 6 and 8. Two transcripts for VASP (Smp_039870 and Smp_171040) were both present in parenchyma cluster 1 and the second also in muscle cluster 1. Collectively, while the desmosomal interaction clearly operates between cells, it is not fully represented at transcript level.

Tight junctions are a second form of intercellular adhesion, frequently associated with epithelia, which are not common in the adult worm body (Fig. 4.11.3). They are characterized by membrane-associated guanylate kinases (MAGUKs), of which there are at least five encoded in the genome. However, only one MAGUK (Smp_309590) is expressed in the two parenchyma clusters. Unfortunately, there appear to be no zona occludens proteins encoded in the genome. In other invertebrates the MAGUKs interact with TSPAN-3, a membrane tetraspanin. There are at least 10 tetraspanins encoded in the genome, but in the absence of experimental evidence it is unclear whether any of them take on the role of TSPAN-3 in schistosomes. The tentative conclusion must be that tight junctions are not important in schistosome muscle or parenchyma.

Of greater interest is the projected occurrence of gap junctions between schistosome cells (Fig. 4.11.4). The differentiation and specialization of cells to form tissues requires instant coordination across large numbers of cells to be effective and gap junctions can serve this role. The key players are a group of proteins called innexins. They have no homology to the connexins of vertebrates but perform the same function in invertebrates, hence innexins. They have four transmembrane segments which form a channel, and two channels lined up in apposing plasma membranes represent a gap junction. Their function is the rapid transport of small molecules (e.g. Ca^{2+}, ATP, inositol triphosphate) between the cytosols of interacting cells. There are 15 innexins encoded in the *S. mansoni* genome and their transcripts are well represented in the worm atlas. However, each gene has a restricted pattern, with Smp_141290 expression confined to parenchyma clusters 1 and 2, while Smp_140860 is present in all eight muscle clusters. Smp_129020 is expressed only in muscle clusters 6, 7 and 8 while Smp_245990 is expressed in muscle clusters 1, 7 and three neuron clusters. It remains to be determined whether the various isoforms allow passage of different solutes but their presence in the muscle sarcolemma provides an explanation for why adjacent myocytes can act together in the generation of peristaltic waves.

There remains only the possibility that schistosomes possess septate desmosomes as a means of firmly anchoring cells. The main feature of septate junctions is that cross-bridges or septa of ladder-like appearance cover the 15–20 nm intermembrane space of cell–cell contact. Certainly, closely apposed membranes can be found in TEMs and one potential function appears to be anchoring sensory nerve bulbs into the cercarial tegument (see Chapter 2 on the cercaria, Section 2.2.4 and Fig. 2.9). Some of the components found in vertebrates are present in the *S. mansoni* genome (e.g. lachesin, neurexin), others are not (e.g. gliotactin, coracle). Lachesin (Smp_300580) is expressed only in muscle clusters 5 and 7. There are three isoforms of the putative neurexin, with N1 (Smp_301990) expressed in muscle clusters 1 and 2, N2 (Smp_123840) in parenchyma cluster 2 and muscle clusters 1, 3, 7 and 8, and N4 (Smp_159570) in parenchyma cluster 1. In vertebrates neurexins act predominantly at the presynaptic terminal in neurons and play essential roles in neurotransmission and differentiation of synapses. The current annotations appear to be based on low homology to *Caenorhabditis elegans* proteins of that name. Quite what role such proteins have at the surface of muscle fibres must for the moment remain a mystery. There is clearly scope for further work on cell adhesion, particularly localization of proteins to specific structures.

4.5 Summary

- Muscle and parenchyma present problems for characterization because of their ubiquitous distribution and the difficulty of isolating individual cells for analysis.
- Morphologically schistosome muscles are of the smooth type. (The pseudo-striated fibres of the cercarial tail are the unique exception.) The individual myocytes have an elongate spindle shape and contract only slowly. Innervations from the nervous system control the waves of peristalsis that pass along the composite muscles. The identification of multiple innexins in the *S. mansoni* genome and their expression in some muscle clusters raises the possibility that myocytes can act together as a single unit without neurogenic input.
- The muscle systems of an adult worm comprise the circular and longitudinal muscles of the body wall, plus the dorsoventral fibres that maintain the flat shape of the male. Distinct muscle systems envelop the oesophagus and gastrodermis. There are muscles associated with male and female reproductive systems, but their layout is poorly understood relative to function. The oral and ventral suckers represent partially autonomous structures, separately innervated to control passage along blood vessels.

- Single-cell sequencing has provided a tantalizing glimpse of the molecular biology underpinning the morphological diversity. Apparently, muscle cell nuclei can be detached sufficiently intact to permit recovery of mRNA transcripts for processing. How this is achieved with the highly branched parenchyma cells is unclear. Eight muscle clusters were identified, three of which were largely restricted to females, one of them surrounding the ovary. Two parenchymal clusters were also identified with widespread body expression of their unique markers. It is an important task to relate these specific gene expression patterns to cell structures.
- The isolation of individual myocytes by tissue digestion for shotgun proteomic analysis, which would inform protein composition, has not so far been deployed. Microdissection has been used to isolate the male oral sucker and might be feasible with the ventral sucker. However, detached cercarial tails can be highly enriched by density gradient centrifugation, and they would make an ideal preparation for proteomic analysis of the 'striated' tail fibres.
- The way that the nervous system interacts with the several muscle systems of adult schistosomes to coordinate the complex processes of locomotion, feeding and reproduction is clearly highly complex. Deciphering the mechanisms involved presents one of the biggest challenges for schistosome cell biology, given the lack of suitable tools for experimentation.

References

Berriman, M., Haas, B.J., LoVerde, P.T., Wilson, R.A., Dillon, G.P. *et al.* (2009) The genome of the blood fluke *Schistosoma mansoni*. *Nature* 460(7253), 352–358. DOI: 10.1038/nature08160

Bexkens, M.L., Mebius, M.M., Houweling, M., Brouwers, J.F., Tielens, A.G.M. *et al.* (2019) *Schistosoma mansoni* does not and cannot oxidise fatty acids, but these are used for biosynthetic purposes instead. *International Journal for Parasitology* 49(8), 647–656. DOI: 10.1016/j.ijpara.2019.03.005

Blair, K.L., Day, T.A., Lewis, M.C., Bennett, J.L. and Pax, R.A. (1991) Studies on muscle cells isolated from *Schistosoma mansoni*: a Ca^{2+}-dependent K^{+} channel. *Parasitology* 102(2), 251–258. DOI: 10.1017/s0031182000062569

Buddenborg, S.K., Tracey, A., Berger, D.J., Lu, Z., Doyle, S.R. *et al.* (2021) Assembled chromosomes of the blood fluke *Schistosoma mansoni* provide insight into the evolution of its ZW sex-determination system. *bioRxiv* 2021.08.13.456314. DOI: 10.1101/2021.08.13.456314

Buddenborg, S.K., Lu, Z., Sankaranarayan, G., Doyle, S.R. and Berriman, M. (2023) The stage- and sex-specific transcriptome of the human parasite *Schistosoma mansoni*. *Scientific Data* 10(1), 775. DOI: 10.1038/s41597-023-02674-2

Bueding, E. and Koletsky, S. (1950) Content and distribution of glycogen in *Schistosoma mansoni*. *Proceedings of the Society for Experimental Biology and Medicine* 73(4), 594–596. DOI: 10.3181/00379727-73-17755

Butler, P.E., Cookson, E.J. and Beynon, R.J. (1985) The turnover of skeletal muscle glycogen phosphorylase studied using the cofactor, pyridoxal phosphate, as a specific label. *Biochimica et Biophysica Acta* 847(3), 316–323. DOI: 10.1016/0167-4889(85)90037-0

Cornford, E.M. and Fitzpatrick, A.M. (1985) The mechanism and rate of glucose transfer from male to female schistosomes. *Molecular and Biochemical Parasitology* 17(2), 131–141. DOI: 10.1016/0166-6851(85)90012-x

Cote, L.E., Simental, E. and Reddien, P.W. (2019) Muscle functions as a connective tissue and source of extracellular matrix in planarians. *Nature Communications* 10(1), 1592. DOI: 10.1038/s41467-019-09539-6

Craig, R. and Woodhead, J.L. (2006) Structure and function of myosin filaments. *Current Opinion in Structural Biology* 16(2), 204–212. DOI: 10.1016/j.sbi.2006.03.006

Day, T.A., Orr, N., Bennett, J.L. and Pax, R.A. (1993) Voltage-gated currents in muscle cells of *Schistosoma mansoni*. *Parasitology* 106(5), 471–477. DOI: 10.1017/s0031182000076769

Day, T.A., Bennett, J.L. and Pax, R.A. (1994) Serotonin and its requirement for maintenance of contractility in muscle fibres isolated from *Schistosoma mansoni*. *Parasitology* 108(4), 425–432. DOI: 10.1017/s0031182000075983

Gobert, G.N., Stenzel, D.J., Jones, M.K., Allen, D.E. and McManus, D.P. (1997) *Schistosoma japonicum*: immunolocalization of paramyosin during development. *Parasitology* 114(1), 45–52. DOI: 10.1017/s0031182096008001

Hahnel, S., Lu, Z., Wilson, R.A., Grevelding, C.G. and Quack, T. (2013) Whole-organ isolation approach as a basis for tissue-specific analyses in *Schistosoma mansoni*. *PLoS Neglected Tropical Diseases* 7(7), e2336. DOI: 10.1371/journal.pntd.0002336

Halton, D.W. (1967) Studies on glycogen deposition in trematoda. *Comparative Biochemistry and Physiology* 23(1), 113–120. DOI: 10.1016/0010-406x(67)90478-1

Holy, J.M., O'Leary, K.A., Oaks, J.A. and Tracy, J.W. (1989) Immunocytochemical localization of the major glutathione S-transferases in adult *Schistosoma mansoni*. *The Journal of Parasitology* 75(2), 181–190.

Kasschau, M.R. and Mansour, T.E. (1982) Serotonin-activated adenylate cyclase during early development of *Schistosoma mansoni*. *Nature* 296(5852), 66–68. DOI: 10.1038/296066a0

Kim, E., Day, T.A., Bennett, J.L. and Pax, R.A. (1995) Cloning and functional expression of a shaker-related voltage-gated potassium channel gene from *Schistosoma mansoni* (Trematoda: Digenea). *Parasitology* 110(2), 171–180. DOI: 10.1017/s0031182000063939

Li, X.-H., Xu, Y.-X., Vance, G., Wang, Y., Lv, L.-B. *et al.* (2015) Evidence that rhesus macaques self-cure from a *Schistosoma japonicum* infection by disrupting worm esophageal function: a new route to an effective vaccine? *PLoS Neglected Tropical Diseases* 9(7), e0003925. DOI: 10.1371/journal.pntd.0003925

MacDonald, K., Buxton, S., Kimber, M.J., Day, T.A., Robertson, A.P. *et al.* (2014) Functional characterization of a novel family of acetylcholine-gated chloride channels in *Schistosoma mansoni*. *PLoS Pathogens* 10(6), e1004181. DOI: 10.1371/journal.ppat.1004181

Mair, G.R., Maule, A.G., Day, T.A. and Halton, D.W. (2000) A confocal microscopical study of the musculature of adult *Schistosoma mansoni*. *Parasitology* 121(2), 163–170. DOI: 10.1017/s0031182099006174

Matsumoto, Y., Perry, G., Levine, R.J., Blanton, R., Mahmoud, A.A. *et al.* (1988) Paramyosin and actin in schistosomal teguments. *Nature* 333(6168), 76–78. DOI: 10.1038/333076a0

Novozhilova, E., Kimber, M.J., Qian, H., McVeigh, P., Robertson, A.P. *et al.* (2010) FMRFamide-like peptides (FLPs) enhance voltage-gated calcium currents to elicit muscle contraction in the human parasite *Schistosoma mansoni*. *PLoS Neglected Tropical Diseases* 4(8), e790. DOI: 10.1371/journal.pntd.0000790

Nuttman, C.J. (1975) The structure and behaviour of the cercaria of *Schistosoma mansoni*. PhD thesis, University of York, York, UK. Available at: https://etheses.whiterose.ac.uk/id/eprint/14197

Parker-Manuel, S.J. and Wilson, R.A. (2022) An atlas of the germ ball–cercaria–schistosomulum transition in *Schistosoma mansoni*, using confocal microscopy and *in situ* hybridisation. *Current Research in Parasitology & Vector-Borne Diseases* 2, 100087. DOI: 10.1016/j.crpvbd.2022.100087

Patocka, N., Sharma, N., Rashid, M. and Ribeiro, P. (2014) Serotonin signaling in *Schistosoma mansoni*: a serotonin-activated G protein-coupled receptor controls parasite movement. *PLoS Pathogens* 10(1), e1003878. DOI: 10.1371/journal.ppat.1003878

Pax, R.A. and Bennett, J.L. (1991) Neurobiology of parasitic platyhelminths: possible solutions to the problems of correlating structure with function. *Parasitology* 102(Suppl.), S31–S39. DOI: 10.1017/s0031182000073273

Pax, R.A., Siefker, C. and Bennett, J.L. (1984) *Schistosoma mansoni*: differences in acetylcholine, dopamine, and serotonin control of circular and longitudinal parasite muscles. *Experimental Parasitology* 58(3), 314–324. DOI: 10.1016/0014-4894(84)90048-1

Porchet, E., McNair, A., Caron, A., Kusnierz, J.P., Zemzoumi, K. *et al.* (1994) Tissue expression of the *Schistosoma mansoni* 28 kDa glutathione *S*-transferase. *Parasitology* 109(5), 565–572. DOI: 10.1017/s0031182000076447

Protasio, A.V., Tsai, I.J., Babbage, A., Nichol, S., Hunt, M. *et al.* (2012) A systematically improved high quality genome and transcriptome of the human blood fluke *Schistosoma mansoni*. *PLoS Neglected Tropical Diseases* 6(1), e1455. DOI: 10.1371/journal.pntd.0001455

Reger, J.F. (1976) Studies on the fine structure of cercarial tail muscle of *Schistosoma* sp. (Trematoda). *Journal of Ultrastructure Research* 57(1), 77–86. DOI: 10.1016/s0022-5320(76)80057-3

Reissig, M. (1970) Characterization of cell types in the parenchyma of *Schistosoma mansoni*. *Parasitology* 60(2), 273–279. DOI: 10.1017/s0031182000078100

Riengrojpitak, S. (1987) *Schistosoma mansoni*: localisation of schistosome antigens using antibodies raised against adult worm tegument membranes. PhD thesis, University of York, York, UK. Available at: https://etheses.whiterose.ac.uk/id/eprint/10942

Rumjanek, F.D. and Simpson, A.J. (1980) The incorporation and utilization of radiolabelled lipids by adult *Schistosoma mansoni in vitro*. *Molecular and Biochemical Parasitology* 1(1), 31–44. DOI: 10.1016/0166-6851(80)90039-0

Schmidt, J., Bodor, O., Gohr, L. and Kunz, W. (1996) Paramyosin isoforms of *Schistosoma mansoni* are phosphorylated and localized in a large variety of muscle types. *Parasitology* 112(5), 459–467. DOI: 10.1017/s0031182000076927

Silk, M.H. and Spence, I.M. (1969) Ultrastructural studies of the blood fluke – *Schistosoma mansoni*. II. The musculature. *The South African Journal of Medical Sciences* 34(1), 11–20.

Skelly, P.J., Da'dara, A.A., Li, X.H., Castro-Borges, W. and Wilson, R.A. (2014) Schistosome feeding and regurgitation. *PLoS Pathogens* 10(8), e1004246. DOI: 10.1371/journal.ppat.1004246

Smith, J.H., Reynolds, E.S. and Von Lichtenberg, F. (1969) The integument of *Schistosoma mansoni*. *The American Journal of Tropical Medicine and Hygiene* 18(1), 28–49.

Sweeney, H.L. and Hammers, D.W. (2018) Muscle contraction. *Cold Spring Harbor Perspectives in Biology* 10(2), a023200. DOI: 10.1101/cshperspect.a023200

Threadgold, L.T. and Gallagher, S.S. (1966) Electron microscope studies of *Fasciola hepatica*: I. The ultrastructure and interrelationship of the parenchymal cells. *Parasitology* 56(2), 299–304. DOI: 10.1017/s0031182000070888

Tielens, A.G. and Van den Bergh, S.G. (1987) Glycogen metabolism in *Schistosoma mansoni* worms after their isolation from the host. *Molecular and Biochemical Parasitology* 24(3), 247–254. DOI: 10.1016/0166-6851(87)90156-3

Tielens, A.G., Celik, C., Van den Heuvel, J.M., Elfring, R.H. and Van den Bergh, S.G. (1989) Synthesis and degradation of glycogen by *Schistosoma mansoni* worms *in vitro*. *Parasitology* 98(1), 67–73. DOI: 10.1017/s0031182000059692

Verjovski-Almeida, S., DeMarco, R., Martins, E.A.L., Guimarães, P.E.M., Ojopi, E.P.B. *et al.* (2003) Transcriptome analysis of the acoelomate human parasite *Schistosoma mansoni*. *Nature Genetics* 35(2), 148–157. DOI: 10.1038/ng1237

Wendt, G., Zhao, L., Chen, R., Liu, C., O'Donoghue, A.J. *et al.* (2020) A single-cell RNA-seq atlas of *Schistosoma mansoni* identifies a key regulator of blood feeding. *Science* 369(6511), 1644–1649. DOI: 10.1126/science.abb7709

Wilson, R.A. (2012) The cell biology of schistosomes: a window on the evolution of the early metazoa. *Protoplasma* 249(3), 503–518. DOI: 10.1007/s00709-011-0326-x

Wilson, R.A. and Barnes, P.E. (1979) Synthesis of macromolecules by the epithelial surfaces of *Schistosoma mansoni*: an autoradiographic study. *Parasitology* 78(3), 295–310. DOI: 10.1017/s0031182000051167

Wilson, R.A., Langermans, J.A.M., van Dam, G.J., Vervenne, R.A., Hall, S.L. *et al.* (2008) Elimination of *Schistosoma mansoni* adult worms by rhesus macaques: basis for a therapeutic vaccine? *PLoS Neglected Tropical Diseases* 2(9), e290. DOI: 10.1371/journal.pntd.0000290

Yeh, Y.-T., Del Álamo, J.C. and Caffrey, C.R. (2024) Biomechanics of parasite migration within hosts. *Trends in Parasitology* 40(2), 164–175. DOI: 10.1016/j.pt.2023.12.001

Zhang, S., Skinner, D., Joshi, P., Criado-Hidalgo, E., Yeh, Y.-T. *et al.* (2019) Quantifying the mechanics of locomotion of the schistosome pathogen with respect to changes in its physical environment. *Journal of the Royal Society, Interface* 16(150), 20180675. DOI: 10.1098/rsif.2018.0675

5

The Nervous System

5.1 Overview

The layout of the nervous system and remarkable diversity of associated sensory endings in the infective miracidium and cercaria was covered in the Chapters 1 and 2, respectively. Chapter 5 focuses primarily on the nervous system in the adult worms, resident in the bloodstream, seeking generalities around structure and function. The layout of central ganglia and extensive peripheral nervous network contrast with the limited diversity of adult sensory endings. The information comes initially from early ultrastructural studies, followed by experimentation on the very mobile and rather intractable solid body of adult worms. Most recently, the emphasis has moved to disaggregation of tissues and single-cell sequencing, associated with *in situ* hybridization and immunocytochemical observations to characterize expression patterns of genes and proteins associated with the nervous system.

5.2 Layout of the Nervous System

Schistosomes, as members of the Platyhelminthes, have a solid acoelomate body plan. Where to place them in the evolutionary tree of animals is by no means clear (Telford *et al.*, 2015) although it is accepted that they are members of the Lophotrochozoa. The more primitive, radially symmetrical members of the phylum Cnidaria possess a well-developed nervous system and it is worth putting the schistosomes into the cnidarian context. Cnidarians such as *Hydra* have a simple tissue organization comprising only ectoderm and endoderm. *Hydra* attaches to the substratum via a holdfast and possesses tentacles for catching planktonic prey around a mouth that leads to a central gastric cavity. Its nervous system comprises a meshwork, or net, of nerve cells running through the body wall, more concentrated in the oral and holdfast regions than elsewhere, but with no central organizing structures like ganglia. Recently, the complexities have been revealed by confocal and electron microscopy as two unconnected distinct nets in the ectoderm and endoderm (Keramidioti *et al.*, 2024). Sensory neurons are numerous running to the gastric cavity from the endodermal net and to the body surface in the mouth and tentacular regions from the ectodermal net, extending a ciliary projection to the surface to detect its immediate environment. The ectodermal nerve net is more directly associated with muscle processes and is more highly connected than the endodermal net. A salient feature of cnidarian genomes is the extensive use of neuropeptides as transmitters, capable of both excitation and inhibition (Grimmelikhuijzen and Westfall, 1995). They are derived from large precursor proteins and present in dense-cored vesicles associated with both synaptic and non-synaptic release

DOI: 10.1079/9781800625167.0005

sites. The extent to which conventional neurotransmitters are active in the cnidarian nervous system remains uncertain (Sprecher, 2022).

A brief comparison of the nervous system of the other major group of helminth parasites, the Nematoda, members of the Ecdysozoa, highlights our limited knowledge of the schistosome nervous system (Fig. 5.1) (Schafer, 2016). Nematodes are part of a small outlier group that have a circum-pharyngeal nerve ring composed of axonal and dendritic processes, whose cell bodies lie in clusters elsewhere, rather than in cephalic ganglia. A single major nerve cord runs from head to tail, along with other minor cords and transverse commissures. Numerous sensory receptors surround the mouth, with cell bodies anterior to the nerve ring sending a dendrite to the sensory ending and an axon to the nerve ring. There are four multimodal amphids close to the mouth containing chemosensors, touch, osmotic pressure and heat receptors. These have the same arrangement of cell bodies in a ganglion cluster sending dendrites to the sensory endings and an axon to the nerve ring. Perhaps most striking, the hermaphroditic model nematode *Caenorhabditis elegans* has a nervous system of remarkable anatomical simplicity comprising just 302 neurons, while the female of the parasitic *Ascaris lumbricoides* has only 298 neurons in a 30 cm long body. There is an enormous degree of structural and functional conservation between *C. elegans* and *A. lumbricoides*, in spite of an evolutionary distance of several hundred million years. Neuropeptide transmission is extremely well developed with around 250 distinct neuropeptides, 150 peptide receptors and 27 nephrilysin proteases for peptide breakdown in *C. elegans*. The connectome has been mapped at the level of individual neurons and synapses – the only animal so far. For example, its ventral nerve cord contains 57 motor neurons (versus 55 in *Ascaris*), which individually fall into seven subtypes with matching morphology, connectivity and neurotransmitter usage. *C. elegans* can detect a wide range of odorant molecules using only four pairs of amphid sensors, each of which is polymodal, expressing many distinct odorant receptors.

The platyhelminth nervous system is certainly more developed than a simple nerve net or plexus. The layout comprises a central nervous system of paired ganglia connected by a commissure astride the oesophagus, out of which two main nerve cords extend towards anterior and posterior (Fig. 5.2.1) (Halton and Gustafsson, 1996). This arrangement is very much in line with the visualization of the schistosome nervous system using cholinergic staining of whole worms (Fig. 5.2.2) (Fripp, 1967). The main nerves are augmented by minor cords and transverse commissures at intervals down the body. The ventral sucker receives its innervation from the main cords on each side running to its rim (Fig. 5.2.3). In the cercaria (Chapter 2) a bilobed central ganglion occupied all the interior beneath the body wall. Five weeks later in the adult,

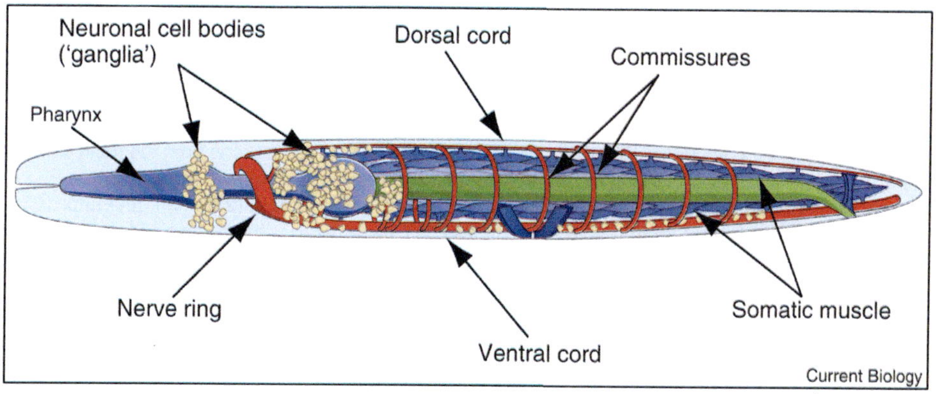

Fig. 5.1. Overview of the nematode nervous system to emphasize the marked differences from the schistosome system. The nerve cell bodies (beige) are separated from the neuropile and nerve cords (red). Muscles are blue and gut is green. (From Schafer, 2016.) Figure used with permission from Elsevier.

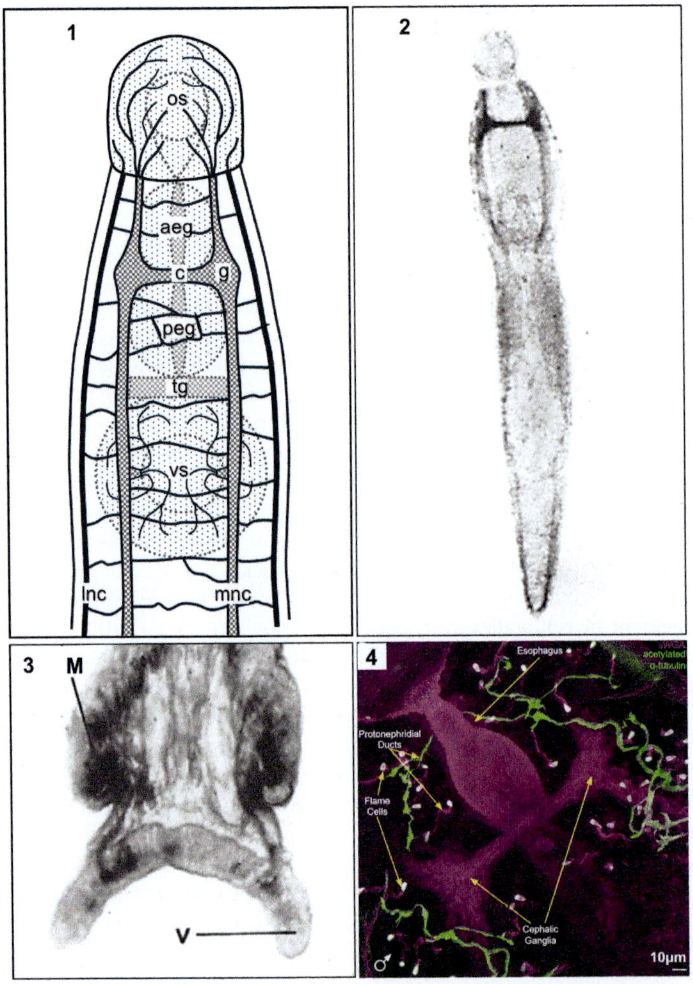

Fig. 5.2. Layout of the adult schistosome nervous system. **1**) Generalized diagram of anterior, dorsal view, with ganglia (g) connected by a commissure (c) located above the junction between anterior and posterior oesophageal glands (aeg, peg). The caecae after the transverse gut (tg) are omitted for clarity. The main and lateral nerve cords (mnc, lnc) and their connections are indicated, plus innervation of the oral and ventral suckers (os, vs). **2**) Pre-adult male ventral view stained for acetylcholinesterase. The paired central ganglia are prominent and main nerve cords run through the parenchyma. **3**) Transverse section at the level of the ventral sucker (V), stained for esterase to reveal neurons from the main cords (M) innervating the muscles. **4**) The paired ganglia connected by a dorsal commissure astride the oesophagus, visualized by lectin staining with wheat germ agglutinin (purple) (**2** and **3** from Fripp, 1967; **4** from Collins *et al.*, 2011.) **1**) Figure author's own. **2** and **3**) Figures used with permission from Elsevier. **4**) Figure used under licence CC-BY-4.0.

the two lobes have become discrete ganglia connected by a wide isthmus of axons astride the oesophagus (Fig. 5.2.4) (Collins *et al.*, 2011).

In the single-cell sequencing study, 31 nerve clusters were identified, all but one expressing a general neural marker, neuroendocrine protein 7b2 (Smp_073270) (Wendt *et al.*, 2020) (see Chapter 4, Fig. 4.6). In addition, the existence of a peripheral nerve net or plexus has recently become apparent (Fig. 5.3.1). It lies beneath the body wall muscles and was identified by confocal imaging of nerve marker SmKK7 (Parker-Manuel

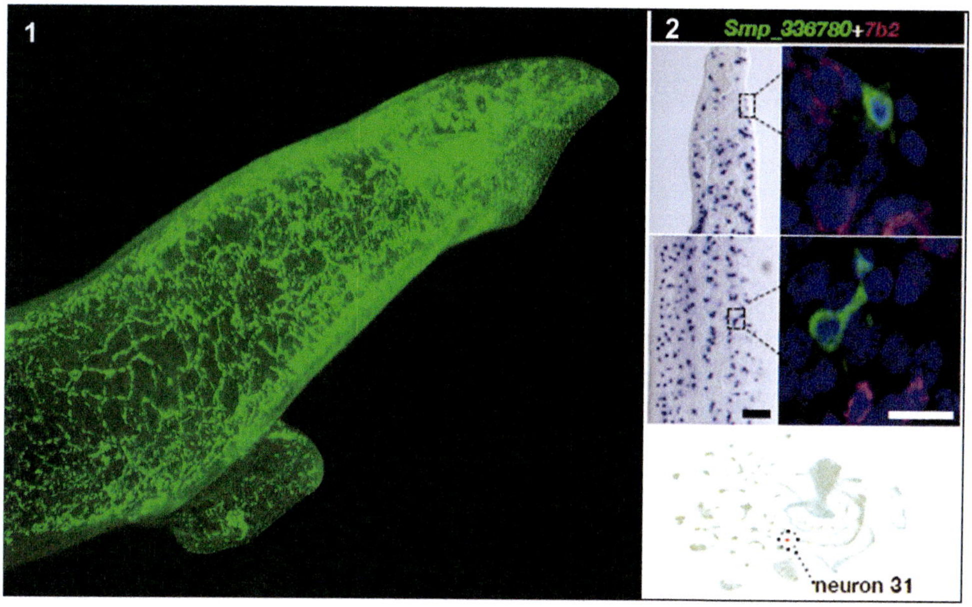

Fig. 5.3. The existence of a peripheral nerve net. **1**) Peripheral nerve net visualized by staining with antibody for SmKK7. The gene is expressed only in neuron cluster 31. **2**) Expression of cluster 31 marker Smp_336780 (green) compared with that of general neural marker 7b2 in head and mid-body. The left panels are whole-mount *in situ* hybridization (WISH) showing numerous 7b2 positive neurons in blue. Scale bar: 100 μm. The right panels show all nuclei visualized with DAPI (blue) and dual fluorescence *in situ* hybridization (FISH) that reveals 7b2 expression (magenta) and Smp_336780 expression (green). Scale bar: 10 μm. There is no apparent overlap in fluorescence suggesting that neuron 31 cluster (bottom panel) has unusual properties. (**1** from Parker-Manuel and Wilson, 2021; **2** is an original image kindly provided by Professor J.J. Collins, UTSouthwestern Medical Center, Dallas, TX, USA, published by Wendt *et al.*, 2020.) Figure used under licence CC-BY-4.0.

and Wilson, 2022). The single-cell sequencing study showed co-expression of SmKK7 only with a hypothetical protein Smp_336780, the marker for neuron cluster 31 (Fig. 5.3.2) (Wendt *et al.*, 2020). The lack of 7b2 expression may indicate that the peripheral plexus has some unique perhaps ancestral properties, setting it apart from the rest of the nervous system. A major task confronting researchers is to relate the diverse neuron clusters identified by single-cell sequencing to specific morphological features within the adult worm body.

In Chapter 1, it was reported that the number of nerve cell bodies in the schistosome miracidium numbered 209, comprising a staggering 57% of the total cell complement (Attenborough *et al.*, 2024). In adult worms by comparison, judging from the results of single-cell sequencing combined with localization of gene expression, there are many hundreds and quite possibly thousands of nerve cells. Figure 5.3.2 provides a glimpse of the distribution of peripheral nerve cells in cluster 31. This alone is far greater than the 298 cells of the entire *Ascaris* nervous system and argues for a great diversity in the neuromuscular coordination needed for locomotion, feeding and reproduction. How is this achieved?

5.3 The Basic Structure of Neurons

The ultrastructure of the paired ganglia and their connecting commissure astride the oesophagus of the adult worm is not well characterized (Silk and Spence, 1969). The ganglia occupy much less volume than in the cercarial stage (see Chapter 2) but the organization is similar. A rind of perikarya surround the ganglia, sending axons and dendrites inwards to form the neuropile. Connections from sensory structures feed into the neuropile and motor nerves exit to the nerve cords, but our knowledge of function is severely limited. The individual neuron cell bodies that surround the neuropile and lie scattered elsewhere along the nerve cords are ovoid in shape (~6 μm × 4 μm), with a prominent nucleus and nucleolus (Silk and Spence, 1969). They may be unipolar or bipolar, i.e. one or two axons may emerge from the cell body. It is important to grasp for what follows about nerve cell types and functions that these cell bodies are the biosynthetic centres where neurotransmitters and the vesicles that contain them are generated. Moreover, the axons (which can be millimetres long in adults) are the conduits along which the vesicles pass to the synapses or sensory endings. The granular cytoplasm of the cell body contains Golgi apparatus, small amounts of endoplasmic reticulum and free ribosomes, plus different types of vesicles which vary with the cell. There are also small mitochondria and glycogen granules as an energy store (Fig. 5.4). There are repercussions for experimental interventions including cell body isolation for single-cell sequencing and gene knock-down by RNA interference (RNAi). It is remarkable that nerve cell bodies can be isolated sufficiently intact by tissue digestion for single-cell sequencing, after they have been detached from their axons. In the intact parasite it is possible to achieve considerable knock-down of gene expression without obtaining an altered phenotype. The gene encoding SmKK7 is a case in point where the abundance of protein detected in the neurons and sensory endings after knock-down is not depleted and no altered phenotype observed.

It is hard to give a sense of the structure of the neuropile and nerve cords, except to say that they appear as a chaotic tangled mass of axons and dendrites (Fig. 5.4) (Dorsey *et al.*, 2002). The axons may only be 0.5 μm in diameter, but depending on the plane of section can run for up to 10 μm, with sparse contents. The scarce mitochondria are only 0.3 μm in diameter and there are occasional aggregates of glycogen or different types of vesicles in transit. Microtubules have been reported, presumably involved in trafficking of vesicles along axons as in higher animals, but they are not numerous. What is apparent in electron micrographs is the tight binding of the axons and processes to each other in the neuropile and nerve cords by what is referred to as a 'cement layer', 12.5 nm thick (Silk and Spence, 1969). This may comprise cadherins or integrins (Fig. 4.12).

There have been attempts to classify the vesicles, by their morphology in transmission electron microscopy (TEM) (Silk and Spence, 1969; Dorsey *et al.*, 2002), but to an extent the descriptions are dependent on fixation and staining techniques. Based on appearance and size there are at least three, possibly four types of vesicle. The smallest and most frequent, with clear contents, are ~20–50 nm in diameter and often

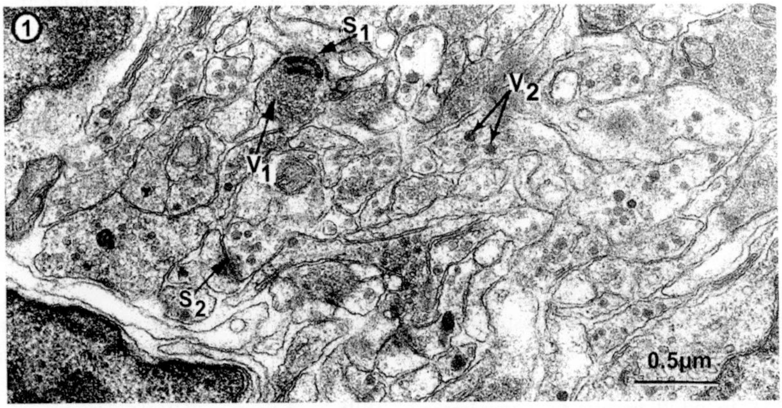

Fig. 5.4. Structure of the ganglia. **1**) A high magnification TEM of the neuropile to show neurons, axons and cytoplasmic inclusions (V1, V2). Two synapses (S) are arrowed. (From Dorsey *et al.*, 2002.) Figure used with permission from Elsevier.

found close to synapses. Slightly larger at 30–90 nm diameter are vesicles with an electron-dense core. The largest, and least frequent, are the vesicles of 100–160 nm diameter, also with a dense core. The fourth type are the clear vesicles 90–110 nm, most apparent in the terminal ciliated bulbs of sensory structures. Potentially, these clear vesicles originate not in the neuropile but in the nerve cell bodies that give rise to the sensory endings. A speculative guess about vesicle contents is that the small vesicles contain acetylcholine, the medium sized ones catecholamines and the large ones neuropeptides. Considering that SmKK7 protein was initially identified as a cercarial 'secretion', released by disruption of sensory endings on the cercarial apical papilla, it is likely to be present in the clear vesicles.

There is relatively little information about schistosome synapses and neuromuscular junctions. Morphologically they appear quite insubstantial, with an accumulation of vesicles in the presynaptic space, adjacent to a 9–17 nm synaptic cleft (Silk and Spence, 1969). One notable feature is the occurrence of '*en passant*' synapses where two neurons form a side-to-side connection (see below) often associated with a physical bulge, termed a varicosity. Within the neurons, the small clear vesicles are usually present, sometimes accompanied by the 30–90 nm vesicles with a dense core, or the larger ~100 nm dense vesicles. Nerve–muscle junctions are essentially similar and there is one report demonstrating apparent colocalization of neuropeptide F and an FMRFamide-related peptide (see below) in the large vesicles, implying their direct role in the modulation of muscle function (Marks *et al.*, 1995). It is also possible that neurosecretory vesicles may be exocytosed from the neuronal membrane directly on to an abutting nerve fibre, fulfilling a neuromodulatory role rather than acting as a direct synaptic transmitter (McVeigh and Maule, 2017).

5.4 Classical Transmitters and Neuropeptides

We saw in Chapter 4, from experiments first on muscle preparations (Pax *et al.*, 1984) and later on isolated muscle cells (Pax and Bennett, 1991), that schistosome motility was inhibited by acetylcholine and stimulated by serotonin. The catecholamine, dopamine, also had a differential effect on longitudinal versus circular muscle fibres (Pax *et al.*, 1984). The other major discovery coming from these studies on muscle preparations was the demonstration that short FMRFamide-like peptides could act via membrane receptors to cause muscle excitation (Day *et al.*, 1994). The conclusion must be that these, and potentially other transmitters, are the products of the nerve cell bodies, delivered via the axons to either the neuromuscular synapses, or to nerve–nerve synapses.

5.4.1 Acetylcholine

Acetylcholine is a major neurotransmitter in both invertebrates and vertebrates and can have both excitatory and inhibitory properties. In *Schistosoma mansoni* it is synthesized by the enzyme choline acetyltransferase (Smp_146910) from metabolic precursors and sequestered in presynaptic vesicles. Its transmitter action in the synaptic cleft is terminated by the enzyme acetylcholinesterase (Smp_125350); this enzyme is distinct from a second acetylcholinesterase recently described at the tegument surface (Skelly and Da'dara, 2023). Acetylcholine signalling is detected by two types of receptor, termed nicotinic and muscarinic (Fig. 5.5). The nicotinic receptor is a homo- or hetero-pentamer in a barrel shape round a central ion-selective pore. Invertebrates have both cation (K^+, Na^+, Ca^{2+}) and anion (Cl^-) selective responses, mediating excitation and inhibition, respectively (MacDonald *et al.*, 2014). Two subunits (out of a possible five to seven Cl^--gated channels in v10 of the *S. mansoni* genome on WormBase) termed ACC-1 (Smp_176310) and ACC-2 (now Smp_306340) have been characterized. Judicious use of nicotinic receptor agonists on 6-day-old schistosomula caused almost complete paralysis, whereas receptor antagonists or the use of RNAi to depress gene expression resulted in parasite hyperactivity.

Immunolocalization revealed the presence of ACC-1 in nerves associated with the muscles of the adult body wall (Fig. 5.6.1) and of ACC-2 in nerve fibres of the day 6 schistosomulum. When the *acc1* gene was expressed in mammalian cells it reconstituted a homomeric channel,

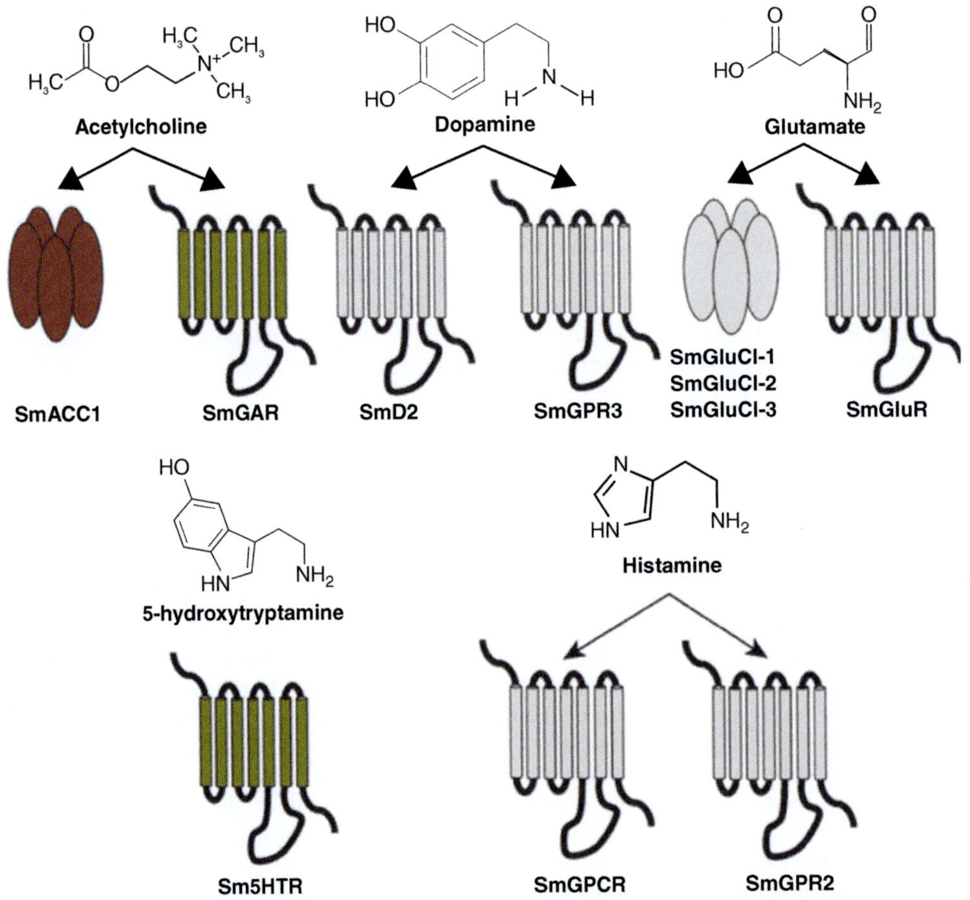

Fig. 5.5. Neuroreceptor signalling. A summary of the ligand-gated (Cl^-) channels and seven-transmembrane GPCR-type receptors for which there is experimental evidence of function, often obtained by expression of the receptor in a heterologous cell system. (Modified from McVeigh and Maule, 2017.) Figure used with permission from Oxford Publishing Ltd.

specific for anions but not Ca^{2+}, which was stimulated by exposure to nicotine. The authors concluded that SmACC-1 and SmACC-2 were present in minor nerve fibres of the submuscular nerve net that innervates the somatic muscles, not the muscles themselves. However, interrogation of the eight muscle clusters identified by single-cell sequencing (Wendt *et al.*, 2020) reveals that while the uncharacterized Smp_142700 and Smp_139330 are expressed in all eight clusters, ACC-1 is expressed in muscle 7 only and ACC-2 is expressed only in neurons. Thus, it seems likely that the flaccid paralysis demonstrated in muscles experimentally is mediated by as yet uncharacterized post-synaptic nicotinic receptors. The situation is made more complicated by the existence of at least two cation-gated nicotinic acetylcholine receptors (Smp_031680 and Smp_139330) (MacDonald *et al.*, 2014). Although again not characterized, but based on function in other animals, these two receptors could well serve an excitatory rather than inhibitory role in muscle activity. The first is expressed in muscle clusters 2 and 7, the second in all eight clusters.

A further layer of complexity in acetylcholine-mediated control of muscle function is added by the identification of three genes encoding muscarinic cholinergic receptors (Smp_145540, Smp_315830 and Smp_336750) in the v10 *S. mansoni* genome. The proteins are members of the seven-membrane-spanning helix receptor

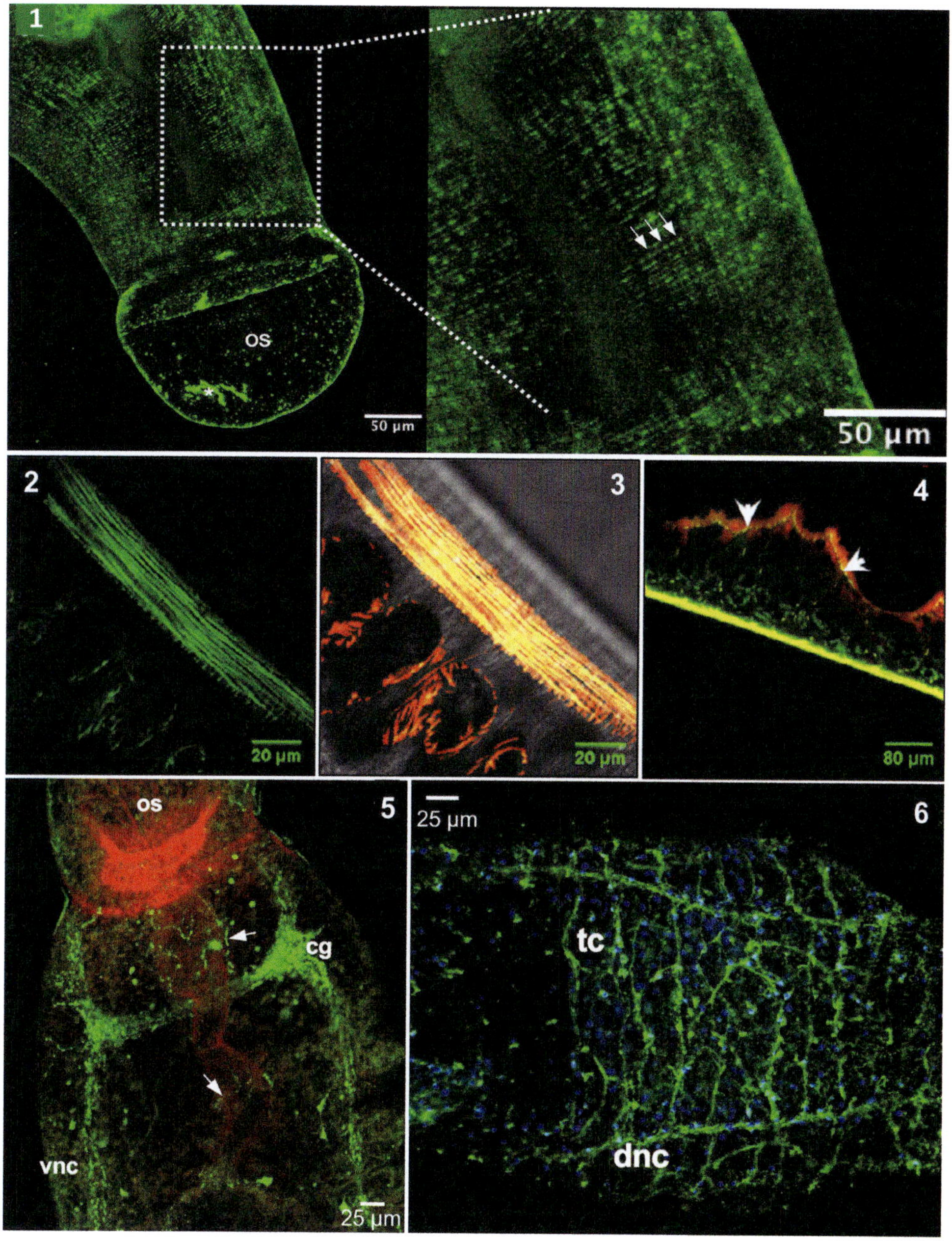

Fig. 5.6. Localization of signalling. **1**) Z-projection of *S. mansoni* acetylcholine receptor 1 (SmACC-1) immunoreactivity in an adult male worm. SmACC-1 is present in both the oral sucker (os) and in minor nerve fibres innervating the body wall. Inset shows the varicose appearance of neurons, resembling a string of beads. **2**) Localization of dopamine receptor 2 (DP2; green) on body wall muscles. **3**) Overlay of receptor (green) on muscle fibres (red, phalloidin) confirms colocalization (yellow). **4**) Higher magnification reveals DP2 is also expressed on the muscles of the gut wall. **5**) Adult male showing localization of 5-hydroxytryptamine (serotonin) receptor (Sm5HT). The central ganglia and main nerve cords are strongly stained. **6**) Dorsal view of male showing Sm5HT in main nerve cords (green), their transverse connections and innervations of the body wall. Note the presence of varicosities (nuclei blue). (**1** from MacDonald *et al.*, 2014; **2–4** from Taman and Ribeiro, 2009; **5** and **6** from Patocka *et al.*, 2014.) **1** and **5**) Figures used under licence CC-BY-4.0. **2–4**) Figures used with permission from Elsevier.

family, mediating their activity by interaction with cytosolic G-proteins, hence abbreviated to GPCRs (G-protein-coupled receptors). They are related to rhodopsin and have been termed GARs (G-protein-coupled acetylcholine receptors) to distinguish them from the several other GPCRs in the nervous system (Fig. 5.5). Ligand binding causes changes to intracellular Ca^{2+} levels or cAMP (MacDonald *et al.*, 2015). In a yeast expression system Smp_145540 protein was significantly activated by acetylcholine but not biogenic amines or glutamate. Its function *in vivo* was also investigated by RNAi gene knock-down applied to newly transformed (3 h) schistosomula and tested in a motility assay at 24 h. Parasite motility was reduced by 70%, compared to controls. This argues for a stimulatory role for this particular muscarinic acetylcholine receptor, at least in schistosomula. Interrogation of the single-cell sequencing data (Wendt *et al.*, 2020) reveals expression of the three muscarinic receptors in 20 neuron clusters, with minimal overlap. Furthermore, one or more muscarinic receptors are expressed in muscle clusters 1, 2, 4, 7 and 8.

5.4.2 Dopamine

The amino acid tyrosine is the starting point for a two-step reaction to generate dopamine. Tyrosine 3-monooxygenase, the first enzyme in the process, has been cloned (Hamdan and Ribeiro, 1998) and is now designated Smp_007690. The second step involves aromatic amino acid decarboxylase, of which three are listed in the v10 *S. mansoni* genome (Smp_135230, Smp_171580 and Smp_342530). Unfortunately, none of these genes is expressed in nerve or muscle clusters (Wendt *et al.*, 2020). Nevertheless, the presence of dopamine has been measured by radiometric assays in the tissues of male and female *S. mansoni*, being highest in the head region of the latter (Gianutsos and Bennett, 1977). Dopamine signalling is mediated by GPCRs, two of which have been characterized in *S. mansoni* (Fig. 5.5). The first, belonging to the D2 family and designated Smp_127310, has been expressed in mammalian cells (Taman and Ribeiro, 2009). It responded only to added dopamine, stimulating cAMP but not Ca^{2+} levels in a dose-dependent manner. An affinity purified polyclonal antibody against two peptides from Smp_127310 bound to the longitudinal and circular fibres of the body wall, and to the muscles investing the gut wall (Fig. 5.6.3–5.6.5). A second uncharacterized D2 type receptor (Smp_315720) is also present in v10 of the genome. The gene encoding Smp_127310 was expressed in six neuron and two parenchyma clusters.

The second type of receptor, also coupled to a G-protein, was termed SmGPR-3 (Smp_043290) (Fig. 5.5) (El-Shehabi *et al.*, 2012). It belongs to a small group of four to five *S. mansoni* receptors which have the rhodopsin-like seven-transmembrane structure. Testing of its function in yeast showed selective activation by dopamine and a dopamine metabolite, epinine, but not other catecholamines. Adult worms probed with purified anti-peptide antibody had high levels of reactivity in the central ganglia and main nerve cords, the muscles around the gut and the peripheral nervous network innervating body wall muscles. The authors concluded that the receptors were more likely to be associated with muscle innervation, rather than on the muscle itself, acting to control motor activity. The situation appears complicated because Smp_043290 gene expression occurs only in one non-neuron cell cluster, whereas three other putative dopamine GPCRs (Smp_127310, Smp_150180 and Smp_326780) were each identified in several neuron clusters (Wendt *et al.*, 2020); in total 15 neuron clusters but only one muscle cluster expressed one or more dopamine receptors.

The termination of dopamine signalling occurs when the transmitter is removed from the synaptic cleft by a membrane-spanning, Na^+-dependent transport protein. One such carrier (Smp_156320, now Smp_333570) has been identified, along with other transmitter transporters (Larsen *et al.*, 2011), and detected by RT-PCR in most life cycle stages.

5.4.3 Glutamate

The first evidence for a Na^+-dependent high-affinity glutamate transporter on the schistosome muscle membranes came from glutamate-induced contractions of isolated muscle fibres (Miller *et al.*, 1996). Glutamate is an important neurotransmitter in both vertebrates and invertebrates, and like dopamine it signals via two types of receptor, termed metabotropic and ionotropic (Fig. 5.5). Three ionotropic receptors (Smp_096480/GluC1, Smp_015630/GluC2 and Smp_104890/GluC3) have been cloned and functionally characterized in *Xenopus* oocytes (Dufour *et al.*, 2013). They have some similarities to the ligand-gated nicotinic acetylcholine channels, comprising a common pentameric structure arranged to form an ion conducting pore, which can be homomeric or heteromeric (Fig. 5.5). Expressed in oocytes, C2 and C3 formed functional homomeric glutamate receptors, while co-expression of C1 and C2 permitted formation of a functional heteromeric channel, which was shown to be permeable to the Cl^- ion. A note of confusion has been added to this work by v10 of the genome, where Smp_096480/GluC1 is annotated as glycine, not glutamine binding, although its role as an ionotropic receptor is not compromised. Between them, the three receptors are expressed on the majority of neuron clusters but only in two muscle clusters, seemingly emphasizing their importance in nerve–nerve interactions. A second group of ionotropic receptors is annotated in the genome and members of the group have been identified by single-cell sequencing (Wendt *et al.*, 2020) but there are no reports of functional characterization. They are classified as belonging to the kainite and *N*-methyl-d-aspartate groups, based on gene annotation.

A metabotropic glutamate receptor has also been cloned and characterized (Smp_128940) (Taman and Ribeiro, 2011). It is a GPCR, which is activated by glutamate (Hamdan and Ribeiro, 1999) when expressed in mammalian cells but not by aspartate or γ-aminobutyric acid (GABA) (Fig. 5.5). Whether it has an excitatory or inhibitory function is unclear but it is immunolocalized in the ganglia, nerve cords and suckers, and perplexingly the antibody reacts with a non-neural component of the female reproductive system. On SchistoCyte (https://www.collinslab.org/schistocyte/) Smp_129840, is expressed only in neuron cluster 1. A second metabotropic receptor, Smp_305430, is annotated in the genome.

5.4.4 Serotonin (5-hydroxytryptamine)

Serotonin is derived from tryptophan in a two-step biosynthetic pathway. The first reaction by the enzyme tryptophan hydroxylase (Smp_174920), converts tryptophan to 5-hydroxytryptophan, which is subsequently decarboxylated to form 5-hydroxytryptamine (serotonin). This is the schistosome neuroexcitatory transmitter (McVeigh and Maule, 2017) but it does not cause direct contraction of *S. mansoni* fibres. However, its action appears to be a prerequisite for depolarization-induced contraction (Day *et al.*, 1994). The majority of serotonin receptors are GPCRs (Fig. 5.5); recent analyses indicate there are at least 126 GPCRs in the *S. mansoni* genome (Hahnel *et al.*, 2018; Kamara *et al.*, 2023). The actual ligand of each GPCR cannot presently be defined by bioinformatic approaches alone but must be backed by experimentation, a process quaintly referred to as deorphanizing. This approach has been used for serotonin in *S. mansoni* (Patocka *et al.*, 2014). Genome searching identified a sequence in the $5HT_7$ clade of serotonin receptors, which was designated Smp_126730 and characterized in a mammalian cell line. Serotonin significantly increased cAMP levels in cells expressing the receptor, compared to controls. The effect was inhibited by co-application of antagonists and enhanced by agonists, but not other biogenic amines such as dopamine, confirming the receptor selectivity for serotonin. The receptor is localized to nerves in the central ganglia, anterior and posterior nerve cords, as well as transverse commissures and elsewhere (Fig. 5.6.5 and 5.6.6).

It is worth recording that the same bioinformatics search (Patocka *et al.*, 2014) identified a sequence (Smp_197700) in the $5HT_{1/5}$ clade and a second (Smp_148210, now Smp_245850) in the $5HT_7$ clade that are also potential serotonin receptors. Moreover, with the caveat that the information is based on bioinformatics, v9 of the genome lists five serotonin receptors, distributed through 29 of the 31 neuron clusters, but no muscle clusters (Wendt *et al.*, 2020). This emphasizes the ubiquity of serotonin signalling, but also its indirect manner of causing muscle excitation. It appears that serotonin can modulate neuronal signalling by regulating the release of other neurotransmitters from presynaptic sites. In vertebrates, the complex array of serotoninergic neurons in the central nervous system impinges on many other neurons and modulates their neurotransmitter release. Conceptual models of varying complexity have been developed to explain the indirect effects of serotonin on nerves and muscles (Fig. 5.7) (Fink and Göthert, 2007). In the much simpler schistosome system it has been suggested that the serotonergic neuron I acts via serotonin receptors on neuron II, which signal via a different transmitter (acetylcholine, dopamine, GABA, peptide) to modulate its effect in the synaptic junction with target III (another nerve or a muscle). Sensory neurons can also feed signals into this complex circuitry. Whatever the molecular details, the outcome of stimulating serotonin release is muscle excitation.

A final consideration is that the serotonin signal is terminated on physical removal from the synapse by a specific re-uptake transporter – incidentally the target of multiple antidepressant drugs in humans (McVeigh and Maule, 2017). A 12-membrane-spanning sodium-dependent symporter from *S. mansoni* has been cloned and partially characterized (Smp_333840 in v10 of the genome) (Patocka and Ribeiro, 2007). Transport inhibitors and RNAi knock-down experiments on schistosomula significantly increased their frequency of movements, compared to controls, suggesting persistence of serotonin action (Patocka and Ribeiro, 2013). Colocalization experiments with specific antibodies revealed that distribution of the symporter closely paralleled that of serotonin in adult worms. Schistosomula showed reactivity in multiple, concentric rings of nerve fibres with a varicose appearance (Fig. 5.8). Such varicosities, common in invertebrate neurons, are multiple presynaptic regions along axons allowing them to form numerous '*en passant*' synaptic connections with their downstream targets (see Section 5.3). At these sites the transmitter is released to exert its effects on the target neuron and then sequestered for destruction or storage (Fig. 5.8).

5.4.5 GABA, histamine, glycine and octopamine

A number of other transmitters may have a lesser role in schistosome nerve function, or a lack of

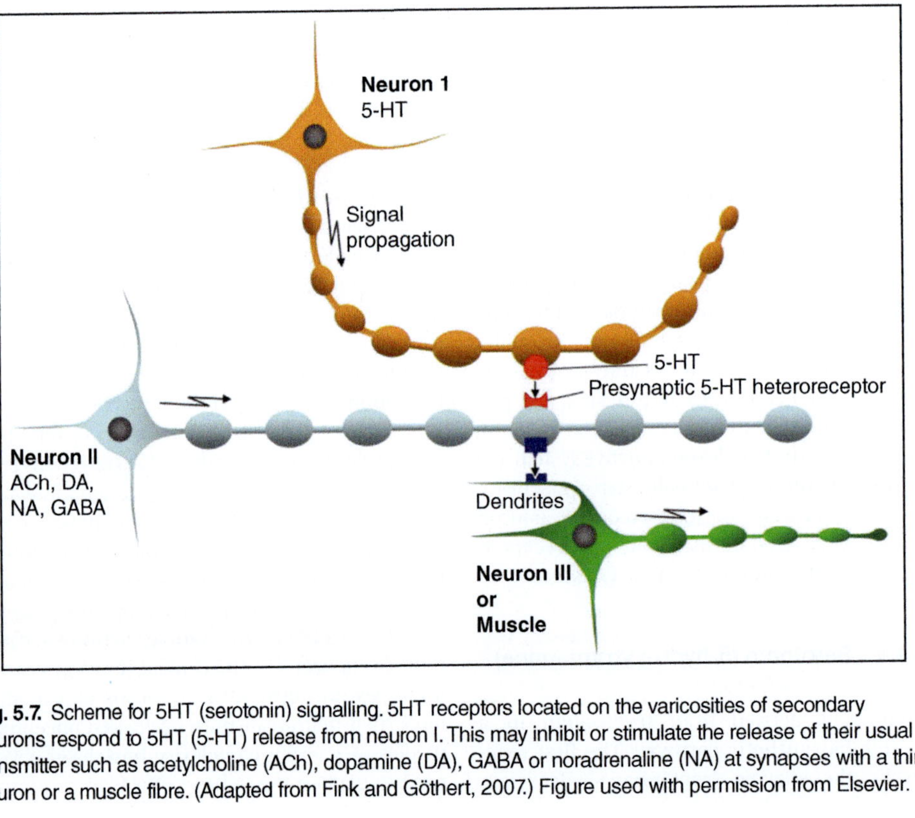

Fig. 5.7. Scheme for 5HT (serotonin) signalling. 5HT receptors located on the varicosities of secondary neurons respond to 5HT (5-HT) release from neuron I. This may inhibit or stimulate the release of their usual transmitter such as acetylcholine (ACh), dopamine (DA), GABA or noradrenaline (NA) at synapses with a third neuron or a muscle fibre. (Adapted from Fink and Göthert, 2007.) Figure used with permission from Elsevier.

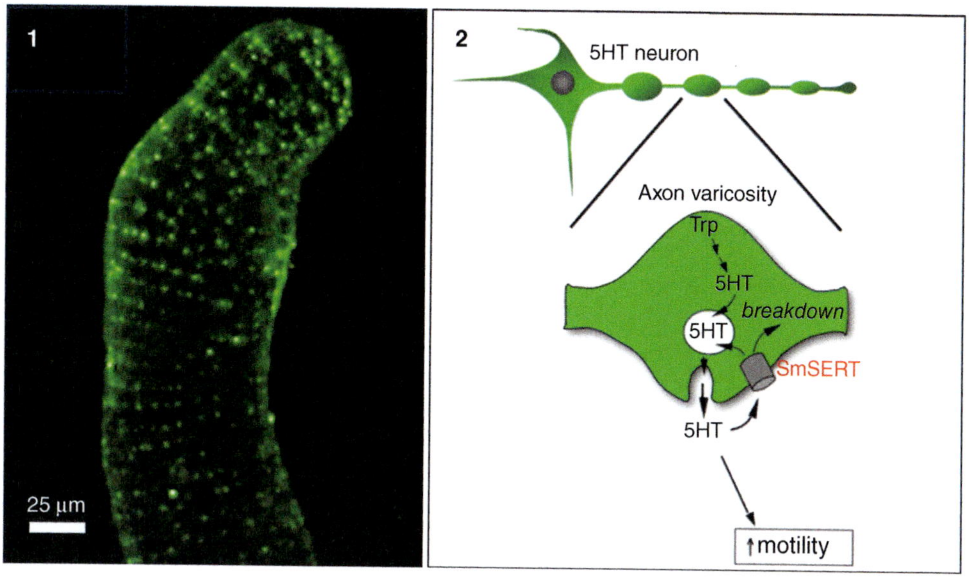

Fig. 5.8. Regulation of 5HT (serotonin) signalling. **1**) The immunoreactivity of serotonin uptake transporter (SmSERT) in multiple, concentric rings of varicose nerve fibres, in proximity to the circular muscle fibres of body wall in 4–6-day-old schistosomula. **2**) Diagram showing how serotonin released from the varicosity may stimulate motility and can be removed from the synapse by SmSERT for recycling or destruction. (From Patocka and Ribeiro, 2013.) Figures used with permission from Elsevier.

evidence may simply mean they are not present – norepinephrine, tyramine and octopamine are cases in point. The enzyme that synthesizes GABA from glutamate has been described (McVeigh and Maule, 2017) but the bioinformatic evidence for GABA receptors is weak. The four genes listed in the single-cell database as GABA receptor subunits (Wendt *et al.*, 2020) are unconvincing when examined on UniProt. Three GABA transporters identified on phylogenetic grounds (Smp_160360, Smp_078930 and Smp_143800, now Smp_244150) (Ribeiro and Patocka, 2013) are eight-membrane-spanning Na/Cl-dependent transporters, but their cargo is yet to be defined.

Two putative GPCR-type histamine receptors have been identified in *S. mansoni*, based on similarity to aminergic receptors in other species. The first, Smp_043260 designated SmGPCR (Fig. 5.5) (Hamdan *et al.*, 2002), certainly encodes a seven-transmembrane-spanning GPCR, but UniProt is non-committal about the ligand. The second, Smp_043340 designated SmGPR2 (Fig. 5.5) (El-Shehabi *et al.*, 2012), has a similar configuration, but just to confuse matters UniProt annotates it as a dopamine receptor. Smp_043260 is expressed in one neuron cluster (Wendt *et al.*, 2020) while Smp_043340 was not detected in the single-cell study, suggesting that the two encoded proteins are not very abundant in the adult stage. Clearly more work is needed to sort out this group of closely related amine receptors. The same is true of two putative glycine transporters (Smp_096480 and Smp_334730) expressed in neuron cluster 1 (Wendt *et al.*, 2020), which UniProt annotates as glutamate-gated Cl^- channels.

The situation with octopamine is equally puzzling. This transmitter, initially described in the octopus, is widespread in molluscs, crustaceans and insects. It has been localized to the nervous system of *S. mansoni* and in an assay of day 7 schistosomular activity, octopamine increased activity 3-fold (compared with 35-fold for serotonin) (El-Sakkary *et al.*, 2018). However, presently no specific receptor has been identified and nearest identity for the synthesizing enzyme, tyramine β-hydroxylase, found in the *S. mansoni* genome, was dopamine β-monooxygenase (Smp_243830). More concrete genetic and molecular evidence is needed for this putative transmitter.

5.4.6 Neuropeptides

Potentially the most novel aspect of neurotransmission in schistosomes is the role played by neuropeptides in muscular coordination, and possibly other processes. Paradoxically it is also the most complex and confusing. The importance of neuropeptide signalling in nematodes like *C. elegans* was mentioned in Section 5.2 above. The ability of heterologous neuropeptides from a mollusc and a cestode to cause dose-dependent contraction of isolated *S. mansoni* muscle fibres appears to be the first demonstration of their potential importance for schistosomes (Day *et al.*, 1994). This study also indicated the presence of peptide receptors on schistosome muscle fibres. There are two broad types of neuropeptide. The short FMRF-like peptides (FLPs) have a C-terminal –RF-NH_2 motif while the longer (36–39 amino acids) neuropeptide Y or neuropeptide F families have an amidated terminal tyrosine or phenylalanine, respectively (McVeigh *et al.*, 2009; Collins *et al.*, 2010). Neuropeptides were identified in other parasitic flatworms before their existence was confirmed in schistosomes (McVeigh *et al.*, 2009). One of the clearest images of their widespread distribution was provided in a study of an FMRFamide-related peptide (Fig. 5.9) (Halton, 2004). Positive staining was present in the central ganglia and transverse commissure as well the nerve cords running forward to invest the muscles of the oral sucker in a finely branching network. Positively stained fibres were also present, running a short distance below the body wall musculature. Two intense centres of staining were associated with and appeared to be the source of axons investing the ventral sucker.

The initial approach taken to identify neuropeptides was essentially bioinformatic, using a strict set of criteria to interrogate expressed

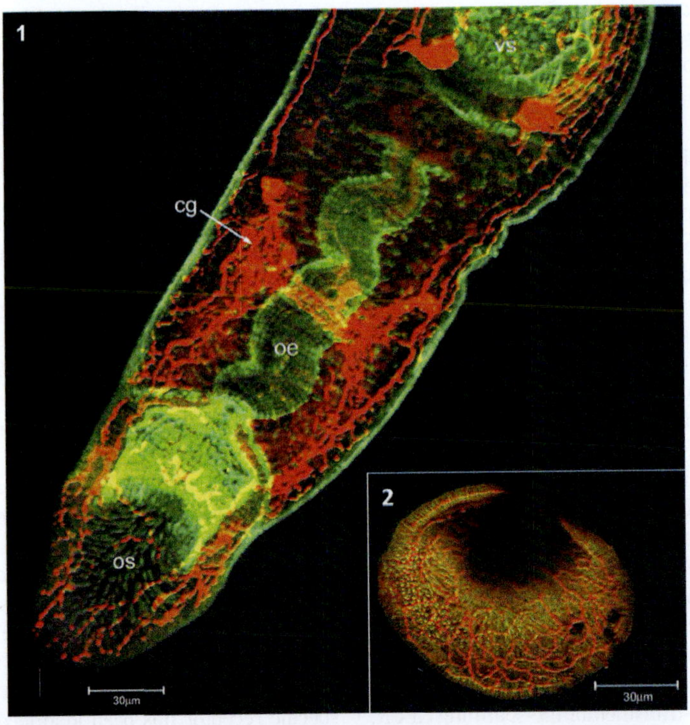

Fig. 5.9. Neuropeptide distribution. **1**) A confocal image of the forebody whole mount of a female schistosome showing immunofluorescence (red) for FMRFamide-related neuropeptide in the central ganglia (cg) and associated neurons, including those innervating the oral (os) and ventral (vs) suckers. oesophagus (oe). **2**) The oral sucker showing the reticulum of fibres (red) innervating the muscles (stained green with FITC-phalloidin). (From Halton, 2004.) Figure used with permission from Elsevier.

sequence tag (EST) sequence data and incipient genome assemblies for free-living and parasitic platyhelminths, using the sequences of known invertebrate neuropeptides. The outcome for *S. mansoni* and *Schistosoma japonicum* is presented in Fig. 5.10.1–5.10.4 (McVeigh *et al.*, 2009). One of the newly identified neuropeptides was subsequently characterized in detail and can be used to illustrate both the ubiquitous reactivity of some peptides and the exquisite specificity of others (McVeigh *et al.*, 2011). The gene Sm*npp1* (Smp_042120) encodes a hormone prepropeptide with signal peptide (Fig. 5.10.3). When the mRNA is translated, this results in the nascent polypeptide entering the lumen of the endoplasmic reticulum. The signal peptide is removed by signal peptidase and the propeptide is then acted on by an endoprotease, mostly likely enriched in the Golgi apparatus. At least one such enzyme is encoded in the genome (neuroendocrine convertase 2; Smp_077980), and potemtially cleaves the prohormone adjacent to KK or KR residues to release the three peptides with a terminal glycine (Fig. 5.10.3). The final step is amidation to generate the bioactive peptide, carried out sequentially by two enzymes. Peptidylglycine α-hydroxylating

1 *gene*	*S. mansoni*	*S. japonicum*
npp-1	AFVRLamide GFVRIamide GFVRIamide	AFVRLamide GFVRLamide GFVRIamide
npp-2	GMIamide	GMIamide GMFamide
npp-5	AAYNDLPWamide AAYIDLPWamide	AAYMDLPWamide AAYIDLPWamide
npp-6	AVRLMRLamide	AVRLMRLamide
npp-14	GLRNMRMamide	GLRNMRMamide
npp-15	VQFLRLamide SAYPYVamide	VQFLRLamide SAYPYVamide
npp-16	NYLWDTRLamide	NYLWDTRLamide SYLWDVRLamide
npp-17	DDFRGamide DHRAFamide	DDFRGamide DHRPFamide
npp-19	FLFNLKDTRWamide NHGSRFamide	FLFNLKDTRWamide NADIYESESGPRHN- IGNRFamide

2 *npp-20*	
Smp_008360	AQALAKLMSLFYTSDAFNKYMENLDAYYMLRGRPRFamide
Smp_159950	AVEIVPPERPFIFETPEALRTYLHKLNEYFAIIGRPRFamide

3 ***npp-1*** **(Smp_042010)**

MTRYSLLGIIQLFISYQIFCLLFICAHGSSRCTTTVNSDGLPILTCDHDRLKVQSHFDIY
NDEQNELIPESDYSNDPLQSQQSAEYIMPSKKAFVRLGKRGFVRIGKRGFVRIGR

4 ***npp-5*** **(Smp_052880 now 340860 hypothetical protein)**

MSLLPPLHIQSKTRYISTYIYIPITLKHFTKLSLFSHCEQIVLRKIVNIVYSHINYQLMN
MLPFQKLSFVILTTLYLSLPWIISMVNTLPATNNNDPNILYRFPPSSSGSLSHQNGVERV
YLPEELLAQLSNDPYFNSMYLPKRAAYMDLPWGKRALAKRAAYIDLPWG

Fig. 5.10. Generation of neuropeptides. **1**) Neuropeptides from *S. mansoni* and *S. japonicum* predicted from neuropeptide precursor (*npp*) genes in the respective genomes. **2**) Longer F/Y family neuropeptides encoded by *npp20* genes. **3**) Processing of the NPP-1 prepropeptide by the removal of the signal peptide (blue) and release of three glycine-terminated peptides (red) by neuroendocrine convertase 2 in the Golgi apparatus, prior to amidation. **4**) Processing of NPP5 protein to release two peptides for amidation. Blue 'KK' and 'KR' are sites of enzyme cleavage. (**1** from McVeigh *et al.*, 2009.) **1**) Figure used with permission from Elsevier. **2–4**) Figures author's own.

monooxygenase (Smp_145300) (Mair *et al.*, 2004) first adds a hydroxyl group to the terminal glycine of the peptide precursor. Then peptidyl α-hydroxyglycine α-amidating lyase (Smp_010820) (Atkinson *et al.*, 2010) converts the hydroxylated intermediate to the α-amidated neuropeptide (Fig. 5.10.1) and free glyoxylate. Just to confuse matters, v10 of the *S. mansoni* genome contains a gene annotated as peptidylglycine monooxygenase (Smp_333880) which, based on the process in higher animals, could potentially perform the amidation in a single step, but has not been investigated. Given this process is occurring within the Golgi apparatus, it is likely that the three peptides are then packaged into vesicles, not for direct secretion from the neuron cell body, but for transport along the axon towards a synapse.

The repertoire of neuropeptides in schistosomes may be quite large, with 15 neuropeptide genes listed in 2017 (McVeigh and Maule, 2017), some of their preproteins giving rise to more than one peptide. The shorter peptides may have L/I, FMRP, L/M/I or PW amide signatures. The neuropeptide F/Y family is represented by at least two genes in *S. mansoni* (Smp_088360 and Smp_159950), possibly more (Fig. 5.10.2). They encode proteins which are processed to produce longer neuropeptides of around 36–38 amino acids, with a C-terminal GRPRFamide motif. Invertebrate F/Y neuropeptides signal via G-protein receptors and multiple receptors of this type are annotated in the v10 *S. mansoni* genome. Peptide binding to the receptor is transmitted to the cytosol via the $G_{i/o}$ subunit inhibiting accumulation of cAMP, but none of the putative *S. mansoni* versions has been functionally characterized (McVeigh and Maule, 2017).

The localization of the pentapeptide GFVRIamide from NPP-1 has been compared with that of FMRFamide on permeabilized whole worms and schistosomula. FMRFamide serves as a marker for the extensive peptidergic nervous system, present in cell bodies and axons of the central ganglia and main nerve cords (Fig. 5.11.1); it also strongly stained the wall of the female ootype. In contrast, the GFVRIamide was detected in just two bipolar neurons, on either side of the central ganglia, and their emergent axons going forward and backward along the main nerve trunks (Fig. 5.11.2). The FMRF and GFVRI staining does not overlap, indicating their expression in separate cells and axons. No peripheral innervation of organ systems or the submuscular plexus was identified so the target of GFVRIamide remains a mystery. However, application of GFRVIamide to adult worms in culture induced a clear reduction in motility. The authors point out that direct inhibition of muscle fibres has yet to be demonstrated. The AAYMDLPWamide peptide encoded by the Sm*npp5* gene (Smp_340860) appears in peripheral nerves innervating the somatic musculature, oral and ventral suckers (Fig. 5.11.3 and 5.11.4).

A different angle on schistosome neuropeptides was provided by a study seeking a role for peptide hormones in controlling reproductive physiology in the free-living planarian *Schmidtea mediterranea* (Collins *et al.*, 2010). The authors used the vertebrate analogy of a neuroendocrine axis involving peptide hormone signalling between the brain and the gonads that controls the maturation and long-term maintenance of reproductive development and function. A bioinformatic approach was initially used to screen the *Schmidtea* genome, supplemented by peptidomic approaches to characterize the worm's peptide hormone complement. This analysis identified 51 prohormone genes and detected peptides from 40 of these by mass spectrometry. It should be emphasized that these were free peptides extracted from homogenates of whole worms, not involving tryptic digestion of parent proteins. Mass spectrometry confirmed multiple distinct peptides from a single prohormone, with biochemical validation for 10 prohormones previously predicted from the *S. mediterranea* genome. An expanded family of genes predicted to encode both NPY-like and NPF-like peptides was found and the requirement for prohormone convertase 2 in prohormone processing was also confirmed.

Extensive *in situ* hybridization results revealed that in asexual planarians, 85% of prohormone genes were expressed in the central nervous system, frequently with differential distributions. A subset of prohormones in the sexual strain of *S. mediterranea* were localized in the oviducts, the copulatory apparatus, gland cells surrounding the copulatory apparatus and the testes, implying the involvement of neuropeptides in reproduction. The authors used the data on validated prohormones from *Schmidtea* to interrogate the genomes of *S. mansoni* and *S. japonicum*. At least four genes encoding preprohormones were

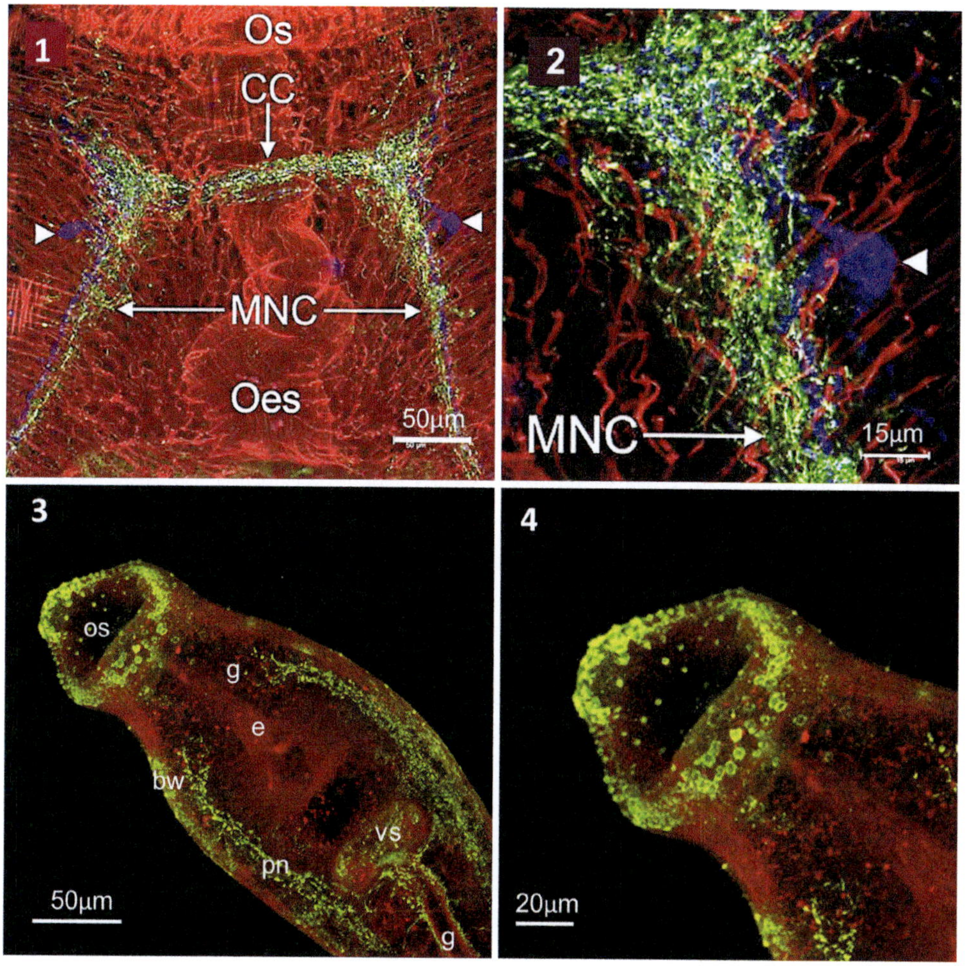

Fig. 5.11. Examples of specific neuropeptide localization. **1**) Male anterior showing distribution of FMRFamide-like peptides (green) and muscle actin (red). The main nerve cords (MNC) ganglia and central commissure (CC) are all positive, while GFVRIamide (blue) is confined to two bipolar cell bodies (arrowed) and their axons. Os, oral sucker; Oes, oesophagus. **2**) Higher magnification of GFVRI distribution. **3**) Distribution of AAYMDLPWamide in peripheral nerves (pn) innervating the body wall (bw) muscles, oral sucker (os) region and the gut wall (gu), but not oesophageal (e) muscles, ventral (vs) sucker or ganglia (g). **4**, Higher magnification of the oral sucker showing AAYMDLPWamide-positive cells are arranged around the lips, suggestive of a role in sensory perception, not muscle contraction. (**1** and **2** from McVeigh *et al.*, 2011; **3** and **4** from McVeigh *et al.*, 2009.) Figures used with permission from Elsevier.

present in *S. mansoni* (Smp_071050, Smp_134550, Smp_188580 and Smp_043650), none of which is annotated in genome v10. However, they all contain the KR or KK cleavage site for the convertase and the predicted hormones for *npp26*, *npp27*, *npp23* and *npp28* are similar or identical to the hormones isolated from *Schmidtea*. The peptidomics approach has been applied to schistosome cercariae (Fogarty *et al.*, 2022) and 11 neuropeptide precursor proteins identified. Synthetic neuropeptides were tested in assays of cercarial swimming behaviour in water, and both short- and long-term changes recorded. Given the apparent impermeability of the cercarial surface provided by the glycocalyx, interpretation of these observations is problematic.

The involvement of neuropeptides in schistosome reproductive biology has recently been highlighted (Li *et al.*, 2024). An RNA sequencing analysis of paired versus unpaired males, females and their gonads identified a differentially expressed GPCR from the rhodopsin family, which was named SmGPCR20 (Smp_084270) (Hahnel *et al.*, 2018). A yeast two-hybrid system was then used to identify two potential ligands for this receptor, SmNPP26 (Smp_071050) and SmNPP40 (Smp_004710) (Li *et al.*, 2024). Expression sites were localized by *in situ* hybridization, and RNAi was used to explore potential functions. These were primarily associated with reduced egg production due to alterations in ovary structure in paired worms. Conversely, no obvious changes were detected along the body of paired males, their testes or seminal vesicle. It was concluded that SmGPCR20 played a multifaceted role in concert with SmNPP26 and SmNPP40 in the growth of females after first pairing, their oogenesis and egg production.

The way in which neuropeptides signal at synapses and neuromuscular junctions is not well explored. One receptor from the planarian *Girardia* (*Dugesia*) has been cloned and partially characterized (Omar *et al.*, 2007). It has an orthologue in *S. mansoni* (Smp_118040) annotated as a neuropeptide Y receptor but nothing else is known. The *Girardia* neuropeptide receptor is a GPCR, which signals through the $G\alpha_{i/o}$ subunit and adenylate cyclase (Zamanian *et al.*, 2012). A different mechanism was proposed for YIRFamide's effect on *S. mansoni* muscle fibres, mediated through a protein kinase C-dependent pathway, triggering cytosolic calcium influx through sarcolemmal voltage-operated Ca^{2+} channels (Novozhilova *et al.*, 2010).

One aspect of neuropeptide signalling appears not to have been considered, namely how the process is terminated. In the model nematode *C. elegans*, where the neuropeptide system is highly developed, over 250 different neuropeptides have been identified. Its genome contains over 150 putative neuropeptide receptors and 27 distinct proteases, termed neprilysins, which degrade neuropeptides (Schafer, 2016). Blasting of *C. elegans* neprilysins 1 and 2 into the WormBase *S. mansoni* repository recovers at least four orthologues with ~50% identity at the amino acid level, annotated either as neprilysins or M8 class proteases. This strongly suggests that schistosomes regulate neuropeptide signalling in the same way as *C. elegans*.

When the expression of neuropeptide preproteins and their receptors is interrogated in the single-cell sequencing study on adult worms (Wendt *et al.*, 2020), a more complicated picture emerges. This comes with the caveat that identities are based largely on electronic annotation, not the much more arduous experimental work. A total of 22 neuropeptide receptors is annotated, in several categories. One of these, the FMRFamide-activated amiloride-sensitive Na^+ channel with seven Smp annotations has not hitherto attracted attention. It provides an alternative pathway for FMRFamide signalling to the GPCR route, and in molluscs mediates fast neuronal transmission (Lingueglia *et al.*, 1995). The seven amiloride-sensitive channel genes are expressed in 23 out of 31 neuron clusters, compared to 21 clusters for the GPCR-type receptor so there is clearly a lot of overlap. It is also worth recording that neuropeptide receptors are expressed in all eight muscle clusters (see Chapter 4), which corresponds with the limited evidence that neuropeptides can mediate muscle contraction (Day *et al.*, 1994). Some of the clusters (1 and 7) express several receptors so clearly the capacity for differential signalling must be considerable.

5.5 Summary

- The solid acoelomate body of schistosomes seriously limits the techniques that might be applied to determine nervous system function. There have been no electrophysiology recordings or dye injections into single nerves that have allowed pathways and connectivity maps to be made, as in nematodes and molluscs. Those groups have a remarkable consistency of neuron size, position, chemistry and connectivity. Furthermore, molluscs are also members of the Lophotrochozoa so similarities might be anticipated.
- Publication of the *S. mansoni* transcriptome in 2003 and the genome in 2009 facilitated biochemical studies, although the lack of a schistosome cell line meant these were in heterologous cell systems. These have produced a reasonable appreciation of classical neurotransmitters and their receptors although, no doubt due to the labour involved, the approach has declined in popularity.
- The identification of neuropeptide transmitters and their potential receptors has

revealed the enormous complexity of the schistosome nervous system. The single-cell sequencing approach, even with caveats, has reinforced the diversity of neuron types.

- Although immunochemistry, and *in situ* hybridization for gene expression, have been used to localize potential activities, making the link between nervous system morphology, motor activity and sensory cell function is a formidable task.
- The miracidial and cercarial stages are equipped with multiple receptor types to detect a wide range of sensory modalities. It seems unlikely that the simple ciliated ending identified on the adult worm surface is the sole means of detecting external signals in the bloodstream. It is inevitable that a highly structured nervous system exists in all life cycle stages – we have simply not come close to defining it yet.

References

Atkinson, L.E., McVeigh, P., Kimber, M.J., Marks, N.J., Eipper, B.A. *et al.* (2010) A PAL for *Schistosoma mansoni* PHM. *Molecular and Biochemical Parasitology* 173(2), 97–106. DOI: 10.1016/j.molbiopara.2010.05.009

Attenborough, T., Rawlinson, K.A., Diaz Soria, C.L., Ambridge, K., Sankaranarayanan, G. *et al.* (2024) A single-cell atlas of the miracidium larva of *Schistosoma mansoni* reveals cell types, developmental pathways, and tissue architecture. *eLife* 13, RP95628. DOI: 10.7554/eLife.95628

Collins, J.J., Hou, X., Romanova, E.V., Lambrus, B.G., Miller, C.M. *et al.* (2010) Genome-wide analyses reveal a role for peptide hormones in planarian germline development. *PLoS Biology* 8(10), e1000509. DOI: 10.1371/journal.pbio.1000509

Collins, J.J., King, R.S., Cogswell, A., Williams, D.L. and Newmark, P.A. (2011) An atlas for *Schistosoma mansoni* organs and life-cycle stages using cell type-specific markers and confocal microscopy. *PLoS Neglected Tropical Diseases* 5(3), e1009. DOI: 10.1371/journal.pntd.0001009

Day, T.A., Maule, A.G., Shaw, C., Halton, D.W., Moore, S. *et al.* (1994) Platyhelminth FMRFamide-related peptides (FaRPs) contract *Schistosoma mansoni* (Trematoda: Digenea) muscle fibres *in vitro*. *Parasitology* 109(4), 455–459. DOI: 10.1017/s0031182000080707

Dorsey, C.H., Cousin, C.E., Lewis, F.A. and Stirewalt, M.A. (2002) Ultrastructure of the *Schistosoma mansoni* cercaria. *Micron* 33(3), 279–323. DOI: 10.1016/s0968-4328(01)00019-1

Dufour, V., Beech, R.N., Wever, C., Dent, J.A. and Geary, T.G. (2013) Molecular cloning and characterization of novel glutamate-gated chloride channel subunits from *Schistosoma mansoni*. *PLoS Pathogens* 9(8), e1003586. DOI: 10.1371/journal.ppat.1003586

El-Sakkary, N., Chen, S., Arkin, M.R., Caffrey, C.R. and Ribeiro, P. (2018) Octopamine signaling in the metazoan pathogen *Schistosoma mansoni*: localization, small-molecule screening and opportunities for drug development. *Disease Models & Mechanisms* 11(7), dmm033563. DOI: 10.1242/dmm.033563

El-Shehabi, F., Taman, A., Moali, L.S., El-Sakkary, N. and Ribeiro, P. (2012) A novel G protein-coupled receptor of *Schistosoma mansoni* (SmGPR-3) is activated by dopamine and is widely expressed in the nervous system. *PLoS Neglected Tropical Diseases* 6(2), e1523. DOI: 10.1371/journal.pntd.0001523

Fink, K.B. and Göthert, M. (2007) 5-HT receptor regulation of neurotransmitter release. *Pharmacological Reviews* 59(4), 360–417. DOI: 10.1124/pr.107.07103

Fogarty, C.E., Suwansa-Ard, S., Phan, P., McManus, D.P., Duke, M.G. *et al.* (2022) Identification of putative neuropeptides that alter the behaviour of *Schistosoma mansoni* cercariae. *Biology* 11(9), 1344. DOI: 10.3390/biology11091344

Fripp, P.J. (1967) Histochemical localization of esterase activity in schistosomes. *Experimental Parasitology* 21(3), 380–390. DOI: 10.1016/0014-4894(67)90098-7

Gianutsos, G. and Bennett, J.L. (1977) The regional distribution of dopamine and norepinephrine in *Schistosoma mansoni* and *Fasciola hepatica*. *Comparative Biochemistry and Physiology Part C: Comparative Pharmacology* 58(2C), 157–159. DOI: 10.1016/0306-4492(77)90097-1

Grimmelikhuijzen, C.J. and Westfall, J.A. (1995) The nervous systems of cnidarians. *EXS* 72, 7–24. DOI: 10.1007/978-3-0348-9219-3_2

Hahnel, S., Wheeler, N., Lu, Z., Wangwiwatsin, A., McVeigh, P. *et al.* (2018) Tissue-specific transcriptome analyses provide new insights into GPCR signalling in adult *Schistosoma mansoni*. *PLoS Pathogens* 14(1), e1006718. DOI: 10.1371/journal.ppat.1006718

Halton, D.W. (2004) Microscopy and the helminth parasite. *Micron* 35(5), 361–390. DOI: 10.1016/j.micron.2003.12.001

Halton, D.W. and Gustafsson, M.K.S. (1996) Functional morphology of the platyhelminth nervous system. *Parasitology* 113(S1), S47–S72. DOI: 10.1017/S0031182000077891

Hamdan, F.F. and Ribeiro, P. (1998) Cloning and characterization of a novel form of tyrosine hydroxylase from the human parasite, *Schistosoma mansoni. Journal of Neurochemistry* 71(4), 1369–1380. DOI: 10.1046/j.1471-4159.1998.71041369.x

Hamdan, F.F. and Ribeiro, P. (1999) Characterization of a stable form of tryptophan hydroxylase from the human parasite *Schistosoma mansoni. The Journal of Biological Chemistry* 274(31), 21746–21754. DOI: 10.1074/jbc.274.31.21746

Hamdan, F.F, Abramovitz, M., Mousa, A., Xie, J., Durocher, Y. *et al.* (2002) A novel *Schistosoma mansoni* G protein-coupled receptor is responsive to histamine. *Molecular and Biochemical Parasitology* 119(1), 75–86. DOI: 10.1016/s0166-6851(01)00400-5

Kamara, I.K., Thao, J.T., Kaur, K., Wheeler, N.J. and Chan, J.D. (2023) Annotation of G-protein coupled receptors in the genomes of parasitic blood flukes. *MicroPublication Biology* 2023, 000704. DOI: 10.17912/micropub.biology.000704

Keramidioti, A., Schneid, S., Busse, C., Cramer von Laue, C., Bertulat, B. *et al.* (2024) A new look at the architecture and dynamics of the *Hydra* nerve net. *eLife* 12, RP87330. DOI: 10.7554/eLife.87330

Larsen, M.B., Fontana, A.C.K., Magalhães, L.G., Rodrigues, V. and Mortensen, O.V. (2011) A catecholamine transporter from the human parasite *Schistosoma mansoni* with low affinity for psychostimulants. *Molecular and Biochemical Parasitology* 177(1), 35–41. DOI: 10.1016/j.molbiopara.2011.01.006

Li, X., Weth, O., Haimann, M., Möscheid, M.F., Huber, T.S. *et al.* (2024) Rhodopsin orphan GPCR20 interacts with neuropeptides and directs growth, sexual differentiation, and egg production in female *Schistosoma mansoni. Microbiology Spectrum* 12(1), e0219323. DOI: 10.1128/spectrum.02193-23

Lingueglia, E., Champigny, G., Lazdunski, M. and Barbry, P. (1995) Cloning of the amiloride-sensitive FMRFamide peptide-gated sodium channel. *Nature* 378(6558), 730–733. DOI: 10.1038/378730a0

MacDonald, K., Kimber, M.J., Day, T.A. and Ribeiro, P. (2015) A constitutively active G protein-coupled acetylcholine receptor regulates motility of larval *Schistosoma mansoni. Molecular and Biochemical Parasitology* 202(1), 29–37. DOI: 10.1016/j.molbiopara.2015.09.001

MacDonald, K., Buxton, S., Kimber, M.J., Day, T.A., Robertson, A.P. *et al.* (2014) Functional characterization of a novel family of acetylcholine-gated chloride channels in *Schistosoma mansoni. PLoS Pathogens* 10(6), e1004181. DOI: 10.1371/journal.ppat.1004181

Mair, G.R., Niciu, M.J., Stewart, M.T., Brennan, G., Omar, H. *et al.* (2004) A functionally atypical amidating enzyme from the human parasite *Schistosoma mansoni. FASEB Journal* 18(1), 114–121. DOI: 10.1096/fj.03-0429com

Marks, N.J., Halton, D.W., Maule, A.G., Brennan, G.P., Shaw, C. *et al.* (1995) Comparative analyses of the neuropeptide F (NPF)- and FMRFamide-related peptide (FaRP)-immunoreactivities in *Fasciola hepatica* and *Schistosoma* spp. *Parasitology* 110(4), 371–381. DOI: 10.1017/s0031182000064714

McVeigh, P., Mair, G.R., Atkinson, L., Ladurner, P., Zamanian, M. *et al.* (2009) Discovery of multiple neuropeptide families in the phylum *Platyhelminthes. International Journal for Parasitology* 39(11), 1243–1252. DOI: 10.1016/j.ijpara.2009.03.005

McVeigh, P. and Maule, A.G. (2017) Structure and function of the helminth neuromuscular system. In: Byrne, J.H. (ed.) *The Oxford Handbook of Invertebrate Neurobiology*. Oxford University Press, Oxford, pp. 219–244.

McVeigh, P., Mair, G.R., Novozhilova, E., Day, A., Zamanian, M. *et al.* (2011) Schistosome I/Lamides – a new family of bioactive helminth neuropeptides. *International Journal for Parasitology* 41(8), 905–913. DOI: 10.1016/j.ijpara.2011.03.010

Miller, C.L., Day, T.A., Bennett, J.L. and Pax, R.A. (1996) *Schistosoma mansoni*: l-glutamate-induced contractions in isolated muscle fibers; evidence for a glutamate transporter. *Experimental Parasitology* 84(3), 410–419. DOI: 10.1006/expr.1996.0129

Novozhilova, E., Kimber, M.J., Qian, H., McVeigh, P., Robertson, A.P. *et al.* (2010) FMRFamide-like peptides (FLPs) enhance voltage-gated calcium currents to elicit muscle contraction in the human parasite *Schistosoma mansoni. PLoS Neglected Tropical Diseases* 4(8), e790. DOI: 10.1371/journal.pntd.0000790

Omar, H.H., Humphries, J.E., Larsen, M.J., Kubiak, T.M., Geary, T.G. *et al.* (2007) Identification of a platyhelminth neuropeptide receptor. *International Journal for Parasitology* 37(7), 725–733. DOI: 10.1016/j.ijpara.2006.12.019

Parker-Manuel, S.J. and Wilson, R.A. (2022) An atlas of the germ ball–cercaria–schistosomulum transition in *Schistosoma mansoni*, using confocal microscopy and *in situ* hybridisation. *Current Research in Parasitology & Vector-Borne Diseases* 2, 100087. DOI: 10.1016/j.crpvbd.2022.100087

Patocka, N. and Ribeiro, P. (2007) Characterization of a serotonin transporter in the parasitic flatworm, *Schistosoma mansoni*: cloning, expression and functional analysis. *Molecular and Biochemical Parasitology* 154(2), 125–133. DOI: 10.1016/j.molbiopara.2007.03.010

Patocka, N. and Ribeiro, P. (2013) The functional role of a serotonin transporter in *Schistosoma mansoni* elucidated through immunolocalization and RNA interference (RNAi). *Molecular and Biochemical Parasitology* 187(1), 32–42. DOI: 10.1016/j.molbiopara.2012.11.008

Patocka, N., Sharma, N., Rashid, M. and Ribeiro, P. (2014) Serotonin signaling in *Schistosoma mansoni*: a serotonin-activated G protein-coupled receptor controls parasite movement. *PLoS Pathogens* 10(1), e1003878. DOI: 10.1371/journal.ppat.1003878

Pax, R.A. and Bennett, J.L. (1991) Neurobiology of parasitic platyhelminths: possible solutions to the problems of correlating structure with function. *Parasitology* 102(Suppl.), S31–S39. DOI: 10.1017/s0031182000073273

Pax, R.A., Siefker, C. and Bennett, J.L. (1984) *Schistosoma mansoni*: differences in acetylcholine, dopamine, and serotonin control of circular and longitudinal parasite muscles. *Experimental Parasitology* 58(3), 314–324. DOI: 10.1016/0014-4894(84)90048-1

Ribeiro, P. and Patocka, N. (2013) Neurotransmitter transporters in schistosomes: structure, function and prospects for drug discovery. *Parasitology International* 62(6), 629–638. DOI: 10.1016/j.parint.2013.06.003

Schafer, W. (2016) Nematode nervous systems. *Current Biology* 26(20), R955–R959. DOI: 10.1016/j.cub.2016.07.044

Silk, M.H. and Spence, I.M. (1969) Ultrastructural studies of the blood fluke – *Schistosoma mansoni*. 3. The nerve tissue and sensory structures. *The South African Journal of Medical Sciences* 34(4), 93–104.

Skelly, P.J. and Da'dara, A.A. (2023) A novel, non-neuronal acetylcholinesterase of schistosome parasites is essential for definitive host infection. *Frontiers in Immunology* 14, 1056469. DOI: 10.3389/fimmu.2023.1056469

Sprecher, S.G. (2022) Neural cell type diversity in cnidaria. *Frontiers in Neuroscience* 16, 909400. DOI: 10.3389/fnins.2022.909400

Taman, A. and Ribeiro, P. (2009) Investigation of a dopamine receptor in *Schistosoma mansoni*: functional studies and immunolocalization. *Molecular and Biochemical Parasitology* 168(1), 24–33. DOI: 10.1016/j.molbiopara.2009.06.003

Taman, A. and Ribeiro, P. (2011) Glutamate-mediated signaling in *Schistosoma mansoni*: a novel glutamate receptor is expressed in neurons and the female reproductive tract. *Molecular and Biochemical Parasitology* 176(1), 42–50. DOI: 10.1016/j.molbiopara.2010.12.001

Telford, M.J., Budd, G.E. and Philippe, H. (2015) Phylogenomic insights into animal evolution. *Current Biology* 25(19), R876–87. DOI: 10.1016/j.cub.2015.07.060

Wendt, G., Zhao, L., Chen, R., Liu, C., O'Donoghue, A.J. *et al.* (2020) A single-cell RNA-seq atlas of *Schistosoma mansoni* identifies a key regulator of blood feeding. *Science* 369(6511), 1644–1649. DOI: 10.1126/science.abb7709

Zamanian, M., Agbedanu, P.N., Wheeler, N.J., McVeigh, P., Kimber, M.J. *et al.* (2012) Novel RNAi-mediated approach to G protein-coupled receptor deorphanization: proof of principle and characterization of a planarian 5-HT receptor. *PLoS ONE* 7(7), e40787. DOI: 10.1371/journal.pone.0040787

6

Protonephridia

6.1 Overview

Even the tiny miracidium, 120 μm long, possesses a protonephridial system comprising four flame cells and paired collecting tubules. The system is more extensive in other larval stages and permeates the whole body of adult worms. The assumption must be that in these flatworms with a solid body plan, simple diffusion is not sufficient to void unwanted metabolites. An auxiliary system is needed to drain the interstitial spaces deep inside the body, transferring potentially toxic substances to the exterior. This chapter deals with the structure of the flame cells, which provide the motive force for the system, and their collecting ducts that transfer fluid towards the excretory pore(s). There has been minimal experimental investigation of processes that occur along those tubules. We must therefore rely on anecdotal reports, often the result of immunocytochemical approaches that highlight tubule cytosol or surface membranes, for hints about biochemical processes.

6.2 Osmoregulation in Schistosomes

It is worth taking a moment to consider the osmotic forces that schistosomes are subjected to during their complex life cycle. The adult worms within the bloodstream are osmoconformers – they live in a virtually constant osmotic and ionic environment provided by the human host. However, it is apparent from studies on blood ingestion (Chapter 8) that the adult female takes in an estimated 0.48 nl of blood per day, equivalent to 4.4 body volumes (Lawrence, 1973). How does the worm deal with this influx of fluid and ions, given that it has a tidal gut, and does not appear to become bloated as it feeds? It is possible that the protonephridial system plays a role in draining significant volumes of fluid from the interstitial spaces, but experimental evidence is lacking. What is apparent from proteomic analyses of the tegument membranes is the abundance of aquaporin at the tegument surface (Castro-Borges *et al.*, 2011). Its molecular characterization revealed a role in lactate excretion as well as water balance (Faghiri and Skelly, 2009; Faghiri *et al.*, 2010). The presence of Na/K transporters, most likely localized in the basal tegument plasma membrane, may also contribute to the ionic equilibrium. These observations suggest that the protonephridia are not involved in volume control in adults.

In complete contrast, the miracidium and cercaria live in freshwater and are subjected to strong osmotic forces. How do they control their internal environment to prevent influx of water and loss of ions? For the cercaria, the best guess

 The Cell Biology of Schistosomes: Implications for Diagnostics and Vaccines (Wilson)
DOI: 10.1079/9781800625167.0006

is the use of the 1 μm thick glycocalyx as a physical barrier. We can infer this because during *in vitro* transformation, loss of the glycocalyx immediately confers susceptibility to osmotic forces; in hypotonic conditions the larvae swell up and die. For the miracidium, there is no equivalent for obvious reasons – a thick glycocalyx would impede beating of the propulsive cilia. Nevertheless, the thin coat of mucus over the miracidium and the cytosol of the ciliated epithelia must provide osmoprotection (see Chapter 1), because when these cells are lost during transformation, the mother sporocyst becomes susceptible to osmotic forces. It is therefore possible that the protonephridial system of the miracidium and cercaria assists in expulsion of water that has entered down the osmotic gradient, and in retention of ions, but we have no direct experimental evidence for this.

6.3 The Flame Cell

6.3.1 The composite structure

Flame cells are just one example of the terminal structures found in the protonephridial systems of different invertebrate phyla. Whether they represent an evolutionary sequence or are examples of convergent evolution remains an open question. Flame cells with the general structure described below are found in trematodes, cestodes and possibly free-living species, although not all platyhelminth protonephridia fit the definition (Wilson and Webster, 1974). They have a uniform size, ~10 μm × 3 μm, throughout the Trematoda and their ultrastructure was first described in the liver fluke (*Fasciola hepatica*) miracidium (Kümmel, 1958). The realization that the flame cell was actually a composite structure, comprised of a cap cell and the first tubule cell, only came a decade later in trematodes (Wilson, 1969) and tapeworms (Howells, 1969). None the less, the flame cell has been treated as one entity up to the present day in single-cell sequencing studies because it can be isolated from tissue digests minus its tubule cell body (Wendt *et al.*, 2020; Attenborough *et al.*, 2024).

The cap cell has a large, rounded nucleus, and bears at one pole a tuft of flagella, each anchored by a prominent rootlet in the cytoplasm (Fig. 6.1.1). The flagella are closely packed and beat with an undulatory motion that gives the illusion of a flickering flame, hence the name. They number around 100 in *Schistosoma japonicum* (Pan, 1980), around 60 in *Schistosoma mansoni* (de Water *et al.*, 1987) and the number reduces in cross-section down the barrel as the flame tapers. The other principal feature of the cap cell is a circle of finger-like 'rods', ~1 μm diameter, surrounding and curving outwards from the flagellar tuft for ~4 μm (Fig. 6.1.2) (Wilson and Webster, 1974). The first tubule cell makes a complimentary contribution to the barrel of the flame cell. Its cytoplasm is drawn out into a deep cup shape, and the rim of the cup is extended by a matching circle of externally positioned, flattened rods, 1 μm × 4 μm. The cap and tube rods interpolate but only make contact at their margins, which are joined by a continuous zipper of extracellular desmosomal material (Fig. 6.1.2, inset). The broader external rods of the cap cell give the barrel a ridged appearance over the 4 μm region of overlap.

An added level of complexity is provided by short projections of cytoplasm from the rods, termed leptotrichs (Kümmel, 1958). The inner ones from the cap rods protrude into the space around the base of the flagella tuft. The larger outer rods bear one to three leptotrichs each, up to 6 μm long, extending out into the interstitial space. Each leptotrich has a single microtubule running down its centre, presumably to provide stiffness rather than mobility. This function is very apparent for the external ring of leptotrichs, which surround the ridged region on the barrel, and create a fluid-filled lacuna. A layer of flocculent material is discernible between the broad external rods but none is not visible within the barrel (Fig. 6.2.1 and 6.2.2). It is a plausible hypothesis that the extracellular desmosomal zipper binding the rods together provides a filter to hold back macromolecules above a certain size (see below). Anecdotally, it was observed that the compound leucomethylene blue paralysed the epidermal cilia of miracidia contracting the posterior, which occluded the excretory pores. The flame cells continued to beat, and the tubules became enormously dilated; finally, the reagent paralysed them too and the tubules immediately collapsed (Wilson and Webster, 1974). This provided visual confirmation that the beating of the flame created a significant hydromotive force.

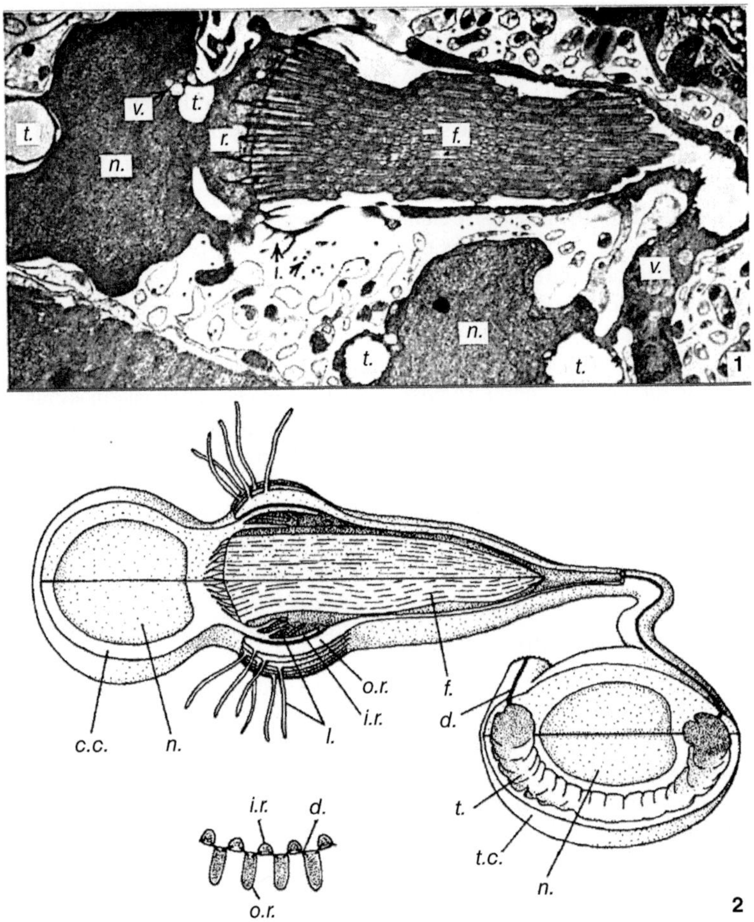

Fig. 6.1. The flame cell is a composite structure. **1**) Longitudinal section of a *Fasciola* cap cell and first tubule cell. t, tubule; n, nucleus; v, vesicles; r, rootlets; l, leptotrichs; f, flagella. **2**) Diagram of the composite structure. c.c., cap cell; o.r., outer rod; i.r., inner rod; d, desmosome; t, tubule; t.c., tubule cell. (**1** from Wilson, 1969; **2** from Wilson and Webster, 1974.) Figures used with permission from **1**) Cambridge University Press and **2**) John Wiley & Sons.

The biochemical nature of the cell-junction proteins that hold the interdigitating rods in place is clearly a key determinant of what is retained or let through.

6.3.2 Mode of action

There is no intrinsic structural distinction between cilia and eukaryotic flagella. However, flagella typically enable propulsion by driving fluid continuously in parallel to the flagellar axis while cilia push fluid orthogonally to their axis, and tangentially to their attachment surface (Gilpin *et al.*, 2020). On that definition, the flame is composed of flagella which synchronize their beating via hydrodynamic or direct mechanical coupling (Fig. 6.2.3). Despite these functional differences, cilia and flagella have identical ultrastructure and nearly identical composition. Beating of flagella/cilia arises from coupled chemical and mechanical processes occurring in the axoneme. This tube-shaped structure contains an arrangement of nine microtubule doublets (each ~25 nm in diameter) surrounding a central pair of microtubules, all of them composed of α- and β-tubulins (Fig. 6.2.4). The outer microtubule doublets are mechanically coupled to one other

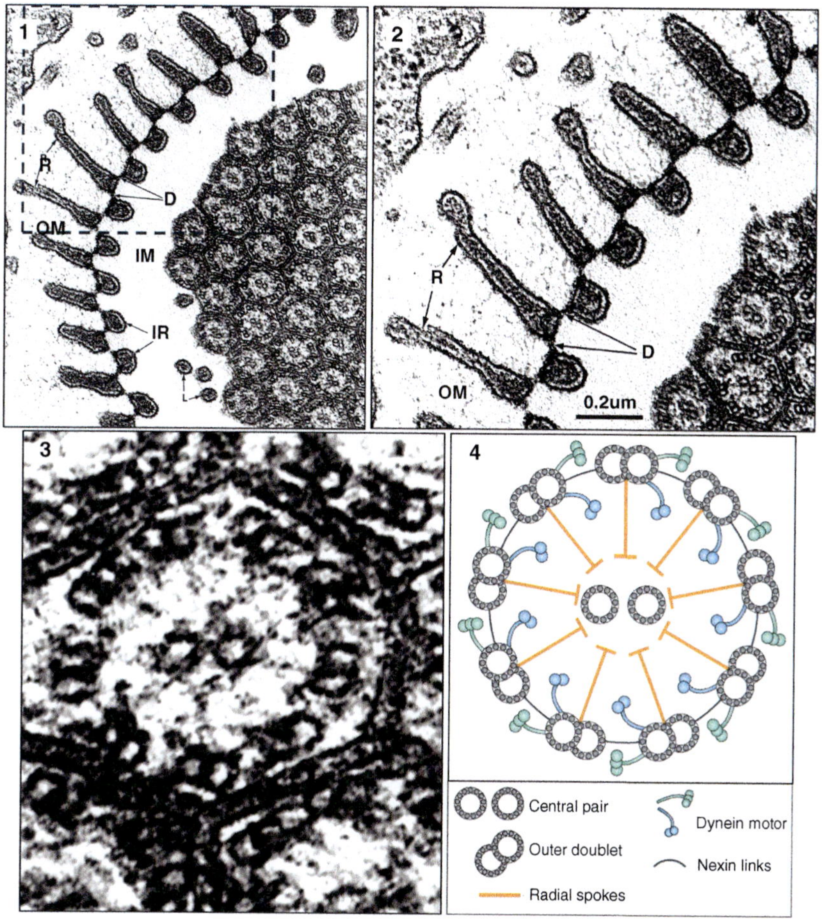

Fig. 6.2. Transverse section of flame cell barrel at the level of the rods. **1**) Ring of broad outer rods (R) contributed by the tube cell interdigitated with rounded trapezoid-shaped rods (IR) from the cap cell. Leptotrichs (L) are visible in cross-section. **2**) Enlargement of the rods (R) showing location of the desmosomal zipper (D). There is a reticulum of fine fibres (OM) lying between the outer rods. **3**) High magnification of a single flagellum showing the nine double plus two single microtubule arrangement. The space between adjacent flagella contains dense material that could indicate they are adherent. **4**) Diagram explaining the molecular organization of a flagellum. (**1–3** courtesy of Dr Roger Pullin; **4** from Gilpin *et al.*, 2020.) **4**) Figure used with permission from Springer Nature.

via nexin links, and 'radial spokes' extend towards the central pair. The orientation of the inner doublet pair breaks the symmetry of the filament to define the bending axis, so that *en masse* the flagella of the flame all appear in register (Fig. 6.2.1) and beat synchronously.

Beating arises from the collective effects of dyneins, the molecular motors that convert the chemical energy of ~10^5 ATP molecules per beat into a relative sliding motion among the nine microtubule doublets comprising the axonemal sheath; at the molecular level the mechanisms are still a matter of conjecture (Gilpin *et al.*, 2020). The synchronized beating of 60–100 flagella, 10 times per second, is an energy-expensive process that generates significant power. Considering that the beating of a single flagellum propels a spermatozoan forward through fluid, we can visualize the synchronous beating of around 100 stationary flagella within the flame cell barrel as driving the enclosed fluid from base to tip. Thus, a suction pressure is created, which draws in fluid across the filter between the rods. How efficient is filtration by suction pressure compared to filtration by positive pressure in the glomerulus of the mammalian kidney? An estimate of ΔP, the pressure difference across the top of the flame cell barrel, was calculated as 1.21×10^3 N/m^2, equivalent to a pressure of 12.4 cmH_2O (Wilson and Webster, 1974), based on the equation for the rate of flow of a liquid through a porous membrane (Pappenheimer, 1953). We can put this into the context of glomerular filtration in the mammalian kidney. There, the hydrostatic pressure in the tuft of capillaries (60 mmHg) is opposed by the colloid osmotic pressure of blood (32 mmHg) plus the back pressure of Bowmans capsule (18 mmHg), resulting in a net filtration pressure of 10 mmHg (Dr L. Webster, personal communication). This converts to 13.6 cmH_2O, almost identical to the estimate for the suction pressure created within the flame cell barrel by the beating flagella.

Indeed, we can make a morphological analogy with the glomerulus of the mammalian kidney (Fig. 6.3) (Mundel and Kriz, 1995; Mundel, 2017). The capillaries projecting into Bowman's capsule have a fenestrated endothelium lying on

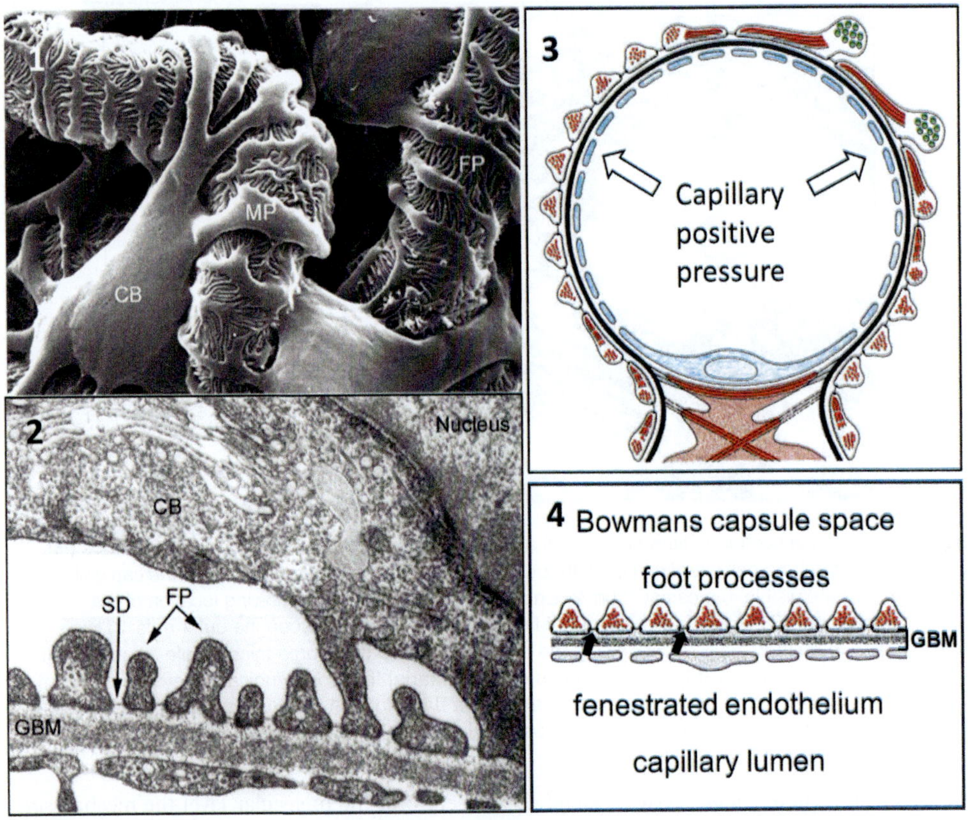

Fig. 6.3. Glomerular filtration in the mammalian kidney. **1**) SEM of a glomerular capillary invested by podocyte cell bodies (CB) from which major processes (MP) extend like tentacles giving rise to interdigitating foot processes (FP) around the vessel wall, termed filtration slits. **2**) TEM of the filtration barrier consisting of fenestrated capillary endothelium, triple-layered glomerular basement membrane (GBM) and podocyte foot processes. These are bridged by the slit diaphragm (SD) which provides the real barrier to passage of plasma proteins into urine. **3**) Diagram of a glomerular capillary showing direction of plasma flow (arrowed) through the fenestrated capillary endothelium into the overlying extracellular basal lamella. **4**) Higher magnification of the podocyte feet adherent to the basal lamella with the slit diaphragm barrier arrowed. (Based on Mundel and Kriz, 1995 and Mundel, 2017.) Figures used with permission from Springer Nature.

a multilayered glomerular basement membrane. Each is enveloped by a single layer of cells on the capsule side, called podocytes because their connections with the capillaries are made via interdigitating foot processes (Fig. 6.3.1 and 6.3.2). The spaces between the interdigitations, known as slit diaphragms or pores, provide the actual molecular barrier retaining proteins in plasma but permitting solutes to enter Bowman's capsule. The pore size and structure of the mammalian slit diaphragm were established by high-resolution electron microscopy, using protein tracers, as being no larger than serum albumin (68 kDa) (Rodewald and Karnovsky, 1974). The proteins of the slit diaphragm include ZO-1 guanylate kinase, nephrin and protocadherin FAT1 (Pavenstädt and Bek, 2002; Greka and Mundel, 2012). The positive pressure of the capillary is the driving force at its centre (Fig. 6.3.3), while the fenestrated endothelium and glomerular basement membrane are permeable, the slit diaphragm between the foot processes provides the filtration barrier (Fig. 6.3.4).

In the flame cell the whole system works in reverse order. The inner and outer rods on the flame cell barrel form the equivalent of the interdigitating feet of the podocytes. There is no exact equivalent to the glomerular basement membrane but the flocculent material between the outer rods may serve an exclusion function (Fig. 6.4.2). The extracellular desmosomal zipper that holds the interdigitating rods of the flame cell barrel in place becomes the real molecular filtration barrier. Suction pressure, equivalent in magnitude to the positive pressure of the glomerular capillary then draws in interstitial fluids and solutes but excludes macromolecules. Two single-cell studies have isolated schistosome flame cells and sequenced their transcriptome (Wendt *et al.*, 2020; Attenborough *et al.*, 2024). Remarkably, a nephrin (Smp_130070), cadherins (Smp_336370 and Smp_165520) and a membrane-associated guanylate kinase (Smp_337580) were identified. It is important not to take this analogy too far, but it does appear that glomerular filtration based on positive pressure and flame cell function based on suction pressure may have much in common.

Immunocytochemical staining unsurprisingly reveals that tubulins are abundant within the flagella of the flame, but also that the barrel itself stains strongly with phalloidin, indicating the presence of an F-actin cytoskeleton (Fig. 6.4.1) (Bahia *et al.*, 2006; Collins *et al.*, 2011). The actin neatly explains the very dense core inside the bounding plasma membrane of both inner and outer rods, providing a basis for their rigidity (Fig. 6.2.2). Another feature of the rod region is that it binds labelled peanut agglutinin very strongly (Fig. 6.4.2). The molecular target of the lectin is Gal-β(1–3)-GalNAc, a core structure in *O*-glycosylated mucins. These molecules form

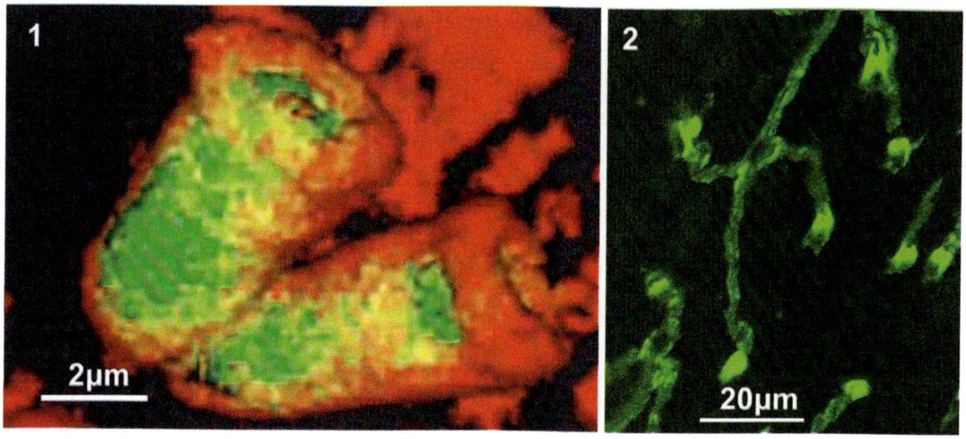

Fig. 6.4. Immunocytochemistry of the flame cell. **1**) Flame cell barrel visualized by staining with phalloidin for F-actin (red) and the tuft of flagella stained with α-tubulin (green) in *S. mansoni*. **2**) Flame cell bodies and the proximal tubules stained with FITC-labelled peanut agglutinin lectin. A high concentration of glycans is revealed in the interdigitating rod region. (**1** from Bahia *et al.*, 2006; **2** from Skelly *et al.*, 2014.) **1**) Figure used with permission from Cambridge University Press. **2**) Figure used under license CC-BY-4.0.

viscoelastic barriers at epithelial surfaces resisting the flow of fluids. The intense lectin staining of the flocculent material between the outer rods (Fig. 6.2.2) indicates a mucin-type deposit. It is also worth noting that the putative schistosome nephrin is predicted by the NetOGlyc server (https://services.healthtech.dtu.dk/services/NetOGlyc-4.0) to bear multiple *O*-glycosylation sites.

The two sequenced flame cell transcriptomes (Wendt *et al.*, 2020; Attenborough *et al.*, 2024) contain a rich diversity of α- and β-tubulins, dynein and kinesin motor proteins, intraflagellar transport proteins, centrosome components and ciliary rootletins. This is exactly as expected for cells with functional cilia/flagella. At present no innervation of flame cells has been reported, so it is unclear whether their activity is autonomous, or under physiological control. However, it is intriguing that flame cells isolated from adult worms (Wendt *et al.*, 2020) were found to express transcripts for FMRFamide (Smp_157640 and Smp_153200), glutamate (Smp_153780) and dopamine (Smp_202470) receptors. Does this imply the existence of external control? Note that the observations were not replicated in the miracidial transcriptome (Attenborough *et al.*, 2024).

6.4 The Tubule Cells

6.4.1 Layout

In adult worms the individual flame cells are scattered throughout the parenchyma, perhaps as close as 20 μm or as far as 100 μm from the nearest neighbour (Fig. 6.5.1) (Skelly *et al.*,

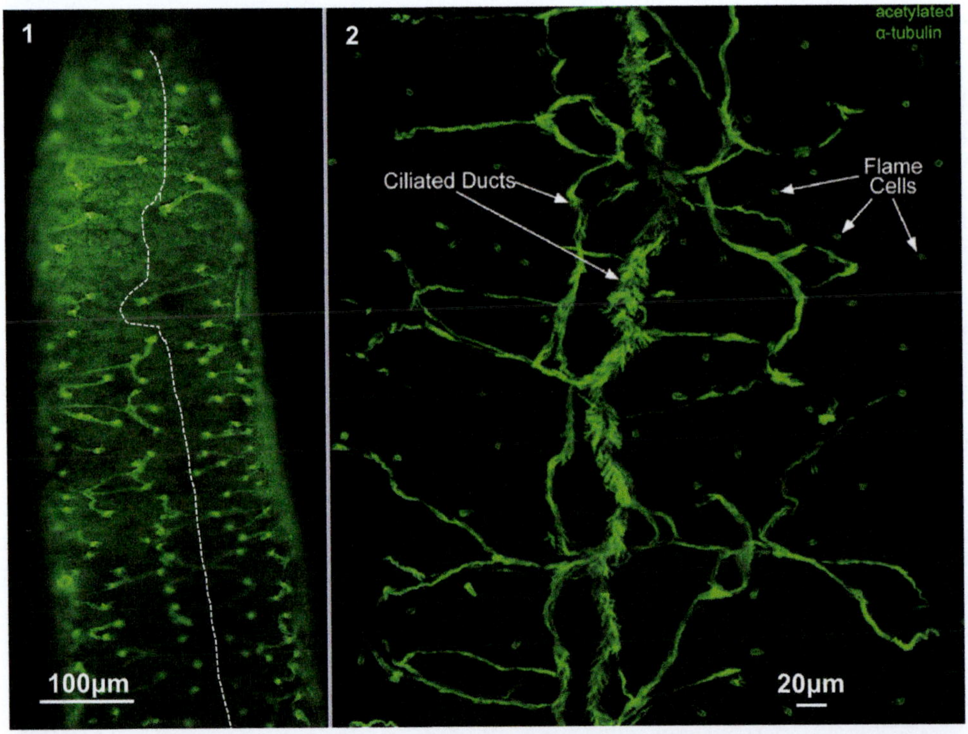

Fig. 6.5. Layout of the system. **1**) Dorsal view of a female *S. japonicum* adult showing the distribution of flame cells and proximal tubules stained with FITC-labelled peanut agglutinin. The dashed line is the boundary between right and left drainage. **2**) Maximum intensity projection depicting anti-acetylated α-tubulin staining of the ciliated (flagellated?) regions of the collecting ducts in the male protonephridial system of *S. mansoni*. Two main ducts appear to run along the longitudinal axis. (**1** courtesy of Dr Xiao-Hong Li, WHO, Geneva, Switzerland; **2** from Collins *et al.*, 2011.)

2014). This density means that the interstitial spaces of males and females are drained by hundreds, even thousands of flame cells in the >1 cm long worms. There is a sharp distinction between the network of tubules immediately downstream of each flame cell, visualized with peanut agglutinin lectin, and the main tubules and collecting ducts which react with antibody to acetylated tubulin (Fig. 6.5.2) (Collins *et al.*, 2011), but the reason for the dichotomy is unclear. The walls of these tubules and main ducts also bear ~10 μm flagella projecting into the lumen. Given the small tubule dimensions, it seems likely that they beat with an undulatory rather than orthogonal motion.

6.4.2 Structure

The first tubule cell, which contributes to the cytoplasmic cup and interdigitating rods of the flame cell wrapped around the tuft of flagella, is sealed at its margins by a desmosome. Similarly, the tubules themselves are flattened cytoplasmic projections arising from the tubule cell, joined where their tips meet by a desmosome (Fig. 6.6.1). The lumen of the tubule is thus extracellular, which must have implications for tubule biochemical processes. Certainly, in this position the luminal projections are rudimentary and numerous small vesicles are present in the cytoplasm, perhaps indicative of secretion of macromolecules into the lumen. The desmosome runs like a zipper along the whole length of the tubule, at least until another tubule cell is reached (Fig. 6.6.2). Here, the images are not clear enough to settle the question, but the tubule cell cytoplasm contains aggregates of small vesicles with dense contents, which could be further indication of macromolecule secretion. In the larger collecting ducts (~5 μm diameter), the luminal surface is extended by numerous lamellae (~1 μm long), plus scattered flagella projecting into the lumen (Fig. 6.6.3). It was suggested that in the liver fluke (*F. hepatica*) the collecting ducts were syncytial (Gallagher and Threadgold, 1967) but the situation in schistosomes is unclear. These ducts, with a surface area extended by lamellae, appear more suited to transmembrane transport of solutes rather than vesicular secretion. The function of the flagella is presumably to drive the fluid towards the major ducts and the terminal excretory pore, essential because unlike the alimentary tract and reproductive system, the nephridial tubules do not have any associated musculature. In cross-section, microtubules can be seen distributed throughout the cytoplasm of the collecting duct wall (Fig. 6.6.3), their longitudinal orientation presumably providing elasticity and support to maintain a circular profile. The main longitudinal ducts are much wider (~20 μm diameter) (Fig. 6.6.4 and 6.6.5) with numerous projecting lamellae up to 2 μm long, while the flagella appear to be grouped into tufts in the duct wall. The very thinness of the wall (~0.5 μm) means little space for synthetic processes, suggesting the ducts have a mainly fluid conduction role. As is evident in the tapeworm *Hymenolepis diminuta* (Webster, 1971), the peristaltic movements reported for *S. mansoni in vivo* (Yeh *et al.*, 2024) (see Chapter 4) probably have a considerable impact on excretory fluid movement down the main canals. Analogies have been drawn between the main ducts and the proximal tubule of the mammalian kidney (Sato *et al.*, 2002) but there is no morphological equivalent of a brush border to support the idea.

6.4.3 Inferences about function

The actions of the flame cell to filter fluid from the interstitial spaces of the schistosome body and propel it down the barrel towards the tubules provides the context for the next question. What are the functions of the tubules and collecting ducts and how are they performed? An obstacle to answering this is a lack of established techniques for exploring the excretory activity of the protonephridia (Sato *et al.*, 2002). There are marked differences in morphology from the larger tubules of the tapeworm *H. diminuta*, which bear short microvilli. The importance of these tubules in regulating glucose resorption by a carrier-mediated mechanism, and lactate and urea levels by passive diffusion, has been demonstrated in the tapeworm (Webster, 1972). We have no similar information for schistosomes and, given the fact that they are bathed in and feed on isotonic nutrient-rich medium, a major role in the regulation of ion and nutrient balance seems unlikely. There is one other function of mammalian proximal tubules that might be

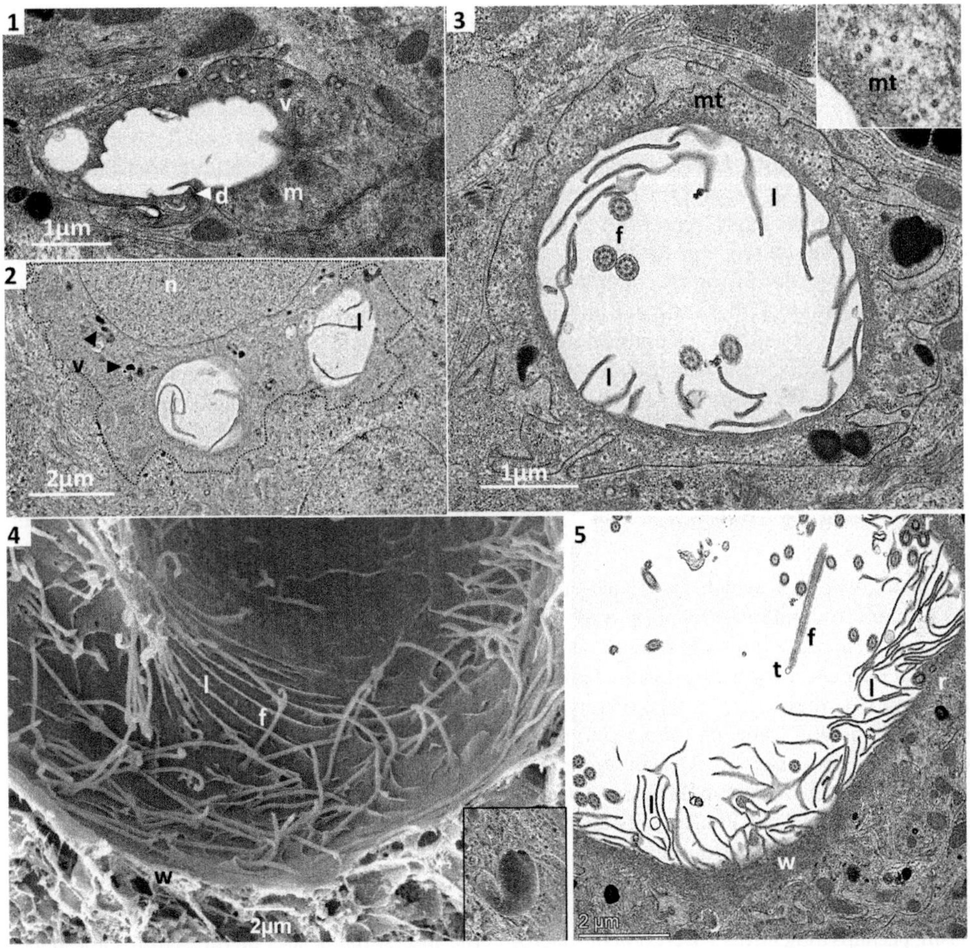

Fig. 6.6. Ultrastructure of the *S. japonicum* nephridial canals. **1**) Tubule leading from a flame cell with cytoplasm containing mitochondria (m) and numerous vesicles (v). A desmosome (d) is visible, confirming that the lumen is extracellular. **2**) A portion of a tubule cell further down the system, with nucleus (n), tubules with surface lamellae (l) and clusters of vesicles (arrowed) with dense contents. **3**) A larger collecting duct with luminal lamellae and flagella. The dense layer cytoplasm beneath the luminal membrane may represent a cytoskeleton, while the remainder of the wall is reinforced by microtubules (inset at high magnification). **4**) SEM looking down a main collecting duct in the anterior of a male, revealing the thin wall (w), surface lamellae and flagella with hooked tips. **5**) TEM through a thin collecting duct wall showing the insertion of lamellae. The flagella rootlets are grouped in tufts on the duct wall (r) and a flagellum with a hollow tip (t) is visible. Figure author's own.

relevant, and for which there is some experimental evidence, namely the excretion of toxic chemicals inimical to life, sometimes referred to as xenobiotics. In the mammalian renal tubule cell this is a two-step process mediated by uptake transporters on basal and lateral membranes, and efflux transporters on the luminal membranes. Multidrug resistance protein 1 (MDR-1; also known as P-glycoprotein) is one such efflux transporter and multidrug resistance protein 2 (MRP-2) is a second; both are ATP-binding cassette exporters (George *et al.*, 2017).

The functional presence of a schistosome MDR-1 was investigated in adult worms using a fluorescent marker resorufin (235 Da) as a potential substrate (Sato *et al.*, 2002). The compound was taken up across the tegument and became concentrated in the excretory tubules

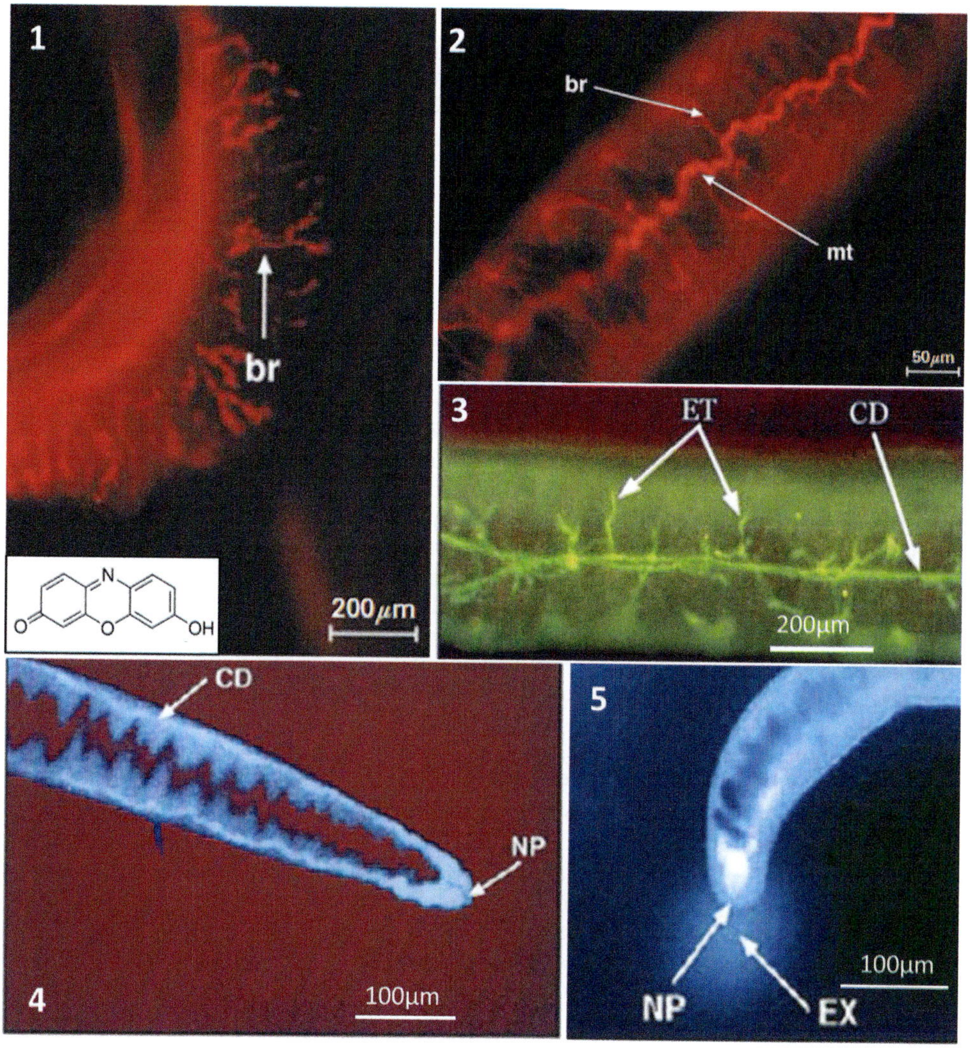

Fig. 6.7. Functional properties of the tubules. **1**) Adult male incubated with resorufin (inset). The branched collecting ducts (br) have become positive as the compound is cleared from the tissues. **2**) Adult female showing the main collecting ducts (mt) are strongly positive. **3**) Male worm exposed to CFDA, showing accumulation of the fluorescent dye in the side excretory tubules (ET) and main collecting ducts (CD). **4**) Female worm exposed to monochlorobimane that has become fluorescent after conjugation to glutathione. The main collecting ducts (CD) are clearly visible. **5**) Female after the same treatment showing the terminal bladder, with a puff of fluorescence being expelled (EX) from the nephridiopore (NP). (**1** and **2** from Sato *et al.*, 2002; **3–5** from Sato *et al.*, 2004.) Figures used with permission from Cambridge University Press.

(Fig. 6.7.1 and 6.7.2) and by an energy-dependent mechanism, before excretion via the nephridiopore. Moreover, a variety of modulators known to interfere with MDR-1 activity also perturbed resorufin excretion from male adult schistosomes, including cyclosporin A, Ro11-2933, verapamil and nifedipine. It was notable that when carbachol was added to paralyse worms in culture, the excretion of resorufin from the protonephridial system was inhibited, leading to the conclusion that contractions of the body musculature drive fluid expulsion. Without muscular paralysis, resorufin was concentrated in the tubules and periodically ejected through the excretory pore. In a second study (Sato *et al.*, 2004) the functional existence of an MRP efflux pump that expels organic anions, including glutathione conjugates, was tested using monochlorobimane (227 Da). The conjugate of this compound with glutathione is brightly fluorescent and serves as a marker for efflux. Worms incubated with monochlorobimane became strongly fluorescent within 1 h; subsequently the main collecting ducts of both males and females were clearly delineated by glutathione bimane, indicating the presence of the MRP pump (Fig. 6.7.4). The tiny vesicular bladder became visible, and periodically a cloud of fluorescence was emitted from the excretory pore (Fig. 6.7.5). It is worth recording that a second substrate of MRP, 5(6)-carboxyfluorescein diacetate (CFDA), also delineated the main collecting ducts and some side channels but did not reach upstream to the flame cells, suggesting a restricted distribution for the MRP pump (Fig. 6.7.3).

It is important to stress that the above functional studies on *S. mansoni* were performed before publication of transcriptome or genome assemblies (Verjovski-Almeida *et al.*, 2003; Berriman *et al.*, 2009). However, interrogation of the current versions of the genome and UniProt database identifies five genes with plausible annotations to MDR-1 or MRP-2 (Smp_089200, Smp_137080, Smp_055780, Smp_063000 and Smp_336100). Expression of these genes is recorded in a variety of tissues after single-cell sequencing (Wendt *et al.*, 2020; Attenborough *et al.*, 2024), although not in flame cells. It seems unlikely that the nephridial tubules, given their ramifying structure, were recovered intact for sequencing. The above genes provide a good starting point for *in situ* hybridization and immunocytochemical studies that would enlarge our scant knowledge of protonephridial tubule function.

There is one other aspect of tubule function that deserves investigation. Mammalian nephron tubules primarily function to salvage small and large molecules from the filtrate, rather than behaving as secretory cells. However, two studies have highlighted a potential protein secretion process by the main protonephridial tubules. In the first, the demonstration of protein disulfide isomerase mRNA expression in the gastrodermis and protonephridial tubules of adult worms provided a strong biomarker for the occurrence of protein synthesis and export in both tissues (Fig. 6.8.1) (Finken *et al.*, 1994). The function of the enzyme is to catalyse isomerization of intramolecular disulfide/sulfhydryl bonds, required for correct folding of nascent polypeptides in the endoplasmic reticulum, prior to their packaging in the Golgi apparatus for secretion. It was also discovered that *S. mansoni* expresses a second member of the protein disulfide isomerase family, namely ER-60 cysteine protease (Fig. 6.8.2) (Finken-Eigen and Kunz, 1997). This protein is also retained in the lumen of the endoplasmic reticulum, where it serves as a protein degradation system. These observations provide biochemical evidence for protein export or surface plasma membrane turnover, by the tubules.

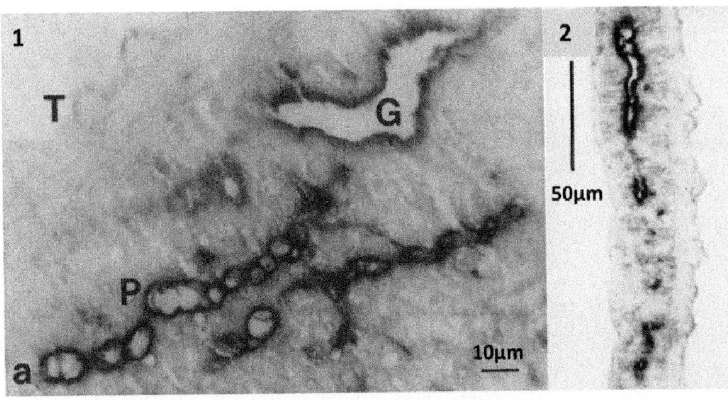

Fig. 6.8. Evidence for protein synthesis in the tubules. **1**) Localization of protein disulfide isomerase mRNA in the protonephridial canals (P) and the gastrodermis (G) of a male schistosome, by *in situ* hybridization. **2**) Localization of ER-60 cysteine protease mRNA in the main canals by *in situ* hybridization. (**1** from Finken *et al.*, 1994; **2** from Finken-Eigen and Kunz, 1997.) Figures used with permission from Elsevier.

6.5 Summary

- The solid body structure of schistosomes, through which the protonephridial system ramifies in all stages, makes experimentation even more difficult than for the nervous system.
- Morphologically the system has three components: (i) the 'flame cell', a composite structure made from a cap cell and the first tubule cell; (ii) the finer tubules which appear to have a desmosomal zipper, plus their associated cells, and (iii) the thin-walled, flagellated collecting ducts terminating in a minuscule bladder and nephridiopore.
- To understand the mechanism of filtration, analogies can be made with glomerular filtration in the mammalian kidney, but in reverse. Synchronous undulatory beating of the flagellar tuft drives fluid from base to tip creating a suction pressure inside the barrel. The extracellular desmosomal zipper that binds the interdigitations of cap cell and tube cell together is the equivalent of the slit diaphragm in the glomerulus, providing the molecular filter. It is potentially aided by the external layer of polysaccharide around the barrel, forming a hydration barrier.
- The vesicular cytoplasm of the finer tubules is suggestive of secretory process adding material to the lumen. The much thinner wall in the main ducts, extended by projecting luminal lamellae, is more indicative of solute transport processes potentially recovering valuable salts and metabolic intermediates.
- Early experiments with fluorescent substrates strongly support a detoxifying role for the protonephridia in adults, mediated by multidrug resistance proteins. This deserves reinvestigation using confocal microscopy to localize expression of genes and proteins at high resolution.
- A method for collecting protonephridial fluids for analysis, uncontaminated by alimentary tract or tegument products is very desirable but represents a real challenge.

References

Attenborough, T., Rawlinson, K.A., Diaz Soria, C.L., Ambridge, K., Sankaranarayanan, G. *et al.* (2024) A single-cell atlas of the miracidium larva of *Schistosoma mansoni* reveals cell types, developmental pathways, and tissue architecture. *eLife* 13, RP95628. DOI: 10.7554/eLife.95628

Bahia, D., Avelar, L.G.A., Vigorosi, F., Cioli, D., Oliveira, G.C. *et al.* (2006) The distribution of motor proteins in the muscles and flame cells of the *Schistosoma mansoni* miracidium and primary sporocyst. *Parasitology* 133(3), 321–329. DOI: 10.1017/S0031182006000400

Berriman, M., Haas, B.J., LoVerde, P.T., Wilson, R.A., Dillon, G.P. *et al.* (2009) The genome of the blood fluke *Schistosoma mansoni*. *Nature* 460(7253), 352–358. DOI: 10.1038/nature08160

Castro-Borges, W., Simpson, D.M., Dowle, A., Curwen, R.S., Thomas-Oates, J. *et al.* (2011) Abundance of tegument surface proteins in the human blood fluke *Schistosoma mansoni* determined by QconCAT proteomics. *Journal of Proteomics* 74(9), 1519–1533. DOI: 10.1016/j.jprot.2011.06.011

Collins, J.J., King, R.S., Cogswell, A., Williams, D.L. and Newmark, P.A. (2011) An atlas for *Schistosoma mansoni* organs and life-cycle stages using cell type-specific markers and confocal microscopy. *PLoS Neglected Tropical Diseases* 5(3), e1009. DOI: 10.1371/journal.pntd.0001009

de Water, R., Fransen, J.A., Schut, D.W. and Deelder, A.M. (1987) Three monoclonal antibodies with specific binding activity to the excretory system of *Schistosoma mansoni*: an immunoelectron microscopic study using the gold labeling technique. *The American Journal of Tropical Medicine and Hygiene* 37(2), 345–352. DOI: 10.4269/ajtmh.1987.37.345

Faghiri, Z. and Skelly, P.J. (2009) The role of tegumental aquaporin from the human parasitic worm, *Schistosoma mansoni*, in osmoregulation and drug uptake. *FASEB Journal* 23(8), 2780–2789. DOI: 10.1096/fj.09-130757

Faghiri, Z., Camargo, S.M.R., Huggel, K., Forster, I.C., Ndegwa, D. *et al.* (2010) The tegument of the human parasitic worm *Schistosoma mansoni* as an excretory organ: the surface aquaporin SmAQP is a lactate transporter. *PLoS ONE* 5(5), e10451. DOI: 10.1371/journal.pone.0010451

Finken, M., Sobek, A., Symmons, P. and Kunz, W. (1994) Characterization of the complete protein disulfide isomerase gene of *Schistosoma mansoni* and identification of the tissues of its expression. *Molecular and Biochemical Parasitology* 64(1), 135–144. DOI: 10.1016/0166-6851(94)90141-4

Finken-Eigen, M. and Kunz, W. (1997) *Schistosoma mansoni*: gene structure and localization of a homologue to cysteine protease ER 60. *Experimental Parasitology* 86(1), 1–7. DOI: 10.1006/expr.1996.4123

Gallagher, S.S.E. and Threadgold, L.T. (1967) Electron-microscope studies of *Fasciola hepatica* II. The interrelationship of the parenchyma with other organ systems. *Parasitology* 57(4), 627–632. DOI: 10.1017/S0031182000073091

George, B., You, D., Joy, M.S. and Aleksunes, L.M. (2017) Xenobiotic transporters and kidney injury. *Advanced Drug Delivery Reviews* 116, 73–91. DOI: 10.1016/j.addr.2017.01.005

Gilpin, W., Bull, M.S. and Prakash, M. (2020) The multiscale physics of cilia and flagella. *Nature Reviews Physics* 2(2), 74–88. DOI: 10.1038/s42254-019-0129-0

Greka, A. and Mundel, P. (2012) Cell biology and pathology of podocytes. *Annual Review of Physiology* 74, 299–323. DOI: 10.1146/annurev-physiol-020911-153238

Howells, R.E. (1969) Observations on the nephridial system of the cestode *Moniezia expansa* (Rud., 1805). *Parasitology* 59(2), 449–459. DOI: 10.1017/s0031182000082408

Kümmel, G. (1958) The terminal organ of protonephridia, fine structure & explanation of their function. *Zeitschrift für Naturforschung. Teil B, Chemie, Biochemie, Biophysik, Biologie und Verwandte Gebiete* 13B(10), 677–679.

Lawrence, J.D. (1973) The ingestion of red blood cells by *Schistosoma mansoni*. *The Journal of Parasitology* 59(1), 60–63. DOI: 10.2307/3278572

Mundel, P. (2017) Podocytes and the quest for precision medicines for kidney diseases. *Pflügers Archiv* 469(7–8), 1029–1037. DOI: 10.1007/s00424-017-2015-x

Mundel, P. and Kriz, W. (1995) Structure and function of podocytes: an update. *Anatomy and Embryology* 192(5), 385–397. DOI: 10.1007/BF00240371

Pan, S.C. (1980) The fine structure of the miracidium of *Schistosoma mansoni*. *Journal of Invertebrate Pathology* 36(3), 307–372. DOI: 10.1016/0022-2011(80)90040-3

Pappenheimer, J.R. (1953) Passage of molecules through capillary walls. *Physiological Reviews* 33(3), 387–423. DOI: 10.1152/physrev.1953.33.3.387

Pavenstädt, H. and Bek, M. (2002) Podocyte electrophysiology, *in vivo* and *in vitro*. *Microscopy Research and Technique* 57(4), 224–227. DOI: 10.1002/jemt.10078

Rodewald, R. and Karnovsky, M.J. (1974) Porous substructure of the glomerular slit diaphragm in the rat and mouse. *The Journal of Cell Biology* 60(2), 423–433. DOI: 10.1083/jcb.60.2.423

Sato, H., Kusel, J.R. and Thornhill, J. (2002) Functional visualization of the excretory system of adult *Schistosoma mansoni* by the fluorescent marker resorufin. *Parasitology* 125(6), 527–535. DOI: 10.1017/s0031182002002536

Sato, H., Kusel, J.R. and Thornhill, J. (2004) Excretion of fluorescent substrates of mammalian multidrug resistance-associated protein (MRP) in the *Schistosoma mansoni* excretory system. *Parasitology* 128(1), 43–52. DOI: 10.1017/s0031182003004177

Skelly, P.J., Da'dara, A.A., Li, X.H., Castro-Borges, W. and Wilson, R.A. (2014) *Schistosome* feeding and regurgitation. *PLoS Pathogens* 10(8), e1004246. DOI: 10.1371/journal.ppat.1004246

Verjovski-Almeida, S., DeMarco, R., Martins, E.A.L., Guimarães, P.E.M., Ojopi, E.P.B. *et al.* (2003) Transcriptome analysis of the acoelomate human parasite *Schistosoma mansoni*. *Nature Genetics* 35(2), 148–157. DOI: 10.1038/ng1237

Webster, L.A. (1971) The flow of fluid in the protonephridial canals of *Hymenolepis diminuta*. *Comparative Biochemistry and Physiology Part A: Physiology* 39(4), 785–793. DOI: 10.1016/0300-9629(71)90200-3

Webster, L.A. (1972) Absorption of glucose, lactate and urea from the protonephridial canals of *Hymenolepis diminuta*. *Comparative Biochemistry and Physiology Part A: Physiology* 41(4), 861–868. DOI: 10.1016/0300-9629(72)90348-9

Wendt, G., Zhao, L., Chen, R., Liu, C., O'Donoghue, A.J. *et al.* (2020) A single-cell RNA-seq atlas of *Schistosoma mansoni* identifies a key regulator of blood feeding. *Science* 369(6511), 1644–1649. DOI: 10.1126/science.abb7709

Wilson, R.A. (1969) The fine structure of the protonephridial system in the miracidium of *Fasciola hepatica*. *Parasitology* 59(2), 461–467. DOI: 10.1017/s003118200008241x

Wilson, R.A. and Webster, L.A. (1974) Protonephridia. *Biological Reviews of the Cambridge Philosophical Society* 49(2), 127–160. DOI: 10.1111/j.1469-185x.1974.tb01572.x

Yeh, Y.-T., Del Álamo, J.C. and Caffrey, C.R. (2024) Biomechanics of parasite migration within hosts. *Trends in Parasitology* 40(2), 164–175. DOI: 10.1016/j.pt.2023.12.001

7

The Tegument and Immune Evasion

7.1 Overview

The tegument is one of the two major interfaces between the adult worms and the host bloodstream. It is a living syncytial layer of cytoplasm, a few microns thick, covering the entire surface. Since schistosomes are long lived in their mammalian host, the tegument must have some very special properties that enable them to survive in such a potentially hostile environment. It is not simply a matter of effective disguise. Paradoxically, especially in male worms, the tegument surface is also an important site of nutrient uptake and fluid regulation. In this chapter, the way in which the parasite balances these conflicting demands is examined in detail. Cellular organization, the structure and composition of the syncytial surface, transport processes and evasion strategies are considered. Attention is also given to controversies and gaps in our knowledge.

7.2 Layout of the Tegument

7.2.1 The contribution of ultrastructural investigations

Historically, the surface of adult trematodes was described as covered by a secreted cuticle, synthesized by mesenchymal cells lying beneath the muscles of the body wall (Hyman, 1951). The development of the electron microscope and associated tissue preparation techniques radically changed perceptions. In 1963, the surface of the liver fluke (*Fasciola hepatica*) was described as a layer of 'protoplasm', an extension of nucleated cell bodies lying deep in the parenchyma, for which the term 'tegument' was adopted (Threadgold, 1963). A detailed investigation of the *Schistosoma mansoni* tegument followed, establishing important features of the tegument cytoplasm, the associated cell bodies, and the microtubule-lined cytoplasmic connections between the two (Fig. 7.1.1 and 7.1.2) (Morris and Threadgold, 1968). Scanning electron microscopy also revealed that the surface of the tegument was pitted in both sexes. The male dorsal surface was covered with spiny tubercles (see Chapter 4) but the male ventral surface and the entire female were much less spiny. The spines were entirely contained within the tegument plasma membranes (Fig. 7.1.3), and the tips appeared deformable on contact with another worm or a blood vessel. The first accounts of the tegument noted nothing unusual about the outer surface plasma membrane of the syncytium but recorded that the basal membrane was highly invaginated, lying over a fibrous basal lamella (Morris and Threadgold, 1968). The dense glycan-rich cytoplasm contained two membrane-bound inclusions, given various names

DOI: 10.1079/9781800625167.0007

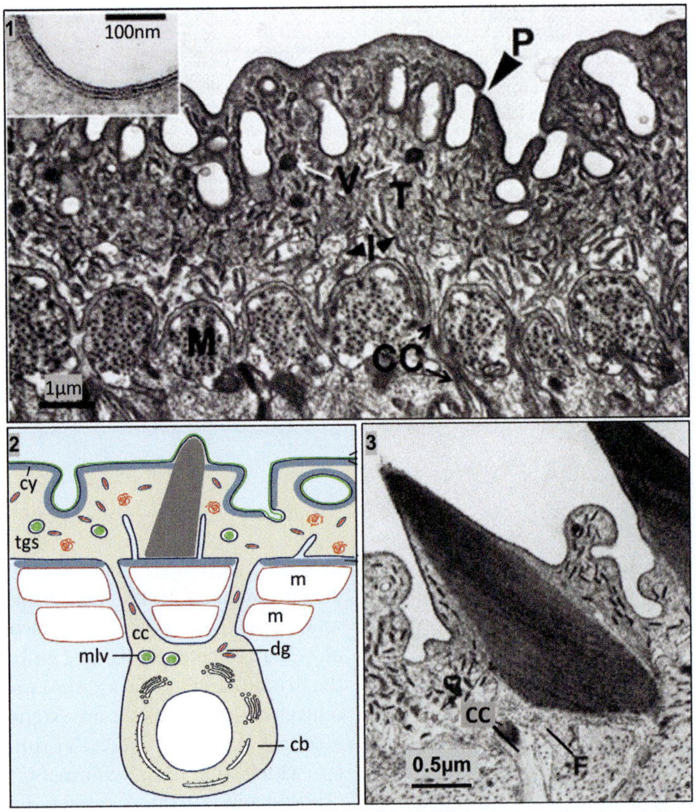

Fig. 7.1. Layout of the tegument. **1**) TEM of male ventral surface. T, tegument cytosol; P, surface pits; V, vesicles; I, basal invaginations; CC, cytoplasmic connections; M, muscle. Inset, multilaminate surface. **2**) Diagram showing the relationship of the tegument syncytium to the cell bodies beneath the body wall muscles. mlv, multilaminate vesicle; dg, discoid granule; cy, cytoskeleton; tgs, tegument ground substance. **3**) Tegument spine entirely enclosed within the syncytium and anchored basally on an extracellular fibrous layer, F. CC, cytoplasmic connection. (**1** from Skelly *et al.*, 2014; **3** from Morris and Threadgold, 1968.) **1**) Figure used under license CC-BY-4.0. **2**) Figure author's own. **3**) Figure used with permission from KGL.

by researchers, but hereafter referred to as discoid bodies and multilaminate vesicles (Wilson and Barnes, 1974). Additionally, a few scattered mitochondria were present but there was no evidence for ribosomes or protein synthetic machinery. Two important points related to current controversies, are that worm pairs fixed immediately after recovery by dissection (not perfusion) showed no evidence of vesicle secretion. Similarly, while tracer molecules, used *in vivo* and *in vitro*, readily filled the tegument surface pits, they did not enter the cytoplasm by endocytosis (Morris and Threadgold, 1968; Smith and von Lichtenberg, 1974; Ernst, 1975; Carlisle and Weisberg, 1978).

The irregularly ovoid tegumental cell bodies (3–6 μm × 6–12 μm) lying beneath the body wall muscles, contained several Golgi bodies usually associated with one or other type of inclusion, while rough endoplasmic reticulum was sparse (Fig. 7.2.1) (Wilson and Barnes, 1974). Free ribosomes were present in the cytosol and bound to the outer nuclear membrane. This is not the structure commonly associated with classical secretory cells producing quantities of protein for export, but the frequency of Golgi bodies does indicate the packaging of material into the inclusions for transit to the tegument syncytium. It is worth emphasizing that in the absence of macromolecule biosynthetic capacity in the tegument, all the contents and membranes must derive from the cell bodies. The layout of cell bodies and syncytium is easiest to appreciate on the male ventral surface because the cytoplasmic connections, ~3 μm long, run through just two layers of muscle; on the dorsal surface they are from 8 to 30 μm long and follow a more tortuous path due to the multiple layers of longitudinal muscle they traverse. Sections tangential to the tegument surface through the underlying muscle layer indicate that the cytoplasmic connections are very abundant, relative to the cell bodies, perhaps as many as 50 per cell (Wilson and Barnes, 1974). The occurrence of the peripheral ring of microtubules in each connection is assumed to keep the lumen open for free passage of solutes, macromolecules and inclusions, and could also assist movement of inclusions using kinesin or dynein motors.

7.2.2 The multilaminate surface and the membranocalyx hypothesis

A keynote article in 1973 revealed that both larval and adult worms had an unusual multilaminate tegument surface, which the authors termed a heptalaminate membrane (Hockley and McLaren, 1973) (see Chapter 3 on cercarial metamorphosis). Importantly, this was revealed by the inclusion of uranyl acetate as part of worm fixation, which also stabilized the contents of the multilaminate vesicles. The obvious conclusion was that the multilaminate vesicles contributed to the multilaminate surface but the way in which they did this was not clear. One possibility considered was for a conveyer belt system, whereby the vesicles formed the inner surface, moving outwards to be sloughed off into the external environment. Importantly, the action of uranyl acetate revealed a differential stability between the multiple surface layers. In its absence, the organic solvents normally used for transmission electron microscopy (TEM) specimen preparation leached out most contents of the multilaminate vesicles but left its bounding membrane intact.

Based on the differing properties of vesicle contents and bounding membrane, an alternative interpretation of the complex tegument surface organization was developed (Wilson and Barnes, 1974). It was proposed that the syncytium was bounded by a conventional plasma membrane, over which the contents of the multilaminate vesicles were secreted as a 'membranocalyx', the equivalent of the glycocalyx in most animal cells. Given knowledge of the amphipathic nature of phospholipids in the eucaryotic plasma membrane then current, the authors argued that the tegument surface should be interpreted as a conventional lipid bilayer, overlain by a second secreted bilayer, also composed of amphipathic lipids (see Chapter 2 on metamorphosis). The fluid mosaic model (Singer and Nicolson, 1972) remains the best explanation for how lipids and proteins are organized in the plasma membrane of eucaryotic cells. The model incorporated integral membrane-spanning proteins (including transport channels), peripheral proteins associated with only one lipid layer, proteins with a lipid anchor and glycolipids. When originally proposed, the emphasis was on the freedom of these components to move laterally in the plane of the bilayer. Inevitably the model has been extended to accommodate membrane-associated cytoskeletal assemblies, extracellular matrix interactions, transmembrane signalling and specialized lipid-protein domains (Nicolson and Ferreira de Mattos, 2023). The model is now less fluid and more mosaic and dense than originally proposed. Nevertheless, it provides a suitable framework to interpret the surface plasma membrane of the schistosome tegument.

The 'membranocalyx' secreted over the plasma membrane is also a bilayer, but it has a fundamentally different origin. The fact that it can flow over the surface and be shed into the bloodstream suggests a considerable fluidity in the lateral plane, and that it also lacks the integral proteins that give a plasma membrane stability. In the rest of this chapter the membranocalyx model is used as a framework to explore tegument surface function. As a footnote, the two bilayers, and the gap between them are taken to constitute five layers, not the supposed seven of a heptalaminate surface.

7.2.3 The cytology of cell bodies and tegument syncytium

There are still many unanswered questions about the way in which the tegument cell bodies function, whether there may be one or two types

(Wilson and Barnes, 1974), or even a series of developmental stages as part of a turnover process (Wendt *et al.*, 2020). One thing was clear from early TEM studies, there were two types of Golgi body. One had a sprawling appearance and was involved in producing the multilaminate vesicles, the other was more compact and produced the discoid bodies; the two were seldom if ever observed in the same section. The scarcity of endoplasmic reticulum in the vicinity of either Golgi body type argues for a relatively subdued synthesis of secretory proteins for export (cf. gastrodermis; Chapter 8). The Golgi bodies themselves comprise the usual stack of cisternae and it must be assumed that the functions of glycan synthesis and lipid transport are more dominant than protein processing (Fig. 7.2.1). There are currently multiple models of Golgi function, such a cisternal progression versus stable compartments; it is unclear which best explains their role in the tegument cell body. Leaving that aside, each Golgi body is surrounded by a cloud of 30–70 nm transport vesicles responsible for moving products to vacuoles, which gradually increase in volume. The final step in vesicle formation is condensation that reduces the size to produce the mature inclusion for transport to the syncytium. This process is well illustrated for the multilaminate vesicle (Fig. 7.2.2–7.2.4). The early structural studies also provided some

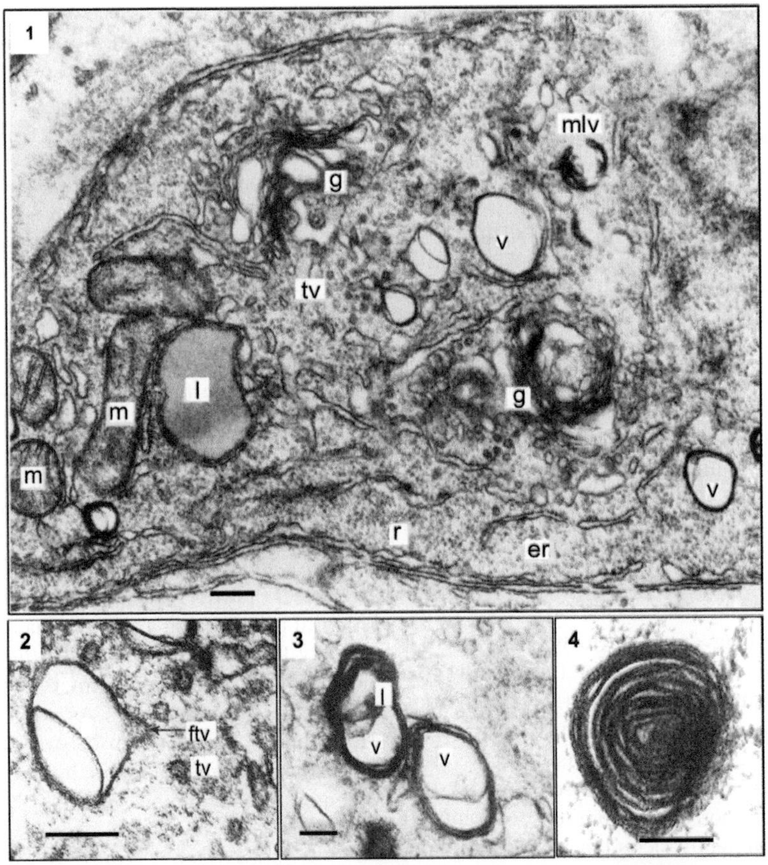

Fig. 7.2. Formation of multilaminate vesicles in a tegument cell body. **1**) TEM of cell body with sparse endoplasmic reticulum (er) and free ribosomes (r). Several mitochondria (m) and a lipid droplet (l) are also visible. Most of the region is occupied by two Golgi bodies (g), their associated transfer vesicles (tv) enlarging vacuoles (v) and one mature multilaminate vesicle (mlv). **2**) Higher magnification of an enlarging vacuole with a fusing transfer vesicle (ftv). **3**) Two much larger vacuoles (v) with whorls of lamellae (l), before condensation. **4**) A mature multilaminate vesicle with distinct and dense lamellae. Scale bars: 0.1 μm. (From Wilson and Barnes, 1974.) Figures used with permission from Cambridge University Press.

information about the multilaminate vesicle contents (Wilson and Barnes, 1974). The lamellae were 50% thicker than the leaflets of a normal plasma membrane, suggesting that they were not simple phospholipids, and they also had a greater electron density than plasma membrane leaflets. In contrast the contents had a slight reactivity for the PATCO (periodic acid–thiocarbohydrazine–osmium) technique, indicating the presence of some endogenous glycan. This was most apparent in vesicles leached with organic solvents and is consistent with the ability of the lectin concanavalin A to inhibit membranocalyx turnover (see below).

The second type of Golgi body associated with discoid body formation is more compact (Fig. 7.3.1). The stack of cisternae is still associated with the cloud of small transfer vesicles and fewer larger vacuoles that represent the nascent discoid bodies. When mature, these have a characteristic flattened appearance comprising a bounding plasma membrane beneath which lies a finely granular layer (Fig. 7.3.2). When tissues are prepared using the PATCO technique, their contents are strongly positive, as is glycogen in the neighbouring parenchyma cells (Fig. 3.3.3). However, while glycogen is removed by pre-treatment with α-amylase, the contents of the discoid bodies are not, emphasizing their glycan composition. There have been no reports of the discoid bodies closely associated with the surface plasma membrane of the tegument that might indicate the external secretion of their contents. Conversely, light microscope histochemistry has revealed that the whole tegument cytosol reacts strongly to periodic acid–Schiff (PAS) reagent, indicating abundant polysaccharide composition (Wheater and Wilson, 1976). As well as discoid bodies, there are also looser blobs of dense material 0.15–0.2 µm in diameter in the tegument, which likely derive from discoid bodies that have lost their bounding membranes and expanded their contents (Wilson and Barnes, 1974). The function of the discoid bodies would thus appear to be maintenance of the glycan-rich tegument cytosol. Since production of discoid bodies is continuous, a turnover process is implied. Despite recent biochemical and proteomic analyses, we still have little idea of the tegument glycan composition, which would provide an avenue to investigate such a process. It is worth recording that discoid bodies outnumber multilaminate vesicles by a ratio of 15:1 so this means a major aspect of tegument function is poorly understood.

7.2.4 Formation and turnover of the membranocalyx

The fusion of multilaminate vesicles with the tegument surface is a transient process that proved difficult to demonstrate. It occurs deep at the base of the tegument surface pits when a side channel briefly forms. The contained lamellae unfold into the channel, adhere to the membranes lining the pits and gradually slide up their sides (Fig. 7.4.1) (Wilson and Barnes, 1977).

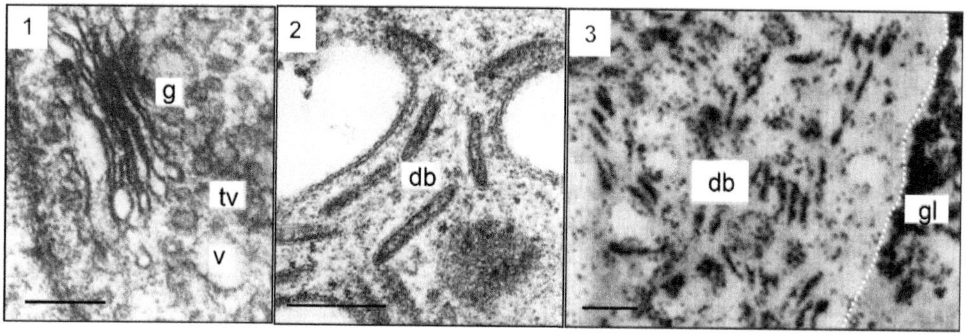

Fig. 7.3. Formation of discoid bodies. **1**) TEM of the more compact Golgi body (g) where discoid bodies are formed, with transfer vesicles (tv) and a forming vacuole (v). **2**) High magnification of mature discoid bodies (db) in the tegument syncytium, showing a dense layer beneath the membrane. **3**) Discoid bodies (db) in a tegument cell body stained by the PATCO technique for detection of glycans. Glycogen in a neighbouring parenchyma cell also stains intensely. Scale bars: 0.25 µm. (From Wilson and Barnes, 1974.) Figures used with permission from Cambridge University Press.

This arrangement has been most clearly described in the tegument of *Schistosoma mekongi* (Fig. 7.4) (Sobhon *et al.*, 1984). Here an additional feature, lucent vesicles with small peripheral membrane fragments, was interpreted as the spent remains of laminate vesicles that had discharged their contents. The question then remains as to how these spent vesicles are eliminated. Are the bounding membranes degraded in a manner suggested for the discoid body membranes, or are they recycled back to the Golgi bodies from which they originated?

The potential secretion of the membranocalyx over the surface of the tegument plasma membrane prompted the first experiments to measure its rate of turnover. The modified iron-containing protein complex, cationized ferritin, which binds stably to negative charges on *ex vivo* schistosomes, was used to measure the rate of shedding (Fig. 7.5.1–7.5.3) (Wilson and Barnes, 1977). Over a 4-h chase period at 37°C, fresh membranocalyx was secreted to displace the bound ferritin/membranocalyx complex up the pits, over the surface and spines, to be sloughed off into the medium. The estimated half-life of 2–3 h for this process must represent a maximum rate of turnover. The lectin concanavalin A, which also binds to the worm surface, had the opposite effect, 'freezing' the lamellae within the vesicles so that they failed to unroll and spread over the surface pits. The result was an accumulation of up to eight aggregated vesicle contents in a single pit (Fig. 7.5.4). This observation confirms the presence of endogenous α-d-mannosyl and/or α-d-glucosyl residues on the external surfaces of the membranocalyx, before contact with host plasma/cells. The ability of the membranocalyx to acquire host components (see Section 7.2.6) was also used in a solid phase radioimmune assay to measure its turnover (Saunders *et al.*, 1987). Adult worms from mice were surgically transferred to the portal vein of hamsters and then subsequently recovered at intervals to measure the rate of loss of mouse components from the tegument surface; the half-life was 5.4 days. The turnover of the membranocalyx suggests a mechanism for ridding the surface of bound immune components or cells. However, *in vivo*, the tegument surface does not bind host leucocytes (Keating *et al.*, 2006) and it has proved difficult to get antibodies to bind to known surface membrane proteins in living undamaged worms, even though a surface localization can be demonstrated on cryosections.

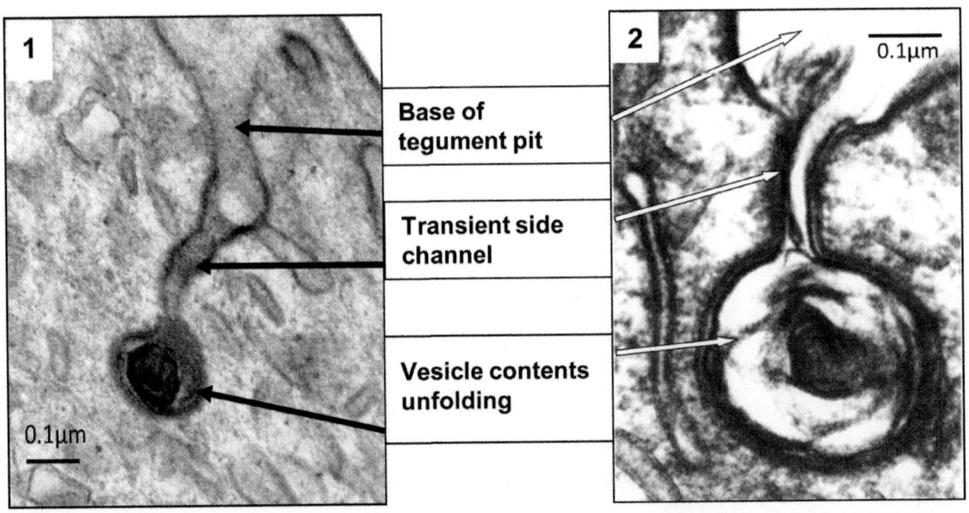

Fig. 7.4. Secretion of the membranocalyx. **1**) *S. mansoni* transient channel lined with membranocalyx as it flows to the base of a tegument pit. **2**) *S. mekongi* multilaminate vesicle with lamellae unfolding into the side channel and flowing up into the pit. (**1** from Wilson and Barnes, 1977, **2** from Sobhon *et al.*, 1984.) Figures used with permission from Cambridge University Press.

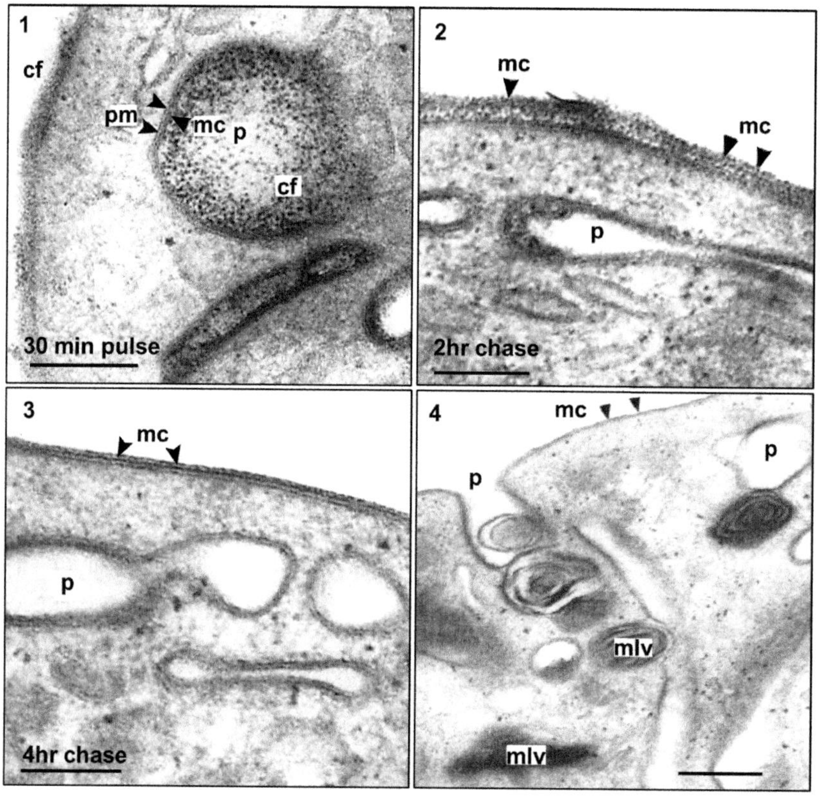

Fig. 7.5. Stimulated shedding of the membranocalyx. **1**) Labelling of the tegument surface and pits (p) with a 30-min pulse of cationized ferritin (cf). Plasma membrane (pm). **2**) A 2-h chase incubation in culture medium. Label is clearing from the pits (p) and layers of membranocalyx (mc) are visible on the surface. **3**) A 4-h chase incubation by which time the pits and surface are covered in fresh membranocalyx. **4**) Incubation of worms with the lectin concanavalin A has the opposite effect, preventing vesicles contents from unfolding so that turnover is blocked. Scale bars: 0.25 μm. (from Wilson and Barnes, 1977.) Figures used with permission from Cambridge University Press.

Perhaps we should view the membranocalyx as a relatively inert protective layer; definitive knowledge of its composition would be invaluable in this context.

7.2.5 Does internalization of the plasma membrane occur?

In general, following fusion of the bounding membrane of a vesicle with the plasma membrane, many secretory cells recycle the excess membrane back to the Golgi bodies for reuse or destruction in lysosomes (Farquhar, 1982). The failure to detect endocytosis of tracers at the tegument surface, mentioned in Section 7.2.1, seems to rule this out. Additionally, in the tegument syncytium there is no obvious or demonstrable continuity between surface and basal membranes that would allow for membrane flow. Consequently, membrane internalization would require a transient link between surface and basal compartments. A hint that this might occur was provided by experiments to label worms with the non-permeant styryl dye FM 1-43 (Ribeiro *et al.*, 1998). The dye appears to insert into the plasma membrane and was rapidly internalized into vesicles in a temperature-dependent process. This contrasted with the lipid compounds, amino fluorescein AF18 and BIODIPY FL sphingomyelin, which inserted only into the membranocalyx and were not internalized (Redman and Kusel, 1996). These experiments were performed before the availability of confocal microscopes and membrane internalization is a topic that would repay a new investigation.

7.2.6 Acquisition of host molecules on the surface

The first evidence that adult worms in the bloodstream were coated in host molecules (confusingly called host antigens) came from worm transfer experiments in rhesus macaques (Smithers *et al.*, 1969). When adult worms recovered from mice were transferred to the portal system of monkeys, previously immunized against mouse tissues, very few survived. This 'protection' was mediated by antibodies and led to the suggestion that schistosomes might disguise themselves with host molecules, thus preventing their rejection by the immune defences (Smithers *et al.*, 1969). Similar transfer experiments were also performed in hamsters immunized with mouse erythrocytes, with virtually all recipient mouse worms eliminated (Boyer *et al.*, 1977). The search was on for the molecular nature of these acquired host molecules. The high lipid content of the membranocalyx was noted above (see Section 7.2.2) and the amphipathic properties of the membranocalyx may thus provide a substratum for the acquisition of lipophilic components from the plasma, blood cells or vascular endothelium. The uptake of host glycolipid blood group antigens was demonstrated using *in vitro* co-culture of schistosomula with erythrocytes, but not the uptake of membrane-spanning glycoprotein blood groups (Goldring *et al.*, 1976). To date there has been no direct compositional demonstration of host glycolipids at the tegument surface, but after a 30-year interlude, proteomic analysis of the isolated surface membranes has revealed a list of host proteins, some with glycosylphosphatidylinositol (GPI) anchors but also the single membrane-spanning CD44 protein (see Section 7.4). The author's currently favoured hypothesis is that a lipid bilayer barrier overlying the plasma membrane, with its enzyme and transport capacities, provides both physical protection AND a substratum for acquisition of mixture of host molecules as an effective disguise. There are some intrinsic implications in this model that need to be resolved.

7.3 Transport Functions at the Tegument Surface

The importance of the tegument surface in nutrient uptake, especially in males, has long been appreciated. The female has a much greater capacity to ingest blood than the male, and it has been estimated that no cell in *S. mansoni* is more than ~40 μm from either gastrodermis or tegument syncytium. No part of the male body is more than ~40 μm from the tegument surface but the extreme edges of the flattened body are ~400 μm from the gastrodermis. Nutrient acquisition across the tegument must therefore dominate in the male (Skelly *et al.*, 2014). Conventional biochemical methods demonstrated the uptake of glucose across the tegument (Skelly *et al.*, 1998) and two glucose transporter proteins were characterized. The surface glucose transporter SGTP-4 mediates the facilitated diffusion across the surface and SGTP-1 across the basal plasma membrane of the tegument syncytium, taking glucose from the bloodstream into the syncytial cytosol and then onwards into the internal tissues (Skelly *et al.*, 1994) (see Table 7.1 for Smp annotations). In a similar approach, the uptake of a range of amino acids across the tegument was demonstrated (Chappell, 1974; Asch and Read, 1975), and one covalently linked heterodimer permease 1 (SPRM-1) has been characterized (Skelly *et al.*, 1999; Krautz-Peterson *et al.*, 2007). It consists of a 72 kDa heavy chain possessing a single transmembrane domain and a 55 kDa, multimembrane spanning, light chain (Smp_083990). When the system was reconstituted in *Xenopus* oocytes, the heavy chain was required for the surface localization of the light chain, which in turn controlled the specificity of amino acid uptake, particularly of basic amino acids (Skelly *et al.*, 1999; Krautz-Peterson *et al.*, 2007). The permease is present in the tegument surface complex, but also in other tissues and life cycle stages.

The potential involvement of aquaporins in the regulation of water balance was covered in Chapter 6 but to complete the picture, the characterization of an aquaporin (now Smp_300990) was reported in the tegument surface by biochemical techniques. The protein was predicted to contain six transmembrane domains as well as the conserved asparagine–proline–alanine motifs that are important in the formation of a water channel in a tetrameric confirmation. Both the N- and C-termini are predicted to be intracellular (Faghiri and Skelly, 2009) and the protein is localized to the surface membrane complex of the tegument syncytium (see Section 7.4.5), but not apparently the protonephridia. Reconstitution of the transport system in *Xenopus* oocytes revealed the capacity of the schistosome aquaporin pore to transport lactate, suggesting that this end-product of glycolysis is eliminated directly across the tegument into the bloodstream, especially across the male dorsal but not ventral surface (Faghiri *et al.*, 2010). Other transporters have been identified in tegument preparations by proteomics, especially ATPase-associated Na/K, calcium and cation transporters, as well as anion and potassium voltage-gated channels (see Section 7.4.5). However, functional studies are required to confirm that the actual transport processes occur across the tegument (Skelly *et al.*, 2014). The presence of exposed phosphohydrolases (see Section 7.6.2) that cleave exogenous nucleotide phosphates may be linked to the salvage of purines and pyrimidines as it appears they are not synthesized *de novo* (Levy and Read, 1975a, b). The identity of appropriate transporters in the tegument surface has yet to be established.

7.4 Isolation of the Tegument Surface and Analysis of Its Composition

With the realization that the tegument was a living syncytial layer, not an inert cuticle, attempts to isolate it began. The absence of lateral connections between the surface and basal membranes meant sheets of surface should be detachable from the worm body. The method eventually settled on in this author's laboratory was based on a freeze–thaw technique (Kusel, 1972), avoiding detergents in the initial steps that would leach proteins. The material released by this physical technique did indeed consist of sheets of membrane that could be purified by differential and density gradient centrifugation, standard techniques for membrane isolation at the time (Roberts *et al.*, 1983). The membrane preparation obtained was enriched 130 times in the surface enzyme marker alkaline phosphatase. However, there were limitations in the approach. Although the protein composition on one-dimensional electrophoretic separations was very different from whole worm homogenate, two-dimensional electrophoresis revealed the presence of tens to hundreds of components. Even more problematic, there was no simple way to obtain their identity. TEM of denuded worm bodies revealed a second drawback, namely that the freeze–thaw method also cleanly sliced off the basal invaginations, which co-purified with the surface membranes.

With the advent of molecular cloning techniques, a number of schistosome tegument proteins were characterized using mRNA isolation, the creation of cDNA libraries and their screening for protein expression, often with serum from supposedly immune hosts. This approach too had its pitfalls, not least rather uncritical choice of sera and imaginative localization techniques. However, it is fair to say that a number of putative surface constituents from *S. mansoni* identified by direct cloning are a testament to the hard slog of the researchers who persisted with their characterization (see Table 7.1 for Smp annotations). One of the first was an ATP-diphosphohydrolase (apyrase), detected on the tegument surface using enzymatic assays and immuno-electron microscopy (Vasconcelos *et al.*, 1993). The gene was eventually cloned and its protein product characterized (DeMarco *et al.*, 2003). A second enzyme, calpain, a Ca^{2+}-dependent cysteine protease not confined to the surface (Karcz *et al.*, 1991; Siddiqui *et al.*, 1993), is now a major vaccine candidate. A third enzyme, a novel ADP-ribosyl cyclase (a $NAD(P)^+$ catabolizing enzyme termed NACE) was a GPI-linked protein detected at the surface of adult schistosomes, which appeared not to be capable of generating cyclic nucleotides (Goodrich *et al.*, 2005). Lastly, a series of 'orphan' tegument proteins, Sm200, Sm25 (now Smp_346910), Sm13 and Sm29 were identified, the function of which remains largely unknown. Sm200, a GPI-anchored protein, not normally exposed in the intact worm, was unmasked after praziquantel treatment (Hall *et al.*, 1995). Sm25, a 25 kDa glycoprotein (Ali *et al.*, 1991), was unusual in being covalently modified by attachment of palmitic acid at the C-terminus to provide a stable interaction with the cytoplasmic leaflet of the lipid bilayer (Pearce *et al.*, 1991). Sm13 was suggested as an integral membrane protein of the tegument (Abath *et al.*, 2000). Finally, Sm29, identified in a transcriptome screen (Cardoso *et al.*, 2006a, b), was a membrane-linked surface glycoprotein, with 20 cysteine residues, suggesting up to 10 disulphide bridges and a tightly folded conformation. To varying degrees, these tegument surface proteins provided useful markers for later tegument surface membrane characterization.

7.4.1 The impact of proteomics – the key to compositional analysis

In the early 2000s technical developments in several fields converged to make protein identification much more straightforward (Ashton *et al.*, 2001). Advances in electrophoresis made the production of detailed maps of the hundreds to thousands of protein isoforms in a mixture possible, and developments in mass spectrometry meant that the protein in a gel spot could be identified. Initially this involved a diagnostic peptide mass fingerprint of a tryptic digest, which cleaves proteins at arginine (R) or lysine (K) residues, generated by matrix-assisted laser desorption and ionization-time of flight mass spectrometry (MALDI-ToF) (Curwen *et al.*, 2004). This was quickly superseded by the introduction of electrospray tandem mass spectrometers (MS/MS), where individual peptides in the fingerprint were subjected to fragmentation in a collision cell to produce a peptide sequence tag. Complex software then allowed the unequivocal identification of the tags by database searching. Fortuitously, in 2003 the transcriptomes of *S. mansoni* (Verjovski-Almeida *et al.*, 2003) and *Schistosoma japonicum* (Hu *et al.*, 2003) were published providing databases that made tegument proteomics possible. Two other developments have greatly augmented the impact of proteomics on schistosome cell biology, although it still lags behind transcriptome analysis in terms of sensitivity. The publication of the genome assemblies in 2009 and the use of high-performance liquid chromatography-electrospray MS/MS have meant that identification of thousands of proteins in a single sample is now possible. With this level of analytical power. Careful sample preparation is a paramount concern, or the data generated will differ little from an extract of the schistosome cytosol.

The first publication based on these technical advances used the freeze–thaw method (Roberts *et al.*, 1983) to generate a stripped tegument preparation and compared its protein composition with that of the stripped body (van Balkom *et al.*, 2005). A total of 740 proteins was identified, 222 in the tegument, 386 in the stripped bodies, 179 shared between the two and 43 enriched in the tegument only. Unfortunately, many of the proteins were annotated using databases that are no longer available so only those with GenBank accession numbers can be verified. What this initial study told us was that, as might be anticipated, most cellular processes occurring in the tegument are the same as those in the rest of the worm tissues. A second report used the same stripping approach, augmented by membrane purification on a density gradient to enrich for the surface marker alkaline phosphatase (Braschi *et al.*, 2006).

Initial analysis of the gradient pellet disappointingly revealed that cystosolic and cytoskeletal proteins were the most prominent constituents of the freeze–thaw preparation. Pellets were therefore subjected to differential extraction in a three-step process of increasing solubilizing power (Tris buffer; urea and thiourea; urea and thiourea plus detergents). The final pellet after these extractions, split and fractioned by gel electrophoresis or liquid chromatography, was highly enriched in membrane proteins (Braschi *et al.*, 2006). This fractionation study was annotated using the transcriptome database (Verjovski-Almeida *et al.*, 2003), which is also no longer available but the membrane protein lists were later reannotated by Smp number and augmented (Wilson, 2012), while soluble and cytoskeletal components were identified using GenBank (Table 7.1).

Proteomic analysis of the purified fractions from the freeze–thaw preparation (Braschi *et al.*, 2006) revealed that the buffer extract was enriched in glycolytic enzymes, but note that glyceraldehyde 3-phosphate dehydrogenase (GAPDH) appears to be associated with the final membrane pellet (see Chapter 9 on vaccines). Several

Table 7.1. Membrane and membrane-associated proteins identified by proteomic analysis of fractionated tegument gradient pellets

Protein	Smp	Protein	Smp
Enzymes		**Defence proteins**	
Alkaline phosphatase	Smp_155890	Ly6/CD59 glycoprotein	Smp_166340
ATP-dpp-hydrolase 1	Smp_042020	Ly6/CD59 glycoprotein	Smp_081920
Phosphodiesterase	Smp_153390	T cell immunomodulatory protein	Smp_194920
Calpain	Smp_157500	**Membrane structure**	
Carbonic anhydrase 4	Smp_168730	Dysferlin	Smp_141010
Acetylcholinesterase	Smp_136690	Otoferlin	Smp_163750
Transporters		Tetraspanin	Smp_167930
Glucose transport protein GTP1	Smp_012440	Tetraspanin	Smp_131840
Glucose transport protein GTP4	Smp_105410	Tetraspanin Sm-TSP-2	Smp_181530
Amino acid transporter SPRMhc	Smp_037540	Tetraspanin	Smp_194970
Cationic amino acid transporter	Smp_176940	Tetraspanin	Smp_140000
Neutral amino acid transporter	Smp_147070	Tetraspanin	Smp_017430
Na/Cl dep glycine transporter	Smp_131890	Annexin	Smp_045560
Na/Cl dep taurine transporter	Smp_143800	Annexin	Smp_077720
Multidrug resistance protein	Smp_170820	Annexin	Smp_045500
Aquaporin-3	Smp_005740	Annexin	Smp_045550
Aquaporin-3	Smp_005720	Annexin	Smp_074140
High-affinity Cu uptake protein	Smp_048230	**Trematode specific**	
Voltage-dep anion-channel	Smp_091240	Sm200 surface glycoprotein	Smp_017730
Voltage-dep anion- channel	Smp_022990	Sm29	Smp_072190
Voltage-gated potassium channel	Smp_151810	Sm25	Smp_195180
Membrane-associated ATPases		Sm13	Smp_195190
Na+/K+ ATPase alpha subunit	Smp_015020	Sm8.7 LMWP	Smp_194860
Na+/K+ ATPase beta subunit	Smp_124240	**Small G proteins**	
Na+/K+ ATPase beta subunit	Smp_033550	Rab 1 GTP-binding GTPase	Smp_169460
Cation/phospholipid trans ATPase	Smp_091650	Rab-27B GTP-binding	Smp_139340
Cation-transporting ATPase	Smp_175360	Rac GTPase	Smp_062300
Calcium-transporting ATPase	Smp_176130	Rho GEF domain	Smp_126600
Calcium-transporting ATPase	Smp_137170	Rho GTPase, Cdc42,	Smp_167030
Aminophospholipid trans ATPase	Smp_104500	Rho2 GTPase	Smp_072140
Phospholipid transporting ATPase	Smp_192080	Rap-1b, Ras-related protein	Smp_071250
		Rap-1b, Ras-related protein	Smp_142450

Smp annotations are v4 or v5 of the *S. mansoni* genome. Adapted from Wilson 2012

proteins protecting against oxidative stress (thioredoxin peroxidase; superoxidase dismutase) and at least five heat shock chaperones were present in the Tris buffer extract suggesting a defence of the tegument cytoplasm against external insult. A cohort of mitochondrial membrane and matrix proteins confirmed the presence of mitochondria in the tegument cytosol, while actins and myosin in both the buffer and urea/thiourea extracts confirmed the presence of cytoskeletal elements. Dynein light chains involved in vesicle motility were also identified, together with a group of EF-hand calcium-binding proteins: Sm22.6, Sm21.7 and Sm20.8 (now renamed as tegument allergen-like (TAL)-1, -2 and -3) (Fitzsimmons *et al.*, 2012). However, there was one obvious absence that remains unsolved. Histochemistry revealed the tegument to be strongly PAS-positive (Wheater and Wilson, 1976), while electrophoretic separations identified a broad glycan band in the range 28–37 kDa (Roberts *et al.*, 1988), postulated as the likely contents of the discoid bodies. No matching tegument glycoproteins have been found by proteomics or glycomics in Tris buffer extracts to date.

Analysis of the final membrane pellet, subsequently repeated with much larger pellets of starting material, revealed approximately 60 constituents, comprising enzymes, transporters, membrane structural, and schistosome-specific proteins (Table 7.1) (Wilson, 2012). This rich diversity of membrane-associated proteins indicates the occurrence of numerous biological processes across the tegument. Questions arise as to where precisely these proteins are located and how they fit into a conceptual framework of tegument surface function. The magnitude of the task is well illustrated by the two glucose transporters, SGTP-1 and SGTP-4, both present in the membrane pellet. From functional studies we know that SGTP-4 is in the surface complex and SGTP-1 in the basal membranes (Skelly *et al.*, 1994). Thus, more discriminating analytical approaches are required to pin down the precise locations if we are to understand tegument functions.

7.4.2 Detection of surface-exposed proteins on live worms by biotinylation

One such approach used in several studies was the incubation of live worms with biotinylation reagents (e.g. Sulfo-NHS-LC-Biotin) that tag exposed primary amine groups on proteins. These can then be retrieved from worm fractions using streptavidin agarose beads and identified by tandem MS. As with other approaches, there are caveats. The labelling must be carried out in a balanced salt solution to avoid quenching by free amino acids, but that can affect surface integrity (labelling at 4 C for 30 min) (Braschi and Wilson, 2006). The extent of supposedly impermeant reagent penetration into the tissues also needs to be tightly controlled to minimize labelling of internal constituents. When short-form and long-form sulfo-NHS-biotin were compared, it was apparent that the short-form reagent was the more permeable and labelled a small number of internal components (Braschi and Wilson, 2006; Wilson, 2012). The distribution of biotin label on/in worms can be visualized by the reaction of worms with FITC-conjugated streptavidin before confocal microscopy at high magnification (see Section 7.4.5). The proteins listed in Table 7.2 are those most accessible and hence present in the surface membrane complex. A subsequent biotinylation experiment with live *S. japonicum* in an identical protocol found a broadly similar range of labelled proteins, notably including the *S. japonicum* homologues of aquaporin, SGTP-4, the amino acid permease heavy chain and a calcium-transporting ATPase (Mulvenna *et al.*, 2010).

Points to note about this list are first, the presence of host immunoglobulins and complement factor C3, even though the adult worm surface is not susceptible to opsonization or lysis, and also host CD44. Second, the three phosphohydrolases and carbonic anhydrase are labelled, strong confirmation that they are externally facing components of the surface. Third, presumed cytosolic GAPDH was labelled but not the abundant cytosolic proteins enolase, aldolase and glutathione *S*-transferase. Is this evidence for a location on the external face of the plasma membrane or just a close but internal position? Lastly, the chaperone HSP70 was labelled together with three likely spine constituents. Since we know that the plasma membrane is closely apposed over the surface of spines, this was interpretated as evidence for permeation of the labelling reagent through the plasma membrane into the proximal cytosol. Later studies using the biotinylation approach identified more cytosolic components, as well as numerous cytoskeletal proteins, indicating greater penetration of the reagent. In some this was confirmed by detection of the biotin probe in deeper tissues (for an appraisal, see Wilson and Jones, 2021)). The interpretation of these biotinylation studies is crucial to the question of whether schistosomes in the bloodstream are coated in glycolytic enzymes (see Section 7.6).

7.4.3 Enzymatic shaving

The gentle enzymatic treatment of adherent cells to detach them from the culture vessel is a common technique in cell culture. It has been adapted to characterize the surface of live schistosomes using phosphatidylinositol-phospholipase C (PiPLC) and trypsin (Castro-Borges *et al.*, 2011a). (Note that is quite different from the enzymatic treatment of fixed schistosomes;

Table 7.2. Proteins biotinylated by incubation of live worms (reaction with sulfo-NHS-biotin and recovery by streptavidin beads)

Host proteins		**Schistosome specific**	
IgM heavy chain	GI:2995714	Sm200	Smp_017730
IgG1 heavy chain	GI:121038	Sm29	Smp_072190
IgG3 heavy chain	GI:558122	**Adhesion**	
Complement C3	GI:387114	TCIP Integrin	Smp_194920
CD44	GI:85540468	Fasciclin	Smp_141680
Membrane structure		**Transporters**	
Tetraspanin, TE736	Smp_194970	Anion channel	Smp_092120
Tetraspanin, TSP-2	Smp_181530	Na/K transporter	Smp_015020
Tetraspanin, CD63r	Smp_140000	**Spine matrix**	
Annexin	Smp_077720	Actin	Smp_091710
Dysferlin	Smp_141010	Fimbrin	Smp_037230
Plasmolipin	Smp_046290	Severin	Smp_008640
Enzymes		**Cytosol**	
Carbonic anhydrase	Smp_168730	GAPDH	Smp_121990
Calpain	Smp_137410	HSP70	Smp_106930
Alkaline phosphatase	Smp_155890		
ATP-diphosphohydrolase	Smp_042020		
Phosphodiesterase	Smp_153390		

Smp annotations are v4 or v5 of the *S. mansoni* genome assembly. Adapted from Wilson 2012.

Pérez-Sánchez *et al.*, 2008). Provided the membrane anchor is accessible to the enzyme (28 kDa), GPI-anchored exposed proteins should be recoverable by incubation with PiPLC. In practice, when worms were incubated in buffered RPMI medium for 1 h, cytosolic proteins were detected by proteomics, whether the enzyme was present or not. Therefore, iTRAQ (isobaric tagging for relative and absolute quantitation) was used to determine the degree of enrichment due to addition of the enzyme (Ross *et al.*, 2004).

It is worth making a digression to understand what this approach offers because the data provide important information about the integrity of worms *in vitro*. Adult worms were incubated with or without the PiPLC enzyme for 1 h, proteins accumulating in the medium were then processed, and their peptides released by trypsin digestion. Replicates were labelled with one of the iTRAQ tags (test tags 116 or 117 Da; control tags 114 or 115 Da). The four samples were then combined and subjected to liquid chromatography-MS-MS. Fragmentation spectra of the most abundant peptides were generated, each with signature peaks for the four reporter tags. For most, these yielded four peaks of approximately equal area and a ratio near unity (Fig. 7.6.1). In a minority of cases the four reporter tag peaks were unequal, with test samples of 2–10-fold greater intensity, revealing that the parent protein was preferentially released by the PiPLC treatment (Fig. 7.6.2). In descending order these were, Sm29, CD59a, Sm200, carbonic anhydrase, CD59b, alkaline phosphatase and ADP-ribosyl cyclase, plus two host proteins, CD48 and CD90 (Thy1.2) (Fig. 7.6.3). These data confirm their accessibility to the external bloodstream environment but their precise location in the membranocalyx or plasma membrane cannot be inferred. Equally important was the group of more than 30 proteins released from worms in the control cultures without enzyme, which had identical tag ratios (Fig. 7.6.3) (for the full list, see Castro-Borges *et al.*, 2011b). Gut-derived proteins regurgitated during incubation (saposin, α_2-macroglobulin) might be anticipated, but were not abundant. The identification of glycolytic enzymes (enolase, aldolase), chaperones (14-3-3, HSP70) and cytoskeletal proteins (actin, Sm20.8) were interpreted as indicators of protein leakage. These identities align with a proteomic analysis of the cytosol in adult worms, where just 18 proteins comprised half the total mass (Neves *et al.*, 2015). Ten of those abundant cytosolic proteins were among the 30 detected by the iTRAQ method. The conclusion must be that worm integrity is easily impaired, even with careful handling *in vitro*, resulting in leakage of cytosol.

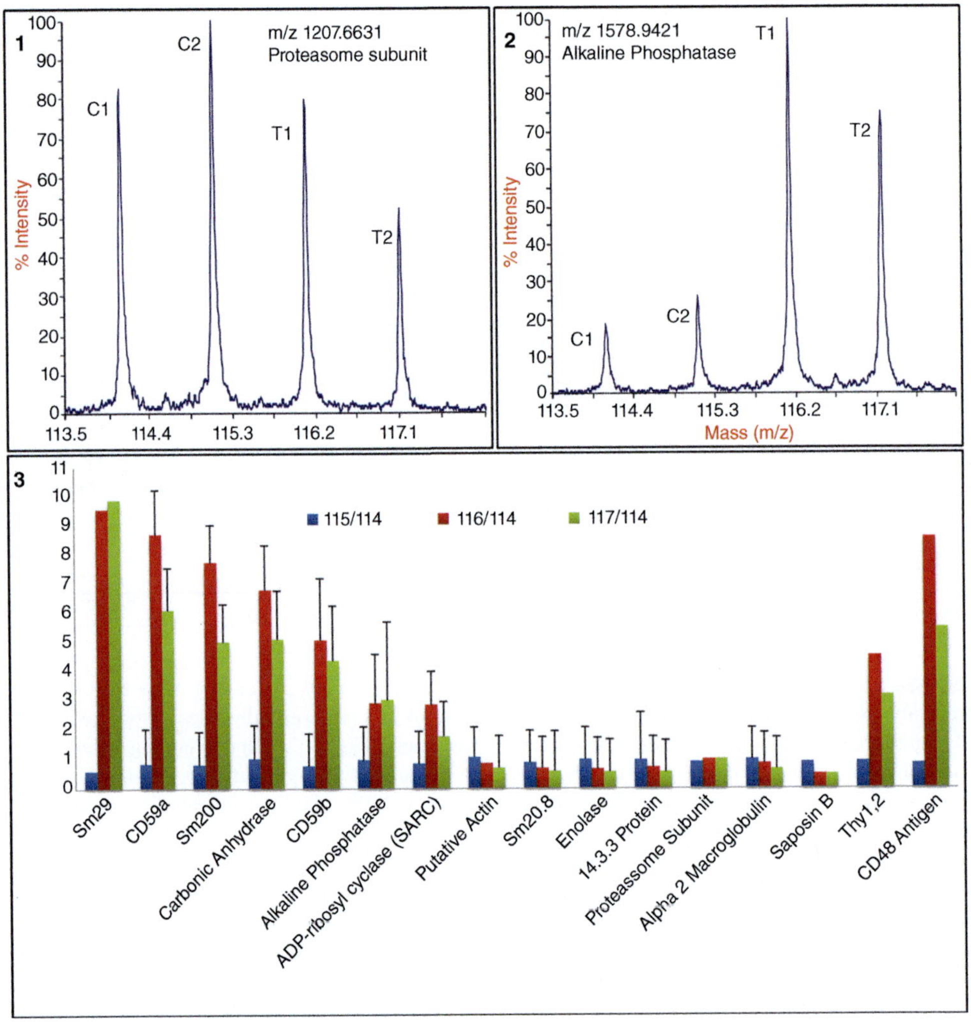

Fig. 7.6. Proteins released by PiPLC shaving of live worms, highlighted by the iTRAQ technique. **1**) Duplicate tagged samples of peptides derived from a proteome subunit show no difference in labelling between control (C) and test (T) samples, whether the PiPLC enzyme was present or not. **2**) Peptides derived from alkaline phosphatase show highly significant labelling in the test samples (T) incubated with PiPLC enzyme. **3**) The fold enrichment of test (116, 117) and control peptides (115) compared to the control 114 Da tag. (From Castro-Borges *et al.*, 2011a.) Figures used under license CC-BY-4.0.

When worms were subjected to gentle trypsinization at one hundredth the concentration used to detach cells in culture, a very select cohort of proteins was identified (Castro-Borges *et al.*, 2011a). Again, cytosolic proteins were detected and taken as evidence of surface damage facilitating leakage. Trypsinization released three annexins (Smp_074140, Smp_074150 and Smp_077720), calpain and a 68 kDa glycoprotein predicted to possess 24 *O*-glycosylation sites. (This is too large to be the PAS-positive protein detected in one-dimensional electrophoretic separations; Roberts *et al.*, 1988). Two tegument-specific proteins, Sm200 and Sm25, were also released, together with two endophilin BAR (bin, amphiphysin and Rvs161/167) domain proteins. Endophilins are normally located on the cytosolic surface of plasma membranes, promoting membrane curvature in exo- and endocytosis (Gallop and McMahon, 2005). Intriguingly, the trypsin did not appear to access plasma membrane proteins on the external surface so was perhaps excluded by the membranocalyx. Indeed, a feasible explanation for the specific pattern of release is that trypsin is accessing the narrow tubules, located at the base of tegument pits, where multilaminate vesicle fusion with the tegument plasma membrane occurs, a situation where protection by overlying membranocalyx is limited. Moreover, calpain lacks a signal peptide and may well function in membrane fusion events (Halliday *et al.*, 2021). The release of Sm25 and the 68 kDa glycoprotein by trypsin place them in the same location. It is notable that both calpain and Sm25 were found to be among the most antigenic tegument peptides in a recent epitope mapping study (Farias *et al.*, 2020), suggesting that neither protein has been subjected to immune silencing.

7.4.4 QconCAT quantification

The question of protein abundance in the surface complex, comprising the plasma membrane and overlying membranocalyx, was tackled using the QconCAT technique (Beynon *et al.*, 2005) The method relies on the production of a concatemer comprising R- or K-terminated peptides generated with 6-^{13}C-labelled lysine/arginine amino acids. (It follows that you can only quantify the proteins you have selected for inclusion, and they must differ in molecular mass.) The artificial protein, produced in a microbial system, is then added to the biological sample and the mixture processed for MALDI-ToF MS. Pairs of peptides separated by a m/z ratio of 6 units (^{12}C versus ^{13}C) are then identified, and the amount in the sample estimated by reference to the added ^{13}C standard. The method was applied to a gradient pellet of freeze–thaw tegument membranes and to a PiPLC fraction released by incubation of live worms. (Castro-Borges *et al.*, 2011b). In summary, the solute transporter aquaporin was the dominant membrane protein. Of the three phosphohydrolases, alkaline phosphatase and ATP-diphosphohydrolase were relatively more abundant than phosphodiesterase. Dysferlin was the most abundant protein contributing to membrane structure, along with two tetraspanins. Analysis of the PiPLC fraction, containing GPI-anchored schistosome proteins, showed that Sm200 was by far the most abundant constituent, compared to alkaline phosphatase and Sm29.

7.4.5 Immunocytochemistry

Theoretically, immunocytochemistry using monospecific antibodies should give useful data on tegument localization but in practice turns out to be fraught with difficulties. These stem from a combination of two factors, the thinness of the tegument cytoplasm (0.9 × 3.0 μm) coupled with the production of low magnification fluorescence images. The result is that many researchers conflate a positive reaction around the exterior of a worm acquired using a ×10 objective with the conclusion that a protein is 'on the tegument surface'. Using the highest possible magnifications (×600–1000), it is possible to distinguish between tegument cytosol and surface membrane complex. Nevertheless, the combined thickness of plasma membrane and membranocalyx at ~25 nm is well below the resolution of the light microscope so discriminating between the two structures is not feasible. The same goes for the multilaminate vesicle and discoid body inclusions, which are too small to resolve in the light microscope (~0.3 μm). Techniques like immunogold labelling for cryoelectron microscopy have also not produced convincing images of localization to subtegument compartments. Indeed, at 10–15 nm diameter, the gold particles used to label detecting antibodies probably cannot discriminate between the plasma membrane and overlying membranocalyx.

A recent study using a panel of antibodies reacted with cryosections of adult worms and imaged at high magnification has examined what is feasible (Fig. 7.7) (Wilson and Jones, 2021). The mouse monoclonal antibody D7.2, a marker for the tegument cytosol and tegument cell bodies (Riengrojpitak *et al.*, 1989) (A), has a uniform distribution. In contrast (B), the reactivity of anti-CD59 antibody for the surface membrane complex clearly lies external to that for Sm22.6 EF-hand Ca^{2+} binding protein (TAL-1), confirming the latter's cytosolic location.

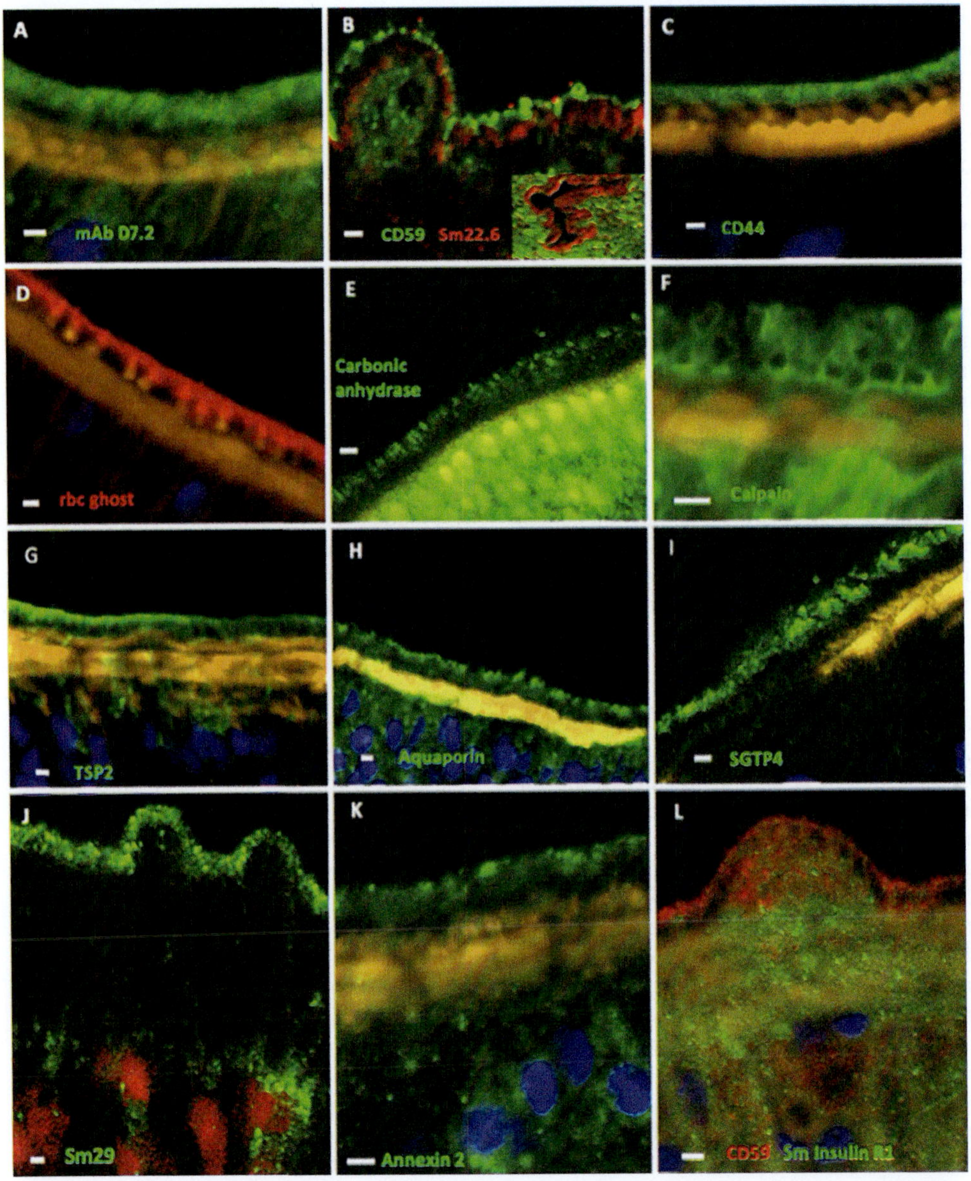

Fig. 7.7. Localization of tegument proteins at high magnification. Colour key: muscle and tegument spines are stained amber (AF555 phalloidin); tegument proteins are red (AF647) or green (AF488 or FITC); nuclei are blue (DAPI). **A**) Anti-glycan D7.2. **B**) CD59, Sm22.6 (TAL-1), inset gastrodermis. **C**) host CD44. **D**) mouse erythrocyte membrane. **E**) Carbonic anhydrase. **F**) Calpain. **G**) Tetraspanin TSP-2. **H**) Aquaporin. **I**) SGTP-4. **J**) Sm29. **K**) Annexin Smp_077720. **L**) CD59 versus Sm insulin receptor 1. Scale bars: 2 μm. (From Wilson and Jones, 2021.) Figure used with permission from Elsevier.

The inset also reveals that the supposed tegument allergen is abundant in the gastrodermis. Host markers CD44 (C) and anti-mouse erythrocyte ghosts (D) are exclusive to the surface membrane complex (i.e. not internalized) but highlight the problem of resolution. In both images the spines, which span the full width of the tegument, are visualized but the antibody staining is confined to the outer half of the tegument. This suggests that the acquired host molecules can access the membranes of surface pits, but do not reach the deeper side channels where multilaminate vesicle fusion occurs. The enzyme carbonic anhydrase (E) has an intriguing distribution since although the surface membrane complex is positive, the underlying tegument cytoplasm is negative, but the individual muscle fibres are strongly positive. This surface enzyme is thus not tegument-specific, having a broad distribution and function in the worm. The same is true of a second enzyme, calpain (F), where the cytosol is positive but vacuoles at the base of the surface pits are clearly demarcated; internal body tissues are also strongly positive for calpain. Tetraspanin TSP-2 (G) appears tegument-specific, being located only in the surface membrane complex and the subtegumental cell bodies where it is synthesized.

Among transporters, the surface membrane complex is positive for aquaporin (H) but not the tegument cytosol, while all tissues internal to the muscle fibres show widespread reactivity. However, the glucose transporter SGTP-4 (I) appears much more specific, with the surface membrane complex staining positive, while all internal tissues appear unreactive. The schistosome-specific Sm29 (J) shows a highly punctate reactivity at the surface, with tegument cell bodies similarly reactive, but the intervening muscle layer is negative apart from cytoplasmic connections (nuclei are red). This confirms the tegument specificity of Sm29. The same appears true for annexin Smp_077720 (K), where reactivity is confined to the surface membrane complex and also the tegument cell bodies. Several claims have been made that adult schistosomes in the bloodstream are capable of detecting and responding to host cytokines like transforming growth factor (TGF)-β, tumour necrosis factor (TNF)-α and insulin. However, no receptors have been identified in the surface membranes by proteomics. The concept of surface location was tested by comparing the distribution of CD59, as the surface marker, with that for insulin receptor 1 (L) (Khayath *et al.*, 2007). The latter is clearly associated with muscle fibres and to a lesser extent the parenchyma, but not the tegument or its cytoplasm. A technique with molecular-level resolution is needed if we are to understand fully the interrelationships of proteins and lipids in the surface complex. Perhaps cryoelectron microscope tomography might be applicable for this?

7.5 The Contribution of Single-cell Sequencing

The development of tissue disaggregation methods for RNA sequencing (RNA-Seq) on single cells from adult worms led ultimately to characterization of 68 molecularly distinct clusters (Wendt *et al.*, 2020), already extensively referenced in earlier chapters. As with other tissues the situation with the tegument is complex, especially due to the extensive previous characterization of proteins using diverse proteomic approaches.

7.5.1 Neoblasts, adult stem cells and tegument cell turnover

The first intimations that the tegument cell bodies might have unusual properties came from investigations of germinal cells. The 'germ cell' theory of schistosome development is well established (see Chapter 1), whereby a stock of undifferentiated cells is maintained throughout the life cycle, while their somatic progeny give rise to the succession of body phenotypes. However, it was only in 2013 that this was given a sound foundation in developmental molecular biology (Collins *et al.*, 2013; Wang *et al.*, 2013). Briefly, free-living planarian flatworms are capable of wound healing and tissue regeneration, regulated by totipotential proliferating cells, termed neoblasts (Newmark and Sánchez Alvarado, 2002). Schistosomes can repair damaged tissues but lack the regenerative capacity of free-living relatives (Popiel *et al.*, 1985; Shaw and Erasmus, 1987). Nevertheless, schistosomes were shown to possess both totipotent stem cells, which control embryogenesis in the molluscan host (Wang *et al.*, 2013), and adult stem cells distributed throughout the soma of males and females (Collins *et al.*, 2013). The work ensuing from this stem cell characterization had profound implications for our understanding of tegument cell biology.

A powerful suite of techniques was developed to investigate these stem cells, based on long-term *in vitro* culture of *ex vivo* mature worms. Dividing cells were labelled with the thymidine analogue 5-ethynyl-2′-deoxyuridine (EdU), coupled with whole-mount *in situ* hybridization and transcriptional profiling to characterize gene expression patterns. These were augmented by γ-irradiation to inhibit cell division capabilities and RNA interference to deplete transcript levels. The principal revelation was that stem cell progeny contribute to the adult worm tegument in a process of continuous renewal (Collins *et al.*, 2016). A group of genes being expressed normally 2 days after worm irradiation were found to be severely depleted at 7 days post-treatment in a non-neoblast population and were designated as delayed irradiation sensitivity (DIS) genes. Double fluorescence *in situ* hybridization showed that the cells expressing the *tsp2*⁺ tegument marker, present just beneath the body wall muscles (Fig. 7.8.1), also expressed a series of other known tegument markers: *sm25*, *sm29*, *sm13*, *endophilin b*, *amino acid transporter*, *dysferlin* and *cd59*. One explanation for this delayed sensitivity is that the *tsp2*⁺ cells represent a brief development stage en route to terminally differentiated tegument cell bodies (Fig. 7.8.2).

The next procedure in this complex saga was a bold innovation, which the authors acknowledged results in surface damage (Wendt and Collins, 2020). Brief incubation of worms in a hypotonic solution containing 10 kDa fluorescent dextran labelled the tegument cytosol, cytoplasmic connections and tegument cell bodies (Fig. 7.8.3 and 7.8.4). The procedure confirmed the interconnectedness of all tegument compartments, discrete from the rest of the body. Furthermore, the cell bodies appeared sufficiently intact for *in situ* hybridization and transcriptional profiling to be applied.

A group of dextran-positive cells, termed definitive tegument cells was characterized by expression of *calpain* (Smp_214190), phosphodiesterase (*npp5*, Smp_153390), *annexin* Smp_077720 and Sm*gtp4* but not *tsp2* (Wendt *et al.*, 2018). Conversely, EdU was incorporated into *tsp2*⁺ cells that were dextran-negative so not connected to the tegument system. They did not express the definitive tegument cell markers, but coexpressed *sm13*. Pulse–chase experiments with EdU injected into mice confirmed that it was first incorporated into *tsp2*⁺ cells before peaking ~10 days later in definitive tegument cells, indicating a process of maturation over an extended time period (Fig. 7.8.5). This raises an interesting question since proteins identified by proteomic analysis (see Section 7.4.1) of the tegument surface membrane complex are coexpressed yet their transcripts appear not to be. This suggests a phased maturation of the cell bodies and their inclusions or distinct maturation pathways (see below). Note that it appears that while the *tsp2* mRNA is downregulated, the TSP-2 protein remains stable.

These observations led to the first tissue disaggregation experiments and the isolation, by cell sorting, of neoblasts, TSP-2⁺ cells and IR rest cells (non-dividing differentiated cells) (Fig. 7.9.1 and 7.9.2). RNA-Seq was performed on these populations, followed by cluster analysis (Wendt *et al.*, 2018). The TSP-2⁺ cells were enriched in *sm13*, *sm25*, *cationic amino acid transporter* and *dysferlin* transcripts, but also included markers of definitive tegument cells (*calp*, *npp5*, *annexin* and *gtp4*) (Fig. 7.9.3). Two transcripts encoding endophilins were expressed at high levels in a subset of mature tegumental cell bodies. These are the same endophilins detected by proteomics of the tegument fraction released by trypsin shaving of live worms (Castro-Borges *et al.*, 2011a). The heterogeneity in gene expression between clusters was taken to represent populations of cells at different stages of commitment to the tegumental lineage (see below).

Intriguingly, further experiments using RNA interference treatment to knock-down expression of gene *zfp1-1*, encoding a zinc finger DNA-binding transcription factor, led to an almost complete block in the ability of new cells to be added to the tegument. This led the authors to conclude that *zfp1-1* represents a critical and specific regulator of tegumental cell body formation (Wendt *et al.*, 2018). Since the two endophilin-encoding genes were only expressed in a subset of mature tegumental cells, the authors also concluded that discrete molecular and functionally distinct cell bodies may exist (see Section 7.2.1). Thus, different types of *tsp2*⁺ cells may give rise to different classes of tegumental cell bodies. Alternatively, a mechanism for tegument cell renewal, independent of *tsp2*⁺ cells, may also exist. A note of caution about the emphasis of TSP-2 protein as a marker is warranted since in this author's laboratory, a rabbit anti-TSP-2 antibody proved to be promiscuous, recognizing

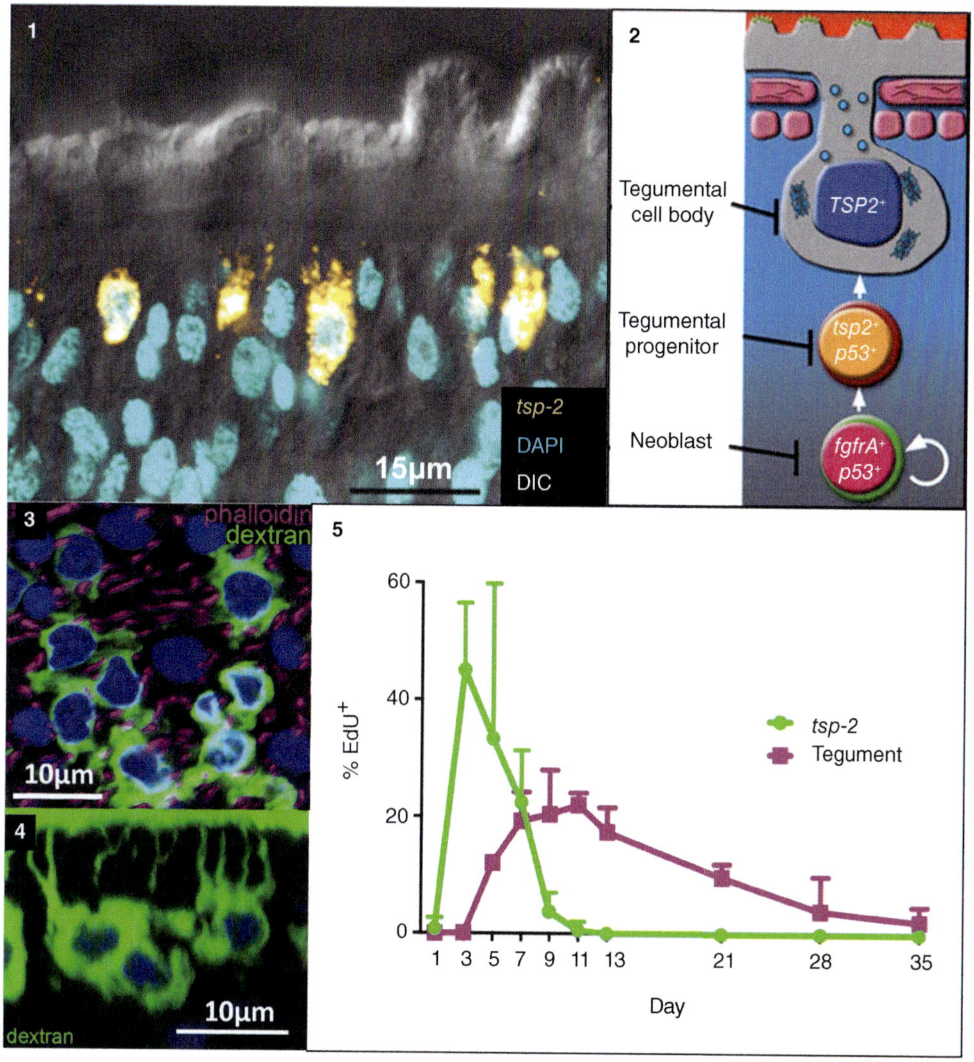

Fig. 7.8. Evidence for tegument cell body turnover. **1**) Fluorescence *in situ* hybridization of *tsp2*⁺ cells and DAPI-labelled nuclei overlaid on a differential interference contrast (DIC) image showing their distribution relative to the tegument. **2**) One model of tegument cell maturation from self renewing neoblasts. **3**) Transverse plane through the subtegument with phalloidin-labelled muscle fibres and fluorescent dextran-labelled tegument cell bodies. **4**) Side view of dextran-labelled tegument, cytoplasmic connections and tegumental cell bodies. **5**) Quantification of EdU incorporation into *tsp2*⁺ cells and subsequently into definitive tegumental cells, consistent with short-lived *tsp2*-expressing progenitors going on to become mature tegumental cells. (**1** and **2** from Collins *et al.*, 2016; **3–5** from Wendt *et al.*, 2018.) Figures used under licence CC-BY-4.0.

a conserved epitope that is also shared with approximately 10 other schistosome tetraspanins (50–62% homology at the amino acid level). It is possible that a heterogeneous population of somatic stem cells is being recovered by fluorescence activated cell sorting of TSP-2⁺ cells, although the specificity of *in situ* hybridization should not be affected.

Eight of the 68 clusters identified by single-cell sequencing expressed tegument markers: neoblast progeny; early *tsp2*⁺, *egc*⁺, *meg1*⁺, *zfp1-1*⁺, *sm13*⁺, *tegument 1* and *tegument 2* (see Chapter 4,

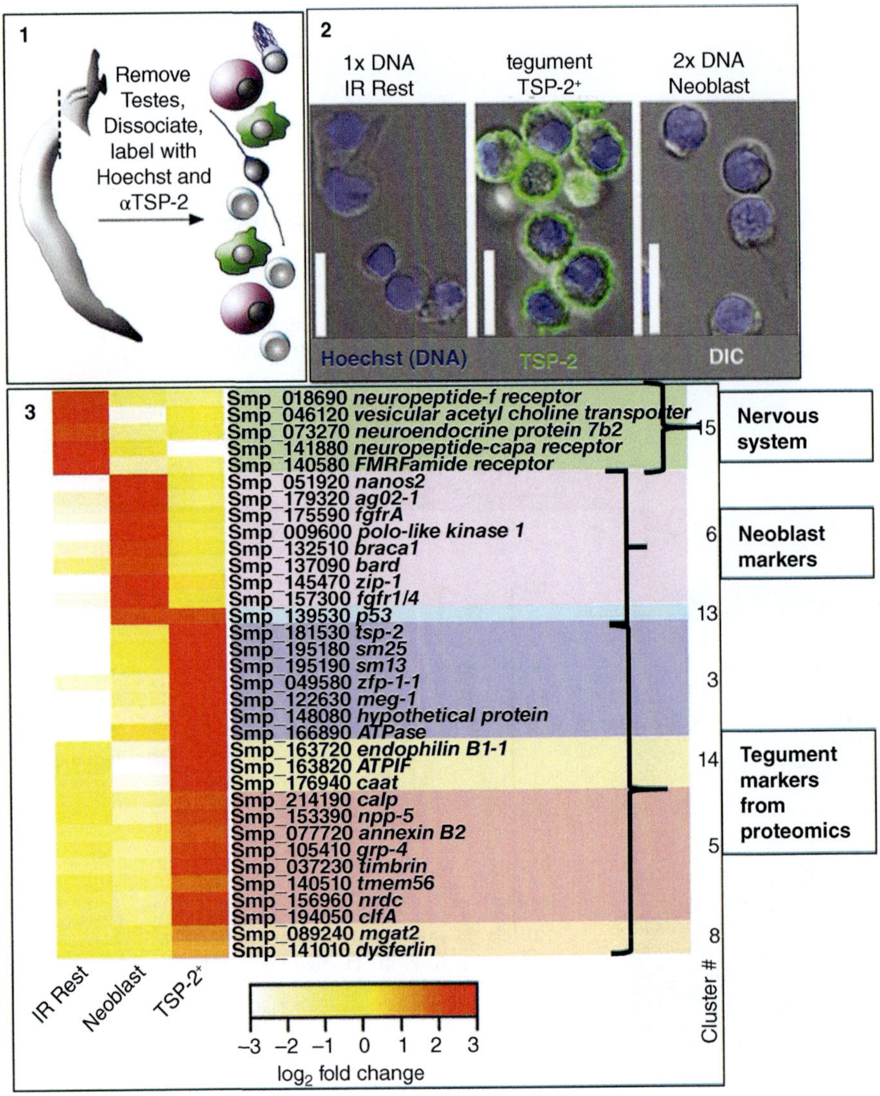

Fig. 7.9. Maturation of tegument cell bodies. **1**) Schema for cell isolation. Worms were minced, digested with trypsin and liberated cells recovered by 500 × *g* spin. DNA was labelled with Hoechst and tegument marker with antibody to TSP-2, before sorting into three populations to determine gene expression patterns. **2**) Representative cells from the three populations: radiation-resistant (IR) non-dividing cells, TSP-2$^+$ tegument cell bodies, and neoblasts with 2× DNA at the G_2/M phase of the cell cycle. Scale bars: 10 µm. **3**) Representative genes upregulated in the three populations. The IR resting cells are nerve cell bodies. Many of the genes in the TSP-2$^+$ cells encode known tegument markers. (From Wendt *et al.*, 2018.) Figures used under licence CC-BY-4.0.

Fig. 4.6). Do these clusters represent different stages in the maturation of a single type of tegument cell body or indicators for a diversity of cell types? The level of expression of genes encoding tegument proteins can be evaluated in all clusters at a website: https://www.collinslab.org/schistocyte/search (Wendt *et al.*, 2021). The site has been interrogated using selected tegument markers (Wilson and Jones, 2021). Expression of some genes was restricted to the eight tegument clusters while others were widely dispersed through many tissue clusters. Most of the membrane-spanning transporters and tetraspanins appear to be dominant in the tegument 1 cluster, while schistosome-specific *sm13*, *sm29*, *sm25* and *dysferlin* are more abundant in other tegument clusters. It is notable that the two endophilins appear to have a reciprocal distribution between the seven clusters. Does this imply a different morphological location for their respective membrane interactions? SchistoCyte threw up a couple of surprises, including the gene for *lmwp*, encoding an 8.7 kDa low-molecular-weight protein, which was expressed solely in a parenchyma cluster, suggesting it was a leakage product in proteomic analyses. The biggest puzzle was provided by Sm200, previously described as a tegument surface protein, and readily removed from live worms by PiPLC treatment; SchistoCyte has the gene expressed in all clusters.

The projected recruitment of new tegument cell bodies requires the removal of existing cell bodies to maintain the steady state. Presumably this is achieved by autophagy, which is poorly researched in schistosomes. A search of SchistoCyte tegument clusters for expression of potential early autophagy genes revealed their presence in all clusters at varying intensities. However, no morphological evidence for autophagic cells has been reported in TEM studies of the tegument. This topic of tegument cell body recruitment and turnover clearly merits further investigation.

7.6 Immune Evasion at the Tegument Surface

The longevity of adult worms in the bloodstream, despite exposing a living syncytial layer of cytoplasm to the full gamut of blood components, is a testament to the tegument's protective capacity. A better understanding of the evasion mechanisms deployed may be the key to development of a successful vaccine.

7.6.1 The membranocalyx as a physical barrier

It is more than 50 years since the presence of the membranocalyx, external to the bounding plasma membrane of the tegument, was described but it remains poorly understood.

Its predominantly lipid composition has been inferred from its instability in organic solvents, but it clearly lacks the structural proteins that give stability to a plasma membrane. An analogy has been made with the multilamellar bodies of the type II pneumocyte in the mammalian lung that generate alveolar surfactant (Wilson and Jones, 2021). There are superficial similarities such the bounding membrane of a multilamellar body creating a fusion pore with the pneumocyte plasma membrane through which its lamellae are extruded and unpack to form the surfactant layer of an alveolus. However, this cell system is 10 times the scale of the tegument, while the lamellae comprise densely packed stacks of phospholipid bilayers (75% phosphatidylcholine) narrower than a conventional 9 nm plasma membrane. In contrast, the more robust appearance and greater electron density of the schistosome multilaminate vesicle contents and secreted membranocalyx argues strongly that they are not simple phospholipid bilayers.

We know that the outer surface of the adult schistosome is highly lipophilic from its ability to acquire host glycolipids, GPI-anchored proteins and single membrane-spanning CD44. The question remains as to what are the lipids of the secreted bilayer that give it these properties and also allow it both to adhere to the plasma membrane beneath and to flow laterally over its surface? What can best be described as hints about composition can be found in the literature.

Sphingomyelin was found to be enriched up to 24% in the stripped worm surfaces versus 7–8% in the worm body but it is unclear where the sphingomyelin was located (Allan *et al.*, 1987). A novel fatty acid, eicosanoic acid [C20:1] was also identified. A second study analysed the lipid composition of membranes released by the freeze–thaw method (Brouwers *et al.*, 1998), confirming the abundance of sphingomyelin (14%) in the surface, and another unusual fatty acid, 5-octadecenoic acid [C18:1(5)], associated with phosphatidyl choline. The problem with these lipid studies is that they fail to distinguish between plasma membrane and membranocalyx, treating them as equivalent when they are not. A quite different approach to estimate the rigidity of the surface layers of lung stage and adult worms has used QUENS (quasielastic neutron scattering) (Migliardo *et al.*, 2014). This is a technique from solid-state physics, normally applied to model membrane systems (Qian *et al.*, 2020); literature on live cells is sparse so the significance of the observations is hard to assess. The principal suggestion from these observations was that the presence of a hydrogen bond barrier around larvae and adult schistosomes would provide resistance to immune attack.

Clearly, a method is needed to generate a preparation enriched in membranocalyx that will facilitate detailed compositional analysis. Only then will we understand/appreciate how its presence protects the intravascular stages against immune attack. As the information on lipid composition shows, our knowledge is meagre. The binding of cationized ferritin confirms a negative charge at physiological pH, while the ability of concanavalin A to inhibit release of vesicle contents has revealed the presence of endogenous α-d-mannosyl and/or α-d-glucosyl residues. Does this indicate the presence of glycosphingolipids? A single cationized ferritin shedding experiment suggests the presence of Sm13, Sm29, Sm200 and SmTSP-2 in the membranocalyx. It is pure speculation that the tegument-specific annexin, Smp_077720, is the best candidate to provide the 'Velcro' to hold the membranocalyx and plasma membrane in close apposition. Another conundrum is that if the membranocalyx is the proposed inert protective barrier, then how do the substrates of the ectoenzymes and solutes for uptake by transporters reach their respective targets? Only with an accurate molecular model of the membranocalyx can this be solved.

7.6.2 The purinergic halo

In the mammalian host, purinergic signalling by purine nucleotides and nucleosides (e.g. adenosine, ATP) is mediated by several families of purinergic receptors on target cells to regulate cellular functions. It has been established that ATP acts as a co-transmitter in nerves of the central and peripheral nervous system, and has a prominent role in vascular system physiology. This natural release of ATP in neurotransmission also intersects with host defence mechanisms of innate immunity. Pattern recognition receptors are host receptors on, for example, leucocytes, that detect molecules typical of a pathogen and initiate the innate response. Additionally, pathogens can damage or kill host cells; the release of normally intracellular solutes then serves as a danger signal (alarmin). The solutes have been termed 'damage associated molecular patterns' (DAMPs) and prominent among them are the cyclic nucleotides (ATP, ADP, AMP, UTP, adenosine), whose extracellular presence as a purinergic halo can be detected by purinergic receptors.

The relevance of these pathways to intravascular schistosomes is envisaged as follows. First, schistosomula squeezing through capillary beds (Chapter 3) interact with the vessels and leucocytes but appear to evade direct cytological damage. Second, adult worms progressing up portal venules (or through the vesical plexus) have the potential to damage host endothelia, especially using spines, yet they do not attract a focus of leucocytes *in vivo* in the portal vessels (Keating *et al.*, 2006). Indeed, the margination of leucocytes on to primate vascular endothelium in the vicinity of a worm attests to vascular damage, yet the entire worm in section had only a single adherent leucocyte. How does the parasite deal with this nascent purinergic halo? This raises a second question regarding the absence of blood clotting in the vicinity of intravascular schistosomes if endothelial damage is occurring. During blood clotting, ADP is crucial in the activation and recruitment of platelets and also ensures the structural integrity of thrombi. These effects are modulated by purinergic receptors on platelets and their activation is necessary to achieve sustained haemostasis.

The identification of alkaline phosphatase, ATP-diphosphohydrolase and phosphodiesterase-5, plus ADP-ribosyl cyclase/SmNACE as tegument ectoenzymes, by biochemical and proteomic approaches, was set out in Section 7.4 above. It has recently been persuasively advocated that these four enzymes give the intravascular schistosomes a powerful anti-inflammatory defence (Fig. 7.10) (Skelly *et al.*, 2022). SmNACE cleaves nicotine adenine dinucleotide to generate nicotinamide and ADP-ribose. The function of the three phosphohydrolases is the catabolism of cyclic nucleotides from ATP to AMP and adenosine. In this they mimic precisely the host enzyme orthologues that drive extracellular cyclic nucleotide catabolism to regulate purinergic signalling. The result of their action is the generation

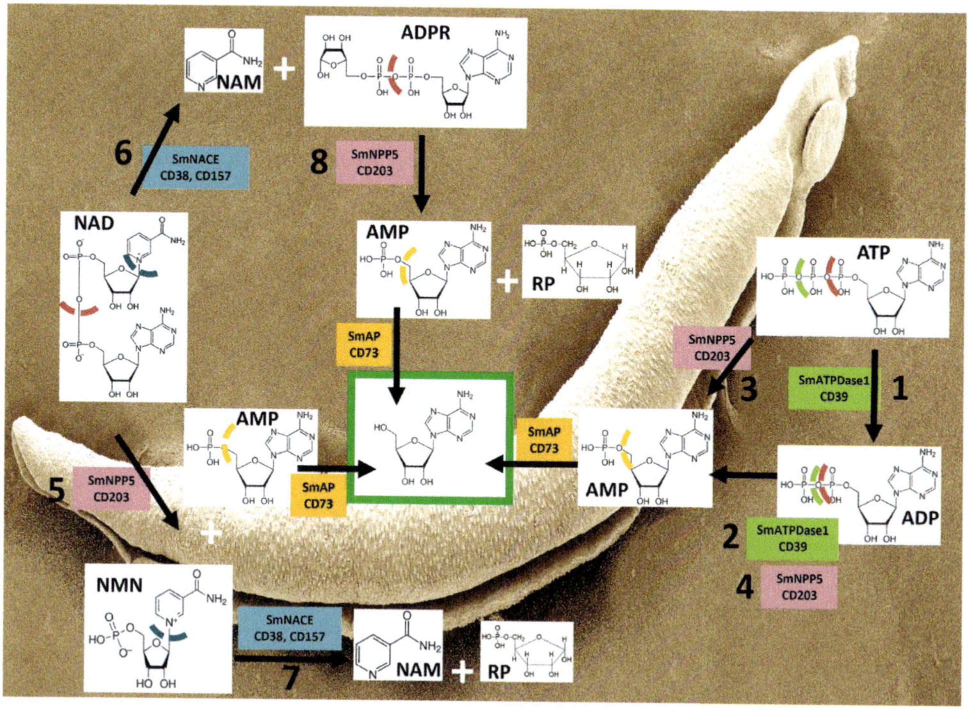

Fig. 7.10. The purinergic halo. Chemical structures of key purinergic metabolites are depicted along with, in coloured boxes, the names of the following key *S. mansoni* tegumental ectoenzymes (and functional host homologues): ATP-diphosphohydrolase I, SmATPDase1 (CD39) ( ); nucleotide pyrophosphatase/ phosphodiesterase 5, SmNPP5 (CD203) ( ); alkaline phosphatase, SmAP (CD73) ( ); NAD-catabolizing enzyme, SmNACE (CD38, CD157) ( ). Colour-coded lines indicate sites of cleavage by the various enzymes. The green box encloses adenosine, a terminal product of several pathways. ADP, adenosine diphosphate; ADPR, adenosine diphosphate ribose; AMP, adenosine monophosphate; ATP, adenosine triphosphate; NAD, nicotinamide adenine dinucleotide; NAM, nicotinamide; NMN, nicotinamide mononucleotide; RP, ribose phosphate. (Image courtesy of Professor P. Skelly, from Skelly *et al.*, 2022.) Figure used with permission from Elsevier.

of adenosine, which has anti-inflammatory properties, and can also be removed by uptake across the tegument surface as a nutrient. The authors also point out that the phosphohydrolase activity efficiently removes the potently prothrombotic molecule ADP, which promotes platelet activation and aggregation. This could block any resulting thrombus formation in the vicinity of the worms. These conclusions add another dimension to the remarkable ability of schistosomes to thrive in the host bloodstream.

7.6.3 Inhibition of complement fixation

Proteomic analyses have identified antibodies of several isotypes and complement factors C3 and C4 in adult tegument surface membranes (Braschi and Wilson, 2006; Castro-Borges *et al.*, 2011a). However, the failure to find factors C5 to C9, the elements of the culminating membrane attack complex (MAC), suggests that the cascade is inhibited at an intermediate step. It is also surprising that the antibodies and complement factors do not trigger leukocyte adherence to parasites in blood vessels (Keating *et al.*, 2006). In the context of complement fixation, the identification of four orthologues of human CD59 (a potent inhibitor of the MAC) at the tegument surface by proteomics, appeared to offer a potential explanation for complement inhibition. There were six genes encoded in the *S. mansoni* genome and the proteins showed 20–30% identity with the human counterparts, rising to >40% if conservative amino acid substitutions were included. The consensus CCXXXCN sequence was also displayed at the C-terminus. Accordingly, these CD59 orthologues were suggested as candidates for inhibition of complement fixation at the tegument surface (Wilson and Coulson, 2009).

The observations prompted a comprehensive molecular characterization of these SmCD59-like genes, and the putative biological functions of two isoforms were investigated (Farias *et al.*, 2013). The study identified seven genes but one Smp has vanished in v10 of the *S. mansoni* genome, so the total remains at six (nine are present in *S. japonicum* and six in *Schistosoma haematobium*). They all contain a three-fingered protein domain, but the conserved amino acid residues involved in complement recognition in humans could not be identified.

As indicated by proteomic analysis (Castro-Borges *et al.*, 2011a), at least some of the SmCD59-like proteins are localized on the tegument surface. However, expression was also detected in internal tissues of adult worms, which argues against a role in complement fixation.

The properties of CD59.1 (Smp_019350) and CD59.2 (Smp_105220) were evaluated in complement inhibition assays (Farias *et al.*, 2013). Soluble forms of the two proteins in a range of concentrations were probed in a haemolytic assay by incubation with normal human serum. Both lacked the ability to inhibit haemolysis of rabbit erythrocytes by the alternative pathway or antibody-sensitized sheep erythrocytes by the classical pathway. In a second assay, Chinese hamster ovary cells expressing the GPI-anchored versions of the two proteins were unable to inhibit lysis by antibodies directed against intrinsic cell membrane proteins. In a third assay, suppression of SmCD59.1 and SmCD59.2 by small interfering RNA (siRNA) was induced in schistosomula before their culture for 5 days (to the lung stage). They were then sensitized by 30 min treatment with heat-inactivated immune or naïve rat serum, before overnight incubation with normal human serum as a source of complement, and viability was assessed by uptake of Hoechst 33258 dye. The significant decrease of protein levels in siRNA-suppressed schistosomula did not enhance *in vitro* parasite killing by human complement beyond 20%, even in the presence of immune serum, when compared to the control groups. From these results the authors concluded that SmCD59.1 and SmCD59.2 are not complement regulatory proteins; their function in schistosomes remains to be determined. That leaves open a major question of why the intravascular parasites do not elicit complement fixation at the tegument surface.

7.7 Current 'Controversies'

The multiple controversies that remain about the way in which the schistosome tegument functions have been covered in two recent publications (Wilson and Jones, 2021; Castro-Borges and Wilson, 2022) but the salient features are summarized here. It must be emphasized that the arguments depend on differences of opinion about how data might be interpreted. What follows are the author's own convictions, held with varying degrees of certainty.

7.7.1 The 'leakyome' and glycolytic enzymes

The difficulty of handling schistosomes *in vitro* was set out in a preceding section (see Section 7.4.3). It has been suggested that the detection of cytosolic components in the culture medium was the result of superficial damage to the surface membrane complex and the term 'leakyome' was coined to distinguish these proteins from the true secretome (Castro-Borges and Wilson, 2022). One of the strongest arguments supporting this was that the leaked proteins like enolase and GAPDH were prominent in a total cytosol extract of adult worms (Neves *et al.*, 2015). The results of the tegument proteomic studies have been interpreted in exactly the opposite way to suggest that schistosome coat themselves in glycolytic enzymes (Pirovich *et al.*, 2019). This is an important distinction because of the proposed capability of GAPDH and enolase in enhancing binding and activation of plasminogen on the tegument surface (Ramajo-Hernández *et al.*, 2007; Figueiredo *et al.*, 2015). This would require the enzymes to be accessible on the external worm surface to generate the potent fibrinolytic agent plasmin, which could degrade blood clots forming around the worms *in vivo*. A problem with this hypothesis is that the two enzymes are strongly antigenic so their exposure would provide targets for antibody-mediated attack, which is not observed *in vivo*.

7.7.2 The release of vesicles from the tegument surface and the 'disintegrome'

The integrity of the schistosome surface membrane complex has been emphasized throughout this chapter, along with the lack of morphological evidence for the release of conventional secretory vesicles across the plasma membrane. Indeed, the fusion of multilaminate vesicles at the base of the pits, via transitory side channels, to release their membranocalyx contents seems explicitly intended to minimize exposure of plasma membrane targets to the immune system. Against this background, it is surprising to discover multiple publications describing the production of extracellular vesicles by the tegument (reviewed by Wilson and Jones, 2021). The suggestion here is that they are not normal feature of tegument cytology but rather evidence of damage resulting from *in vitro* conditions, for which the term 'disintegrome' was coined (Castro-Borges and Wilson, 2022). The ultrastructure of vesicles has been reported by electron microscopy (Sotillo *et al.*, 2015; Liu *et al.*, 2018) but the integrity of the worms from which they originated has not been considered. The handling conditions of *ex vivo* worms are a cause for concern, ranging from multiple washes in PBS (Liu *et al.*, 2019) to culture for 10 days in a complex but serum-free medium (Kifle *et al.*, 2020b). These considerations are crucial because the vesicle preparations containing tegumental markers (SmTSP-2, Sm29 and annexins), as well as cytosolic proteins (Sm22.6 and dynein light chains) (Sotillo *et al.*, 2015) have been used to stimulate reactivity in various monocyte and endothelial cell lines (Kifle *et al.*, 2020a; Liu *et al.*, 2019). If the vesicles are an artefact of technique, the findings are irrelevant to the interplay between the live worm and its host. It was observed decades ago that *ex vivo* day 21 liver worms, incubated for 24 h in defined Minimal Eagle's Medium,

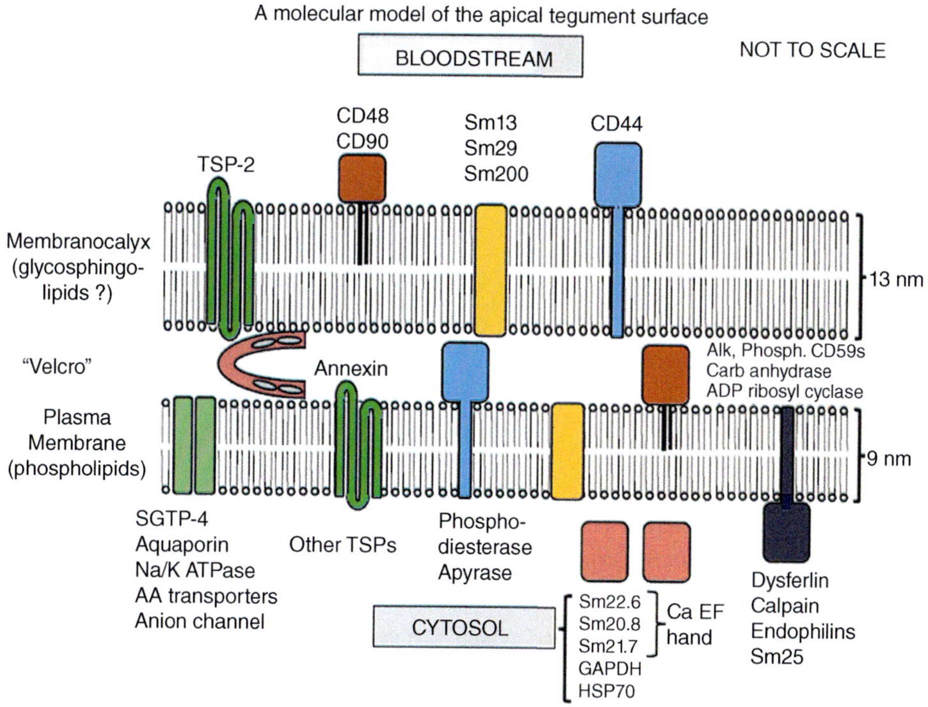

Fig. 7.11. The latest iteration of a molecular model for the tegument surface complex. (From Wilson and Jones, 2021.) Figure used with permission from Elsevier.

exhibited small patches of tegument damage readily detected by fluorescence microscopy (Riengrojpitak, 1987; Castro-Borges and Wilson, 2022). Today, with more sophisticated instruments and reagents (Wendt and Collins, 2020), it is now feasible to explore routinely the integrity of the entire surface of worms maintained *in vitro* to look for signs of damage. It is incumbent on the proponents of vesicle production from the tegument surface to show that it occurs without detectable surface damage. Better still they need to show that worms producing such vesicles are viable when transplanted back into the portal vein of a host.

7.8 A Molecular Model of the Tegument Surface

The first attempt to place tegument proteins into a model of the molecular architecture of the tegument surface was based on the results of proteomic analyses (Braschi and Wilson, 2006). This has been updated through later iterations (Wilson, 2012; Wilson and Jones, 2021) but is very much work in progress (Fig. 7.11). Note that a different model of the multilaminate tegument surface has just been proposed that is at odds with many of the propositions put forward in this chapter (Da'Dara and Skelly, 2025). The point of such models is to pull together numerous disparate observations in the hope that it will point up inconsistencies that stimulate further experiments.

7.9 Summary

- After more than 50 years of research many questions remain to be answered about tegument composition, dynamics and means of immune evasion.
- Uppermost of these must be a better understanding of the molecular composition and organization of the secreted membranocalyx bilayer, which endow it with special properties. If it represents a physical barrier then how do substrates and nutrients access the underlying plasma membrane? Does it contain pores that could serve that function? Sm200 is the only large constituent that could play such a role.
- The composition of the discoid bodies, their projected role in providing the tegument cytoplasm and the dynamics of their turnover are largely unexplored.
- Does recycling of the surface plasma membrane occur, potentially via transient links to the basal invaginations permitting membrane flow of components back to the cell bodies?
- The clearly demonstrated turnover of tegument cell bodies, their developmental sequence and equally senescence, e.g. via autophagy, are major questions. Whether the two types of Golgi body represent two distinct cell populations still has no clear answer.
- The co-incubation of worms with host polypeptide 'hormones' such as insulin, TNF-α and TGF-β has been reported to induce changes in gene expression, via postulated host receptors expressed on the tegument surface. Such receptors have not been identified in proteomic analyses, and it is difficult to envisage how they might signal to the interior, especially given how dextran permeation has revealed the tegument to be such a tight system.

References

Abath, F.G., Xavier, E.M., Allen, R., Gomes, Y.M., Lucena-Silva, N. *et al.* (2000) Characterization of Sm13, a tegumental antigen of *Schistosoma mansoni*. *Parasitology Research* 86(9), 745–752. DOI: 10.1007/pl00008562

Ali, P.O., Jeffs, S.A., Meadows, H.M., Hollyer, T., Owen, C.A. *et al.* (1991) Structure of Sm25, an antigenic integral membrane glycoprotein of adult *Schistosoma mansoni*. *Molecular and Biochemical Parasitology* 45(2), 215–222. DOI: 10.1016/0166-6851(91)90088-N

Allan, D., Payares, G. and Evans, W.H. (1987) The phospholipid and fatty acid composition of *Schistosoma mansoni* and of its purified tegumental membranes. *Molecular and Biochemical Parasitology* 23(2), 123–128. DOI: 10.1016/0166-6851(87)90147-2

Asch, H.L. and Read, C.P. (1975) Transtegumental absorption of amino acids by male *Schistosoma mansoni*. *The Journal of Parasitology* 61(2), 378–379. DOI: 10.2307/3279026

Ashton, P.D., Curwen, R.S. and Wilson, R.A. (2001) Linking proteome and genome: how to identify parasite proteins. *Trends in Parasitology* 17(4), 198–202. DOI: 10.1016/s1471-4922(00)01947-4

Beynon, R.J., Doherty, M.K., Pratt, J.M. and Gaskell, S.J. (2005) Multiplexed absolute quantification in proteomics using artificial QCAT proteins of concatenated signature peptides. *Nature Methods* 2(8), 587–589. DOI: 10.1038/nmeth774

Boyer, M.H., Kalfayan, L.J. and Ketchum, D.G. (1977) The host antigen phenomenon in experimental murine schistosomiasis. III. Destruction of parasites transferred from mice to hamsters. *The American Journal of Tropical Medicine and Hygiene* 26(2), 254–257. DOI: 10.4269/ajtmh.1977.26.254

Braschi, S. and Wilson, R.A. (2006) Proteins exposed at the adult schistosome surface revealed by *biotinylation*. *Molecular & Cellular Proteomics* 5(2), 347–356. DOI: 10.1074/mcp.M500287-MCP200

Braschi, S., Curwen, R.S., Ashton, P.D., Verjovski-Almeida, S. and Wilson, A. (2006) The tegument surface membranes of the human blood parasite *Schistosoma mansoni*: a proteomic analysis after differential extraction. *Proteomics* 6(5), 1471–1482. DOI: 10.1002/pmic.200500368

Brouwers, J.F., Versluis, C., van Golde, L.M. and Tielens, A.G. (1998) 5-Octadecenoic acid: evidence for a novel type of fatty acid modification in schistosomes. *Biochemical Journal* 334(2), 315–319. DOI: 10.1042/bj3340315

Cardoso, F.C., Pacífico, R.N., Mortara, R.A. and Oliveira, S.C. (2006a) Human antibody responses of patients living in endemic areas for schistosomiasis to the tegumental protein Sm29 identified through genomic studies. *Clinical and Experimental Immunology* 144(3), 382–391. DOI: 10.1111/j.1365-2249.2006.03081.x

Cardoso, L.S., Oliveira, S.C., Pacífico, L.G., Góes, A.M., Oliveira, R.R. *et al.* (2006b) *Schistosoma mansoni* antigen-driven interleukin-10 production in infected asthmatic individuals. *Memórias do Instituto Oswaldo Cruz* 101(Suppl. 1), 339–343. DOI: 10.1590/S0074-02762006000900055

Carlisle, S. and Weisberg, L.S. (1978) *Schistosoma mansoni*: tracer studies in mice. *Experimental Parasitology* 44(1), 124–135. DOI: 10.1016/0014-4894(78)90088-7

Castro-Borges, W. and Wilson, R.A. (2022) Schistosome proteomics: updates and clinical implications. *Expert Review of Proteomics* 19(4–6), 247–261. DOI: 10.1080/14789450.2022.2142565

Castro-Borges, W., Dowle, A., Curwen, R.S., Thomas-Oates, J. and Wilson, R.A. (2011a) Enzymatic shaving of the tegument surface of live schistosomes for proteomic analysis: a rational approach to select vaccine candidates. *PLoS Neglected Tropical Diseases* 5(3), e993. DOI: 10.1371/journal.pntd.0000993

Castro-Borges, W., Simpson, D.M., Dowle, A., Curwen, R.S., Thomas-Oates, J. *et al.* (2011b) Abundance of tegument surface proteins in the human blood fluke *Schistosoma mansoni* determined by QconCAT proteomics. *Journal of Proteomics* 74(9), 1519–1533. DOI: 10.1016/j.jprot.2011.06.011

Chappell, L.H. (1974) Methionine uptake by larval and adult *Schistosoma mansoni*. *International Journal for Parasitology* 4(4), 361–369. DOI: 10.1016/0020-7519(74)90043-5

Collins, J.J., III, Wang, B., Lambrus, B.G., Tharp, M.E., Iyer, H. *et al.* (2013) Adult somatic stem cells in the human parasite *Schistosoma mansoni*. *Nature* 494(7438), 476–479. DOI: 10.1038/nature11924

Collins, J.J., III, Wendt, G.R., Iyer, H. and Newmark, P.A. (2016) Stem cell progeny contribute to the schistosome host-parasite interface. *eLife* 5, e12473. DOI: 10.7554/eLife.12473

Curwen, R.S., Ashton, P.D., Johnston, D.A. and Wilson, R.A. (2004) The *Schistosoma mansoni* soluble proteome: a comparison across four life-cycle stages. *Molecular and Biochemical Parasitology* 138(1), 57–66. DOI: 10.1016/j.molbiopara.2004.06.016

Da'Dara, A.A. and Skelly, P.J. (2025) The enigmatic heptalaminate surface membrane of intravascular schistosomes. *Trends in Parasitology* 41(3), 177–187. DOI: 10.1016/j.pt.2025.01.005

DeMarco, R., Kowaltowski, A.T., Mortara, R.A. and Verjovski-Almeida, S. (2003) Molecular characterization and immunolocalization of *Schistosoma mansoni* ATP-diphosphohydrolase. *Biochemical and Biophysical Research Communications* 307(4), 831–838. DOI: 10.1016/s0006-291x(03)01268-3

Ernst, S.C. (1975) Biochemical and cytochemical studies of digestive-absorptive functions of esophagus, cecum, and tequment in *Schistosoma mansioni*: acid phosphatase and tracer studies. *The Journal of Parasitology* 61(4), 633–647. DOI: 10.2307/3279456

Faghiri, Z. and Skelly, P.J. (2009) The role of tegumental aquaporin from the human parasitic worm, *Schistosoma mansoni*, in osmoregulation and drug uptake. *FASEB Journal* 23(8), 2780–2789. DOI: 10.1096/fj.09-130757

Faghiri, Z., Camargo, S.M.R., Huggel, K., Forster, I.C., Ndegwa, D. *et al.* (2010) The tegument of the human parasitic worm *Schistosoma mansoni* as an excretory organ: the surface aquaporin SmAQP is a lactate transporter. *PLoS ONE* 5(5), e10451. DOI: 10.1371/journal.pone.0010451

Farias, L.P., Krautz-Peterson, G., Tararam, C.A., Araujo-Montoya, B.O., Fraga, T.R. *et al.* (2013) On the three-finger protein domain fold and CD59-like proteins in *Schistosoma mansoni*. *PLoS Neglected Tropical Diseases* 7(10), e2482. DOI: 10.1371/journal.pntd.0002482

Farias, L.P., Vance, G.M., Coulson, P.S., Vitoriano-Souza, J., Neto, A.P. da S. *et al.* (2020) Epitope mapping of exposed tegument and alimentary tract proteins identifies putative antigenic targets of the attenuated schistosome vaccine. *Frontiers in Immunology* 11, 624613. DOI: 10.3389/fimmu.2020.624613

Farquhar, M.G. (1982) Membrane recycling in secretory cells: pathway to the Golgi complex. *Ciba Foundation Symposium* (92), 157–183. DOI: 10.1002/9780470720745.ch9

Figueiredo, B.C., Da'dara, A.A., Oliveira, S.C. and Skelly, P.J. (2015) Schistosomes enhance plasminogen activation: the role of tegumental enolase. *PLoS Pathogens* 11(12), e1005335. DOI: 10.1371/journal.ppat.1005335

Fitzsimmons, C.M., Jones, F.M., Stearn, A., Chalmers, I.W., Hoffmann, K.F. *et al.* (2012) The *Schistosoma mansoni* tegumental-allergen-like (TAL) protein family: influence of developmental expression on human IgE responses. *PLoS Neglected Tropical Diseases* 6(4), e1593. DOI: 10.1371/journal.pntd.0001593

Gallop, J.L. and McMahon, H.T. (2005) BAR domains and membrane curvature: bringing your curves to the BAR. *Biochemical Society Symposium* (72), 223–231. DOI: 10.1042/bss0720223

Goldring, O.L., Clegg, J.A., Smithers, S.R. and Terry, R.J. (1976) Acquisition of human blood group antigens by *Schistosoma mansoni*. *Clinical and Experimental Immunology* 26(1), 181–187.

Goodrich, S.P., Muller-Steffner, H., Osman, A., Moutin, M.-J., Kusser, K. *et al.* (2005) Production of calcium-mobilizing metabolites by a novel member of the ADP-ribosyl cyclase family expressed in *Schistosoma mansoni*. *Biochemistry* 44(33), 11082–11097. DOI: 10.1021/bi050704r

Hall, T.M.T., Joseph, G.T. and Strand, M. (1995) *Schistosoma mansoni*: molecular cloning and sequencing of the 200-kDa chemotherapeutic target antigen. *Experimental Parasitology* 80(2), 242–249. DOI: 10.1006/expr.1995.1030

Halliday, C., de Castro-Neto, A., Alcantara, C.L., Cunha-e-Silva, N.L., Vaughan, S. *et al.* (2021) Trypanosomatid flagellar pocket from structure to function. *Trends in Parasitology* 37(4), 317–329. DOI: 10.1016/j.pt.2020.11.005

Hockley, D.J. and McLaren, D.J. (1973) *Schistosoma mansoni*: changes in the outer membrane of the tegument during development from cercaria to adult worm. *International Journal for Parasitology* 3(1), 13–25. DOI: 10.1016/0020-7519(73)90004-0

Hu, W., Yan, Q., Shen, D.-K., Liu, F., Zhu, Z.-D. *et al.* (2003) Evolutionary and biomedical implications of a *Schistosoma japonicum* complementary DNA resource. *Nature Genetics* 35(2), 139–147. DOI: 10.1038/ng1236

Hyman, L.H. (1951) *The Invertebrates: II Platyhelminthes and Rhyncocoela. The Acoelomate Bilateria*. McGraw-Hill, New York.

Karcz, S.R., Podesta, R.B., Siddiqui, A.A., Dekaban, G.A., Strejan, G.H. *et al.* (1991) Molecular cloning and sequence analysis of a calcium-activated neutral protease (calpain) from *Schistosoma mansoni*. *Molecular and Biochemical Parasitology* 49(2), 333–336. DOI: 10.1016/0166-6851(91)90078-k

Keating, J.H., Wilson, R.A. and Skelly, P.J. (2006) No overt cellular inflammation around intravascular schistosomes *in vivo*. *The Journal of Parasitology* 92(6), 1365–1369. DOI: 10.1645/GE-864R.1

Khayath, N., Vicogne, J., Ahier, A., BenYounes, A., Konrad, C. *et al.* (2007) Diversification of the insulin receptor family in the helminth parasite *Schistosoma mansoni*. *The FEBS Journal* 274(3), 659–676. DOI: 10.1111/j.1742-4658.2006.05610.x

Kifle, D.W., Chaiyadet, S., Waardenberg, A.J., Wise, I., Cooper, M. *et al.* (2020a) Uptake of *Schistosoma mansoni* extracellular vesicles by human endothelial and monocytic cell lines and impact on vascular endothelial cell gene expression. *International Journal for Parasitology* 50(9), 685–696. DOI: 10.1016/j.ijpara.2020.05.005

Kifle, D.W., Pearson, M.S., Becker, L., Pickering, D., Loukas, A. *et al.* (2020b) Proteomic analysis of two populations of *Schistosoma mansoni*-derived extracellular vesicles: 15k pellet and 120k pellet vesicles. *Molecular and Biochemical Parasitology* 236, 111264. DOI: 10.1016/j.molbiopara.2020.111264

Krautz-Peterson, G., Camargo, S., Huggel, K., Verrey, F., Shoemaker, C.B. *et al.* (2007) Amino acid transport in schistosomes: characterization of the permease heavy chain SPRM1hc. *The Journal of Biological Chemistry* 282(30), 21767–21775. DOI: 10.1074/jbc.M703512200

Kusel, J.R. (1972) Protein composition and protein synthesis in the surface membranes of *Schistosoma mansoni*. *Parasitology* 65(1), 55–69. DOI: 10.1017/s0031182000044231

Levy, M.G. and Read, C.P. (1975a) Purine and pyrimidine transport in *Schistosoma mansoni*. *The Journal of Parasitology* 61(4), 627. DOI: 10.2307/3279455

Levy, M.G. and Read, C.P. (1975b) Relation of tegumentary phosphohydrolase to purine and pyrimidine transport in *Schistosoma mansoni*. *The Journal of Parasitology* 61(4), 648. DOI: 10.2307/3279457

Liu, J., Zhu, L., Wang, L., Chen, Y., Giri, B.R. *et al.* (2018) Isolation and characterization of extracellular vesicles from adult *Schistosoma japonicum*. *Journal of Visualized Experiments* 135. DOI: 10.3791/57514

Liu, J., Zhu, L., Wang, J., Qiu, L., Chen, Y. *et al.* (2019) *Schistosoma japonicum* extracellular vesicle miRNA cargo regulates host macrophage functions facilitating parasitism. *PLoS Pathogens* 15(6), e1007817. DOI: 10.1371/journal.ppat.1007817

Migliardo, F., Tallima, H. and El Ridi, R. (2014) Rigidity and resistance of larval- and adult schistosomes-medium interface. *Biochemical and Biophysical Research Communications* 446(1), 255–260. DOI: 10.1016/j.bbrc.2014.02.100

Morris, G.P. and Threadgold, L.T. (1968) Ultrastructure of the tegument of adult *Schistosoma mansoni*. *The Journal of Parasitology* 54(1), 15–27. DOI: 10.2307/3276867

Mulvenna, J., Moertel, L., Jones, M.K., Nawaratna, S., Lovas, E.M. *et al.* (2010) Exposed proteins of the *Schistosoma japonicum* tegument. *International Journal for Parasitology* 40(5), 543–554. DOI: 10.1016/j.ijpara.2009.10.002

Neves, L.X., Sanson, A.L., Wilson, R.A. and Castro-Borges, W. (2015) What's in SWAP? Abundance of the principal constituents in a soluble extract of *Schistosoma mansoni* revealed by shotgun proteomics. *Parasites & Vectors* 8, 337. DOI: 10.1186/s13071-015-0943-x

Newmark, P.A. and Sánchez Alvarado, A. (2002) Not your father's planarian: a classic model enters the era of functional genomics. *Nature Reviews Genetics* 3(3), 210–219. DOI: 10.1038/nrg759

Nicolson, G.L. and Ferreira de Mattos, G. (2023) The fluid-mosaic model of cell membranes: a brief introduction, historical features, some general principles, and its adaptation to current information. *Biochimica et Biophysica Acta. Biomembranes* 1865(4), 184135. DOI: 10.1016/j.bbamem.2023.184135

Pearce, E.J., Magee, A.I., Smithers, S.R. and Simpson, A.J. (1991) Sm25, a major schistosome tegumental glycoprotein, is dependent on palmitic acid for membrane attachment. *The EMBO Journal* 10(10), 2741–2746. DOI: 10.1002/j.1460-2075.1991.tb07822.x

Pérez-Sánchez, R., Valero, M.L., Ramajo-Hernández, A., Siles-Lucas, M., Ramajo-Martín, V. *et al.* (2008) A proteomic approach to the identification of tegumental proteins of male and female *Schistosoma bovis* worms. *Molecular and Biochemical Parasitology* 161(2), 112–123. DOI: 10.1016/j.molbiopara.2008.06.011

Pirovich, D., Da'dara, A.A. and Skelly, P.J. (2019) Why do intravascular schistosomes coat themselves in glycolytic enzymes? *BioEssays* 41(12), e1900103. DOI: 10.1002/bies.201900103

Popiel, I., Irving, D.L. and Basch, P.F. (1985) Wound healing in the trematode *Schistosoma*. *Tissue & Cell* 17(1), 69–77. DOI: 10.1016/0040-8166(85)90016-3

Qian, S., Sharma, V.K. and Clifton, L.A. (2020) Understanding the structure and dynamics of complex *biomembrane* interactions by neutron scattering techniques. *Langmuir* 36(50), 15189–15211. DOI: 10.1021/acs.langmuir.0c02516

Ramajo-Hernández, A., Pérez-Sánchez, R., Ramajo-Martín, V. and Oleaga, A. (2007) *Schistosoma bovis*: plasminogen binding in adults and the identification of plasminogen-binding proteins from the worm tegument. *Experimental Parasitology* 115(1), 83–91. DOI: 10.1016/j.exppara.2006.07.003

Redman, C.A. and Kusel, J.R. (1996) Distribution and biophysical properties of fluorescent lipids on the surface of adult *Schistosoma mansoni*. *Parasitology* 113(2), 137–143. DOI: 10.1017/s0031182000066385

Ribeiro, F., Coelho, P.M., Vieira, L.Q., Powell, K. and Kusel, J.R. (1998) Membrane internalization processes in different stages of *Schistosoma mansoni* as shown by a styryl dye (Frei Mao1-43). *Parasitology* 116(1), 51–59. DOI: 10.1017/s0031182097001960

Riengrojpitak, S. (1987) *Schistosoma mansoni*: localisation of schistosome antigens using antibodies raised against adult worm tegument membranes. PhD thesis, University of York, York, UK. Available at: https://etheses.whiterose.ac.uk/id/eprint/10942

Riengrojpitak, S., Vojvodic, M., Boot, C. and Wilson, R.A. (1989) Reactivity of anti-tegument monoclonal antibodies with target epitopes in different worm tissues and developmental stages of *Schistosoma mansoni*. *Parasitology* 98(2), 213–225. DOI: 10.1017/s0031182000062120

Roberts, S.M., MacGregor, A.N., Vojvodic, M., Wells, E., Crabtree, J.E. *et al.* (1983) Tegument surface membranes of adult *Schistosoma mansoni*: development of a method for their isolation. *Molecular and Biochemical Parasitology* 9(2), 105–127. DOI: 10.1016/0166-6851(83)90104-4

Roberts, S.M., Boot, C. and Wilson, R.A. (1988) Antibody responses of rodents to a tegument membrane preparation from adult *Schistosoma mansoni*. *Parasitology* 97(3), 425–435. DOI: 10.1017/S0031182000058832

Ross, P.L., Huang, Y.N., Marchese, J.N., Williamson, B., Parker, K. *et al.* (2004) Multiplexed protein quantitation in *Saccharomyces cerevisiae* using amine-reactive isobaric tagging reagents. *Molecular & Cellular Proteomics* 3(12), 1154–1169. DOI: 10.1074/mcp.M400129-MCP200

Saunders, N., Wilson, R.A. and Coulson, P.S. (1987) The outer bilayer of the adult schistosome tegument surface has a low turnover rate *in vitro* and *in vivo*. *Molecular and Biochemical Parasitology* 25(2), 123–131. DOI: 10.1016/0166-6851(87)90001-6

Shaw, M.K. and Erasmus, D.A. (1987) *Schistosoma mansoni*: structural damage and tegumental repair after *in vivo* treatment with praziquantel. *Parasitology* 94(2), 243–254. DOI: 10.1017/s0031182000053920

Siddiqui, A.A., Zhou, Y., Podesta, R.B., Karcz, S.R., Tognon, C.E. *et al.* (1993) Characterization of Ca^{2+}-dependent neutral protease (calpain) from human blood flukes, *Schistosoma mansoni*. *Biochimica et Biophysica Acta* 1181(1), 37–44. DOI: 10.1016/0925-4439(93)90087-h

Singer, S.J. and Nicolson, G.L. (1972) The fluid mosaic model of the structure of cell membranes. *Science* 175(4023), 720–731. DOI: 10.1126/science.175.4023.720

Skelly, P.J., Kim, J.W., Cunningham, J. and Shoemaker, C.B. (1994) Cloning, characterization, and functional expression of cDNAs encoding glucose transporter proteins from the human parasite *Schistosoma mansoni*. *The Journal of Biological Chemistry* 269(6), 4247–4253. DOI: 10.1016/S0021-9258(17)41770-4

Skelly, P.J., Tielens, A.G. and Shoemaker, C.B. (1998) Glucose transport and metabolism in mammalian-stage schistosomes. *Parasitology Today* 14(10), 402–406. DOI: 10.1016/s0169-4758(98)01319-2

Skelly, P.J., Pfeiffer, R., Verrey, F. and Shoemaker, C.B. (1999) SPRM1lc, a heterodimeric amino acid permease light chain of the human parasitic platyhelminth, *Schistosoma mansoni*. *Parasitology* 119(6), 569–576. DOI: 10.1017/s0031182099005181

Skelly, P.J., Da'dara, A.A., Li, X.H., Castro-Borges, W. and Wilson, R.A. (2014) Schistosome feeding and regurgitation. *PLoS Pathogens* 10(8), e1004246. DOI: 10.1371/journal.ppat.1004246

Skelly, P.J., Nation, C.S. and Da'Dara, A.A. (2022) *Schistosoma mansoni* and the purinergic halo. *Trends in Parasitology* 38(12), 1080–1088. DOI: 10.1016/j.pt.2022.09.001

Smith, J.H. and von Lichtenberg, F. (1974) Observations on the ultrastructure of the tegument of *Schistosoma mansoni* in mesenteric veins. *The American Journal of Tropical Medicine and Hygiene* 23(1), 71–77. DOI: 10.4269/ajtmh.1974.23.71

Smithers, S.R., Terry, R.J. and Hockley, D.J. (1969) Host antigens in schistosomiasis. *Proceedings of the Royal Society of London. Series B, Biological Sciences* 171(1025), 483–494. DOI: 10.1098/rspb.1969.0007

Sobhon, P., Upatham, E.S. and McLaren, D.J. (1984) Topography and ultrastructure of the tegument of adult *Schistosoma mekongi*. *Parasitology* 89(3), 511–521. DOI: 10.1017/s0031182000056730

Sotillo, J., Pearson, M., Becker, L., Mulvenna, J. and Loukas, A. (2015) A quantitative proteomic analysis of the tegumental proteins from *Schistosoma mansoni* schistosomula reveals novel potential therapeutic targets. *International Journal for Parasitology* 45(8), 505–516. DOI: 10.1016/j.ijpara.2015.03.004

Threadgold, L.T. (1963) The tegument and associated structures of *Fasciola hepatica*. *Journal of Cell Science* 104(68), 505–512. DOI: 10.1242/jcs.s3-104.68.505

van Balkom, B.W.M., van Gestel, R.A., Brouwers, J.F., Krijgsveld, J., Tielens, A.G.M. *et al.* (2005) Mass spectrometric analysis of the *Schistosoma mansoni* tegumental sub-proteome. *Journal of Proteome Research* 4(3), 958–966. DOI: 10.1021/pr050036w

Vasconcelos, E.G., Nascimento, P.S., Meirelles, M.N., Verjovski-Almeida, S. and Ferreira, S.T. (1993) Characterization and localization of an ATP-diphosphohydrolase on the external surface of the tegument of *Schistosoma mansoni*. *Molecular and Biochemical Parasitology* 58(2), 205–214. DOI: 10.1016/0166-6851(93)90042-v

Verjovski-Almeida, S., DeMarco, R., Martins, E.A., Guimarães, P.E., Ojopi, E.P.B. *et al.* (2003) Transcriptome analysis of the acoelomate human parasite *Schistosoma mansoni*. *Nature Genetics* 35(2), 148–157. DOI: 10.1038/ng1237

Wang, B., Collins, J.J., III and Newmark, P.A. (2013) Functional genomic characterization of neoblast-like stem cells in larval *Schistosoma mansoni*. *eLife* 2, e00768. DOI: 10.7554/eLife.00768

Wendt, G. and Collins, J.J. (2020) Labeling of the *Schistosoma mansoni* tegument. *Methods in Molecular Biology* 2151, 65–74. DOI: 10.1007/978-1-0716-0635-3_6

Wendt, G., Zhao, L., Chen, R., Liu, C., O'Donoghue, A.J. *et al.* (2020) A single-cell RNA-seq atlas of *Schistosoma mansoni* identifies a key regulator of blood feeding. *Science* 369(6511), 1644–1649. DOI: 10.1126/science.abb7709

Wendt, G.R., Collins, J.N., Pei, J., Pearson, M.S., Bennett, H.M. *et al.* (2018) Flatworm-specific transcriptional regulators promote the specification of tegumental progenitors in *Schistosoma mansoni*. *eLife* 7, e33221. DOI: 10.7554/eLife.33221

Wendt, G.R., Reese, M.L. and Collins, J.J., III (2021) SchistoCyte Atlas: a single-cell transcriptome resource for adult schistosomes. *Trends in Parasitology* 37(7), 585–587. DOI: 10.1016/j.pt.2021.04.010

Wheater, P.R. and Wilson, R.A. (1976) The tegument of *Schistosoma mansoni*: a histochemical investigation. *Parasitology* 72(1), 99–109. DOI: 10.1017/s0031182000043237

Wilson, R.A. (2012) Proteomics at the schistosome–mammalian host interface: any prospects for diagnostics or vaccines? *Parasitology* 139(9), 1178–1194. DOI: 10.1017/S0031182012000339

Wilson, R.A. and Barnes, P.E. (1974) The tegument of *Schistosoma mansoni*: observations on the formation, structure and composition of cytoplasmic inclusions in relation to tegument function. *Parasitology* 68(2), 239–258. DOI: 10.1017/S0031182000045765

Wilson, R.A. and Barnes, P.E. (1977) The formation and turnover of the *membranocalyx* on the tegument of *Schistosoma mansoni*. *Parasitology* 74(1), 61–71. DOI: 10.1017/s0031182000047533

Wilson, R.A. and Coulson, P.S. (2009) Immune effector mechanisms against schistosomiasis: looking for a chink in the parasite's *armour*. *Trends in Parasitology* 25(9), 423–431. DOI: 10.1016/j.pt.2009.05.011

Wilson, R.A. and Jones, M.K. (2021) Fifty years of the schistosome tegument: discoveries, controversies, and outstanding questions. *International Journal for Parasitology* 51(13–14), 1213–1232. DOI: 10.1016/j.ijpara.2021.11.002

8

The Alimentary Tract: Oesophageal Glands and Gastrodermis

8.1 Overview

The alimentary tract is the second major interface between the adult worms and the host bloodstream. It becomes active during intravascular migration of the schistosomulum, but erythrocytes are not ingested until after transformation in the liver. It is blind-ending so must function as a tidal system, with blood taken in and waste products expelled through the mouth situated at the base of the oral sucker. The tract comprises two functional regions, an oesophagus where blood is initially processed, and an elongate gut where digestion and absorption take place. In this chapter, the structure, functional activity and secretions of the anterior and posterior oesophageal glands are covered in detail. This includes a consideration of the numerous micro-exon gene (MEG)-encoded proteins, their evolution in the family Schistosomatidae and putative roles in blood processing. The structure of the gastrodermis, the processing of haemoglobin for absorption and of the haem group into non-toxic insoluble haemozoin are covered. The characterization of gastrodermal secretions revealed via proteomic analysis of worm vomitus and single-cell sequencing of gastrodermal and oesophageal gland clusters provides a comprehensive inventory of luminal processes. This contrasts with our paucity of knowledge about epithelial transporters on the gastrodermal surface compared to the tegument. The evidence for an ability to endocytose material at the gastrodermal surface is set out and the enigmatic nature of digestion at an acid pH is also covered.

8.2 Layout of the Alimentary Tract

Detailed reviews of the alimentary tract (Skelly *et al.*, 2014; Li and Wilson, 2017) form the basis of this chapter and an overview of its layout is summarized below. One of the best ways to appreciate the relative proportions of the tract in males and females is by viewing the distribution of the dark brown haemozoin (β-haematin) pigment residue from haemoglobin digestion (Fig. 8.1.1 and 8.1.2). The females are much darker in appearance than males due to their greater ingestion of blood (see below) but the organization is similar. The oesophagus, a short muscular tube, connects the mouth to a transverse region of the gut, and the junction of the two is marked by a desmosome, suggesting an abrupt change in functions and distinct embryological origins. The transverse gut then bifurcates in both sexes to run in parallel around the reproductive system before uniting to form a single caecum (so termed because it ends blindly), which passes to the extreme posterior. The structure of the gastrodermis and its overlying musculature (see Chapter 4) is uniform along its length in both

DOI: 10.1079/9781800625167.0008

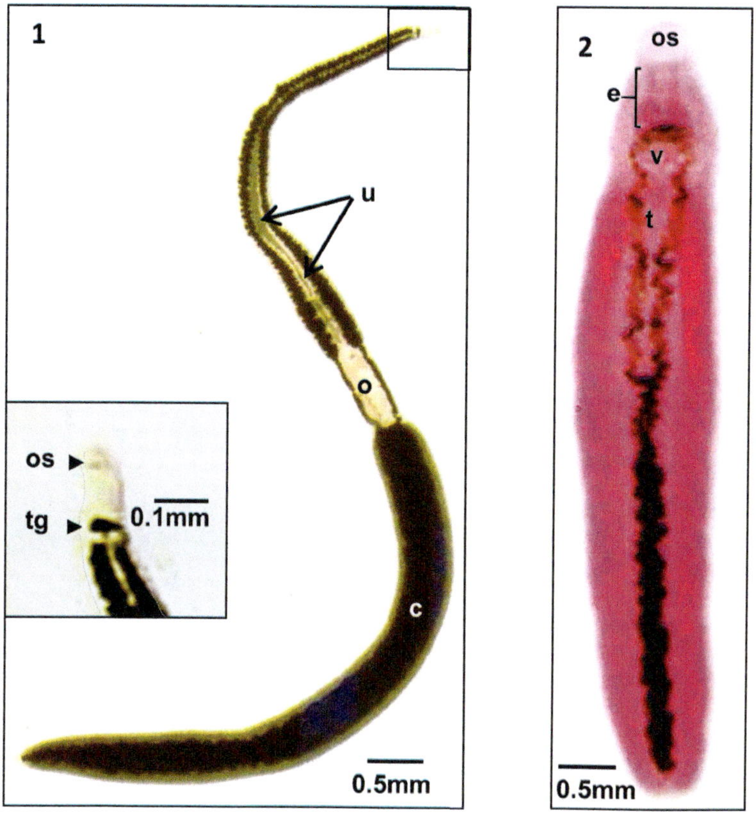

Fig. 8.1. Layout of the alimentary tract. **1**) Female *S. japonicum* from rabbit. The oesophagus (inset; e) is minute compared to the length of the female body. Haemozoin pigment delineates extent of the caecum (c). The transverse gut (tg) bifurcates after the oesophagus with parallel branches running around the uterus (u) and ovary (o) before uniting in a single channel. **2**) A juvenile 28-day male *S. mansoni* worm showing a proportionally larger oral sucker and oesophagus (e). The layout is similar to the female with the transverse gut bifurcating at the level of the ventral sucker (v) to run around the testes (t) before uniting in a single channel one-third of the way along the body. Haemozoin is present at a lower intensity. (**1** from Skelly and Wilson, 2014; **2** from Li and Wilson, 2017.) **1**) Figure used under license CC-BY-4.0. **2**) Figure used with permission from CRC Press.

sexes, with ingested markers rapidly reaching the extreme posterior due to waves of peristalsis. The organization of the oesophagus, with anterior and posterior glands surrounding the lumen, is identical in both sexes but in the female is only one-fifth the size of that in the male (Skelly *et al.*, 2014). This disparity is a major puzzle because the function of the combined contractions of the oral sucker and oesophageal muscles is to pump blood from mouth to gut. On the basis of size and feeding dynamics, the pump in females must move 8.5 times the volume of blood as males, so needs to work 40 times as hard. How is this achieved? Plausibly, females feed continuously with short interruptions for regurgitation of hemozoin, whereas males feed intermittently (the male cannot ingest blood while using his oral sucker to transport a female along a blood vessel). A feeding/digestion/regurgitation cycle in males would explain why they come in various shades of brown while females are more uniformly black.

8.3 The Oesophagus

The structure of the oesophagus and its associated glands was examined by transmission electron microscopy (TEM) more than 50 years ago (Dike, 1971), but then largely forgotten until the localization of a MEG gene expression (Antigen 10.3) to the posterior gland reignited interest (Dillon *et al.*, 2007). The oesophageal lining is contiguous with the tegument syncytium of the oral sucker but with a highly differentiated surface. The equivalents of tegument cell bodies are clustered outside the muscle layer and aggregated into two multicellular glands (Fig. 8.2.1), which deliver their inclusions into the oesophageal lining. Thus, based on their cytological organization, we might anticipate similarities of function between oesophagus and tegument. There is presently no information on whether oesophageal gland cell bodies turnover in the manner of tegument cell bodies. Emphatically, recent discoveries on the cytology, secretions and putative functions of the glands have provided new insights about the way worms feed on blood and added an extra dimension to the search for effective vaccine candidates.

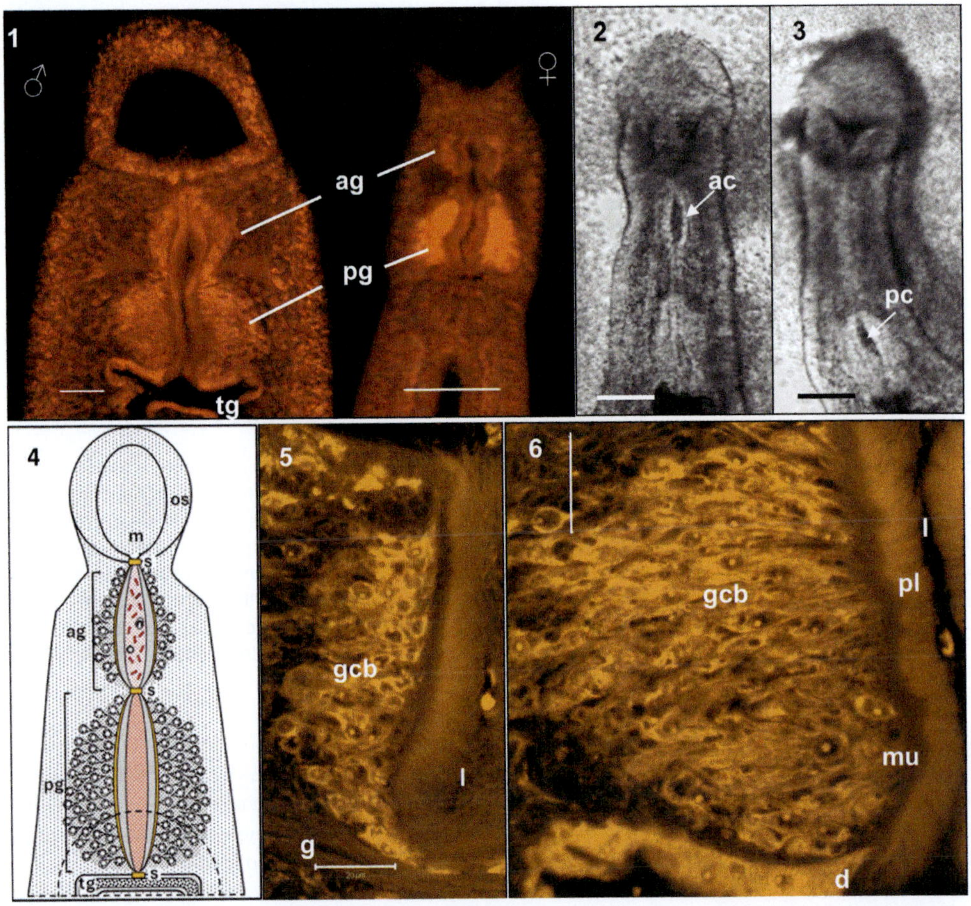

Fig. 8.2. Layout of the oesophageal glands. **1**) The position of the glands in male and female *S. japonicum*. **2** and **3**) Single video frames from a male worm feeding *in vitro*. **4**) Diagram of the oesophageal region. **5**) Anterior gland showing distribution of cell bodies, muscle layer and luminal plates. **6**) The larger posterior gland showing the same arrangement plus the desmosomal junction with the gastrodermis. ac, anterior compartment; ag, anterior gland; d, desmosome; g, central ganglion; gcb, gland cell bodies; l, lumen; m, mouth; mu, muscle; pg, posterior gland; pl, plates; s, sphincters; tg, transverse gut. Scale bars: **1**, 50 μm; **2** and **3**, 100 μm; **5** and **6**, 50 μm. (**1–3**, **5** and **6** from Li *et al.*, 2013.) **1–3**, **5** and **6**) Figures used under license CC-BY-4.0. **4**) Figure author's own.

8.3.1 The feeding process

To appreciate how the oesophageal glands operate, we need to consider the task that males and females undertake. The ideal experimental situation would be observation of worms feeding *in vivo* in blood vessels and one study did attempt this (Bloch, 1980). Visibility in the bloodstream is a problem and the parameter selected was the opening and closing of the oral sucker (presumably of males). This occurred approximately once every 1–2 s, accompanied by flexion and extension movements. Feeding might be continuous for up to an hour or in intermittent 10 min bursts. Worms remained stationary during feeding, but non-feeding worms moved a few hundred microns along a vessel. More detailed *in vitro* information was obtained from video analysis of male *Schistosoma mansoni* worms feeding at 37°C on a diluted suspension of erythrocytes (Li *et al.*, 2013). In this situation, the grabbing motion of the oral sucker could be as rapid as 4 times per second. The oesophageal lumen was shown to comprise two separate compartments. During feeding, erythrocytes accumulated in the lumen of the anterior compartment (Fig. 8.2.2) before a wave of peristalsis drove the bolus into the posterior compartment (Fig. 8.2.3), and finally into the transverse gut. The process in females is similar but proved difficult to analyse, due to their small size and greater motility. It is worth noting that regurgitation did not involve reverse peristalsis of the oesophageal muscles. Rather, vomiting was preceded by intense muscular activity in the anterior gut, followed by relaxation of the oesophageal wall. A thin dark line of vomitus travelled towards the mouth and a stream of pigment particles was ejected from the oral sucker (Li *et al.*, 2013).

As described in Chapter 4, the oesophagus has its own set of outer longitudinal and inner circular muscles, capable of propagating waves of peristalsis, under independent neuronal control. An extra level of complexity, which ties in with the presence of separate functional compartments is that three groups of circular fibres act as sphincters, at the junction with the oral sucker/mouth, centrally between anterior and posterior compartments, and at the junction of the oesophagus with the transverse gut (Fig. 8.2.4). The inference must be that these sphincters are under separate control, but their relaxation/contraction cycle must be synchronized with the interrupted waves of peristalsis that propel blood through the anterior and posterior compartments.

Our knowledge of the dynamics of blood feeding derives from a single pioneering *in vivo* study in mice using ^{51}Cr-labelled erythrocytes (Lawrence, 1973). Loss of label from the erythrocytes was trivial over the 24 h time course and the γ-emissions provided estimates of counts associated with both cells and worms. Label accumulated rapidly in worms and a steady state was reached after ~8 h when the amount ingested equalled the amount excreted. The maximum number of erythrocytes in a pair was estimated at 1.33×10^6, acquired at a rate of 3.32×10^5 per hour, so complete exchange of caecal contents would take ~4 h. The distinction in feeding capacity between females and males was very marked at 330,000 versus 39,000 erythrocytes per hour, which equates to daily intakes of 880 and 105 nl of whole blood, respectively. The relative values for haem content of paler males versus much darker females confirm these differences in blood intake (Oliveira *et al.*, 2000). There are quite large disparities in the body fluid volume (111 versus 290 nl) and gut volume (15 versus 7.5 nl) between females and males (Li and Wilson, 2017). When these values are taken into account and the blood intake is adjusted for packed cell volume, the female ingests 484 nl of plasma fluids per day, equivalent to 32.3 gut volumes, or 4.4 body volumes. The values for the male are 58 nl of plasma fluids equivalent to 7.7 gut volumes and, emphasizing his larger size, only 0.2 body volumes of fluid (Skelly *et al.*, 2014). Since vomiting by worms is infrequent and of low volume, this leads to another conclusion. We must infer that there is a major flux of salts and water from the worm gut to the bloodstream across the tegument surface. This in turn provides a context for the importance of aquaporin at the tegument surface (see Chapter 7), and a prediction that its abundance should be greater in the female than the male.

8.3.2 The structure of anterior and posterior glands

Initial observations on oesophageal structure by confocal microscopy and TEM (Li *et al.*, 2013) ignored the existence of an anterior gland, focusing only on the larger posterior gland. Subsequently, the smaller and morphologically distinct anterior gland was described in *Schistosoma japonicum* (Li *et al.*, 2014); a similar anterior gland exists in *S. mansoni* but has not been formally described, due to a lack of publication quality images. The distinction between males and females, and in the size of anterior and posterior glands, is readily appreciated from longitudinal images of whole worms (Fig. 8.2.1). The number of cells contained in the anterior cluster of male worms was estimated from consecutive confocal slices through a Z-stack as 750 in both *S. japonicum* and *S. mansoni*. The comparable numbers for the larger posterior cluster were 1400 cells for *S. japonicum* males and 1000 cells for *S. mansoni*. The close packing of gland cells (Fig. 8.2.5) means some are positioned up to 80 μm from the lining syncytium of the oesophagus, each connected by a microtubule-lined extension for passage of secretory vesicles. Although the lining of the oesophagus is an extension of the tegument, when viewed in the confocal microscope, in both anterior and posterior compartments it is many times thicker (Fig. 8.2.5 and 8.2.6). Additionally, the lumen of the anterior compartment appears to have numerous wispy threads at the limit of resolution.

Examination of the posterior gland by TEM reveals the cells to be typical secretory cells with dense granular cytoplasm, Golgi bodies and a special type of inclusion termed a crystalloid vesicle (0.23 × 0.27 μm) (Fig. 8.3.1) (Li *et al.*, 2013). Its dense contents arranged in parallel rows were considered potentially membranous in nature (Bogitsh and Carter, 1977), but see Section 8.3.7. The most remarkable feature of the syncytium is its extension into long narrow plates of cytoplasm up to 25 μm from base to tip, each with a central invagination of the basal membrane that runs almost to the tip (Fig. 8.3.2). The plates are loosely separated and orientated longitudinally over the full length of the posterior compartment. They are too closely spaced to admit entry of host cells between them, but the crystalloid vesicles appear to be secreted at sites part way along and their contents remain as visibly aggregated structures after release (Fig. 8.3.2). It was estimated that the plates increased the surface area of the lumen 26-fold, compared to a smooth prolate spheroid (Li *et al.*, 2013). This combination of the plate extensions of the luminal membrane with the very elongate invaginations of the basal membrane raises the possibility that the enormous surface area is an adaptation to generate massive ion fluxes into or out of the posterior oesophageal lumen, linked in some way to blood processing. Numbers of tegumental discoid bodies are also evident in the plates right out to their tips. The organization of the gland, wall and lumen of the posterior oesophageal compartment in transverse section is summarized in Fig. 8.3.4.

Preparation of transverse ‘steaks’ from male worms for viewing by scanning electron microscopy (SEM) revealed an equally complex but distinct organization for the anterior oesophageal compartment (Fig. 8.4.1) (Li *et al.*, 2014). Similar to the posterior gland, there is an arrangement of closely spaced vertical plates (Fig. 4.8.2), with central invaginations of the basal membrane, but these plates terminate in what can only be described as a central ‘mass of spaghetti’ virtually filling the whole lumen. At higher magnification, this can be seen to comprise long narrow threads of cytoplasm interspersed with flattened discs, each containing numerous tiny pits 50 nm in diameter (Fig. 8.4.3; see Chapter 9 for their potential role in immunity). When viewed using TEM, the basic layout of cell bodies close-packed outside the muscle layer is similar to the posterior ball of cells (Fig. 8.4.4). However, in the anterior oesophagus of *S. japonicum* the inclusions are quite distinct, with light flocculent contents, very different from the crystalloid vesicles in the posterior (Fig. 8.4.5 and 8.4.7). In addition, some light vesicles possess marginal membranous layers (Fig. 8.4.5) which contribute to the membranous coating layers of the surface plates, as might be anticipated for a layer contiguous with the tegument (Li *et al.*, 2014). The luminal extensions appear to be even longer in the anterior oesophagus, up to 20 μm in males, and sinuous with bifurcations. Another difference from the posterior plates is that while some light vesicles certainly secrete their contents at points along the extensions (Fig. 8.4.5), they also travel out to the threads and plates, accumulating there, awaiting discharge of their contents (Fig. 8.4.6–8.4.8).

What might this remarkable cellular architecture achieve? Clearly the corrugations expand enormously the surface area of the anterior

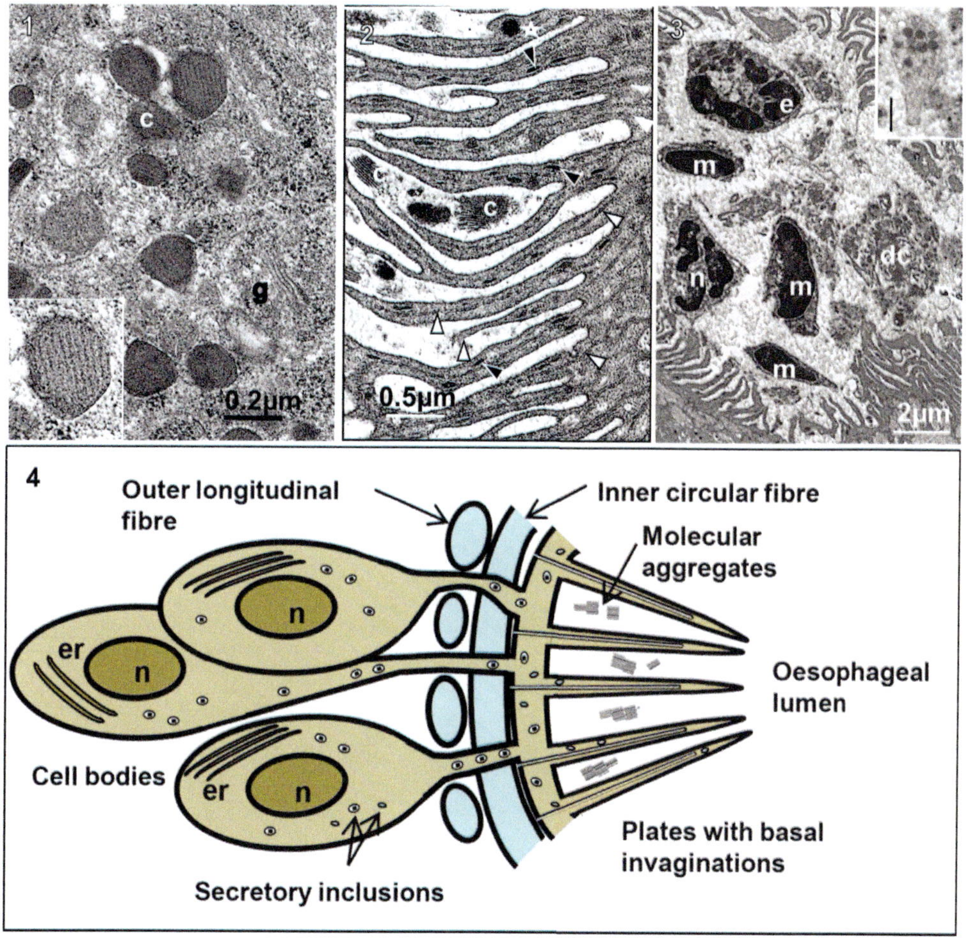

Fig. 8.3. Posterior oesophageal gland. **1**) Cytoplasm of a gland cell body with Golgi body (g), mitochondria (m) and crystalloid vesicles (c). Inset shows regular arrangement of contents. **2**) Luminal plates with central basal invaginations (white arrowheads), discoid bodies (black arrowheads) and aggregates of crystalloid vesicle contents in the lumen. The star indicates a site of vesicle fusion. **3**) The plug in the posterior lumen, comprised of macrophages (m), neutrophils (n), eosinophils (e) and disintegrating cells (dc). The inset is a platelet with granules. **4**) Diagram of the various elements of the gland and their relationship to the oesophageal muscle layer. (From Li *et al.*, 2013.) Figures used under license CC-BY-4.0.

oesophagus while the fringe of threads extends still further the potential interaction surface with ingested blood (no attempt was made to calculate the amplification factor). Indeed, it is possible, especially in the males, that the spaghetti-like threads intruding into the lumen are intended to entangle cells and retard erythrocyte passage, allowing more time for interaction with oesophageal secretions. The dissimilarity in structural appearance of light and crystalloid vesicles argues for marked differences in composition of their contents, hence different roles in the processing of ingested blood (see below).

8.3.3 The uncoating of erythrocytes and tethering of leucocytes

The scarcity of recognizable erythrocytes in TEM images of the oesophagus is the best evidence that they are lysed during passage through the anterior and posterior compartments. Additionally,

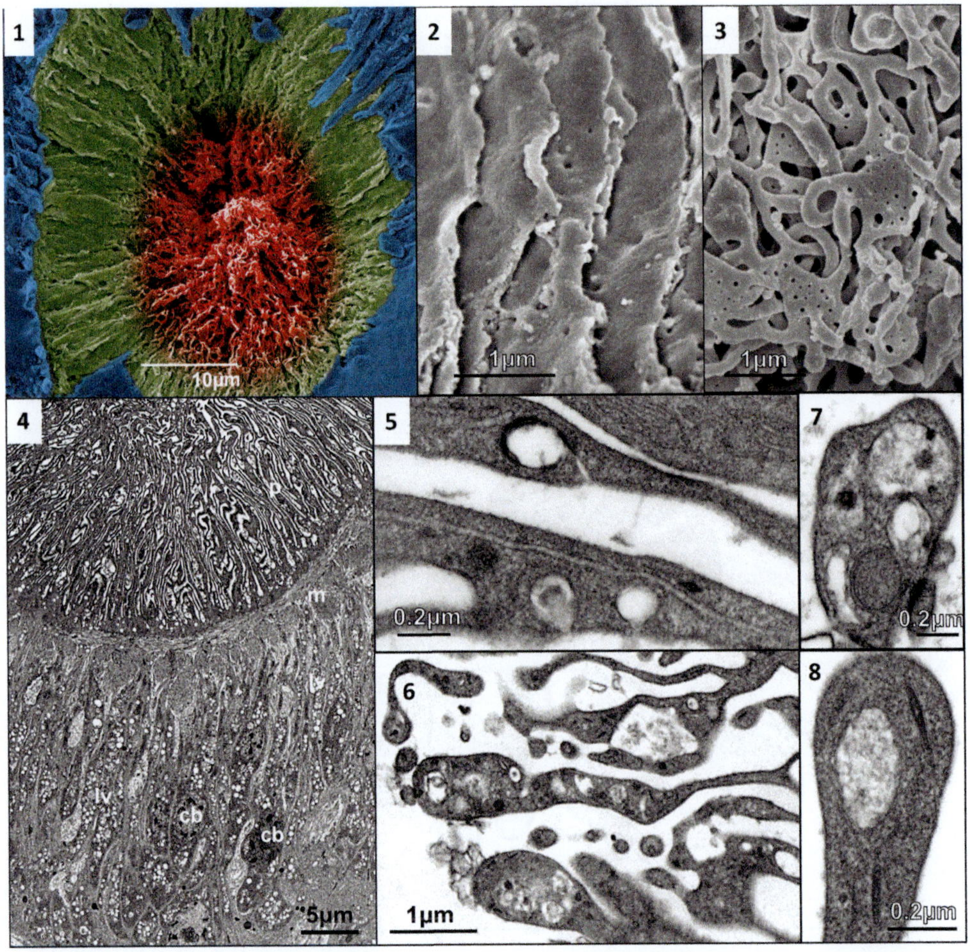

Fig. 8.4. The anterior oesophageal gland of *S. japonicum* (**1–3**, SEM; **4–8**, TEM). **1**) False colour slice across the anterior of a male with gland tissue (blue) luminal plates (green) and spaghetti-like extensions (red). **2**) The thin luminal plates with smooth surfaces. **3**) Long narrow threads of cytoplasm interspersed with flattened, pitted plates. **4**) Transverse slice through the cell bodies (cb) of the gland and sinuous luminal plates (p) separated by the circular and longitudinal muscle fibres (m). **5**) Section through parallel luminal plates showing central basal invagination and several light vesicles in the act of releasing contents. One contains marginated membranous layers. **6**) The expanded leading edges of plates, filled with light vesicles awaiting secretion. **7**) Higher magnification of a single expanded tip containing light vesicles with dense spots. **8**) A single tip with a vesicle and three discoid bodies. (From Li *et al.*, 2014.)

an *in vitro* feeding experiment using erythrocytes pre-labelled with the fluorescent membrane dye PKH2 has provided direct evidence for the interaction of gland secretions with incoming blood. Previously starved worms were stimulated to feed avidly when labelled erythrocytes were added to the culture medium. Within 15 min the anterior, and to a much greater extent the posterior regions, had acquired the PKH2 label as erythrocytes lysed and the freed dye transferred to the membranes of the oesophageal lining (Fig. 8.5.1) (Hall *et al.*, 2011). The second aspect of function is the presence of a stationary plug, composed of leucocytes, in the posterior lumen (Li *et al.*, 2013). Analysis of consecutive video frames at high magnification shows that a bolus of material arriving from the anterior compartment streams as a dark current around the plug (Fig. 8.5.2).

The final act in this process is the transit of material into the transverse gut, presumably when the posterior sphincter relaxes. The mechanism for sequestration of leucocytes appears to involve their binding by gland secretions (see Section 8.3.7). From Z-stacks of consecutive confocal images through *S. mansoni* fixed *in vivo*, the mean number of tethered leucocytes present in the lumen of the posterior oesophagus was estimated at 29 in males and 11 in females (Li *et al.*, 2013). Based on the cellular content of blood, and its rate of ingestion *in vivo* (Lawrence, 1973), the number in males equates to ~30 min of feeding. In contrast, for females the size of the plug equates to only 1–2 min of blood ingestion. How do the secretions of the anterior and posterior glands function to lyse erythrocytes and platelets, at the same time tethering and disabling leucocytes? This is not a trivial question to answer, given the minute size of the glands. The first step in finding answers was to discover what proteins the glands secreted.

8.3.4 Gland isolation by microdissection for subtractive RNA sequencing

The approach taken to characterize the pattern of gene expression relied on the fact that the anterior and posterior glands are unique to the oesophageal region. A microdissection method was developed to isolate these tissues from male worms by transection of the body at the level of the transverse gut. Their pattern of gene expression was then compared with that in the posterior third of the male body (which excluded the testes) (Wilson *et al.*, 2015). Ion torrent sequencing of the DNA fragments from two technical replicates of head and tail mRNA extracts yielded between 0.86 and 1.8 million reads, ~65% of which mapped to predicted genes in v5 of the *S. mansoni* genome. Differences in expression between heads and tails were compared using the RPKM statistic (reads per kilobase transcript per million mapped reads) (Mortazavi *et al.*, 2008) and the fold change visualized on log base 2 plots (Fig. 8.6). A total of 5010 genes was

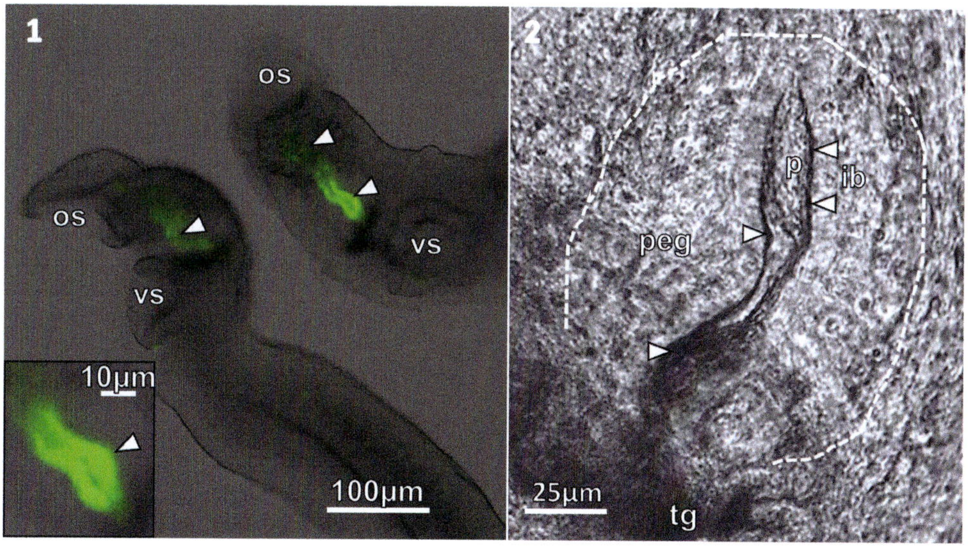

Fig. 8.5. Functional processes in the oesophageal lumen. **1**) The uncoating of PKH2-labelled erythrocytes revealed in a feeding experiment by transfer of the marker to the plates of the oesophageal lining, beginning in the anterior and completing in the posterior compartment. Inset: posterior plates. os, oral sucker; vs, ventral sucker. **2**) Composite image of more than 40 video frames showing ingested blood (ib, white arrows) passing around a plug (p) of leucocytes in the lumen of the posterior oesophageal gland (peg) to reach the transverse gut (tg). (**1** from Hall *et al.*, 2011; **2** from Li *et al.*, 2013.) **1**) Figure used with permission from Elsevier. **2**) Figure used under license CC-BY-4.0.

identified, 2583 more highly expressed in the heads and 2427 in the tails. Setting a threshold of 4-fold difference either side of the equivalence line $x = 0$ ultimately delineated 92 genes differentially expressed in the head (1.95%) and 67 in the tail (1.6%) (Fig. 8.6.1). Of these, 23 genes were expressed in the heads only and 10 in the tails only (the points lying along the 45° line). The identities of differentially expressed genes were first interrogated using a panel of around 250 signature genes from different tissues. Only four potential tegument genes encoding annexins and tetraspanins, one saposin from the gut secreted category, and three glycosyl transferases were expressed at 4-fold greater level in the heads, so potentially associated with oesophageal region. With these eight exceptions, the remaining 84 genes included three MEGs already known to be expressed in the oesophageal gland (MEG-4.1, -4.2 and -14) plus a further eight (MEG-8.1, -8.2, -9, -11, -12, -15, -16 and -17), whose site of expression was not previously recorded (Fig. 8.6.2). Some of these, like MEG-4.2, were expressed at up to 1000 times the level of nervous system genes in adjacent tissues. Two further genes (Smp_123100 and Smp_123200) with abundant and differential expression in the heads proved on close inspection to have a central region encoded by micro-exons and were designated MEG-32.1 and -32.2, respectively.

Since a significant number of reads did not map to the genome, a *de novo* assembly of all reads was performed and checked by comparing the abundance and differential expression of 12 known MEGs identified by both methods (the r value for their RPKMs was 0.88 and for their ratio in heads/tails was 0.93). A total of 51 differentially expressed, unannotated contigs was retrieved from the assembly for manual analysis. Their mean RPKM value for abundance ($\bar{x} = 418$) was much lower than for the 92 genes mapped to the genome ($\bar{x} = 3963$), but this might be anticipated, given that the unannotated contigs encode potential genes not detected by conventional methods. Of the 51, 63% were expressed in the heads alone and 16 were identified as encoding unannotated MEGs (Fig. 8.6.2). These included six previously described MEG proteins not in the genome (MEG-8.3, -8.4, -19, -20, -22 and -24) (Almeida *et al.*, 2012), and a further eight that were entirely new, namely MEG-26 to -31, plus two new members of existing families,

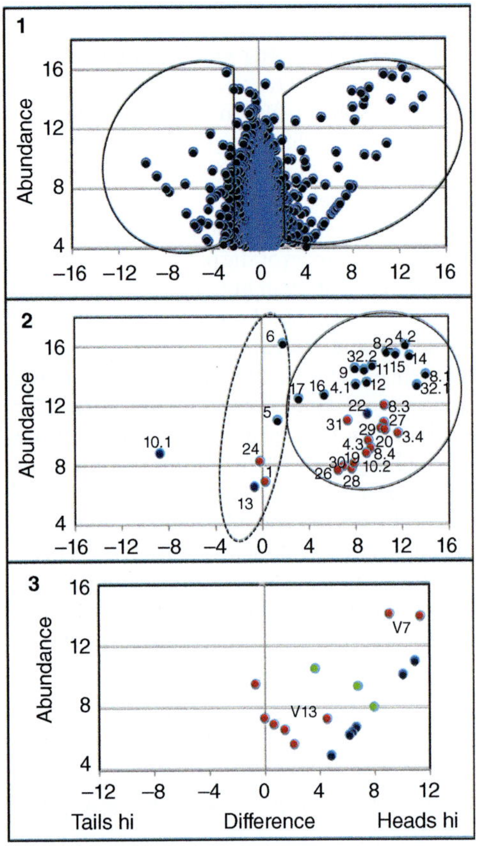

Fig. 8.6. Subtractive RNA-Seq of heads versus tails. **1**) Abundance on the *y*-axis is the $\log_2$ RPKM score of each head-enriched gene or tail-enriched gene. Difference on the *x*-axis is the $\log_2$ ratio of mean RPKM scores. The demarcated areas enclose genes that are expressed at 4-fold higher level. **2**) All MEGs identified: already mapped to the genome (●) or novel (●). **3**) Aspartyl proteases (●), phospholipases (●) and VAL (●) genes. (From Wilson *et al.*, 2015.) Figures used under license CC-BY-4.0.

MEG-10.2 and -4.3. (Thus, a total of at least 28 MEGs are potentially expressed in the oesophageal tissues.) A search for any MEGs not differentially expressed between heads and tails identified a further five (MEG-1, -5, -6, -13 and -24); MEG-5 was previously identified by tegument proteomics and MEG-24 was shown by whole-mount *in situ* hybridization (WISH) to be expressed in tegument cell bodies (Felizatti *et al.*, 2020). This suggests that the five MEGs might all be expressed in the tegument cell bodies throughout the worm. One final MEG (MEG-10.1) appears to be an outlier, expressed in tails only and possibly confined to a very scarce tissue (e.g. bladder).

A second prominent group of genes detected by the mapping to the genome (and confirmed by the Trinity assembly) comprised nine hydrolases (Fig. 8.6.3) (Wilson *et al.*, 2015). Homology searching of NCBInr indicates that these are likely to be of lysosomal origin. The group of six genes, exclusive to the head preparation, encoded closely related aspartyl proteases, referred to as cathepsin D homologues. Transcripts for two other hydrolases, annotated as phospholipase A2, were abundant, and almost exclusively expressed in the heads. The final hydrolase, palmitoyl protein thioesterase 1 enzyme, removes thioester-linked fatty acyl groups from modified cysteine residues in proteins. Finally, the venom-allergen-like (VAL) protein, VAL-7, already known to be expressed in the oesophageal gland (Rofatto *et al.*, 2012), was detected with a high level of expression. It is a member of a large family of secreted proteins potentially important in modifying host responses, encoded in v5 of the genome by two scaffolds whose level of expression was very close on the scatter plot (now annotated in v10 as Smp_300070) (Fig. 8.6.3). Only one further gene for a VAL (VAL-13) came above the >4-fold difference threshold, while five other VALs (VAL-16, -8, -12, -11 and -6) were more evenly distributed between heads and tails so not likely associated with the glands.

8.3.5 Validation of oesophageal gene expression and protein localization

The differential expression of genes in tissues isolated by microdissection needs to be backed up by WISH and/or protein immunocytochemistry, to confirm an oesophageal gland location. The expression of MEG-4.1 (Dillon *et al.*, 2007), MEG-4.2, MEG-14 (Li *et al.*, 2013) and VAL-7 (Rofatto *et al.*, 2012) were the first to be revealed in the posterior oesophageal gland of *S. mansoni* by WISH. In addition, seven proteins (six MEGs and VAL-7) were localized to the posterior oesophageal gland of *S. japonicum* by immunocytochemistry (Li *et al.*, 2013, 2015). The expression of a further 13 selected genes, identified by subtractive RNA sequencing (RNA-Seq), was confirmed in both males (Fig. 8.7.1) and females by WISH (Wilson *et al.*, 2015). Four of the selected genes, those for MEG-12, -16, -17 and phospholipase A2, were revealed as exclusively expressed in the cells surrounding the anterior oesophageal compartment, confirming its status as a distinct gland in *S. mansoni*.

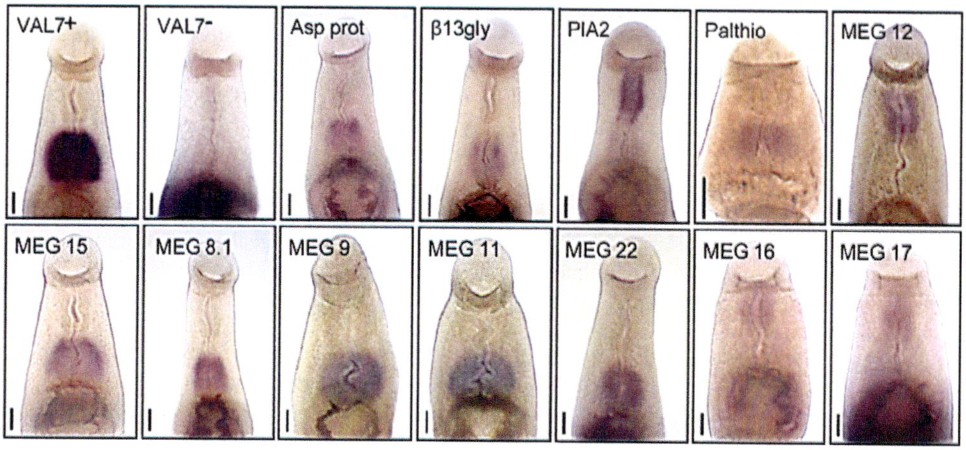

Fig. 8.7. Expression of selected genes in the male head region of *S. mansoni*. Asp prot, aspartyl protease; β13gly, β1,3-galactosyltransferase; PIA2, phospholipase A2; Palthio, palmitoyl thioesterase. The pattern of expression in females (not shown) was identical to that in males. Scale bar: 24 μm. (From Wilson *et al.*, 2015.)

Expression of the remainder, with VAL-7$^+$ as the positive control and VAL-7$^-$ sense strand as the negative control, was confined to the posterior oesophageal gland cell bodies. They comprised two hydrolases (aspartyl protease and palmitoyl thioesterase), five MEGs (MEG-8.2, -9, -11, -15 and -22) plus one of the three glycosyltransferases (β1,3-galactosyltransferase). (For the colocalization of MEG proteins and their interaction with host antibodies in permissive and immune hosts see Chapter 9 on vaccines.)

8.3.6 Oesophageal gland secretions in *Schistosoma japonicum*

The subtractive RNA-Seq approach was subsequently used to characterize the gene expression pattern in the oesophagus of *S. japonicum* males and females (Li *et al.*, 2018). The data obtained was intended to provide a comparison with *S. mansoni*, obtain a better understanding of blood processing in females given the much greater amounts of blood they ingest, and examine the evolution of MEGs, using bioinformatic analysis. A note of caution on this last point is that most MEGs are not annotated in the latest update of the *S. japonicum* genome (Luo *et al.*, 2019), so the reader is referred to the sequence depositions by Li *et al.* (2018). The sequence reads obtained from *S. japonicum* mRNA isolation and library construction were assembled *de novo* using the Trinity platform. Eliminating gene models with trivial read numbers produced a core of 9204 genes, expressed in heads and/or tails, with mapped read numbers ranging over five orders of magnitude. Those genes enriched >8-fold in the head preparation were subjected to detailed bioinformatics analysis.

As with *S. mansoni*, the largest group of genes (24/62) highlighted from the male heads of *S. japonicum* comprised MEGs. With a few exceptions (MEG-16 and -17), orthologues could be identified between the two species and were numbered accordingly (Li *et al.*, 2018). All the MEGs were predicted to encode a signal peptide so were either exported from the glands, or in three cases (MEG-11, -14 and -32.1) predicted to be membrane-anchored. These three membrane proteins were predicted to be heavily *O*-glycosylated, likely forming a glycocalyx to line the oesophageal surface. A further six putatively secreted MEGs were also predicted to be *O*-glycosylated, suggesting that they may have viscous, mucin-like properties in the oesophageal lumen, to assist in leucocyte entrapment (see Section 8.3.7). Further differentially expressed genes in the *S. japonicum* oesophagus included orthologues of the two phospholipases and palmitoyl protein thioesterase 1 present in *S. mansoni*, but only a single aspartyl protease compared with the six in *S. mansoni*. VAL-7 was a prominent product of the *S. japonicum* oesophagus, along with a second abundant transcript encoding a domain shared with a group of venoms termed Natterins. These can act as kininogenases and also as plasminogen activators, triggering plasmin to break down fibrin clots. The occurrence of such enzymatic activity in the oesophageal secretions could partly explain the absence of blood clotting there. An abundant differential transcript in the male heads of *S. mansoni* (Smp_167280), annotated as a hypothetical protein (Wilson *et al.*, 2015), is the orthologue of *S. japonicum* Natterin.

When the pattern of oesophageal gene expression was compared between males and females surprisingly little difference was seen, despite the latter processing much more blood. With the exception of outlier, MEG-11, there was a good association between the transcript levels of all oesophageal genes in the two sexes (correlation coefficient $r = 0.83$). This appears to rule out regulation of oesophageal gland secretions at the level of gene transcription. The most plausible alternative is that secretion is regulated at the level of translation. It was indicated in Section 8.2 that females appear to feed almost continuously; a faster rate of translation would provide the necessary products for more rapid blood processing. A comparison of rates of synthesis of oesophageal proteins in males and females would test this hypothesis.

8.3.7 MEG protein function inferred from sequence analysis

Characterization of the proteins encoded by MEGs presents special challenges. The first reports of their discovery revealed there were at least 45 genes with an unusual micro-exon structure (MEGs) in *S. mansoni* (Berriman *et al.*,

2009; DeMarco *et al.*, 2010). Approximately 75% of the coding sequence comprises exon lengths that are multiples of three bases (from 6 to 36), flanked at the 5′ and 3′ extremes by conventional exons. Other than having shared gene structure, no similarity could be detected between 14 MEG families identified (now 32 families) nor with annotated genes from outside *Schistosoma* spp. They did not possess identifiable motifs or functional domains, apart from a signal peptide at the 5′ end. At the transcript level, RT-PCR has revealed alternative splicing of micro-exons in several families (DeMarco *et al.*, 2010) but only recently has it proved possible to detect sequence variation using proteomics (Neves *et al.*, 2020), possibly because of the lower sensitivity of the latter technique.

In addition to MEG sequences from *S. mansoni* and *S. japonicum*, the availability of genome sequences for *Schistosoma haematobium* and the bird schistosome, *Trichobilharzia regenti* (same family, different genus), meant that for some MEG families it has been possible to search for common motifs and build evolutionary trees. The same caveat about MEG annotation also applies to *S. haematobium* sequence assemblies in the latest version of the genome (Stroehlein *et al.*, 2019), where MEGs are annotated as hypothetical proteins (strictly correct since they lack homology to known proteins). The genes for *meg-9*, *-12*, *-26*, *-27* and *-28* encode short peptides of 20–30 amino acids, preceded by a signal peptide, cleaved when they are secreted. MEG-12 was the first to be analysed using the HeliQuest server and shown to contain a central amphipathic helix with a hydrophobic interaction face (Fig. 8.8.1) (Wilson *et al.*, 2015). The MEG-26 family is a closely related group of genes with seven members (two with duplicated domains), plus three members in *T. regenti* making a total of 21 conserved motifs. Analysis using HeliQuest clearly shows there are distinct hydrophobic and hydrophilic faces (Fig. 8.8.2) (Li *et al.*, 2018). What is the value of releasing a swarm of amphipathic peptides into the oesophageal lumen? The most obvious explanation is that they interact with incoming erythrocytes and leucocytes to destabilize their membranes. MEG-27 strongly affects the fluidity of erythrocyte ghost membranes in an *in vitro* experimental system (Felizatti *et al.*, 2020). We can envisage this potentially increases membrane accessibility to secreted enzymes like the phospholipases and proteases. It is pure conjecture, but the phospholipases could, for example, release acyl chains from membrane phospholipids, destabilizing cell surface integrity. This would give the palmitoyl thioesterase access to the cytosolic leaflet of the lipid bilayer, to detach palmitoyl-linked proteins (e.g. G-protein-coupled receptors). Taken together these observations support the idea that the oesophageal lumen is the graveyard for ingested host cells.

The use of bioinformatic approaches to identify conserved motifs has also been applied to MEG-4 and -8 family proteins secreted into the oesophageal lumen. The C-terminal hydrophobic regions of MEG-4.1 and -4.2, not encoded by micro-exons, are highly conserved in *S. mansoni*, *S. japonicum* and *S. haematobium* (Li *et al.*, 2013). Clustal alignment of all six sequences identifies a region of homology of 22 amino acids (27% identity, 68% conserved residues) suggesting a shared motif executing a common function. The four members of the MEG-8 family similarly have a shared hydrophobic motif largely encoded by the C-terminal long 5′ flanking exon (Fig. 8.8.3). MEG-8.1 and -8.2 display >40% of their length as intrinsically disordered regions that are rich in threonine, serine and proline (TSP) residues, and are predicted to be heavily *O*-glycosylated. MEG-8.3 is also predicted to be *O*-glycosylated but without extensive regions of disorder. Clustal comparisons of MEG-8 family sequences across three species revealed a conserved protein domain with characteristic signatures, which segregate by family member, not schistosome species (Fig. 8.8.4). This indicates that MEG-8 diversity is ancient, arising before speciation of the genus *Schistosoma* occurred. This ancient divergence is further emphasized when data for the bird schistosome is included in the family tree (Li *et al.*, 2018).

Posterior oesophageal gland secretions, including MEG-4.1, -4.2 and -8.2, have been localized in the lumen of the posterior compartment of *S. japonicum* (Li *et al.*, 2015). This is a strong pointer to their potential function in blood processing, but we can only conjecture about their precise role. One possibility is that the conserved motifs of MEG-4 and -8 family members represent ligands for a docking site on ingested leucocytes, potentially via a pan-leucocyte marker such as CD45 (Li *et al.*, 2015). Unfortunately,

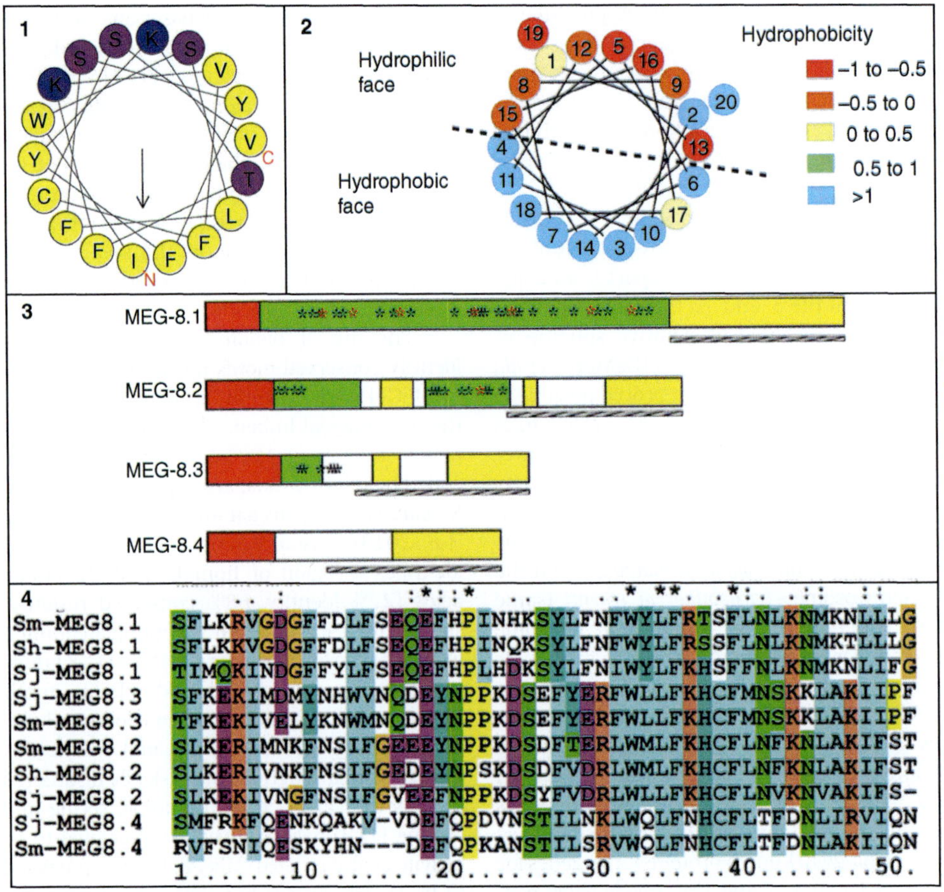

Fig. 8.8. Bioinformatic analysis of MEG proteins. **1**) Diagram of the central helix region of MEG-12 showing its amphipathic character. Amino acids are: (○) hydrophobic, (●) polar, and (●) positively charged and small side-chains. **2**) Helical wheel representation of the amphipathic helix of MEG-26 family members. Numbers represent the sequential order in the primary sequence and the average hydrophobicity for all members in each position of the helix. **3**) Schematic representation of protein products from MEG-8 family members. Key: ■, signal peptide; ■, intrinsically unstructured hydrophilic; ■, hydrophobic; *, predicted *O*-glycosylation; *, *N*-glycosylation; ▨: C-terminal conserved region. **4**) Multiple alignment of the conserved C-terminus of MEG-8 family proteins. (**1**, **3** and **4** from Wilson *et al.*, 2015; **2** from Li *et al.*, 2018.) Figures used under license CC-BY-4.0.

attempts to test the binding of biotinylated synthetic peptide motifs from MEG-4.1 and -4.2 of *S. mansoni* to murine leucocytes have been thwarted by the poor solubility of the constructs, but this is an avenue worth exploring.

An alternative explanation makes a loose analogy with the secreted mucin (MUC) proteins that coat the surfaces of mammalian airways (Wilson *et al.*, 2015). A major role of mucins is to form a mucus layer in the airways to entrap foreign particles and pathogens (Thornton *et al.*, 2008). In common with the *O*-glycosylated MEGs, mucins have central unstructured TSP regions which are heavily glycosylated. They can also polymerize via N- and C-terminal domains and are stored dehydrated within secretory granules; when released they swell to create a mucus gel with viscoelastic proprieties. This is somewhat reminiscent of the crystalloid vesicles (see Section 8.3.2) within the posterior gland cell bodies of schistosomes, whose regular structure could imply polymerization of constituents. When the MEGs are secreted into the posterior oesophageal lumen, they appear to form a net that entangles incoming leucocytes. Certainly, in some images the cells in a plug look as if they are wrapped in a cocoon (Li *et al.*, 2015).

8.4 The Gut

The gut is lined by a thin 'gastrodermis', another enigmatic tissue, with some quite unusual features. It is surrounded by circular muscle fibres responsible for bidirectional peristalsis (cf. oesophagus) and is probably syncytial, like the tegument, but with the nuclei resident in its cytoplasm not in separate cell bodies. The name gastrodermis is shared with the inner layer of members of the diploblastic phylum Cnidaria (*Hydra*, corals) but there it comprises distinct digestive, mucus-secreting and nerve cells, morphologically quite unlike the schistosome syncytium (Davis, 1975; Goldberg and Taylor, 1989). Digestion in the blind-ending sac occurs at pH ~4.5 and this is reflected in the involvement of cathepsin enzymes, typical of lysosomes, in the process (de Duve, 1983). Although the gastrodermis has an absorptive function, it does not bear typical luminal microvilli; instead, its surface is drawn out into thin lamellae. Equally unusual, although it is the source of the luminal enzymes needed for blood digestion, the syncytium contains no obvious vesicles or granules typical of secretory cells. It has been suggested that the best way to make sense of the schistosome gut is as a gigantic phagosome into which gastrodermal lysosomes secrete their contents (Hall *et al.*, 2011).

8.4.1 The structure of the gastrodermis by TEM and SEM

The structure of the gastrodermis was accurately described in the first TEM study (Morris, 1968) (Fig. 8.9.1 and 8.9.2) with subsequent studies adding some further details. Its thickness in both sexes varies between 1.5 and 4.0 μm, probably depending on the state of body contraction. In TEM sections, the luminal surface bears short narrow 1 μm extensions of cytoplasm. When these are visualized in transverse slices of starved worms by SEM, they appear as lamellae several microns long running in no particular direction (Fig. 8.10.1). In both TEM sections and in slices of freshly perfused worms prepared for SEM, the lamellae are covered in adherent spheres of haemoglobin protein (Fig. 8.10.2 and 8.10.3). The gastrodermis is separated from the investing muscles by an extracellular basal lamella of fibrous material, and like the tegument, its basal plasma membrane has invaginations which project a short distance into the cytoplasm (Fig. 8.9.1). The bulk of the cytosol is filled with rough endoplasmic reticulum, indicative of a tissue synthesizing proteins for export (Fig. 8.10.3). Small Golgi bodies are also present, with few cisternae surrounded by numerous small vesicles, and have been visualized by staining for the enzyme thiamine pyrophosphatase (Bogitsh, 1975). Despite all this activity in the protein synthetic and secretory pathway there are no obvious vesicles in proximity to the base of the surface lamellae, where secretion might be expected. Mitochondria and some potential endocytic vesicles are also present in the cytosol. In that context, lipid droplets are numerous in the gut lumen and cytosol, presumably taken up intact by endocytosis although this has not been formally demonstrated by feeding experiments.

Lastly, the luminal surface has a demonstrable filamentous glycocalyx, which has been visualized by TEM using the PATCO (periodic acid–thiocarbohydrazine–osmium) technique (Fig. 8.10.4) (Wilson and Barnes, 1974). Its function is presumably to protect the gastrodermis against the low luminal pH and hydrolytic environment. The glycocalyx is the source of the polysaccharide antigens detected in the host circulation (Berggren and Weller, 1967; Nash, 1974; Nash and Deelder, 1985) and used in diagnostic techniques (see Chapter 12).

It is clear from TEM observations that digestion of haemoglobin, the principal source of dietary protein takes place primarily in the gut lumen, apparently within the spheres anchored to the gastrodermal lamellae (Fig. 8.10.5). The tethering to the gut wall may in fact be a device to prevent wash-out of undigested food when a worm regurgitates. In common with the malaria parasite *Plasmodium*, a primary diet of haemoglobin brings with it problems. The potentially toxic haem prosthetic group (ferriprotoporphyrin IX)

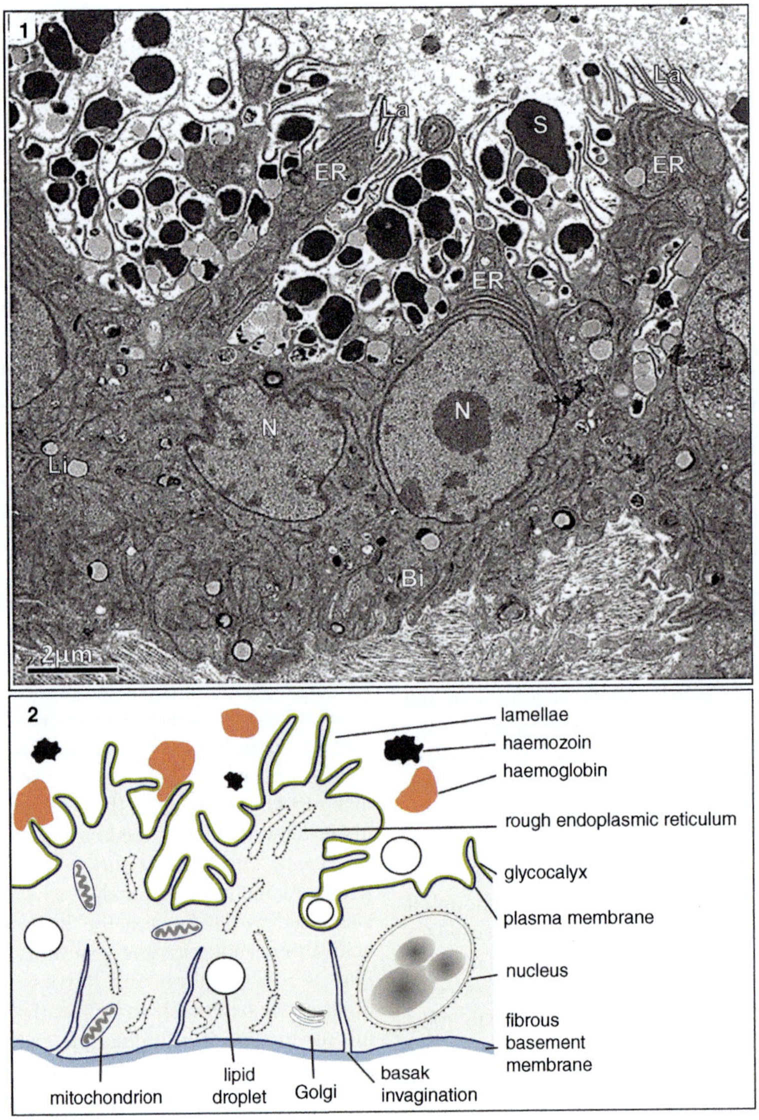

Fig. 8.9. Structure of the gastrodermis. **1**) TEM of the syncytium with nuclei (N) abundant endoplasmic reticulum (ER) and lipid droplets (Li). The luminal surface is extended by thin lamellae (La) of cytoplasm while the basal membrane is highly invaginated (Bi). Large dense spheres (S) of haemoglobin appear to be sequestered adjacent to the lamellae. **2**) Diagram of the layout to aid interpretation. (**1** from Delcroix *et al.*, 2007; **2** is an original diagram drawn by P. Roberts, University of York.) **1**) Figure used with permission from Elsevier.

is released and needs to be quickly rendered harmless. In *Plasmodium* this takes place within the acidic food vacuole, and the released ferriprotoporphyrin IX is combined into insoluble cyclic dimers of haemozoin/β-haematin which aggregate into crystals (Egan, 2008). Although haemozoin is insoluble in aqueous solution, it can partition in acidic environments into lipid compartments. In schistosomes the process of haemozoin formation takes place in the gut lumen, more specifically within the spheres of haemoglobin and as these diminish in size the haemozoin crystals become more prominent. Ultimately, all that remains are clusters of irregularly shaped

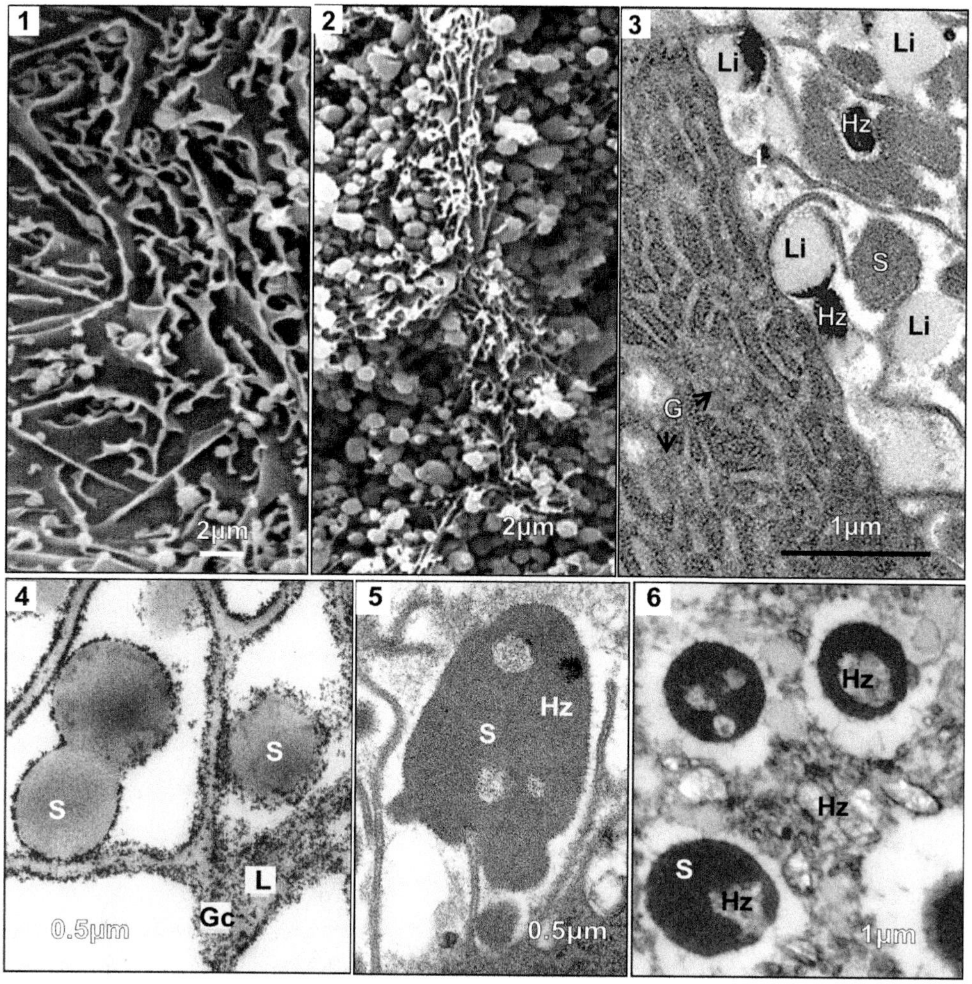

Fig. 8.10. SEM and TEM detail of the gastrodermis. **1**) SEM of a 'steak' from a starved worm showing the surface lamellae running in no particular direction. **2**) SEM of a newly perfused worm showing the adherent spheres of haemoglobin. **3**) TEM of the gastrodermal surface with distended endoplasmic reticulum, and a small Golgi body (arrowed). The lumen contains lipid droplets (Li), haemoglobin spheres and haemozoin (Hz) pigment. **4**) The filamentous glycocalyx coating the lamellae and spheres. **5**) An individual sphere (S) anchored to a lamella, with haemozoin (Hz) forming in the interior. **6**) Spheres (S) of haemoglobin with internal haemozoin (Hz), plus aggregates of free crystals. (**1–3**, **5** and **6** from Hall *et al.*, 2011; **4** from Wilson and Barnes, 1974.) **1–3**, **5** and **6**) Figures used with permission from Elsevier.

insoluble crystals (Fig. 8.10.6) that comprise the dark brown particles in the stream of vomitus. It has been proposed that haemozoin formation in the gut occurs at the surface of lipid vesicles (Oliveira *et al.*, 2005) but a more likely explanation is it naturally partitions there due to its lipophilic properties in an acidic environment (Skelly *et al.*, 2014).

There is relatively little information about the dynamics of secretion of proteins from or uptake of nutrients across the gastrodermis, due to its inaccessibility for experimentation. The rate of synthesis and export of proteins and glycans from the gastrodermis was investigated using isotopically labelled molecules, in pulse–chase experiments, detected by laborious autoradiography on worm sections (Wilson and Barnes, 1979). Both ^{3}H-leucine and ^{3}H-glucosamine were readily incorporated into gastrodermal macromolecules over a 30-min pulse incubation, and labelled proteins were rapidly secreted into the lumen thereafter. The incorporation of glucosamine was highly focal, revealing the restricted distribution of Golgi bodies in the gastrodermis (spaced ~2 μm apart). The pattern of labelled glycan secretion also differed. Transfer of label to the lumen peaked after 4 h, but large amounts were still detectable there after 24 h, presumably reflecting the function of the glycans as constituents of the persistent and adherent glycocalyx.

The occurrence of bulk endocytosis at the gastrodermal surface has been demonstrated in an erythrocyte feeding experiment, with 10 kDa FITC-labelled dextran as the marker (Hall *et al.*, 2011). Within 1 h of feeding, the dextran was uniformly distributed along the entire gut lumen (Fig. 8.11.1), confirming the efficiency of mixing by peristalsis. By 24 h the pattern had completely changed, with no dextran remaining in the lumen (Fig. 8.11.2) while numerous small discrete and intense spots (up to 2 μm diameter) were present in the gastrodermal syncytium, representing endosomes (Fig. 8.11.3). Mining of the *S. mansoni* transcriptome has revealed the requisite elements of receptor-mediated endocytosis (Fig. 8.11.4) (Wilson, 2012), and the uptake of lipid droplets was mentioned above as a potential candidate for endocytosis. Feeding experiments provide an avenue to characterize

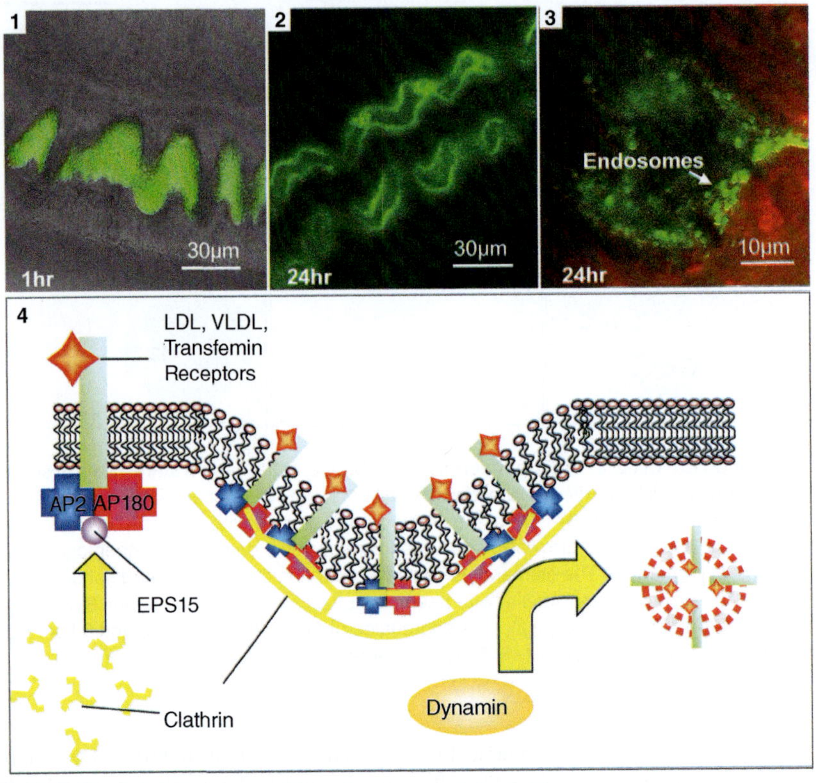

Fig. 8.11. Endocytosis by the gastrodermis. **1**) At 1 h after feeding FITC-dextran is distributed along the entire gastrodermal lumen. **2**) At 24 h the lumen is clear and the dextran confined to the gastrodermis. **3**) At high magnification the dextran is present in small endosomes. **4**) Diagram of the components of receptor-mediated endocytosis identified in the *S. mansoni* transcriptome. (**1–3** from Hall *et al.*, 2011; **4** from Wilson, 2012.) Figures used with permission from **1–3**) Elsevier and **4**) Springer Nature.

the endocytosis pathways of the gastrodermis and are clearly an area amenable to further experimentation.

8.4.2 The dynamics of gastrodermal tissues

The work elucidating the turnover of adult somatic stem cell populations (Collins *et al.*, 2013) proved very informative on the dynamics of gastrodermal tissues. A pulse of the thymidine analogue 5-ethynyl-2′-deoxyuridine (EdU) injected into infected mice will label any schistosome cells in the process of cell division. It was notable that no nuclei in gastrodermal cells of worms recovered 24 h after the pulse were EdU^+, so clearly the gastrodermal cells were not proliferating *in situ*. However, when worms were recovered from mice 7 days after the pulse, ~2.5% of gastrodermal nuclei were EdU^+. The explanation must be that adult stem cells proliferating elsewhere have the capacity to enter the gastrodermis and differentiate. This raises a dilemma since the tissue is a syncytium whose nuclei are not perpetually increasing in number. An equal number of nuclei will thus need to be removed to maintain an equilibrium. As with the tegument, autophagy seems the most likely mechanism but to date there are no reports of this process in gastrodermal tissues. The gastrodermis is not an isolated case because the differentiation of adult stem cells into body wall myocytes was demonstrated in the same experiment. At 24 h after an EdU pulse no muscle nuclei from male worms were labelled, whereas at 7 days ~10% were EdU^+. This strongly indicates that body wall myocytes are also gradually replaced over time from an external source.

8.4.3 Proteomic analysis of vomitus

The proteins and glycans expelled into the host bloodstream are vital signals that the worm cannot avoid making in the course of its biological activity. The identities of the macromolecules released can inform both the search for potential vaccine candidates and provide a source of diagnostic markers of ongoing infection. The intermittent regurgitation of vomitus into the external environment should provide material for proteomic analysis but there is an immediate technical problem. Worm pairs freshly recovered by perfusion are very reluctant to release vomitus. The first attempt used the drastic step of immersing worms in distilled water for 20 min (Delcroix *et al.*, 2007) and identified a relatively small number of host and worm constituents. A temperature shock protocol was subsequently used to produce a longer list of constituents, but these included obvious cytosolic, cytoskeletal and tegument proteins (Hall *et al.*, 2011). Ultimately, the best protocol found to obtain vomitus was aseptic culture of pre-adult (28 day) worms for several days in serum-free medium. A list of proteins identified, together with their Smp identities, is presented in Table 8.1. Additional to worm proteins, several murine proteins were identified in this proteomic analysis, including α and β haemoglobin chains, and serum albumin, but intriguingly, not immunoglobulins.

The proteins found in vomitus were assumed to be those involved in luminal processes and their identities strongly support the hypothesis that the schistosome gut functions as a gigantic lysosome/phagosome. This is especially pertinent for LAMP (lysosome-associated membrane protein) and VAMP (vesicle-associated membrane protein) (Table 8.1) which are involved in lysosome membrane fusion events; why they are found free in vomitus is unclear. The series of cathepsins identified have pH optima towards the acidic end of the spectrum (Caffrey *et al.*, 2004). Some function as endopeptidases and others as exopeptidases removing terminal amino acids. Many are secreted as inactive precursors (zymogens), requiring activation by asparaginyl endopeptidase. The identification of two Pro-X carboxylpeptidases suggests a special capacity for dealing with this type of C-terminal bond. The host version of this enzyme (Walter *et al.*, 1980) inactivates the peptide hormone angiotensin II, which among other properties regulates vascular smooth muscle contraction. Perhaps this enzyme is an intentional constituent of vomitus, intended to cause a relaxation of vessels along which worm pairs travel during

Table 8.1. Proteins of the gastrodermis identified by different approaches

Hydrolases	Smp	1	2	3	**Lysosomal**	Smp	1	2	3
Asparaginyl endopeptidase (Sm32)	075800	V	hi	S	Apoferritin	063530	V	+	
Cathepsin B1 (Sm31)	103610	V	hi	S	Ferritins	047650	V	=	S
Cathepsin B1	067060	V	hi	S	Saposin	194910	V	+	
Cathepsin C	019030	V	=	S	Saposin	014570	V	hi	
Cathepsin K/S	139240	V	hi	S	Saposin	105450	V	?	
Serine carboxypeptidase	172590		hi	S	Saposin	130100	V	=	S
Cathepsin L2	343260		hi	S	Saposin	105420		hi	S
Cathepsin B	085010			S	Saposin	016490		=	S
Cathepsin L	187140			S	Saposin	137720			S
Cathepsin D	013040		hi	S	Saposin	181060			S
Pro-X carboxylpeptidase	002600	V	hi	S	Saposin	202610			S
Pro-X carboxylpeptidase	071610	V	hi	S	NPC2	194840	V	=	S
DJ-1/Park7 protease	082030	V	hi	S	LAMP	162770	V	hi	S
Glucan 1,4 b-glucosidase	043390	V	hi		VAMP	136240	V	=	
Palmitoyl-CoA hydrolase	213510	V	hi		Natterin	035560			S
Phospholipase A2	166530			S	Natterin	006310			S
Inhibitors					**Transporters**				
Serpin	090080	V	+		Permease	131410			S
a2 macroglobulin	089670	V	+		Proton ATPase	330620			S
					Aquaporin	128110			S

1, Hall et al., 2011. Vomitus
2, Neves et al., 2020. RNASeq, comparing back ends versus heads:hi, highly enriched; +, slightly enriched; =, not enriched
3, Wendt et al., 2020. Single cell sequencing of gastrodermal cells

oviposition? The presence of β1,4-glucosidase and palmitoyl-CoA hydrolase is also worth noting. The former enzyme has been tentatively annotated as a xylosidase, and schistosomes possess core-xylosylated *N*-glycans. Does it provide a dietary source of xylose? The palmitoyl-CoA hydrolase is normally a constituent of peroxisomes and may indicate that these organelles also contribute to luminal digestion. The role of the two protease inhibitors, serpin and α_2-macroglobulin, in a hydrolytic environment seems paradoxical unless they have a protective role. The host α_2-macroglobulin is a large molecule with the ability to inhibit proteases from all catalytic classes so protection of the gastrodermal surfaces is an obvious site of action for this schistosome inhibitor. The recent characterization of a serpin, located in the tegument and identical with Smp_090080 (Lee *et al.*, 2024), may indicate that it is not of gut origin.

The vomitus proteome also contained a series of lysosomal carrier proteins (Hall *et al.*, 2011). These included several ferritins potentially involved in iron uptake, only one of which (apoferritin) has a signal peptide. (A calcium-binding calumenin in the original study has been deleted because the SchistoCyte website (Wendt *et al.*, 2021) predicts a parenchymal origin.) Four proteins with saposin motifs were present, possessing a domain comprising four α-helixes separated by two hinges and a loop (Farias *et al.*, 2020). The saposins combine in pairs, unfolding to create a lipid-transporting disc. Host saposins, encoded by a single gene, are lysosomal proteins involved in breakdown of membrane glycosphingolipids (Kishimoto *et al.*, 1992). The role of schistosome proteins with saposin motifs is unclear, especially as sphingolipid hydrolases have not been found in vomitus. Their number (perhaps 12 encoded in the genome, see below) and their diversity points to an important function in nutrition. The NPC-2 protein (Niemann-Pick intracellular cholesterol transporter 2) also detected in vomitus is probably crucial in the acquisition of cholesterol, which schistosomes cannot synthesize. In the mammalian host it binds cholesterol from the lysosomal interior and transfers it to the NPC-1 partner, an integral lysosomal membrane protein, from where it passes to post-lysosomal destinations. The *S. mansoni* genome encodes an orthologue of NPC-1, Smp_039130, which should reside on the luminal surface of the gastrodermis if it follows the same pattern, but has not to date been localized.

8.4.4 Protein enriched in male back ends versus heads

The microdissection approach that successfully identified oesophageal MEGs has also been applied to the back ends of schistosomes but followed by proteomic analysis not RNA-Seq (Table 8.1) (Neves *et al.*, 2020). The implicit assumption was lysosomal proteins enriched in the back ends should be distinguishable from those common to the lysosomes of all worm tissues. This approach assumes that lysosomes are a ubiquitous feature of all schistosome cells. The proteins enriched in the back ends (designated by "hi"), including asparaginyl endopeptidase, cathepsins (B1, K/S, L2), a novel serine carboxypeptidase, LAMP and a saposin, mostly coincided with the ones found in vomitus. Another group enriched by a factor of ≤2 (designated by "+") included cathepsin D, apoferritin, α_2-macroglobulin, serpin and another saposin. The remaining proteins (designated by "=") were distributed evenly between heads and back ends, implying that they are normal components of schistosome lysosome function, not especially implicated in blood feeding. They include the two Pro-X carboxypeptidases, palmitoyl-CoA thioesterase, β-glucosidase, DJ-1/PARK7 protease, NPC-2, VAMP and two more saposins.

8.4.5 Single-cell sequencing

The single-cell sequencing approach provides a different perspective on gastrodermal function, based on the gene expression patterns of isolated cells, clustered on the presence of genes for many of the markers described above (Wendt *et al.*, 2020). As the gut is a syncytium the surmise must be that the cells analysed were yet to merge with the syncytium; the less plausible alternative is that they were fragments of syncytium that had rounded off. The gut cluster comprised 105 cells, in which expression of 81 genes was recorded, including multiple ferritins, at least nine saposins and 13 proteases, many present in vomitus and back ends (Table 8.1). The expression site of three of the proteases, also detected in vomitus, was confirmed as the gastrodermis by WISH (Wendt *et al.*, 2020) but no comparable expression sites for the carrier proteins have been localized. The identification of two Natterin genes, one of them detected in the oesophagus, reinforces the potential role of their proteins in blood processing.

A novel feature of the single-cell approach was the detection of three transporter genes. A BLAST search indicates that one annotated simply as a permease appears is unique to the Schistosomatidae. The second, a proton ATPase (Smp_330620), may be of special relevance, due to the acidic milieu of the gut lumen. Located on the luminal surface such a pump would provide a mechanism to generate the acidic luminal pH. The same is true of an aquaporin (Smp_128110) which, if expressed on either luminal or basal surface of the gastrodermis, could mediate a significant fluid flux from gut lumen into surrounding tissues (see Chapter 7). A study of gene expression using laser capture microdissection (Nawaratna *et al.*, 2011) has provided further clues to transportation (multidrug resistance protein, Smp_115190; calcium-transporting ATPase Smp_137170 and cationic amino acid transporter Smp_004190). Endocytosis was also supported by the detection of scavenger receptor (Smp_128430) and vesicle trafficking protein (Smp_127380), both of them potentially at the luminal surface. However, this short list of membrane proteins really tells us how little we know about the absorptive capacities of the gut. What is needed is a technique that selectively labels the gut surface in the way that biotinylation has been used for the much more accessible tegument.

When the three different approaches are viewed collectively, they provide an overall picture of gut function but also pose questions. Some cathepsin proteases (D1 and L2) were not found in vomitus. Does this mean that the initial part of the proteolytic cascade takes place in the lumen and the final stages in the gastrodermal tissues. This is an important distinction if antibodies are targeted to gut proteins. The presence of iron, lipid and cholesterol binding proteins in the vomitus suggests an involvement in nutrient uptake, but without experimental evidence. Why so many saposin domain-containing proteins? Ferritins are found in vomitus but also expressed in gastrodermal tissue. There is a lot of iron in a worm blood diet. Is the function of ferritins to aid its entry or to sequester it out of harm's way? The apparent ubiquity of the two Pro-X carboxypeptidases in all lysosomes argues against the suggestion above that they might be deliberate products of vomitus designed to affect vascular tone.

8.5 Summary

- The alimentary tract is the major source of products that adult worms must regurgitate into host blood as part of normal feeding activities. Paradoxically, the oesophageal glands and gastrodermis are more inaccessible to experimentation and analysis than the tegument surface. For the oesophageal glands this has in large measure been solved by microdissection and subtractive RNA-Seq, but the gastrodermis remains less well characterized.
- Whole blood entering through the mouth passes through anterior and posterior oesophageal compartments, separated by sphincters before it reaches the gut lumen. Proteins secreted from surrounding anterior and posterior glands interact with incoming cells and plasma proteins, causing lysis of erythrocytes and aggregation of leucocytes into a central plus of disintegrating cells.
- The gastrodermis (probably syncytial) has a very different structure, with a surface extended in thin lamellae to which spheres of haemoglobin adhere. Digestion takes place here within the masses, ultimately leaving behind a residue of insoluble haemozoin pigment that is voided in vomitus. The female has a much more active gut, consuming far more blood than the male, yet has much smaller oesophageal glands.
- The processes in the lumen occur at an acid pH of ~4.5 and the whole of the gut lumen can be considered analogous to a giant lysosome. The gastrodermal cytoplasm is rich in rough endoplasmic reticulum, indicative of protein synthesis, but lacks typical secretory vesicles. Endocytosis has been demonstrated at the luminal surface and may be the point of entry for lipid droplets. Feeding experiments with fluorescent substrates would illuminate this process.
- The presence of ferritins, saposins and NPC-2 in gastrodermal secretions argues for carrier-mediated uptake into the gastrodermis but information about receptors and transporters on the luminal surface is sparse.
- The host generates antibodies against vomitus proteins and these are ingested with whole blood. These could make both oesophageal and gastrodermal secretions important targets of antibody-mediated attack. However, there is minimal information about the stability of such antibodies in the acidic gut environment, or their ability to block alimentary tract function effectively.

References

Almeida, G.T., Amaral, M.S., Beckedorff, F.C.F., Kitajima, J.P., DeMarco, R. *et al.* (2012) Exploring the *Schistosoma mansoni* adult male transcriptome using RNA-seq. *Experimental Parasitology* 132(1), 22–31. DOI: 10.1016/j.exppara.2011.06.010

Berggren, W.L. and Weller, T.H. (1967) Immunoelectrophoretic demonstration of specific circulating antigen in animals infected with *Schistosoma mansoni*. *The American Journal of Tropical Medicine and Hygiene* 16(5), 606–612. DOI: 10.4269/ajtmh.1967.16.606

Berriman, M., Haas, B.J., LoVerde, P.T., Wilson, R.A., Dillon, G.P. *et al.* (2009) The genome of the blood fluke *Schistosoma mansoni*. *Nature* 460(7253), 352–358. DOI: 10.1038/nature08160

Bloch, E.H. (1980) *In vivo* microscopy of schistosomiasis. II. Migration of *Schistosoma mansoni* in the lungs, liver, and intestine. *The American Journal of Tropical Medicine and Hygiene* 29(1), 62–70. DOI: 10.4269/ajtmh.1980.29.62

Bogitsh, B.J. (1975) Cytochemistry of gastrodermal autophagy following starvation in *Schistosoma mansoni*. *The Journal of Parasitology* 61(2), 237–248. DOI: 10.2307/3279000

Bogitsh, B.J. and Carter, O.S. (1977) *Schistosoma mansoni*: ultrastructural studies on the esophageal secretory granules. *The Journal of Parasitology* 63(4), 681–686. DOI: 10.2307/3279570

Caffrey, C.R., McKerrow, J.H., Salter, J.P. and Sajid, M. (2004) Blood 'n' guts: an update on schistosome digestive peptidases. *Trends in Parasitology* 20(5), 241–248. DOI: 10.1016/j.pt.2004.03.004

Collins, J.J., III, Wang, B., Lambrus, B.G., Tharp, M.E., Iyer, H. *et al.* (2013) Adult somatic stem cells in the human parasite *Schistosoma mansoni*. *Nature* 494(7438), 476–479. DOI: 10.1038/nature11924

Davis, L.E. (1975) Histological and ultrastructural studies of the basal disk of *Hydra*. III. The gastrodermis and the mesoglea. *Cell and Tissue Research* 162(1), 107–118. DOI: 10.1007/BF00223266

de Duve, C. (1983) Lysosomes revisited. *European Journal of Biochemistry* 137(3), 391–397. DOI: 10.1111/j.1432-1033.1983.tb07841.x

Delcroix, M., Medzihradsky, K., Caffrey, C.R., Fetter, R.D. and McKerrow, J.H. (2007) Proteomic analysis of adult *S. mansoni* gut contents. *Molecular and Biochemical Parasitology* 154(1), 95–97. DOI: 10.1016/j.molbiopara.2007.03.008

DeMarco, R., Mathieson, W., Manuel, S.J., Dillon, G.P., Curwen, R.S. *et al.* (2010) Protein variation in blood-dwelling schistosome worms generated by differential splicing of micro-exon gene transcripts. *Genome Research* 20(8), 1112–1121. DOI: 10.1101/gr.100099.109

Dike, S.C. (1971) Ultrastructure of the esophageal region in *Schistosoma mansoni*. *The American Journal of Tropical Medicine and Hygiene* 20(4), 552–568. DOI: 10.4269/ajtmh.1971.20.552

Dillon, G.P., Illes, J.C., Isaacs, H.V. and Wilson, R.A. (2007) Patterns of gene expression in schistosomes: localization by whole mount *in situ* hybridization. *Parasitology* 134(11), 1589–1597. DOI: 10.1017/S0031182007002995

Egan, T.J. (2008) Haemozoin formation. *Molecular and Biochemical Parasitology* 157(2), 127–136. DOI: 10.1016/j.molbiopara.2007.11.005

Farias, L.P., Vance, G.M., Coulson, P.S., Vitoriano-Souza, J., Neto, A.P. da S. *et al.* (2020) Epitope mapping of exposed tegument and alimentary tract proteins identifies putative antigenic targets of the attenuated schistosome vaccine. *Frontiers in Immunology* 11, 624613. DOI: 10.3389/fimmu.2020.624613

Felizatti, A.P., Zeraik, A.E., Basso, L.G.M., Kumagai, P.S., Lopes, J.L.S. *et al.* (2020) Interactions of amphipathic α-helical MEG proteins from *Schistosoma mansoni* with membranes. *Biochimica et Biophysica Acta Biomembranes* 1862(3), 183173. DOI: 10.1016/j.bbamem.2019.183173

Goldberg, W.M. and Taylor, G.T. (1989) Cellular structure and ultrastructure of the black coral *Antipathes aperta*: 2. The gastrodermis and its collar cells. *Journal of Morphology* 202(2), 255–269. DOI: 10.1002/jmor.1052020211

Hall, S.L., Braschi, S., Truscott, M., Mathieson, W., Cesari, I.M. *et al.* (2011) Insights into blood feeding by schistosomes from a proteomic analysis of worm vomitus. *Molecular and Biochemical Parasitology* 179(1), 18–29. DOI: 10.1016/j.molbiopara.2011.05.002

Kishimoto, Y., Hiraiwa, M. and O'Brien, J.S. (1992) Saposins: structure, function, distribution, and molecular genetics. *Journal of Lipid Research* 33(9), 1255–1267. DOI: 10.1016/S0022-2275(20)40540-1

Lawrence, J.D. (1973) The ingestion of red blood cells by *Schistosoma mansoni*. *The Journal of Parasitology* 59(1), 60–63. DOI: 10.2307/3278572

Lee, C.N., Hall, B.A., Sanford, L. and Molehin, A.J. (2024) Molecular characterization and functional analysis of a *Schistosoma mansoni* serine protease inhibitor, Smserpin-p46. *Microorganisms* 12(6), 1164. DOI: 10.3390/microorganisms12061164

Li, X.-H., de Castro-Borges, W., Parker-Manuel, S., Vance, G.M., Demarco, R. *et al.* (2013) The schistosome oesophageal gland: initiator of blood processing. *PLoS Neglected Tropical Diseases* 7(7), e2337. DOI: 10.1371/journal.pntd.0002337

Li, X.H., Stark, M., Vance, G.M., Cao, J.P. and Wilson, R.A. (2014) The anterior esophageal region of *Schistosoma japonicum* is a secretory organ. *Parasites & Vectors* 7, 565. DOI: 10.1186/s13071-014-0565-8

Li, X.-H., Xu, Y.-X., Vance, G., Wang, Y., Lv, L.-B. *et al.* (2015) Evidence that rhesus macaques self-cure from a *Schistosoma japonicum* infection by disrupting worm esophageal function: a new route to an effective vaccine? *PLoS Neglected Tropical Diseases* 9(7), e0003925. DOI: 10.1371/journal.pntd.0003925

Li, X.H. and Wilson, R.A. (2017) Alimentary tract of *Schistosoma*. In: Jamieson, B.G.M. (ed.) *Schistosoma: Biology, Pathology and Control*. CRC Press, Boca Raton, FL, chapter 11. DOI: 10.1201/9781315368900

Li, X.-H., DeMarco, R., Neves, L.X., James, S.R., Newling, K. *et al.* (2018) Microexon gene transcriptional profiles and evolution provide insights into blood processing by the *Schistosoma japonicum* esophagus. *PLoS Neglected Tropical Diseases* 12(2), e0006235. DOI: 10.1371/journal.pntd.0006235

Luo, F., Yin, M., Mo, X., Sun, C., Wu, Q. *et al.* (2019) An improved genome assembly of the fluke *Schistosoma japonicum*. *PLoS Neglected Tropical Diseases* 13(8), e0007612. DOI: 10.1371/journal.pntd.0007612

Mortazavi, A., Williams, B.A., McCue, K., Schaeffer, L. and Wold, B. (2008) Mapping and quantifying mammalian transcriptomes by RNA-seq. *Nature Methods* 5(7), 621–628. DOI: 10.1038/nmeth.1226

Morris G.P. (1968) Fine structure of the gut epithelium of *Schistosoma mansoni*. *Experientia* 24(5), 480–482. DOI: 10.1007/BF02144405

Nash, T.E. (1974) Localization of the circulating antigen within the gut of *Schistosoma mansoni*. *The American Journal of Tropical Medicine and Hygiene* 23(6), 1085–1087. DOI: 10.4269/ajtmh.1974.23.1085

Nash, T.E. and Deelder, A.M. (1985) Comparison of four schistosome excretory-secretory antigens: phenol sulfuric test active peak, cathodic circulating antigen, gut-associated proteoglycan, and circulating anodic antigen. *The American Journal of Tropical Medicine and Hygiene* 34(2), 236–241. DOI: 10.4269/ajtmh.1985.34.236

Nawaratna, S.S.K., McManus, D.P., Moertel, L., Gobert, G.N. and Jones, M.K. (2011) Gene atlasing of digestive and reproductive tissues in *Schistosoma mansoni*. *PLoS Neglected Tropical Diseases* 5(4), e1043. DOI: 10.1371/journal.pntd.0001043

Neves, L.X., Wilson, R.A., Brownridge, P., Harman, V.M., Holman, S.W. *et al.* (2020) Quantitative proteomics of enriched esophageal and gut tissues from the human blood fluke *Schistosoma mansoni* pinpoints secreted proteins for vaccine development. *Journal of Proteome Research* 19(1), 314–326. DOI: 10.1021/acs.jproteome.9b00531

Oliveira, M.F, d'Avila, J.C., Torres, C.R., Oliveira, P.L., Tempone, A.J. *et al.* (2000) Haemozoin in *Schistosoma mansoni*. *Molecular and Biochemical Parasitology* 111(1), 217–221. DOI: 10.1016/s0166-6851(00)00299-1

Oliveira, M.F., Kycia, S.W., Gomez, A., Kosar, A.J., Bohle, D.S. *et al.* (2005) Structural and morphological characterization of hemozoin produced by *Schistosoma mansoni* and *Rhodnius prolixus*. *FEBS Letters* 579(27), 6010–6016. DOI: 10.1016/j.febslet.2005.09.035

Rofatto, H.K., Parker-Manuel, S.J., Barbosa, T.C., Tararam, C.A., Wilson, R.A. *et al.* (2012) Tissue expression patterns of *Schistosoma mansoni* venom allergen-like proteins 6 and 7. *International Journal for Parasitology* 42(7), 613–620. DOI: 10.1016/j.ijpara.2012.04.008

Skelly, P.J., Da'dara, A.A., Li, X.H., Castro-Borges, W. and Wilson, R.A. (2014) Schistosome feeding and regurgitation. *PLoS Pathogens* 10(8), e1004246. DOI: 10.1371/journal.ppat.1004246

Stroehlein, A.J., Korhonen, P.K., Chong, T.M., Lim, Y.L., Chan, K.G. *et al.* (2019) High-quality *Schistosoma haematobium* genome achieved by single-molecule and long-range sequencing. *GigaScience* 8(9), giz108. DOI: 10.1093/gigascience/giz108

Thornton, D.J., Rousseau, K. and McGuckin, M.A. (2008) Structure and function of the polymeric mucins in airways mucus. *Annual Review of Physiology* 70, 459–486. DOI: 10.1146/annurev.physiol.70.113006.100702

Walter, R., Simmons, W.H. and Yoshimoto, T. (1980) Proline specific endo- and exopeptidases. *Molecular and Cellular Biochemistry* 30(2), 111–127. DOI: 10.1007/BF00227927

Wendt, G., Zhao, L., Chen, R., Liu, C., O'Donoghue, A.J. *et al.* (2020) A single-cell RNA-seq atlas of *Schistosoma mansoni* identifies a key regulator of blood feeding. *Science* 369(6511), 1644–1649. DOI: 10.1126/science.abb7709

Wendt, G.R., Reese, M.L. and Collins, J.J., III (2021) SchistoCyte Atlas: a single-cell transcriptome resource for adult schistosomes. *Trends in Parasitology* 37(7), 585–587. DOI: 10.1016/j.pt.2021.04.010

Wilson, R.A. (2012) The cell biology of schistosomes: a window on the evolution of the early metazoa. *Protoplasma* 249(3), 503–518. DOI: 10.1007/s00709-011-0326-x

Wilson, R.A. and Barnes, P.E. (1974) The tegument of *Schistosoma mansoni*: observations on the formation, structure and composition of cytoplasmic inclusions in relation to tegument function. *Parasitology* 68(2), 239–258. DOI: 10.1017/S0031182000045765

Wilson, R.A. and Barnes, P.E. (1979) Synthesis of macromolecules by the epithelial surfaces of *Schistosoma mansoni*: an autoradiographic study. *Parasitology* 78(3), 295–310. DOI: 10.1017/s0031182000051167

Wilson, R.A., Li, X.H., MacDonald, S., Neves, L.X., Vitoriano-Souza, J. *et al.* (2015) The schistosome esophagus is a 'hotspot' for microexon and lysosomal hydrolase gene expression: implications for blood processing. *PLoS Neglected Tropical Diseases* 9(12), e0004272. DOI: 10.1371/journal.pntd.0004272

9

Vaccines

9.1 Overview

This chapter seeks to tease out why, after much research effort over the last 60 years, an effective schistosome vaccine is not an imminent prospect. In part this is due to the particular characteristics of helminth infections, especially the considerable longevity of schistosomes within the human bloodstream, surrounded by and feeding on the host humoral and cellular components. It is reinforced by the lack of a useable paradigm for a vaccine based on human responses. Researchers have therefore turned to laboratory animals for testing experimental vaccines and hypotheses about protective mechanisms, but there are still problems and pitfalls in the vaccine testing process. Nevertheless, there are situations where acquired immunity can be demonstrated in laboratory hosts. The radiation-attenuated (RA) cercarial vaccine in rodents and primates, and a self-cure mechanism in the laboratory rat and rhesus macaque are all noteworthy. A gradual shift of emphasis from highly immunogenic internal antigens to more cryptic surface-exposed and secreted targets has followed. In the last decade this has led to a variety of mass screening approaches using the available transcript and proteome data to identify putative targets. Many of these have yet to be tested for vaccine potential. The first tentative human vaccine trials have also begun, and the Controlled Human Infection (CHI) model using volunteers exposed to cercariae of a single sex should accelerate the testing of candidate vaccines.

9.2 Special Considerations for a Schistosome Vaccine

It has been suggested that a schistosome vaccine, both as a prophylactic to prevent infection and as a therapeutic to eliminate existing worm populations, would be invaluable for the control of schistosomiasis if adequate levels of protection could be achieved (Alsallaq *et al.*, 2017). Against this there is the question 'why attempt to develop a vaccine when there is an effective chemotherapeutic agent in the form of praziquantel?' The arguments in favour were summarized in earlier publications (Wilson and Coulson, 1998, 1999). Briefly, praziquantel does not protect against reinfection or kill schistosomula larvae so dosing must be repeated at intervals. Importantly, schistosomiasis is a cryptic disease with morbidity roughly proportional to infection intensity (Andrade *et al.*, 2017) so infected individuals may be unaware of their accumulating worm burden. Even in heavy infections, egg-induced pathology may progress slowly so that the hepatosplenic condition only becomes apparent at a late stage.

DOI: 10.1079/9781800625167.0009

This is equally true of urogenital system pathology induced by *Schistosoma haematobium* infection. Chemotherapy can do little to reverse the progressive fibrotic damage. In addition, current diagnostics for intestinal schistosomiasis are relatively insensitive so fail to detect low-level infections that could still have clinical sequelae (Colley *et al.*, 2017). The immune-depressive nature of a schistosome infection, evident from both human (King *et al.*, 1996; Natukunda *et al.*, 2024) and animal studies (Schramm *et al.*, 2018), provides a further potent argument for a vaccine.

9.2.1 Biological features of helminth parasitism

At the outset we need to be clear that key features of helminths in general and schistosomes specifically mark them out as distinct from other infectious agents. There are certain inescapable parameters with implications for vaccine development. First, unlike viruses, microbes and protozoa, schistosomes do not multiply within the mammalian host but exist as a long-lived resident population in the bloodstream. Their vascular location means that they must possess sophisticated mechanisms of immune evasion (see Section 7.6). In addition, the antigenic signals they send to immune surveillance systems are apparently not adequate to provoke protective immunity. Thus, a vaccine delivering antigens exposed on epithelial surfaces or secreted from intravascular parasites needs to do better than the normal/intrinsic immune response. What is meant by protective immunity in the schistosome context, especially as no vaccine procedure has yet generated sterile immunity? Since pathology is proportional to worm burden, it is implicit that a vaccine eliciting a reduction in that burden would ameliorate disease morbidity. The question then becomes what level of reduction would make the cost and effort of vaccination worthwhile?

The ideal schistosome vaccine would eliminate the infecting larvae in the skin before they enter the vasculature, but that has its own inherent problems. Vaccines normally establish memory, which is then triggered by a rising antigenic signal from the multiplication of a new infection. With incoming schistosome larvae, there is no time to trigger memory so the immune system must be permanently on 'red alert', capable of mounting an instantaneous effector response before transformation to the schistosomulum is complete (<24 h) (Wilson and Coulson, 2009). Equally unfortunate, infection of the human host is largely a sporadic event, with intermittent recruitment to the resident population. In this situation, the antigenic signal delivered by a single penetrating cercaria (~10 ng acetabular gland secretions) at some random point on the skin is unlikely to trigger a memory response that would maintain a high alert over a useful timespan. This would be a hard call for any vaccine to achieve, irrespective of the pathogen. The failure to appreciate these features goes a long way to explaining why progress towards a vaccine has been slow, with so many problems and pitfalls (Wilson *et al.*, 2017).

9.2.2 The lack of a useable vaccine paradigm based on immunity in humans

Data collected in earlier decades indicated that adult schistosomes, once established in the bloodstream, were long lived. This could be >30 years for *Schistosoma mansoni* (Harris *et al.*, 1984), while mean lifespan of 3.4 years was estimated for *S. haematobium* (Wilkins *et al.*, 1984). This longevity suggests that immune responses against adult worms cannot be very effective; indeed, the problem has been to demonstrate the existence of protection, irrespective of parasite stage. The first detailed parasitological studies of *S. mansoni* in human populations were performed in endemic areas of Kenya (Butterworth *et al.*, 1984, 1985), where rates of reinfection of schoolchildren in a high transmission area were characterized (cf. the study on *S. haematobium*; Wilkins *et al.*, 1984). In these reinfection studies, the fall in reinfection rate coincided with the onset of puberty (Fulford *et al.*, 1998), which could implicate host physiology as much as acquired immunity. It was also evident that children most in need of protection, between the ages of 2 and 15 years, showed little evidence of acquired immunity.

These studies of the human immune responses to schistosome infection posited a role for IgE, individuals with high levels of parasite-specific IgE being significantly less likely to become reinfected with *S. haematobium*, *Schistosoma japonicum* or *S. mansoni* (Fitzsimmons *et al.*, 2012). A principal target of IgE was a 22.6 kDa EF-hand calcium-binding protein, localized in the tegument, gastrodermis and nephridial canals (Dunne *et al.*, 1997). Two similar proteins of 21.7 and 20.8 kDa, were also identified and form part of a 13-member group in *S. mansoni*, termed the tegument allergen-like (TAL) family (Fitzsimmons *et al.*, 2012); a similar family has been characterized in *S. haematobium* (Oettle *et al.*, 2023). The consensus is that production of IgE in humans is stimulated by specific allergens released on the death of adult worms due to senility; repeated chemotherapy may hasten the process. Inherent problems with Sm22.6/TAL-1, the principal allergen, are its situation within the tegument cytoplasm of adult worms (see Chapter 7 on the tegument) and a lack of expression in the penetrating cercaria or early schistosomulum. Thus, to act as a target in incoming larvae would require a degree of cross-reactivity between adult and larval TALs to trigger an immediate hypersensitivity response that prevents their establishment (Oettle *et al.*, 2023). Other plausible targets for IgE-mediated dermal hypersensitivity are the three VALs released into host skin during cercarial penetration (Curwen *et al.*, 2006). It is not known if an IgE response to secreted VALs builds up in exposed humans over time, but experimentally SmVAL-4 triggers airway reactivity when given as an intranasal challenge to sensitized animals (Farias *et al.*, 2012). Arming of dermal mast cells gets round the problem of humoral responses needing to be on 'red alert', but it is unclear how mast cell degranulation might work to block or kill larvae. Finally, as recently acknowledged (Oettle *et al.*, 2023), schistosome antigens that stimulate IgE production emphatically cannot be considered as vaccine candidates because of the association between IgE and anaphylactic responses. They need to be avoided at all costs, as the triggering of urticaria by the promising NaASP-2 hookworm (*Necator americanus*) vaccine revealed when administered to volunteers living in an endemic area of Brazil (Diemert *et al.*, 2012); it led to the termination of that project.

9.2.3 Problems and pitfalls of vaccine testing

The schistosome vaccine field has been hampered by misleading concepts that deflected the search for a vaccine (Wilson *et al.*, 2017). The idea of concomitant immunity, borrowed from cancer research, was used to explain self-cure in the rhesus macaque whereby animals with a primary infection were believed to be fully protected against cercarial challenge (Smithers and Terry, 1969). However, this was based on a misinterpretation of the course of an *S. mansoni* infection in rhesus macaques (see Cheever and Powers, 1972). The concept was then applied to human infections with *S. haematobium* in Tanzania as a way to interpret the shape of the age/prevalence curve (Bradley and McCullough, 1973; McCullough and Bradley, 1973). Around the same time, an *in vitro* antibody-dependant cellular cytotoxicity (ADCC) assay was developed to measure the killing of newly transformed schistosomula by host serum and cells, especially eosinophils (Butterworth *et al.*, 1974). Taken together, concomitant immunity and ADCC was a seductive paradigm, and trialling various combinations of sera and cells rapidly became a very active research area. Ultimately, this led to bold conclusions that 'in rat, primate, and human schistosomiasis, [ADCC] is the main mechanism of killing parasite larvae, whereas in mice, cytotoxicity in schistosomiasis requires activated macrophages' (Capron and Capron, 1994). The problem with all of this was an almost complete lack of *in vivo* histopathological evidence for the occurrence of ADCC against skin-stage schistosomes in any host. It is plausible, given the build-up of IgE against schistosome allergens in infected humans over time, that a dermal response might operate there. One possible value of identifying potential allergens in a dermal response would be to eliminate them from vaccine formulations.

Another pitfall for vaccine development came from the advent of molecular biology technologies facilitating screening of bacterial (later, yeast and eucaryotic cell) expression libraries with sera to select highly reactive clones. This facilitated the production of recombinant proteins and their testing for vaccine potential. It appears that abundant internal proteins are highly immunoreactive, precisely because they have not been subjected to immunological pressure in the live worm (Philippsen *et al.*, 2015). The outcome of expression screening was a long list of cytosolic and cytoskeletal proteins with supposed vaccine potential. Such was the groundswell that World Health Organization (WHO) Special Programme for Research and Training in Tropical Diseases (TDR) (around 1990) sponsored independent trials in mice for six candidates (three cytosolic, two cytoskeletal and one transmembrane) in two separate laboratories (Bergquist, 1995). All of them failed to deliver adequate protection, even with a bar set at a quite low 40% (summarized in Wilson and Coulson, 2006). Furthermore, a quantitative proteomic analysis of the soluble proteins in an adult worm homogenate, colloquially called SWAP (soluble worm antigenic proteins), revealed that half the total mass comprised only 18 proteins (Neves *et al.*, 2015). SWAP itself is poorly protective but 11 of these (25% of total mass) had shown supposed protective potential in multiple laboratories, when used singly to vaccinate mice. Perhaps there is a flaw in the mouse model for vaccine testing (Wilson *et al.*, 2016)?

The mouse is a very convenient laboratory host in which to grow schistosomes, but is it optimal for vaccine testing? Migration from the skin to the portal system is entirely intravascular (see Chapter 3). The level of maturation can be estimated from the number of worms recovered by portal perfusion of challenge control mice around 6 weeks post-exposure to a known number of cercariae. Data from two UK research groups gave values of ~32% (Wilson *et al.*, 2016), meaning that of 100 penetrating cercaria, 68 will fail to mature anyway. A vaccination protocol that gives a ~50% level of protection, eliminates only a further 16 parasites. Thus, 84 parasites did not mature, but the vaccine only accounts for (16/84 × 100) ~19% of the total deaths. In larger hosts the maturation in naïve animals is higher, 56–76% in hamster and >80% in baboons (Wilson *et al.*, 2016), which means they automatically provide a better test of vaccine potential. Why is the mouse so problematic?

Passage through capillary beds is a tight squeeze for which larvae become very elongate, with the lungs presenting the greatest obstacle to migration (see Chapter 3). The fragility of pulmonary capillaries, related to animal size, and their susceptibility to a cytokine-induced vascular leak syndrome is well documented (West, 2013). During lung transit in mice, some schistosomula burst into the alveolar spaces (Crabtree and Wilson, 1986; Dean and Mangold, 1992), yet possess only a limited capacity to re-enter tissues. This provides a physical explanation for the low level of maturation (Wilson *et al.*, 2016). The situation for *S. japonicum* may be more complicated but has not been well researched using tracking techniques (see Chapter 3). Levels of maturation in naïve mice have variously been reported as between 43% and 86% depending on mouse and parasite strain (Moloney and Webbe, 1983). A rapid passage of schistosomula through the lungs, accompanied by large numbers of haemorrhages has been noted, and these authors suggested that ‘unlike *S. mansoni*, *S. japonicum* is not heedful in its negotiation of the pulmonary capillary beds’.

Another pitfall with antigen trials in mice has been the practice to shorten the interval between the last antigen boost and cercarial challenge, usually to 2 or 3 weeks and sometimes only 10 days. For the irradiated cercaria vaccine in mice (see Section 9.3.1) it has been customary to leave an interval of 5 weeks between the last vaccination and challenge, precisely to avoid pulmonary responses elicited by the attenuated vaccinating larvae. When the interval between last vaccination and challenge is short, challenge parasites will reach the lungs when both activated T cells and cytokine levels from the preceding vaccination are maximal in the circulation (Wilson *et al.*, 2016). The ‘protection’ in this situation may simply be the result of physiological effects on the pulmonary blood vessels, increasing the proportion of parasites that enter the alveoli. The hypothesis provides an explanation for why internal antigens and even heterologous proteins, reduce the level of maturation in a non-antigen-specific way. This argues for trials in more realistic larger hosts with less fragile pulmonary capillaries and a higher percentage maturation of penetrant cercariae, like the baboon (*S. mansoni*) and rabbit (*S. japonicum*). It is also important to take account of experimental variability in the basic parasitology. Delivery of precise numbers of cercariae to the exposure site is hard to achieve and requires at least five to seven animals per test and control group to minimize the within-group standard deviations and hence obtain a statistical significance of $P < 0.05$.

It is also not a good idea to rely on derived variables such as egg burden, faecal egg output or circulating antigen levels if portal perfusion is ethically permissible.

9.3 Animal Models Where Protection Can Be Demonstrated and the Underlying Mechanism

In the absence of a realistic paradigm based on human responses to schistosome infection, are there laboratory models in which acquired immunity can be demonstrated after infection or vaccination? Can the attenuated cercarial vaccine in rodents and primates or self-cure in the rat (*Rattus norvegicus*) and rhesus macaque (*Macaca mulatta*) provide pointers to the development of a prophylactic or therapeutic vaccine?

9.3.1 The RA cercarial vaccine

The idea of attenuating infectious agents so that they can elicit protective immunity without disease morbidity has a long history but really came to the forefront with the Bacillus Calmette–Guérin (BCG) vaccine against tuberculosis in the 1940s and the poliomyelitis vaccine in the 1950s. The first attenuated anti-helminth vaccine was developed against the lungworm *Dictyocaulus viviparus* in cattle (Cornwell, 1960). Around the same time schistosome cercariae attenuated with γ-rays from a ^{60}Co source or X-rays, were used to elicit immunity in mice (Villella *et al.*, 1961) and rhesus macaques (Hsü *et al.*, 1962). Detailed reviews of the RA vaccine model have been published (James, 1992; Coulson, 1997; Hewitson *et al.*, 2005; Bickle, 2009), with the bulk of information about the dynamics and mechanism coming from mouse experiments. The dose of radiation used is critical. Too little and attenuated parasites reach and develop in the portal system, leading to misinterpretation of results (Fukushige *et al.*, 2015), too much and they are confined to the skin, failing to elicit protection after a single exposure (Constant *et al.*, 1990). A crucial feature of the model is that it allows a large dose of larvae, which would normally be fatal, to be applied. Typically, this is 500 for a mouse, 1000 for a rat and 9000 for a primate like the baboon. The optimal radiation dose (200 Gy/20 krad) allows vaccinating parasites to exit the mouse skin, some via draining lymph nodes, and reach the lungs, where they persist to arm that organ (Coulson and Wilson, 1993). Similar information about mechanism is not available for primate hosts, which must be treated as something of a 'black box'.

All the caveats about vaccine testing in the mouse apply equally to the RA vaccine model. However, it is evident that a single exposure to attenuated parasites arms the lungs by recruiting persistent effector/memory T helper (Th) cells to the pulmonary parenchyma (Coulson and Wilson, 1993). In this situation, the arrival of a single challenge parasite in the lungs is an independent event which triggers a cellular effector focus (Smythies *et al.*, 1996). This blocks onward migration, increasing the probability of deflection into an alveolus. However, it must be emphasized that this trapping of migrating schistosomula in the lungs is not in itself a lethal killing event. An ultrastructural study of such challenge schistosomula found minimal evidence for cytological damage (Crabtree and Wilson, 1986). Moreover, trapped lung schistosomula, which would not mature if left *in situ*, could do so if transferred to the vascular system of naïve mice, confirming their viability (Coulson and Wilson, 1988). Two studies have indicated that this pulmonary phase immunity in mice, induced by a single exposure to the RA vaccine, is reasonably persistent presumably while the effector T cells remain. In the first, challenge at 15 weeks resulted in no reduction in the 78–80% protection (Minard *et al.*, 1978). In the second, protection was around two-thirds of the original level at 6 months but had declined to zero by 1 year (Smith and Clegg, 1984). To replicate such events with an antigen vaccine would require a protocol that generated and then armed the lungs with CD4^{+} memory/effector cells. To date no protocol has attempted to do this BUT it has the attraction of a persisting response (see Section 9.4.4). Perhaps recombinant BCG could have such desirable properties (Marques-Neto *et al.*, 2023).

A single exposure of mice to the RA vaccine elicits a predominant Th1 response while subsequent exposures augment Th2 involvement and the contribution of the antibody as part of the effector response. The Th1:Th2 balance can be deliberately skewed by the exposure of interferon-γ receptor knock-out (IFNγR KO) mice in which the Th1 response is abrogated (Farias *et al.*, 2021a). The antibody titre and the level of protection rise in parallel with successive vaccinations, 57% protection being achieved by three exposures to the RA vaccine. At this point, the IFNγR KO titres were 2.5 times those in comparably treated C57BL/6 mice and protection could be passively transferred to naïve C57BL/6 recipients by administration of immune serum. One feature of antibody-mediated protection is that it is easier to identify the antigenic targets than the targets of effector T cell receptors (see Section 9.4).

The most compelling evidence for the utility of the RA vaccine as a paradigm comes from its administration to primates, in which worm maturation is not a problem, with 82% of penetrating cercariae reaching maturity in vervet monkeys (*Cercopithecus aethiops*) (Yole *et al.*, 1996b) and a mean 80.5% in three baboon (*Papio anubis*) experiments (Yole *et al.*, 1996a). At this level of maturation, less then 20 out of 100 parasites died of 'natural causes' during migration. Three to five exposures elicited strong antibody-mediated protective immunity. This was as high as 86% after five vaccinations, based on recovered worm burden (Kariuki *et al.*, 2004), so a further 69 out of 100 worms died due to the immune effector response. No evidence has been found for arming of the lungs in primates by attenuated parasites, but this could simply be a matter of scale: a 5 kg baboon would need a dose of 1.25×10^5 attenuated cercariae to match the 5×10^2 dose that arms the lungs in a mouse.

The baboon antibody responses highlight a particular problem for schistosome vaccine development (Fig. 9.1). Specific IgM is elicited by exposure to the attenuated cercariae but as

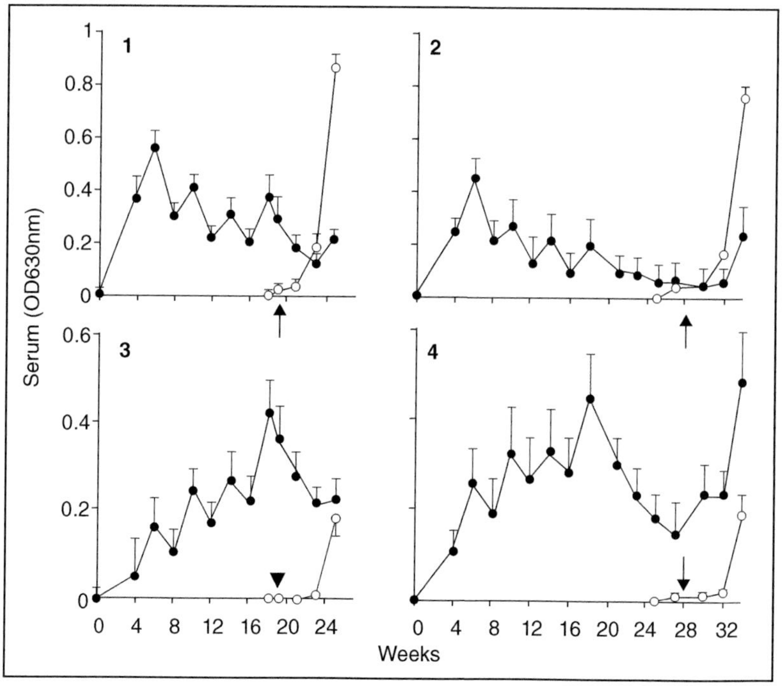

Fig. 9.1. Exposure of two groups of baboons, *Papio anubis*, to multiple doses of the RA cercarial vaccine, followed by a normal cercarial challenge at 3 weeks (**1**, **3**) or 12 weeks (**2**, **4**) after the last vaccination: **1** and **2**) IgM profiles; **3** and **4**) IgG profiles. Open circles are challenge control responses. Arrows denote time of challenge. The important features are that with repeated exposures the IgM profiles gradually subside while the IgG profiles increase. However, the titres peak 2 weeks after each exposure before declining. In the absence of an antigenic stimulus that decline continues steadily. The major stimulus for a response after challenge is the deposition of eggs from ~5 weeks, not the larval antigens. (From Kariuki *et al.*, 2004.) Figures used with permission from American Society for Microbiology.

might be anticipated, with successive vaccinations it declines towards the background (Fig. 9.1.1 and 9.1.2). In contrast, the specific IgG response showed a sawtooth pattern of boost and decline with successive vaccinations (Fig. 9.1.3 and 9.1.4). The titre rose progressively to a maximum at 3 weeks after the fifth exposure and in the experiment illustrated, cercarial challenge at this time of resulted in a 73% reduction in worm burden, compared to the challenge control group. However, the antibody titre began to decline once the antigenic stimulus was removed. When challenge of the vaccinated group was given at 12 weeks, the specific IgG titre had declined by 66% and the reduction in worm burden was 53% (Kariuki *et al.*, 2004). The message from these RA vaccinations in primates is that if the antibody-mediated protection is to be emulated by an antigen vaccine, then a formulation must be found that will maintain high anti-schistosome titres for prolonged periods.

9.3.2 Self-cure in the rat

Exposure of the laboratory rat to schistosome cercariae results in a well-defined infection profile with some differences between strains; the Fischer rat has been especially popular. Parasite tracking revealed that a plateau of ~40% of *S. mansoni* cercariae could be recovered by perfusion at day 21 (Knopf *et al.*, 1986). Other studies show numbers peaking in the portal system at day 28, but all agree on a dramatic decline thereafter, essentially a self-cure response. Note that a few stunted worms can be recovered for weeks to months after infection. Rats which have eliminated their primary burden may be immune to a normal cercarial challenge, but the data is sparse (Maddison *et al.*, 1970). Can this self-cure in the rat inform schistosome vaccine development? Examination of worms recovered from the portal system by confocal microscopy indicates that they suffer a direct insult, presumably immunological in nature (Fig. 9.2) and succumb much faster than the worms in self-curing rhesus macaques that take weeks to die (see Section 9.3.3).

The bad news is that the self-cure process is strongly associated with rapid increases in both total and specific IgE levels (Cutts and Wilson, 1997; Rousseaux-Prevost *et al.*, 1977). Concomitant with worm elimination, a pronounced hepatic mastocytosis was reported (Miller *et al.*, 1994). The majority of recruited mast cells contained mast cell protease-2, and it was released into the bloodstream during the period of worm elimination. It can be argued that juvenile worms arriving in the portal tract are responsible for arming the peri-portal tissues with mast cells in the same way that attenuated larvae arm the lungs. How might mast cell degranulation products kill the adult worms? Direct damage inflicted by the mast cell protease is possible (note

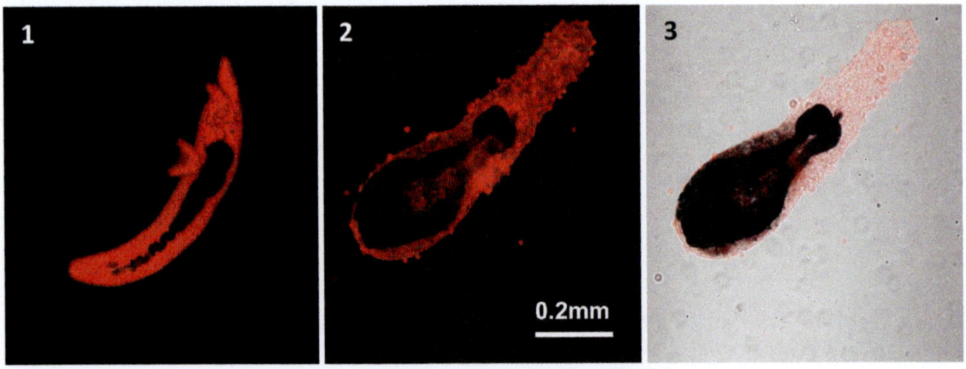

Fig. 9.2. Fate of day 21 liver worms in Fischer strain rats, stained with Langeron's Carmine (LC). **1**) Apparently normal blood feeding worm with gut delineated by black haemozoin pigment. **2**) Worm already showing signs of damage, with leucocytes attached to the tegument surface and the outlines of the gut not clearly defined. **3**) Combined LC and interference contrast image of the same worm shows that it has been damaged from the inside and gut haemozoin is leaking into the surrounding tissues. Figures author's own.

Fig. 9.2.2 – has the worm swallowed something unpleasant?), but also the potential effects of biogenic amines (histamine and serotonin). *S. mansoni* possesses a variety of relevant receptors (see Chapter 5). Worms in the portal tract might suddenly experience hyperstimulation of activity via the nervous system, leading to exhaustion and death.

A different angle on worm elimination has been provided by experiments with *S. japonicum* in rats with the gene for inducible nitric synthase knocked out (iNOS$^{-/-}$) (Shen *et al.*, 2017). Essentially, the lack of NO production allowed for more normal worm development, egg production and granulomatous pathology not seen in wild type rats. There were other immunological changes in the iNOS$^{-/-}$ animals (Shen *et al.*, 2022) and nothing is known about occurrence of hepatic mastocytosis so it is not currently possible to integrate the two proposed mechanisms of hepatic elimination in the rat.

The intimate involvement of IgE class antibodies in the rat self-cure process really does diminish its utility as a paradigm for vaccine development. Not least of the problems is the potentiation of IgE responses against bystander proteins by helminth parasite infections (Orr and Blair, 1969; Jarrett, 1978). It would be useful to identify the specific allergens involved in schistosome elimination in the rat portal system, if only to inform choices about which proteins to include in vaccine formulations (cf. Diemert *et al.*, 2012). Finally, the pattern of gene expression in the individual stunted worms, which survive for long periods in the rat portal system, is worth scrutiny. It is possible that they have particularly high levels of antioxidant (Huang *et al.*, 2012) or other enzymes that provide partial protection against immune attack.

9.3.3 Self-cure in the rhesus macaque

The features of this animal model were established in the 1960s in experiments using small numbers of animals given a variety of treatments. Primary exposures to between 100 and 1600 *S. mansoni* cercariae resulted in a patent infection, judged by faecal egg excretion from 5 weeks. Then, starting around 10 weeks, egg output declined to very low levels. After a large challenge with 2000 cercariae at 21 weeks, previously infected animals were highly protected, compared to single uninfected controls (Smithers and Terry, 1965). These pioneering experiments led, via worm transfer experiments, to the suggestion that host molecules were acquired on the tegument surface as a potential immune evasion mechanism. (Smithers and Terry, 1969). Recent proteomic studies have provided concrete evidence for this, and we now have a much clearer idea of some of their identities (e.g. CD44) (Wilson and Jones, 2021). It is worth emphasizing that the rhesus macaque is unique among primates in developing a self-cure response, occurring from weeks to months after a primary exposure. The olive baboon, for example, neither develops porta-caval shunting that would allow portal worms to escape (Sturrock *et al.*, 1988) nor strong immunity during a chronic infection (Sturrock *et al.*, 1976).

The rhesus macaque model has been revisited using both *S. mansoni* (Wilson *et al.*, 2008) and *S. japonicum* (Li *et al.*, 2015) infections in groups of six animals, with strikingly similar outcomes. In an independent *S. mansoni* experiment with macaques at the same primate facility, an estimated 44–65% of 1000 penetrant cercariae were recovered as adult worms, normal in size and appearance, after 8 weeks (Fallon *et al.*, 2003). In the 18-week *S. mansoni* time course, oviposition began at week 5, but from week 8–10, egg excretion in faeces tailed off. Circulating anodic antigen (CAA) released from the worm gut was used as a surrogate to estimate worm burden. Intriguingly, the decline in faecal egg output preceded that of CAA level in the blood. At perfusion the six macaques fell into three distinct groups, with low, medium and high worm burdens, which were inversely correlated with antibody titre. Strikingly, many recovered worms were pallid and emaciated; they appeared to be starving to death. In the later 22-week *S. japonicum* experiment, the six macaques did not stratify by worm burden or antibody titre. However, a severe size reduction of worms was noted, especially of females, compared to control worms from mice, with shrinkage of ovary and testes, and fewer eggs in the uterus and sperm in the seminal vesicle. These morphological changes in schistosome species were attributed to a generalized immunological pressure, under which it took worms several weeks to die. This was clearly different from the acute worm death in rats occurring over a period of days (see Section 9.3.2). A likely explanation for the slow death is that adult worms acquire nutrients across both their tegument surface and via the gut, the latter being more important in females with their greater needs owing to egg production (Lawrence, 1973). The female's response to cessation of blood feeding appears to be the gradual resorption of non-essential internal organs, leading to shrinkage of the body, while the shrinkage of more muscular males is less marked (Wilson *et al.*, 2008). Ultimately, both sexes succumb to the pressure.

These experiments led to a more comprehensive study of the rhesus model, using a cohort of 12 animals in a standardized protocol with modern immunological and parasitological techniques (Amaral *et al.*, 2021). It produced a wealth of information on the progress of a primary infection and a subsequent challenge with *S. mansoni* cercariae. The first worms were estimated to arrive in the portal system on day 6 and blood feeding began on day 8. Based on peak CAA levels, worm maturation was estimated at between 30% and 70% of penetrating cercariae. The impact of egg deposition on macaque physiology was evident from week 5 onwards, with rapid declines in animal weight a testament to the pathogenicity of the disease. Surprisingly, those animals with the greatest percentage weight loss for a longer period were the ones that dealt most effectively with the primary infection and then with the challenge. These were outbred animals, with a wide variation between individuals – a lesson for human vaccine trials. A pivot point at week 10, was followed by an exponential decline in egg excretion at approximately twice the rate of CAA level. From the decline in CAA, it was possible to calculate a half-life ($t_{1/2}$) of worm death, which varied between 2.8 weeks in the fastest responder and 8.7 weeks in the slowest (Fig. 9.3). The mechanism by which the rhesus macaque deals with a primary infection and the precise targets of immune attack are important questions to answer.

All animals received a challenge of 700 cercariae at 42 weeks when specific IgG levels were a quarter to one-third of the peak values. There was some evidence of a memory response after challenge, particularly in fast responder animals. The CAA levels in fast responder animals remained near background, revealing minimal inception of blood feeding, whereas slow responders showed a clear rise peaking at weeks 4–8, before declining. Apparently, some worms had developed to the blood feeding stage in these animals, but the few worms recovered by portal perfusion

1

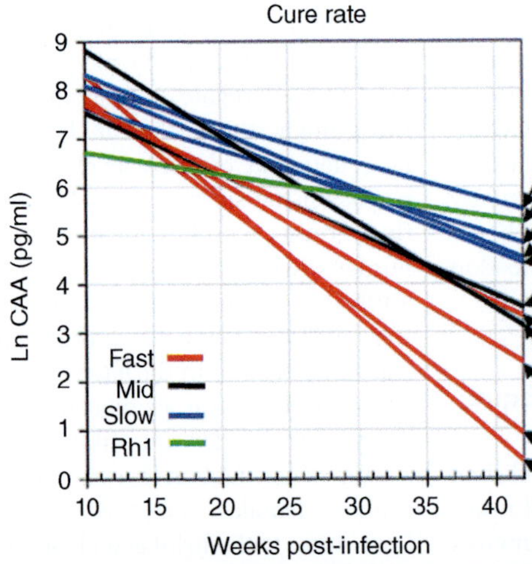

2

	$t^{1/2}$ weeks	R^2
Rh6	8,74	0.95
Rh1	15.47	0.75
Rh5	7.91	0.97
Rh8	5.86	0.90
Rh11	6.06	0.94
Rh7	5.54	0.98
Mean	5.32	
Rh9	5.10	0.90
Rh12	3.91	0.97
Rh4	4.10	0.94
Rh3	3.19	0.92
Rh2	2.79	0.99

Fig. 9.3. The self-cure phase of rhesus macaques infected with *S. mansoni*, between weeks 10 and 42. **1**) Cure rate for each animal from an Ln-transform of CAA levels, where $t_{1/2} = \ln 2/\lambda = 0.693$/regression slope. **2**) Table of $t_{1/2}$ cure rates showing stratification into Fast and Slow responder groups, where R^2 indicates goodness of fit of each regression to the raw data. (From Amaral *et al.*, 2021.) Figure used under license CC-BY-4.0.

at 20 weeks were small and showed no evidence of blood feeding or reproductive activity. Note that this was the result of a bolus challenge, providing a much greater antigenic stimulus than the trickle stimulus in human populations. However, the observations do indicate that although adult worm products initiate the immune responses that bring about self-cure, their targets must also be present and accessible to antibodies in developing worms, thus preventing worm establishment. This makes the replication of the self-cure process with a vaccine a tempting proposition.

The experimental infection of rhesus macaques with *S. japonicum* has provided both morphological and immunocytochemical information about the way in which worm elimination may be achieved (Li *et al.*, 2015). The complex structure of the anterior and posterior oesophageal glands was presented in Chapter 8 (Figs 8.3 and 8.4). Sections of the anterior oesophagus of worms recovered from rhesus macaques at week 22 post-infection stained strongly for deposits of macaque IgG, both intense focal spheroids and smaller fainter spots (Fig. 9.4.1). Under scanning electron microscopy (SEM), the flat pitted plates of cytoplasm that form the oesophageal lining were largely obscured by a deposit of material – it is tempting to conclude that this comprised immune complexes (Fig. 9.4.2). When the region was examined under transmission electron microscopy (TEM) it was apparent that the mechanism for vesicle release into the oesophageal lumen was completely choked up, with vesicles accumulating in the bulging tips (Fig. 9.4.3). These vesicles were 2–3 times the diameter of the 'light vesicles' in the normal anterior oesophageal gland (Fig. 9.4.4) (Li *et al.*, 2014). The inference is that antibodies elicited by the primary infection can bind proteins normally secreted by the glands to block their release. The identity of these anterior gland

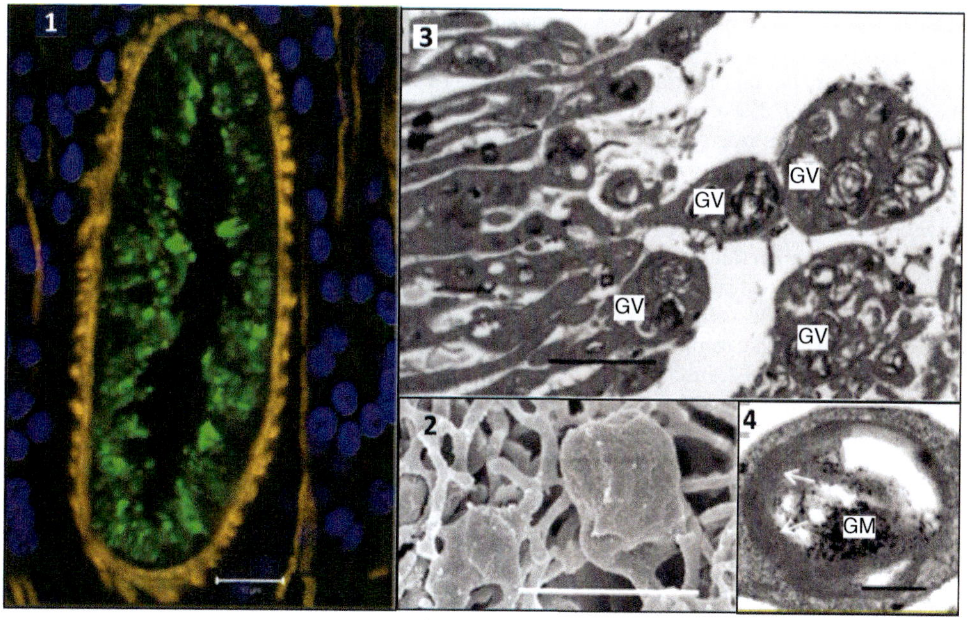

Fig. 9.4. Disrupted vesicle release in the anterior oesophagus of *S. japonicum* worms from rhesus macaques. **1**) Section of a worm head stained with AF488-labelled anti-monkey IgG (green) showing both focal areas and punctuate staining in the lining (nuclei, blue; muscle, orange). Scale bar: 10 µm. **2**) SEM image of a flat plate of cytoplasm in the fringe of the anterior lining, completely obscured by a deposit of material. Scale bar: 200 nm. **3**) TEM of the luminal edge of the anterior lining, showing its tips greatly expanded, and containing giant vesicles (GV). Scale bar: 2 µm. **4**) TEM of a giant vesicle showing the contents of both granular material (GM) and membrane stacks (arrowed). These resemble the membranocalyx coating of the oesophageal surface lining. Scale bar: 200 nm. (From Li *et al.*, 2015.)

products thus becomes important as potential vaccine candidates. There were also features of the posterior gland plates that suggested they had become adherent, again contributing to impaired function. Cumulatively, these observations provide an explanation for why worms might starve to death. Their ability to ingest and process blood is seriously impaired by an antibody response to oesophageal gland secretions.

9.4 Identification of Immune Targets in Animal Models and Humans

The advent of proteomic and RNA sequencing (RNA-Seq) technologies has made possible the characterization of the proteins and glycans that comprise the schistosome interface with its mammalian host, defining the interactome of parasite and host molecules involved in essential biological processes. These parasite products are the Achilles heel that a vaccine attempts to exploit to bring about elimination. The potential cercarial targets were covered in Chapter 2 and those of the intravascular migrating schistosomulum in Chapter 3. For the blood feeding juveniles and adult worms, the potentially accessible proteins of the tegument were considered in Chapter 7 and the extensive products of the oesophageal glands and gastrodermis vomited into the bloodstream in Chapter 8. By definition, the vaccine targets must be accessible in the live worm, and it is from the really quite extensive list that a successful vaccine would emerge.

As proteomic and transcriptomic reports have multiplied, another pitfall has emerged, namely the incautious handling of worms during perfusion and *in vitro* incubation. Consequently, inventories of gut and tegument surface proteins are now heavily infiltrated by the familiar and highly abundant internal proteins. This chapter on vaccines takes a conservative view that adult schistosomes do not have a unique cell biology involving secretion of cytosolic and cytoskeletal proteins. Chapter 7 (Sections 7.7.1 and 7.7.2) dealt with the controversies surrounding the cytosolic proteins of the leakyome and the tegument vesicles of the disintegrome. Those proteins containing an N-terminal signal peptide, denoting export via the classical endoplasmic reticulum and Golgi pathway, are included but qualified by an additional criterion. There should be cytological evidence for expression/secretion at either tegument or alimentary tract interfaces with the host, not at some internal tissue location such as muscle or parenchyma. There are a few exceptions, such as calpain and some annexins, lacking signal peptides but nevertheless demonstrated at the tegument surface by immunocytochemistry, although their accessibility to antibodies in the live worm is presently unclear.

9.4.1 Conventional cloning of targets

What has been achieved using this strict definition of the parasite – host interface? Several tegumental proteins have been cloned and expressed by conventional molecular biology methods and then tested singly for protective capacity in the mouse model. They included TSP-2 (Tran *et al.*, 2006), Sm29 (Cardoso *et al.*, 2008) and the C-terminal portion of Sm200 (Carvalho *et al.*, 2014). The tegument protease Smp80 calpain (Hota-Mitchell *et al.*, 1997) has a long history of vaccine experiments with successful transfer to the baboon model (Siddiqui and Siddiqui, 2017) and is now in human trials (see Section 9.6). Among alimentary tract secretions, gut cathepsins have been shown to elicit protection in the mouse model, and cross-protection against *S. haematobium* in hamsters (El Ridi *et al.*, 2014; Tallima *et al.*, 2017a, b). The cathepsin immunogens need to be enzymatically active, suggesting that a note of caution is required. The fact that papains from plants (El Ridi and Tallima, 2013) and the liver fluke (*Fasciola hepatica*) (El Ridi *et al.*, 2014) are also protective may indicate that the mechanism involves a bystander effect (Wilson *et al.*, 2016). Further evidence for the efficacy of cathepsins has come from a study expressing cathepsin B1 (GenBank M21309.1) in an attenuated *Salmonella* strain (Hassan *et al.*, 2023). When administered orally to mice the vaccine notably elicited specific intestinal IgA responses and a high level of protection. The observation of high mucosal IgA levels could provide a novel route for attack when adult worms migrate to the mucosa to deposit eggs (Dr E. Houlder, personal communication).

9.4.2 Recombinant protein arrays

Even applying strict selection criteria, there are so many potential components in the schistosome host interactome that researchers have turned to mass screening techniques to identify the most reactive antigens in the immune responses of humans or animal model hosts. This has parallels with the expression libraries screened in the 1980s, but with a deterministic choice of proteins (or glycans) to be screened. The first such array was generated using 214 *S. japonicum* and 63 *S. mansoni* potential antigens, chosen by literature and database searching (Driguez *et al.*, 2010). The proteins from an *in vitro* cell-free *Escherichia coli* system were printed directly on to microscope slides for probing with antisera. It was first used with human sera from an *S. mansoni* endemic area of Brazil, classified as putatively resistant (PR) or chronically infected (CI), to search for signatures associated with protected status (Gaze *et al.*, 2014). It identified SmTSP-2 and a calmodulin as recognized strongly by the PR group, but not by CI individuals. The array was also used to screen the responses of sera from humans potentially acquiring drug-induced resistance (DIR) to *S. haematobium* infection, and from rhesus macaques self-curing from *S. japonicum* (Pearson *et al.*, 2015). The one protein identified by the rhesus macaque serum was an extracellular superoxide dismutase, whose *S. mansoni* orthologue has induced protection in the mouse model. The argument that the heterogeneous design would identify proteins cross-reactive between the main schistosome species seems optimistic. SmTSP-2 is now in the early stages of human trials (see Section 9.6).

A more recent recombinant protein library expressed in mammalian cells was based on published proteomics studies and transcriptional data comprising secreted and membrane-tethered *S. mansoni* proteins from the schistosomula stage (Crosnier *et al.*, 2022). Its principal value was that conformational epitopes would be detectable, and a biotin tag permitted coating of ELISA plates. Tested against pooled human sera from an endemic region of Uganda, almost all reacted positively, two-thirds of them strongly. Probing of infected mouse sera identified early markers of infection from the worm gut, with tegument markers detected by 7 weeks. Applied to human sera from the CHI model (see Section 9.6) the reactivity of gut proteins (saposins, cathepsins) was apparent by 8 weeks (Fig. 9.5), with tegument surface proteins at 20 weeks. As a postscript, 96 proteins from this mammalian expression library were employed in a systematic programme of vaccination and challenge experiments in mice. Unfortunately, no strongly protective vaccine candidates were identified (Crosnier *et al.*, 2019).

9.4.3 Shotgun glycan arrays

Many exported schistosome proteins are decorated with highly antigenic glycan moieties shared between life cycle stages such as the cercarial and egg secretions (Jang-Lee *et al.*, 2007). Unfortunately, while high antibody titres are elicited by vaccination of mice with viable eggs, such mice show zero protection against cercarial challenge (Kariuki *et al.*, 2008). This has led to the smokescreen hypothesis that suggests the role of the glycans is to divert antibody responses away from more sensitive peptide epitopes (Eberl *et al.*, 2001). Even with knowledge of glycan structures there is no easy way to synthesize a glycan array *de novo*. Instead researchers have devised *N*-linked (van Diepen *et al.*, 2012b) and *O*-linked (van Diepen *et al.*, 2015) shotgun arrays by isolation of native glycan structures from different life cycle stages, their chromatographic separation, and printing of fractions on to glass slides for screening with host sera (van Diepen *et al.*, 2012b). Reactive glycan structures on such arrays can be tentatively identified by mass spectrometry.

One of the first studies compared the IgM and IgG responses of groups of children in an endemic area of Uganda (van Diepen *et al.*, 2012a). It revealed that anti-glycan responses to both classes were higher in the children, the group more susceptible to reinfection. This suggests an inverse correlation between anti-glycan titres and protective immunity, supporting the smokescreen hypothesis. A note of caution was sounded about specific glycan epitopes because the fractions produced by chromatographic procedures contain more than one glycan structure. In the quest for glycans associated with vaccine-induced protection the shotgun arrays have also been used with sera from rhesus macaques

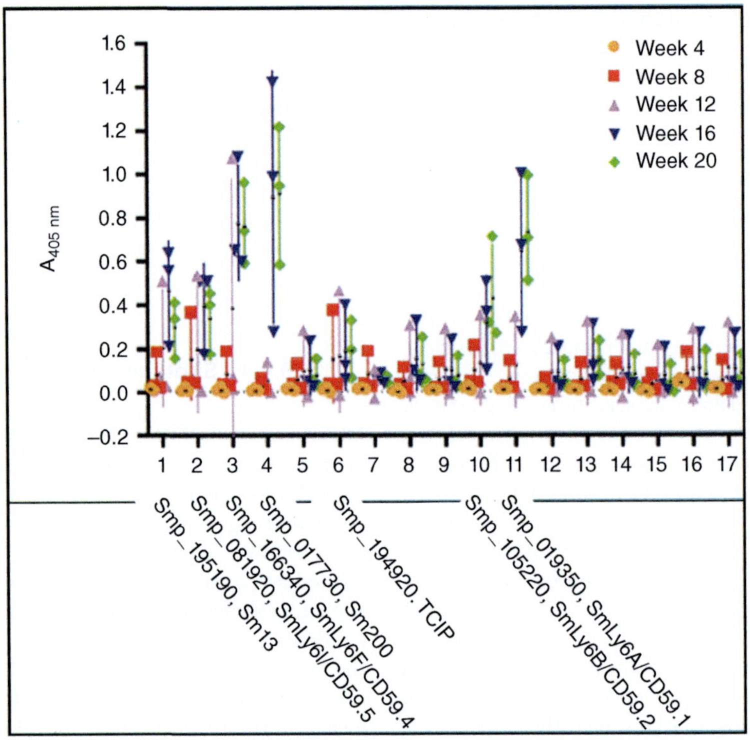

Fig. 9.5. The responses of human volunteers after exposure to 30 male cercariae for a 20-week period. The segment shows a selection of tegument surface proteins, colour-coded by week. (From Crosnier *et al.*, 2022.) Figure used under license CC-BY-4.0.

self-curing from *S. japonicum* infection (Yang *et al.*, 2017). Antibody responses towards schistosome glycans at week 4 post-infection were dominated by IgM while IgG was high at week 8. The profound increase in IgG was observed mainly for antibodies towards a large subset of glycans that contain multi-fucosylated terminal LDN and Lewis X (LeX) motifs. In general, glycans with a higher degree of fucosylation gave rise to stronger antibody responses than non-fucosylated glycans. Although many IgG and IgM responses had declined by week 22 post-infection, IgG towards *O*-glycans with highly fucosylated LDN motifs remained. The authors note that although some oesophageal micro-exon gene (MEG)-encoded proteins are predicted to be *O*-glycosylated, they are secreted in minute amounts, and their *O*-glycans are not yet identified.

An array of cercarial, worm and egg glycans has also been used to screen sera from baboons highly protected by exposure to the *S. mansoni* RA cercarial vaccine, over a 25-week time course (Yang *et al.*, 2019). Anti-glycan IgM responses developed early after the initial vaccination but not after subsequent exposures while anti-glycan IgG responses progressively increased. After challenge, most antibody levels decreased due to the absence of vaccine stimulation, but IgG towards a subset of glycans containing multiple-fucosylated motifs remained high until 6 weeks post-challenge, over the period of parasite elimination. It is possible that protective responses are elicited by multi-fucosylated epitopes, but they pose a significant challenge. The chemical technology presently does not exist to produce such structures synthetically at scale to facilitate either probing of host responses or vaccine experiments in animal models.

9.4.4 Peptide microarrays

Peptide microarrays allow antibody–antigen reactions to be visualized at the level of individual epitopes within a target protein, an altogether higher level of resolution than other screening methods. The concept of high-density peptide microarrays created by combinatorial synthesis was published in 2007 (Beyer *et al.*, 2007), and is now marketed as PEPperPRINT arrays (https://www.pepperprint.com). Hundreds to thousands of short overlapping peptides can be printed, representing panels of individual protein targets determined by the user, and the data obtained can in many cases be mapped on to the three-dimensional structure of the parent protein.

The first small-scale peptide arrays were designed to test the hypothesis that the mechanism of self-cure in macaques involved cessation of feeding, followed by slow starvation to death (see Section 9.3.3). Arrays printed with overlapping 15-mer peptides from 32 *S. japonicum* oesophageal gland proteins (minus signal peptide) screened for reactivity against 22-week serum from six self-curing macaques, four permissive rabbits and four mouse hosts, revealed considerable intra- and interspecies variation (Li *et al.*, 2020). No obvious unique target was associated with macaque self-cure status versus responses of the permissive hosts. MEG-4.1 (C-terminus), -4.2, -11, -12, an unclassified MEG, an aspartyl protease and a tetraspanin loop were prominent across species, while responses to the C-termini of MEG-8.1 and -8.2 were largely confined to macaques. As proof of principal, seven reactive regions from MEG-4.1, -4.2, -8.1, -8.2, -9 and -11 plus VAL-7 were selected for encoding in a synthetic gene. The 27 kDa recombinant protein was used to vaccinate test rabbits, and resulting serum screened for target reactivity. Five of the seven reactive regions elicited high-titre IgG against the target epitopes, confirming that a 'string of pearls' construct may be a way of immunizing simultaneously against multiple targets.

Four larger arrays comprising 15-mer overlapping peptides, with one, two or three amino acid offsets, were used to screen a range of mouse sera (Farias *et al.*, 2021a). This permitted printing of the full-length sequence of 55 alimentary tract and tegument proteins, chosen from published analyses (Fig. 9.6.1; Chapters 7 and 8). Data comparisons were based on a reactivity score for each antigenic target (Fig. 9.6.2). Serum from the multiply vaccinated IFNγR KO mice, capable of conferring protection on naïve recipients was the most reactive. The targets formed four distinct reactivity groups with the oesophageal MEGs lying at the top left the strongest, followed by gastrodermal carriers in the centre and gastrodermal enzymes on the right, all of them more reactive than tegument surface targets. The actual conformation that linear 15-mer peptides take on the arrays is unclear, but the epitope mapping to crystal structures revealed antibody binding to α-helixes and β-sheets, as well as extrinsic loops. The broad conclusions from this murine study are that many potential targets have a quite limited reactivity, and in one way that makes sense. The blood-dwelling stages can only survive if they present a minimal target for immune attack – otherwise they would be eliminated.

In the final peptide array analysis, the same array used in the mouse study was screened with high- and low-responder pools of 18-week sera from rhesus macaques self-curing from *S. mansoni* infection (Wilson *et al.*, 2008), detected using Cy5-labelled secondary antibody on the red channel (Fig. 9.7) (Vance *et al.*, 2024). The two-colour detection allowed the direct comparison of previously identified murine responses with the rhesus macaque reactivities (Fig. 9.8). Mice and macaques respond to similar protein targets but with both identical and distinct reactivities. Overall, in the two macaque pools, the target epitopes were the same but the intensity of response was twice as strong in the high responders. Tegument proteins elicited much weaker responses than those originating in the alimentary tract, exactly as apparent in the murine study (Fig. 9.6.2). However, there were two outliers, Sm25 highly reactive for the tegument and MEG-15 under-reactive for the oesophageal gland. If these are removed from the analysis then again, tegument proteins have a significantly lower reactivity than alimentary tract proteins. In this macaque study, titre not target appears to determine the rate of self-cure.

As a postscript, partly informed by a genome-wide phage display screen (Woellner-Santos *et al.*, 2024) and partly by peptide array data (Vance *et al.*, 2024) the principal reactive regions of several of the alimentary tract and tegument proteins of rhesus macaques have been selected for inclusion in a multiepitope 'string of pearls' construct for vaccine experiments in macaques (Brazilian Patent number: BR 10 2024 002799 0). These are now in progress in Brazil.

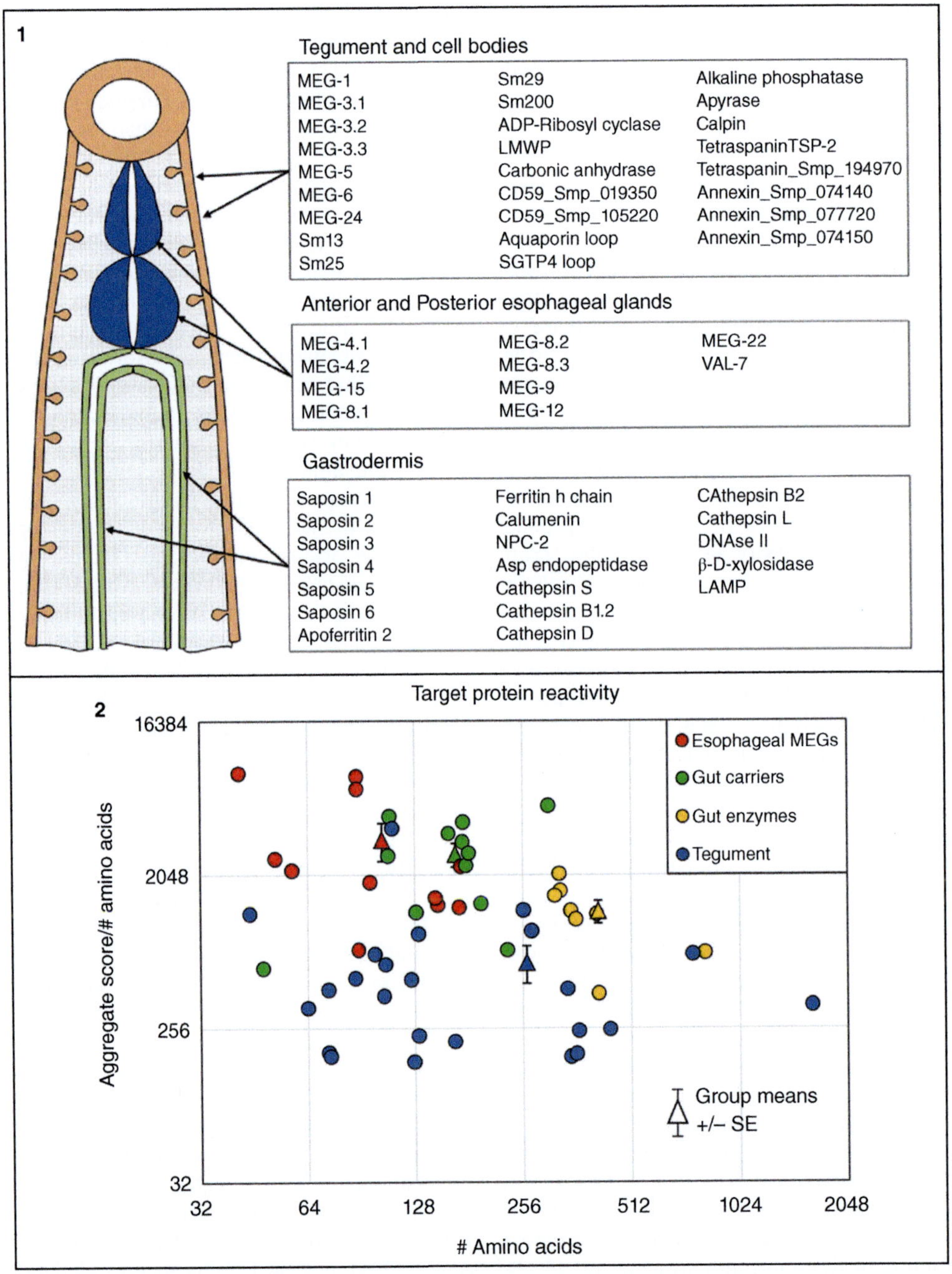

Fig. 9.6. Screening of antibody reactivity using peptide arrays. **1**) Schematic of the 55 proteins printed as 15-mer high-density PEPperPRINT peptide arrays for screening of rodent and primate protective sera to identify potential targets. **2**) The mean reactivity of array proteins for mouse sera, normalized for number of amino acids and segregated into four groups by tissue of origin. Note the log axis scales. (From Farias *et al.*, 2021a.)

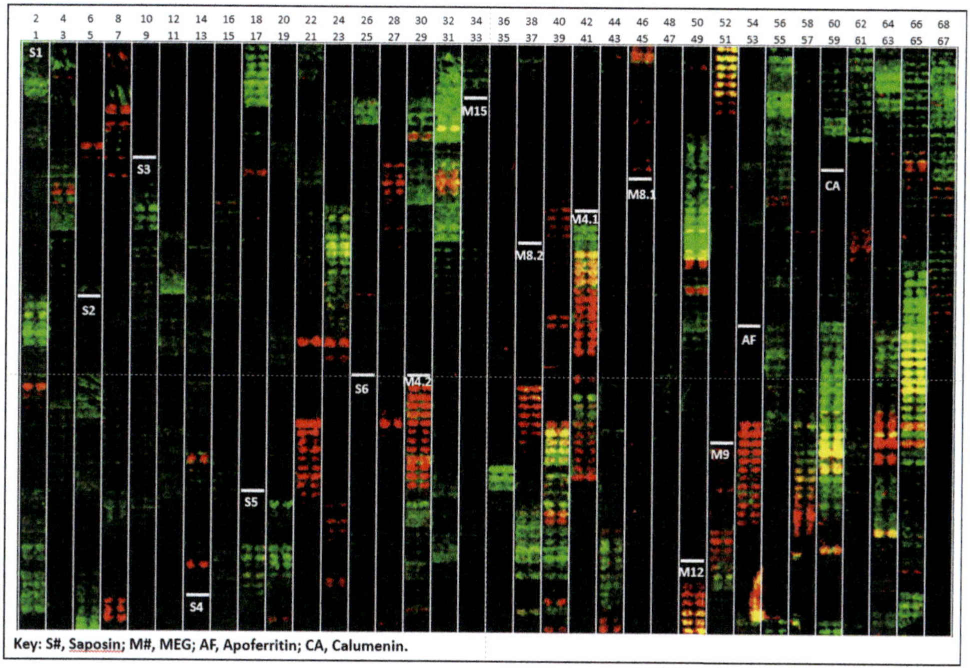

Fig. 9.7. Visual output from an array scanner. Annotated image of a short alimentary tract protein array reacted with sera from IFNγR KO mice in the green (Cy3) channel and a rhesus macaque pool in the red (Cy5) channel. Overlapping reactivities appear yellow. Protein boundaries are indicated by a horizontal line with abbreviated name below. (From Vance *et al.*, 2024.) Figure used under license CC-BY-4.0.

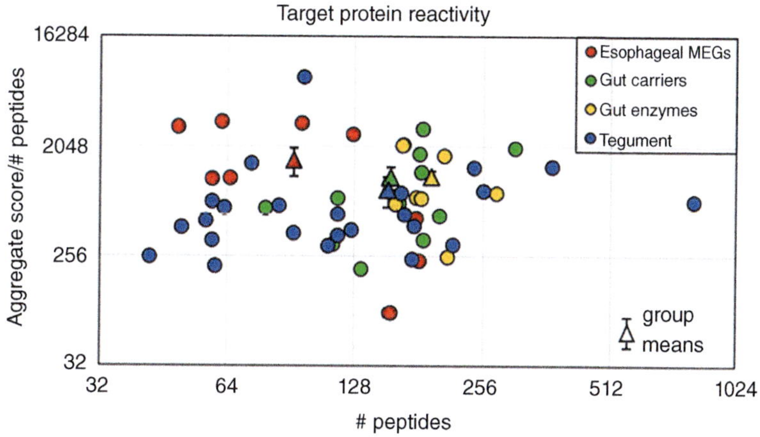

Fig. 9.8. The mean reactivity of array proteins with a pool of serum from hi-responder rhesus macaques. The proteins were normalized for number of peptides printed, which compensates for one, two or three amino acid offsets. The proteins are colour-coded by function. Note the log axis scales. (From Vance *et al.*, 2024.) Figure used under license CC-BY-4.0.

9.5 Systems Biology and the Missing Dimension

Many aspects of vaccine development are empirical. Select antigen(s) and an adjuvant formulation, administer in animal or human trials and then evaluate the outcome as a measure of protection achieved. Some vaccines have proved highly successful but many, perhaps most, attempts have been suboptimal. In part this is due to ignorance about the immune mechanisms the vaccine is trying to emulate in the host, so researchers have turned to Systems Biology in an attempt to supply this missing dimension (Hagan *et al.*, 2015). It involves the study of immune responses to vaccination, combining the measurement of various parameters, analysis of their interaction network and predictive modelling using bioinformatics tools. Examples include analysis of the genes activated in peripheral blood mononuclear cells (PBMCs) to identify molecular signatures that predict the early events in the immunogenicity of the attenuated yellow fever virus vaccine in humans (Querec *et al.*, 2009). The gene networks in humans immunized with inactivated versus attenuated influenza vaccines have also been compared (Nakaya *et al.*, 2011).

The systems biology approach has been applied to PBMC and skin-draining lymph node data from mice exposed to the RA cercarial vaccine or normal cercariae. The analysis was intended to illuminate why attenuated larvae elicit a protective response while normal larvae do not, and additionally why multiple exposures to the RA vaccine change the balance from a Th1 to a Th1/Th2 profile but nevertheless fail to drive protection towards sterile immunity (Farias *et al.*, 2021b). Infected mice showed early upregulation of pathways associated with Th2 skewing and polarization of IgG antibody profiles, while haemostasis pathways were downregulated, correlating with platelet reduction, potentially aiding parasite migration through capillary beds. Conversely, a single exposure to attenuated cercariae showed an early Th1 bias, with genes encoding chemokines and their receptors more prominent, indicating an enhanced capacity for inflammation that would block pulmonary migration. Three vaccinations did not elevate protection greatly but there was a clear shift towards antibody-mediators. However, the persistence of a Th1 response put a limit on expression of antibody-mediated mechanisms and there was also evidence for the development of anergy, which may explain why multiple doses fail to drive protection towards sterile immunity.

A second study has examined gene expression patterns in PBMCs at days 7 and 17 after infection or vaccination, and day 7 post-challenge (Pires da Silva *et al.*, 2024). Co-expression network analysis identified a module (M2) associated with the infection process, grouping genes related to a Th2 immune response and a second module (M6) associated with the vaccination process, displaying pathways related to a Th1 response, $CD8^+$ T cells and natural killer (NK) cells. This is the first time that a potential role for NK cells has been highlighted in the RA vaccine response, operating through the production of IFN-γ orchestrated by the T-bet transcription factor (Tbx21). The network analysis has provided a series of genetic markers as pointers to the response being elicited. The two studies neatly illustrate the dilemma facing vaccine developers in deciding what complexion of response to aim for when seeking to replicate the RA vaccine with an antigen formulation.

9.6 Human Vaccine Trials and the CHI Model

Since the development of molecular biology techniques and the WHO-sponsored independent trials of vaccine candidates in mice (Bergquist, 1995), there has been pressure to move forward to trials of vaccine candidates in humans. This is not a trivial matter as experience with malaria vaccine trials testify (Stanisic and Good, 2023). The use of controlled infection of human volunteers has been widespread in malaria research for the testing of vaccination regimes, at least as far back as the 1970s, with infections being terminated by chemotherapy. Only recently has this practice, the CHI model, been developed for schistosomes (Langenberg *et al.*, 2020). Sometimes the process of vaccine development is driven as much by personality as by science and it becomes hard to distinguish between the two. Vaccines for diseases prevalent in low-income countries need external funding and funders want to pick winners, so are attracted by claims of success that do not hold up in the face of complex and well-adapted parasites. Arguably, malaria is an acute disease with a high mortality in young children so deserves and has received much more attention. Schistosomiasis has a much slower and more insidious time course. It has received only a tiny fraction of the funding for malaria research, so it is really quite remarkable that several schistosome vaccine candidates have been taken forward to human trials by committed teams of individuals. The vaccine candidates undergoing trials are summarized in Table 9.1, based on material extracted from the National Institutes of Health (NIH) website (https://clinicaltrials.gov), searched with schistosomiasis and vaccine. They derive partly from the original WHO trials and partly from the switch in emphasis to secreted and surface-exposed antigens. Few of the antigens identified in large-scale screens (see Sections 9.4.2–9.4.4) has yet reached the stage of an animal, let alone a human trial.

Sm28GST is a very abundant cytosolic protein with a long history of vaccine experimentation; by extension the Sh28GST used in the first and only Phase 3 human trials is similarly abundant. Unfortunately, although the vaccine was well tolerated, no significant difference was observed in the recurrence of urinary schistosomiasis in 84.8% of the vaccinated individuals and in 89.6% of the control group, over the 2 years after vaccination (Riveau *et al.*, 2018). The trial was designed as an anti-pathology vaccine, based on an experiment in Patas monkeys (*Erythrocebus patas*) where a reduction in egg output was observed, although not in worm burdens (Boulanger *et al.*, 1999). It is worth noting that the Sh28GST vaccine trialled against *S. haematobium* infection in mice, using four different vaccine formulations, elicited neither a reduction in worm burden nor female fecundity, relative to controls (R.A. Wilson, unpublished data). In retrospect, despite an enormous volume of research, glutathione *S*-transferase does not appear to be a viable candidate.

Sm14 fatty acid binding protein has a similar long history of vaccine research stretching back decades. It is another abundant cytosolic protein in adult worms, and due to its cross-reactivity between schistosome species, and with the liver fluke (*F. hepatica*), was proposed as a multivalent anti-helminth vaccine (Tendler *et al.*, 1995). In the first human trials in Brazil it was shown to be well tolerated and highly immunogenic (Santini-Oliveira *et al.*, 2016). Phase 2a and 2b trials in adults and children have been completed in Senegal (Table 9.1) (Ly *et al.*, 2025). The authors conclude that the Sm14 vaccine, formulated with glucopyranosyl lipid A (GLA-SE), is safe and highly immunogenic with a clear protective potential against schistosomiasis, supporting progression to Phase 3 clinical trials. Its internal location does not augur well for success.

Table 9.1. Human vaccine trials registered at the NIH website 'https://clinicaltrials.gov'

Group	Candidate	Trial number	Country	Stage	Status
Capron France	ShGST28 Bilhvax	NCT00870649	Senegal	Phase 3	completed 2012
Tendler Brasil		NCT01154049 NCT03041766 NCT03799510 NCT05658614	Brasil Senegal	Phase 1 Phase 2a Phase 2b Phase 2	completed 2014 completed 2017 completed 2019 unclear
was Loukas Australia now Hotez USA	Sm-TSP-2	NCT02337855 NCT03110757 NCT03910972	USA Brasil Uganda	Phase 1 Phase 1b Phase 1/2	completed 2017 completed 2019 ongoing
was Podesta Canada now Siddiqui USA	Smp80 calpain Schistoshield	NCT05292391 NCT05762393 NCT05999825	USA Burkina Faso Madagascar Netherlands	Phase 1 Phase 1b Phase 2	completed 2024 ongoing not started
Roestenberg Leiden	CHI Model CHI Model CHI Model	NCT02755324 NCT04269915 NCT05085470	Netherlands Netherlands Netherlands	NA NA NA	completed 2019 completed 2022 completed 2023

SmTSP-2, a more recent candidate, was identified as exposed on the tegument surface (see Chapter 7 and Section 9.4.2). The vaccine tested in mice comprised the 78 amino acids of the long tetraspanin extracellular loop (Glu107–His184), formulated in Freund's complete (prime) and Freund's incomplete (two boosts) adjuvant, gave a mean 57% reduction in adult worm burden and a 64% reduction in liver egg burdens compared with control animals (Tran *et al.*, 2006). For human administration, this recombinant was formulated on aluminium hydroxide adjuvant (Alhydrogel) with or without 5 mg of glucopyranosyl lipid A (GLA-AF). It was found to be safe and immunogenic well tolerated in a phase 1, dose-escalation trial with adults in the USA (Keitel *et al.*, 2019). The protocol was then essentially replicated in a Phase 1b trial with adults living in a region of Brazil with ongoing *S. mansoni* transmission using the Alhydrogel formulation ± GLA-AF (now known as AP 10-701) (Diemert *et al.*, 2023). Again, the vaccine was well tolerated in this population, and a significant dose–response relationship was seen in those individuals given SmTSP-2/Alhydrogel with AP 10-701. As of September 2024, a Phase 1/2 trial is under way in an endemic area of Uganda and the outcome is eagerly awaited.

The Smp80 calpain vaccine is the one candidate extensively trialled in the baboon model as well as in rodents (Zhang *et al.*, 2020). It too is located in the tegument but more basally than SmTSP-2 (see Chapter 7). The strongest credentials for Smp80 calpain derive from four independent double-blind experiments in baboons, which generated a remarkable data-set (Zhang *et al.*, 2018). Groups of five test and five control animals received a prime and three boosts at 4-week intervals with Smp80 calpain formulated with GLA-SE, or with GLA-SE alone, and then 4 weeks after the last vaccination all animals were challenged with 1000 cercariae. Efficacy, assessed by portal perfusion after 8 weeks, revealed an overall mean protection of 66%. However, there was a marked differential effect on female worms, with a 93% protection versus 44% for the males. In consequence there was also a marked 90% reduction in intestinal and tissue egg load, a 35-fold reduction in faecal egg excretion and an 82% reduction in the capacity of eggs to hatch. The differential susceptibility of females correlates with their greater expression of calpain in the tegument. The first human Phase 1 trial, completed in early 2024, was a dose-escalation study to evaluate the safety, reactogenicity, and immunogenicity of the Smp80 + GLA-SE vaccine formulation in healthy adults, in the USA. No results have been posted but the fact that a Phase 1b trial is under way in Madagascar and Burkina Faso implies that no problems were encountered. The proposed Phase 2 trial in The Netherlands with the CHI model is still pending.

The CHI has to date been used only with varying doses of male or female cercaria, basically to explore the parameters, and the certainty of achieving a complete cure after treatment with one to two doses of praziquantel at the end of an experiment. Worm burden is estimated using the CAA level as a surrogate, with the slight limitation of inability to calibrate against worm number. The first reported trial was a dose escalation with 10, 20 or 30 male cercariae (Langenberg *et al.*, 2020), which might be considered a low exposure. Surprisingly, all but one of the 17 participants developed a mild dermatitis within two days after exposure, with duration proportional to cercarial dose. Equally, the three participants in the 30 cercaria group developed a series of adverse events from 2.5 to 5 weeks after exposure, equivalent to an acute schistosomiasis syndrome of the Katayama fever type. This may be the first report in recent times charting the effects of a deliberate but small exposure to schistosome cercariae and reveals just how insidious this parasite is.

The second study with 13 participants had a similar design, with three exposed to 10 female cercariae and the remaining 10 to 20 (Koopman *et al.*, 2023). Again, there was a skin reaction to exposure, visible for a median 23 days, and five of the participants exposed to 20 cercariae showed adverse systemic events of acute schistosomiasis. In participants exposed to 20 cercariae, six out of 10 had detectable CAA levels but surprisingly although treated twice with praziquantel, four out of 10 did not clear their infection. The authors concluded that there is a decreased susceptibility of single female worms to praziquantel in the human host which limits the use of female cercariae for future vaccine testing but may have important implications for disease control programmes.

The CHI model has also been used to test the hypothesis that partial immunity develops over time and is enhanced by repeated treatment with praziquantel that will release a pulse of antigens into the bloodstream (Koopman *et al.*, 2024). The test group was exposed to 20 male cercariae at weeks 0, 9 and 18, while the control group received two mock exposures at weeks 0 and 9, and a cercarial exposure at week 18. The test group received praziquantel and the control group a placebo at week 8 and week 17, before all participants received praziquantel at week 30. In this study all participants were cured by the praziquantel treatment. Based on CAA levels and boosting of IgG1 titres, two exposure and treatment cycles did not produce any evidence for the development of protective immunity resulting from infection and cure. The CHI model should provide an ideal test environment for new vaccine formulations in humans.

9.7 Miscellanea

9.7.1 Vaccine Value Profile

A Vaccine Value Profile (VVP) for schistosomiasis, commissioned by the WHO and funded by the Bill & Melinda Gates Foundation, has produced an exhaustive assessment of what is required to achieve a worthwhile schistosome vaccine (Yamey *et al.*, 2024). While having some merit, the profile is very far removed from current reality. The desired minimal duration of protection is stated as 2–3 years after the last vaccine dose, and preferably 10 years (this last would be a hard ask for any vaccine). Based on modelling studies, an efficacy of ≥90% is also envisaged, to make the vaccine cost-effective compared to mass drug administration. This is not a fair comparison because, as set out in Section 9.2, vaccines possess attributes that chemotherapy does not. In the schistosome context the efficacy must mean a 90% lower worm burden, compared to non-vaccinated compatriots, persisting over a period of 2–3 years.

A recent scoping review of pre-clinical prophylactic vaccine studies targeting *S. mansoni* in the last 30 years recorded that over 100 vaccine candidates have been tested (Houlder *et al.*, 2025). The median efficacy for all tests, based on worm count, was 35%. Only 10 candidates achieved an efficacy of >60%, and only two of >90%, in any experiment. No candidate tested repeatedly had a median efficacy of >60%, based on worm and egg counts. The persistence of any level of protection was a matter of weeks to a few months, never anywhere near 2–3 years called for in the VVP. Apparently, we are not even in the foothills of the climb needed to reach the summit of a useable vaccine that will impact on the health of the human population in an endemic area.

9.7.2 Novel vaccine constructs

The development of adjuvants and new vaccine vectors, principally designed to generate high antibody titres, is a very active field stimulated by the recent COVID-19 pandemic. The Toll-like receptor agonist GLA, with Alhydrogel, is the mainstay of the Smp80 calpain trials. Another option being used is a nanoparticulate comprising bacterial outer membrane vesicles of *Neisseria lactamica* conjugated with biotin and decorated with expressed recombinant schistosome proteins in fusion with biotin-binding rhizavidin (Barbosa *et al.*, 2021). Virus-like particles are a third approach, already commercialized for hepatitis B and papilloma virus (Brune and Howarth, 2018), that is being explored with schistosome targets (S. Liu, personal communication). These particles can be decorated with antigens using catcher-tag technologies, potentially for delivery of multiple targets. Beyond the schistosome field, the new R21/Matrix-M malaria vaccine (Datoo *et al.*, 2021), licensed for human use, is also a nanoparticle construct comprising saponins (triterpene structures with a variety of glycoside side-chains), cholesterol and phospholipids in a 40 nm cage-like nanoparticle that induces potent humoral and cellular immune responses (Stertman *et al.*, 2023). It is probable that one of these new technologies can be adapted for use in schistosome vaccine development, but the design of realistic experiments is crucial.

9.7.3 Multi-antigen targets

The vaccine value profile appears to be predicated on identifying a single ideal antigenic target. It is possible that researchers might get lucky in finding such a magic bullet, an Achilles heel that makes all schistosomes vulnerable to elimination, but the chances are not high. The variability of the antigen-presenting major histocompatibility complex loci alone makes it unlikely that a human population can be uniformly protected. Add to that the genetic variability of schistosomes and the demonstrable ability of some individual worms to survive the immune environment of rats or slow responder rhesus macaques, as a demonstration of their tenacity. It seems more likely that an antigen cocktail or a multiepitope 'string of pearls' construct will be needed. That is where the novel constructs may ultimately provide a solution.

9.8 Summary

- There is not an obvious pathway to design a successful vaccine based on human responses because any involvement of IgE antibodies must be excluded. Blocking cercarial invasion of the skin appears to be a non-starter since a vaccine formulation that kept the immune response on 'red alert' for a significant period in the absence of continued stimulation probably does not exist. Trapping schistosomula in the lungs or eliminating them during development in the portal tract are the best options from animal models.
- Much past research has centred on finding the right antigenic target, but it seems unlikely that a single magic bullet antigen exists. More likely protection, where it can be demonstrated, is mediated by multiple antigens. Whether targeting lung schistosomula or blood feeding juveniles in the portal tract, there is a cohort of unexplored secreted and surface-exposed proteins that deserve scrutiny.
- An important parameter elicited by the vaccine protocol, independent of the antigen, is to elicit a high-intensity primary response. As a corollary, that response needs to be sustained for a significant period in the absence of restimulation. A rapid decline in intensity after the last vaccination is unlikely to succeed.
- An immunization protocol should generate populations of memory B and/or T cells that can respond rapidly when a new challenge is encountered. This is particularly relevant to developing juveniles in the portal tract whose products need to trigger that memory in the months after priming. Will parasite numbers eventually build up above a threshold where the elicited antibody titre is high enough to cause starvation and death of the newly recruited worms?
- Systems biology analysis applied to self-cure in the rhesus macaque could highlight why some animals respond quickly to both primary infection and challenge that facilitates elimination of adult worms, whereas others struggle to control both exposures. Hopefully someone will compare the gene expression patterns associated with macaque self-cure with those being characterized in the CHI model.
- Identity of target(s), intensity of response, its persistence and the induction of memory are the watchwords. If only researchers knew how to combine these four aspects in an effective formulation, a schistosome vaccine might become a realistic prospect.

References

Alsallaq, R.A., Gurarie, D., Ndeffo Mbah, M., Galvani, A. and King, C. (2017) Quantitative assessment of the impact of partially protective anti-schistosomiasis vaccines. *PLoS Neglected Tropical Diseases* 11(4), e0005544. DOI: 10.1371/journal.pntd.0005544

Amaral, M.S., Santos, D.W., Pereira, A.S.A., Tahira, A.C., Malvezzi, J.V.M. *et al.* (2021) Rhesus macaques self-curing from a schistosome infection can display complete immunity to challenge. *Nature Communications* 12(1), 6181. DOI: 10.1038/s41467-021-26497-0

Andrade, G., Bertsch, D.J., Gazzinelli, A. and King, C.H. (2017) Decline in infection-related morbidities following drug-mediated reductions in the intensity of *Schistosoma* infection: a systematic review and meta-analysis. *PLoS Neglected Tropical Diseases* 11(2), e0005372. DOI: 10.1371/journal.pntd.0005372

Barbosa, M.M.F., Kanno, A.I., Barazzone, G.C., Rodriguez, D., Pancakova, V. *et al.* (2021) Robust immune response induced by *Schistosoma mansoni* TSP-2 antigen coupled to bacterial outer membrane vesicles. *International Journal of Nanomedicine* 16, 7153–7168. DOI: 10.2147/IJN.S315786

Bergquist, N.R. (1995) Controlling schistosomiasis by vaccination: a realistic option? *Parasitology Today* 11(5), 191–194. DOI: 10.1016/0169-4758(95)80157-X

Beyer, M., Nesterov, A., Block, I., König, K., Felgenhauer, T. *et al.* (2007) Combinatorial synthesis of peptide arrays onto a microchip. *Science* 318(5858), 1888. DOI: 10.1126/science.1149751

Bickle, Q.D. (2009) Radiation-attenuated schistosome vaccination – a brief historical perspective. *Parasitology* 136(12), 1621–1632. DOI: 10.1017/S0031182009005848

Boulanger, D., Warter, A., Sellin, B., Lindner, V., Pierce, R.J. *et al.* (1999) Vaccine potential of a recombinant glutathione *S*-transferase cloned from *Schistosoma haematobium* in primates experimentally infected with an homologous challenge. *Vaccine* 17(4), 319–326. DOI: 10.1016/s0264-410x(98)00202-3

Bradley, D.J. and McCullough, F.S. (1973) Egg output stability and the epidemiology of *Schistosoma haematobium*. II. An analysis of the epidemiology of endemic *S. haematobium*. *Transactions of the Royal Society of Tropical Medicine and Hygiene* 67(4), 491–500. DOI: 10.1016/0035-9203(73)90080-1

Brune, K.D. and Howarth, M. (2018) New routes and opportunities for modular construction of particulate vaccines: stick, click, and glue. *Frontiers in Immunology* 9, 1432. DOI: 10.3389/fimmu.2018.01432

Butterworth, A.E., Sturrock, R.F., Houba, V. and Rees, P.H. (1974) Antibody-dependent cell-mediated damage to schistosomula *in vitro*. *Nature* 252(5483), 503–505. DOI: 10.1038/252503a0

Butterworth, A.E., Dalton, P.R., Dunne, D.W., Mugambi, M., Ouma, J.H. *et al.* (1984) Immunity after treatment of human schistosomiasis mansoni. I. Study design, pretreatment observations and the results of treatment. *Transactions of the Royal Society of Tropical Medicine and Hygiene* 78(1), 108–123. DOI: 10.1016/0035-9203(84)90190-1

Butterworth, A.E., Capron, M., Cordingley, J.S., Dalton, P.R., Dunne, D.W. *et al.* (1985) Immunity after treatment of human schistosomiasis mansoni. II. Identification of resistant individuals, and analysis of their immune responses. *Transactions of the Royal Society of Tropical Medicine and Hygiene* 79(3), 393–408. DOI: 10.1016/0035-9203(85)90391-8

Capron, M. and Capron, A. (1994) Immunoglobulin E and effector cells in schistosomiasis. *Science* 264(5167), 1876–1877. DOI: 10.1126/science.8009216

Cardoso, F.C., Macedo, G.C., Gava, E., Kitten, G.T., Mati, V.L. *et al.* (2008) *Schistosoma mansoni* tegument protein Sm29 is able to induce a Th1-type of immune response and protection against parasite infection. *PLoS Neglected Tropical Diseases* 2(10), e308. DOI: 10.1371/journal.pntd.0000308

Carvalho, G.B.F. de, Pacífico, L.G.G., Pimenta, D.L.F., Siqueira, L.M.V., Teixeira-Carvalho, A. *et al.* (2014) Evaluation of the use of C-terminal part of the *Schistosoma mansoni* 200 kDa tegumental protein in schistosomiasis diagnosis and vaccine formulation. *Experimental Parasitology* 139, 24–32. DOI: 10.1016/j.exppara.2014.02.003

Cheever, A.W. and Powers, K.G. (1972) *Schistosoma mansoni* infection in rhesus monkeys: comparison of the course of heavy and light infections. *Bulletin of the World Health Organization* 46, 301–309.

Colley, D.G., Andros, T.S. and Campbell, C.H., Jr (2017) Schistosomiasis is more prevalent than previously thought: what does it mean for public health goals, policies, strategies, guidelines and intervention programs? *Infectious Diseases of Poverty* 6(1), 63. DOI: 10.1186/s40249-017-0275-5

Constant, S.L., Mountford, A.P. and Wilson, R.A. (1990) Phenotypic analysis of the cellular responses in regional lymphoid organs of mice vaccinated against *Schistosoma mansoni*. *Parasitology* 101(1), 15–22. DOI: 10.1017/s0031182000079695

Cornwell, R.L. (1960) The complement-fixing antibody response of calves to *Dictyocaulus viviparus*. II. Vaccination with irradiated larvae. *Journal of Comparative Pathology* 70, 494–498. DOI: 10.1016/s0368-1742(60)80047-1

Coulson, P.S. (1997) The radiation-attenuated vaccine against schistosomes in animal models: paradigm for a human vaccine? *Advances in Parasitology* 39, 271–336. DOI: 10.1016/s0065-308x(08)60048-2

Coulson, P.S. and Wilson, R.A. (1988) Examination of the mechanisms of pulmonary phase resistance to *Schistosoma mansoni* in vaccinated mice. *The American Journal of Tropical Medicine and Hygiene* 38(3), 529–539. DOI: 10.4269/ajtmh.1988.38.529

Coulson, P.S. and Wilson, R.A. (1993) Pulmonary T helper lymphocytes are $CD44^{hi}$, $CD45RB^{-}$ effector/memory cells in mice vaccinated with attenuated cercariae of *Schistosoma mansoni*. *Journal of Immunology* 151(7), 3663–3671. DOI: 10.4049/jimmunol.151.7.3663

Crabtree, J.E. and Wilson, R.A. (1986) The role of pulmonary cellular reactions in the resistance of vaccinated mice to *Schistosoma mansoni*. *Parasite Immunology* 8(3), 265–285. DOI: 10.1111/j.1365-3024.1986.tb01038.x

Crosnier, C., Brandt, C., Rinaldi, G., McCarthy, C., Barker, C. *et al.* (2019) Systematic screening of 96 *Schistosoma mansoni* cell-surface and secreted antigens does not identify any strongly protective vaccine candidates in a mouse model of infection. *Wellcome Open Research* 4, 159. DOI: 10.12688/wellcomeopenres.15487.1

Crosnier, C., Hokke, C.H., Protasio, A.V., Brandt, C., Rinaldi, G. *et al.* (2022) Screening of a library of recombinant *Schistosoma mansoni* proteins with sera from murine and human controlled infections identifies early serological markers. *The Journal of Infectious Diseases* 225(8), 1435–1446. DOI: 10.1093/infdis/jiaa329

Curwen, R.S., Ashton, P.D., Sundaralingam, S. and Wilson, R.A. (2006) Identification of novel proteases and immunomodulators in the secretions of schistosome cercariae that facilitate host entry. *Molecular & Cellular Proteomics* 5(5), 835–844. DOI: 10.1074/mcp.M500313-MCP200

Cutts, L. and Wilson, R.A. (1997) Elimination of a primary schistosome infection from rats coincides with elevated IgE titres and mast cell degranulation. *Parasite Immunology* 19(2), 91–102. DOI: 10.1046/j.1365-3024.1997.d01-184.x

Datoo, M.S., Natama, M.H., Somé, A., Traoré, O., Rouamba, T. *et al.* (2021) Efficacy of a low-dose candidate malaria vaccine, R21 in adjuvant Matrix-M, with seasonal administration to children in Burkina Faso: a randomised controlled trial. *Lancet* 397(10287), 1809–1818. DOI: 10.1016/S0140-6736(21)00943-0

Dean, D.A. and Mangold, B.L. (1992) Evidence that both normal and immune elimination of *Schistosoma mansoni* take place at the lung stage of migration prior to parasite death. *The American Journal of Tropical Medicine and Hygiene* 47(2), 238–248. DOI: 10.4269/ajtmh.1992.47.238

Diemert, D.J., Pinto, A.G., Freire, J., Jariwala, A., Santiago, H. *et al.* (2012) Generalized urticaria induced by the Na-ASP-2 hookworm vaccine: implications for the development of vaccines against helminths. *The Journal of Allergy and Clinical Immunology* 130(1), 169–76. DOI: 10.1016/j.jaci.2012.04.027

Diemert, D.J., Correa-Oliveira, R., Fraga, C.G., Talles, F., Silva, M.R. *et al.* (2023) A randomized, controlled phase 1b trial of the Sm-TSP-2 vaccine for intestinal schistosomiasis in healthy brazilian adults living in an endemic area. *PLoS Neglected Tropical Diseases* 17(3), e0011236. DOI: 10.1371/journal.pntd.0011236

Driguez, P., Doolan, D.L., Loukas, A., Felgner, P.L. and McManus, D.P. (2010) Schistosomiasis vaccine discovery using immunomics. *Parasites & Vectors* 3, 4. DOI: 10.1186/1756-3305-3-4

Dunne, D.W., Webster, M., Smith, P., Langley, J.G., Richardson, B.A. *et al.* (1997) The isolation of a 22 kDa band after SDS-PAGE of *Schistosoma mansoni* adult worms and its use to demonstrate that IgE responses against the antigen(s) it contains are associated with human resistance to reinfection. *Parasite Immunology* 19(2), 79–89. DOI: 10.1046/j.1365-3024.1997.d01-186.x

Eberl, M., Langermans, J.A., Vervenne, R.A., Nyame, A.K., Cummings, R.D. *et al.* (2001) Antibodies to glycans dominate the host response to schistosome larvae and eggs: is their role protective or subversive? *The Journal of Infectious Diseases* 183(8), 1238–1247. DOI: 10.1086/319691

El Ridi, R. and Tallima, H. (2013) Vaccine-induced protection against murine schistosomiasis mansoni with larval excretory-secretory antigens and papain or type-2 cytokines. *The Journal of Parasitology* 99(2), 194–202. DOI: 10.1645/GE-3186.1

El Ridi, R., Tallima, H., Selim, S., Donnelly, S., Cotton, S. *et al.* (2014) Cysteine peptidases as schistosomiasis vaccines with inbuilt adjuvanticity. *PLoS ONE* 9(1), e85401. DOI: 10.1371/journal.pone.0085401

Fallon, P.G., Gibbons, J., Vervenne, R.A., Richardson, E.J., Fulford, A.J.C. *et al.* (2003) Juvenile rhesus monkeys have lower type 2 cytokine responses than adults after primary infection with *Schistosoma mansoni*. *The Journal of Infectious Diseases* 187(6), 939–945. DOI: 10.1086/368130

Farias, L.P., Rodrigues, D., Cunna, V., Rofatto, H.K., Faquim-Mauro, E.L. *et al.* (2012) *Schistosoma mansoni* venom allergen like proteins present differential allergic responses in a murine model of airway inflammation. *PLoS Neglected Tropical Diseases* 6(2), e1510. DOI: 10.1371/journal.pntd.0001510

Farias, L.P., Vance, G.M., Coulson, P.S., Vitoriano-Souza, J., Neto, A.P. da S. *et al.* (2021a) Epitope mapping of exposed tegument and alimentary tract proteins identifies putative antigenic targets of the attenuated schistosome vaccine. *Frontiers in Immunology* 11, 624613. DOI: 10.3389/fimmu.2020.624613

Farias, L.P., Vitoriano-Souza, J., Cardozo, L.E., Gama, L.D.R., Singh, Y. *et al.* (2021b) Systems biology analysis of the radiation-attenuated schistosome vaccine reveals a role for growth factors in protection and hemostasis inhibition in parasite survival. *Frontiers in Immunology* 12, 624191. DOI: 10.3389/fimmu.2021.624191

Fitzsimmons, C.M., Jones, F.M., Stearn, A., Chalmers, I.W., Hoffmann, K.F. *et al.* (2012) The *Schistosoma mansoni* tegumental-allergen-like (TAL) protein family: influence of developmental expression on human IgE responses. *PLoS Neglected Tropical Diseases* 6(4), e1593. DOI: 10.1371/journal.pntd.0001593

Fukushige, M., Mitchell, K.M., Bourke, C.D., Woolhouse, M.E.J. and Mutapi, F. (2015) A meta-analysis of experimental studies of attenuated *Schistosoma mansoni* vaccines in the mouse model. *Frontiers in Immunology* 6, 85. DOI: 10.3389/fimmu.2015.00085

Fulford, A.J.C., Webster, M., Ouma, J.H., Kimani, G. and Dunne, D.W. (1998) Puberty and age-related changes in susceptibility to schistosome infection. *Parasitology Today* 14(1), 23–26. DOI: 10.1016/S0169-4758(97)01168-X

Gaze, S., Driguez, P., Pearson, M.S., Mendes, T., Doolan, D.L. *et al.* (2014) An immunomics approach to schistosome antigen discovery: antibody signatures of naturally resistant and chronically infected individuals from endemic areas. *PLoS Pathogens* 10(3), e1004033. DOI: 10.1371/journal.ppat.1004033

Hagan, T., Nakaya, H.I., Subramaniam, S. and Pulendran, B. (2015) Systems vaccinology: enabling rational vaccine design with systems biological approaches. *Vaccine* 33(40), 5294–5301. DOI: 10.1016/j.vaccine.2015.03.072

Harris, A.R., Russell, R.J. and Charters, A.D. (1984) A review of schistosomiasis in immigrants in Western Australia, demonstrating the unusual longevity of *Schistosoma mansoni*. *Transactions of the Royal Society of Tropical Medicine and Hygiene* 78(3), 385–388. DOI: 10.1016/0035-9203(84)90129-9

Hassan, A.S., Houle, S., Labrie, L., Perera, D.J., Dozois, C.M. *et al.* (2023) *Salmonella typhimurium* expressing chromosomally integrated *Schistosoma mansoni* cathepsin B protects against schistosomiasis in mice. *NPJ Vaccines* 8(1), 27. DOI: 10.1038/s41541-023-00599-w

Hewitson, J.P., Hamblin, P.A. and Mountford, A.P. (2005) Immunity induced by the radiation-attenuated schistosome vaccine. *Parasite Immunology* 27(7–8), 271–280. DOI: 10.1111/j.1365-3024.2005.00764.x

Hota-Mitchell, S., Siddiqui, A.A., Dekaban, G.A., Smith, J., Tognon, C. *et al.* (1997) Protection against *Schistosoma mansoni* infection with a recombinant baculovirus-expressed subunit of calpain. *Vaccine* 15(15), 1631–1640. DOI: 10.1016/s0264-410x(97)00081-9

Houlder, E.L., Da Silva, L.F., Van Diepen, A., Amaral, M.S., Wilson, R.A. *et al.* (2025) Pre-clinical studies of *Schistosoma mansoni* vaccines: a scoping review. *PLoS Neglected Tropical Diseases* 19(6), e0012956. DOI: 10.1371/journal.pntd.0012956

Hsü, H.F., Li Hsü, S.Y. and Osborne, J.W. (1962) Immunization against *Schistosoma japonicum* in rhesus monkeys produced by irradiated cercariæ. *Nature* 194(4823), 98–99. DOI: 10.1038/194098a0

Huang, H.H., Rigouin, C. and Williams, D.L. (2012) The redox biology of schistosome parasites and applications for drug development. *Current Pharmaceutical Design* 18, 3595–3611. DOI: 10.2174/138161212801327220

James, S.L. (1992) Experimental models of immunization against schistosomes: lessons for vaccine development. *Immunological Investigations* 21(5), 477–493. DOI: 10.3109/08820139209069385

Jang-Lee, J., Curwen, R.S., Ashton, P.D., Tissot, B., Mathieson, W. *et al.* (2007) Glycomics analysis of *Schistosoma mansoni* egg and cercarial secretions. *Molecular & Cellular Proteomics* 6(9), 1485–1499. DOI: 10.1074/mcp.M700004-MCP200

Jarrett, E.E. (1978) Stimuli for the production and control of IgE in rats. *Immunological Reviews* 41, 52–76. DOI: 10.1111/j.1600-065x.1978.tb01460.x

Kariuki, T.M., Farah, I.O., Wilson, R.A. and Coulson, P.S. (2008) Antibodies elicited by the secretions from schistosome cercariae and eggs are predominantly against glycan epitopes. *Parasite Immunology* 30(10), 554–562. DOI: 10.1111/j.1365-3024.2008.01054.x

Kariuki, M., Farah, I.O., Yole, D.S., Mwenda, J.M., van Dam, G.J. *et al.* (2004) Parameters of the attenuated schistosome vaccine evaluated in the olive baboon. *Infection and Immunity* 72(9), 5526–5529. DOI: 10.1128/IAI.72.9.5526-5529.2004

Keitel, W.A., Potter, G.E., Diemert, D., Bethony, J., El Sahly, H.M. *et al.* (2019) A phase 1 study of the safety, reactogenicity, and immunogenicity of a *Schistosoma mansoni* vaccine with or without glucopyranosyl lipid A aqueous formulation (GLA-AF) in healthy adults from a non-endemic area. *Vaccine* 37(43), 6500–6509. DOI: 10.1016/j.vaccine.2019.08.075

King, C.L., Medhat, A., Malhotra, I., Nafeh, M., Helmy, A. *et al.* (1996) Cytokine control of parasite-specific anergy in human urinary schistosomiasis. IL-10 modulates lymphocyte reactivity. *The Journal of Immunology* 156(12), 4715–4721. DOI: 10.4049/jimmunol.156.12.4715

Knopf, P.M., Cioli, D., Mangold, B.L. and Dean, D.A. (1986) Migration of *Schistosoma mansoni* in normal and passively immunized laboratory rats. *The American Journal of Tropical Medicine and Hygiene* 35(6), 1173–1184. DOI: 10.4269/ajtmh.1986.35.1173

Koopman, J.P.R., Houlder, E.L., Janse, J.J., Casacuberta-Partal, M., Lamers, O.A.C. *et al.* (2023) Safety and infectivity of female cercariae in schistosoma-naïve, healthy participants: a controlled human *Schistosoma mansoni* infection study. *EBioMedicine* 97, 104832. DOI: 10.1016/j.ebiom.2023.104832

Koopman, J.P.R., Houlder, E.L., Janse, J.J., Lamers, O.A., Roozen, G.V. *et al.* (2024) Clinical tolerance but no protective efficacy in a placebo-controlled trial of repeated controlled schistosome infection. *The Journal of Clinical Investigation* 135(4), e185422. DOI: 10.1172/JCI185422

Langenberg, M.C.C., Hoogerwerf, M.-A., Koopman, J.P.R., Janse, J.J., Kos-van Oosterhoud, J. *et al.* (2020) A controlled human *Schistosoma mansoni* infection model to advance novel drugs, vaccines and diagnostics. *Nature Medicine* 26(3), 326–332. DOI: 10.1038/s41591-020-0759-x

Lawrence, J.D. (1973) The ingestion of red blood cells by *Schistosoma mansoni*. *The Journal of Parasitology* 59(1), 60–63. DOI: 10.2307/3278572

Li, X.H., Stark, M., Vance, G.M., Cao, J.P. and Wilson, R.A. (2014) The anterior esophageal region of *Schistosoma japonicum* is a secretory organ. *Parasites & Vectors* 7, 565. DOI: 10.1186/s13071-014-0565-8

Li, X.-H., Xu, Y.-X., Vance, G., Wang, Y., Lv, L.-B. *et al.* (2015) Evidence that rhesus macaques self-cure from a *Schistosoma japonicum* infection by disrupting worm esophageal function: a new route to an effective vaccine? *PLoS Neglected Tropical Diseases* 9(7), e0003925. DOI: 10.1371/journal.pntd.0003925

Li, X.-H., Vance, G.M., Cartwright, J., Cao, J.-P., Wilson, R.A. *et al.* (2020) Mapping the epitopes of *Schistosoma japonicum* esophageal gland proteins for incorporation into vaccine constructs. *PLoS ONE* 15(2), e0229542. DOI: 10.1371/journal.pone.0229542

Ly, A.T., Diop, D., Diop, M., Schacht, A.M, *et al.* (2025) The Sm14+GLA-SE recombinant vaccine against *Schistosoma mansoni* and *S. haematobium* in adults and school children: phase II clinical trials in West Africa. *Vaccines* 13, 316. DOI: 10.3390/vaccines13030316

Maddison, S.E., Norman, L., Geiger, S.J. and Kagan, I.G. (1970) *Schistosoma mansoni* infection in the rat. I. Worm burden and serological response in infected, reexposed, and antigen-sensitized animals. *The Journal of Parasitology* 56(6), 1058. DOI: 10.2307/3277547

Marques-Neto, L.M., Trentini, M.M., Kanno, A.I., Rodriguez, D. and Leite, L.C.C. (2023) Recombinant BCG expressing the LTAK63 adjuvant increased memory T cells and induced long-lasting protection against *Mycobacterium tuberculosis* challenge in mice. *Frontiers in Immunology* 14, 1205449. DOI: 10.3389/fimmu.2023.1205449

McCullough, F.S. and Bradley, D.J. (1973) Egg output stability and the epidemiology of *Schistosoma haematobium*. I. Variation and stability in *Schistosoma haematobium* egg counts. *Transactions of the Royal Society of Tropical Medicine and Hygiene* 67(4), 475–490. DOI: 10.1016/0035-9203(73)90079-5

Miller, H.R.P., Newlands, G.F.J., McKellar, A., Inglis, L., Coulson, P.S. *et al.* (1994) Hepatic recruitment of mast cells occurs in rats but not mice infected with *Schistosoma mansoni*. *Parasite Immunology* 16(3), 145–155. DOI: 10.1111/j.1365-3024.1994.tb00334.x

Minard, P., Dean, D.A., Jacobson, R.H., Vannier, W.E. and Murrell, K.D. (1978) Immunization of mice with cobalt-60 irradiated *Schistosoma mansoni* cercariae. *The American Journal of Tropical Medicine and Hygiene* 27(1), 76–86. DOI: 10.4269/ajtmh.1978.27.76

Moloney, N.A. and Webbe, G. (1983) The host–parasite relationship of *Schistosoma japonicum* in CBA mice. *Parasitology* 87(2), 327–342. DOI: 10.1017/S0031182000052677

Nakaya, H.I., Wrammert, J., Lee, E.K., Racioppi, L., Marie-Kunze, S. *et al.* (2011) Systems biology of vaccination for seasonal influenza in humans. *Nature Immunology* 12(8), 786–795. DOI: 10.1038/ni.2067

Natukunda, A., Zirimenya, L., Nkurunungi, G., Nassuuna, J., Nkangi, R. *et al.* (2024) Pre-vaccination *Schistosoma mansoni* and hookworm infections are associated with altered vaccine immune responses: a longitudinal analysis among adolescents living in helminth-endemic islands of Lake Victoria, Uganda. *Frontiers in Immunology* 15, 1460183. DOI: 10.3389/fimmu.2024.1460183

Neves, L.X., Sanson, A.L., Wilson, R.A. and Castro-Borges, W. (2015) What's in SWAP? Abundance of the principal constituents in a soluble extract of *Schistosoma mansoni* revealed by shotgun proteomics. *Parasites & Vectors* 8(1), 337. DOI: 10.1186/s13071-015-0943-x

Oettle, R.C., Dickinson, H.A., Fitzsimmons, C.M., Sacko, M., Tukahebwa, E.M. *et al.* (2023) Protective human IgE responses are promoted by comparable life-cycle dependent tegument allergen-like expression in *Schistosoma haematobium* and *Schistosoma mansoni* infection. *PLoS Pathogens* 19(5), e1011037. DOI: 10.1371/journal.ppat.1011037

Orr, T.S. and Blair, A.M. (1969) Potentiated reagin response to egg albumin and conalbumin in *Nippostrongylus brasiliensis* infected rats. *Life Sciences* 8(20), 1073–1077. DOI: 10.1016/0024-3205(69)90459-7

Pearson, M.S., Becker, L., Driguez, P., Young, N.D., Gaze, S. *et al.* (2015) Of monkeys and men: immunomic profiling of sera from humans and non-human primates resistant to schistosomiasis reveals novel potential vaccine candidates. *Frontiers in Immunology* 6, 213. DOI: 10.3389/fimmu.2015.00213

Philippsen, G.S., Wilson, R.A. and DeMarco, R. (2015) Accelerated evolution of schistosome genes coding for proteins located at the host–parasite interface. *Genome Biology and Evolution* 7(2), 431–443. DOI: 10.1093/gbe/evu287

Pires da Silva, A., Vitoriano-Souza, J., Khouri, M.I., Favaro, R.D., Wilson, R.A. *et al.* (2024) Co-expression gene module analysis in response to attenuated cercaria vaccine reveals a critical role for NK cells in protection against *Schistosoma mansoni*. *Parasites & Vectors* 17(1), 476. DOI: 10.1186/s13071-024-06505-0

Querec, T.D., Akondy, R.S., Lee, E.K., Cao, W., Nakaya, H.I. *et al.* (2009) Systems biology approach predicts immunogenicity of the yellow fever vaccine in humans. *Nature Immunology* 10(1), 116–125. DOI: 10.1038/ni.1688

Riveau, G., Schacht, A.-M., Dompnier, J.-P., Deplanque, D., Seck, M. *et al.* (2018) Safety and efficacy of the rSh28GST urinary schistosomiasis vaccine: a phase 3 randomized, controlled trial in Senegalese children. *PLoS Neglected Tropical Diseases* 12(12), e0006968. DOI: 10.1371/journal.pntd.0006968

Rousseaux-Prevost, R., Bazin, H. and Capron, A. (1977) IgE in experimental schistosomiasis. I. Serum IgE levels after infection by *Schistosoma mansoni* in various strains of rats. *Immunology* 33(4), 501–505.

Santini-Oliveira, M., Coler, R.N., Parra, J., Veloso, V., Jayashankar, L. *et al.* (2016) Schistosomiasis vaccine candidate Sm14/GLA-SE: phase 1 safety and immunogenicity clinical trial in healthy, male adults. *Vaccine* 34(4), 586–594. DOI: 10.1016/j.vaccine.2015.10.027

Schramm, G., Suwandi, A., Galeev, A., Sharma, S., Braun, J. *et al.* (2018) Schistosome eggs impair protective Th1/Th17 immune responses against *Salmonella* infection. *Frontiers in Immunology* 9, 2614. DOI: 10.3389/fimmu.2018.02614

Shen, J., Lai, D.-H., Wilson, R.A., Chen, Y.-F., Wang, L.-F. *et al.* (2017) Nitric oxide blocks the development of the human parasite *Schistosoma japonicum*. *Proceedings of the National Academy of Sciences of the United States of America* 114(38), 10214–10219. DOI: 10.1073/pnas.1708578114

Shen, J., Yu, S.-F., Peng, M., Lai, D.-H., Hide, G. *et al.* (2022) iNOS is essential to maintain a protective Th1/Th2 response and the production of cytokines/chemokines against *Schistosoma japonicum* infection in rats. *PLoS Neglected Tropical Diseases* 16(5), e0010403. DOI: 10.1371/journal.pntd.0010403

Siddiqui, A.A. and Siddiqui, S.Z. (2017) Sm-p80-based schistosomiasis vaccine: preparation for human clinical trials. *Trends in Parasitology* 33(3), 194–201. DOI: 10.1016/j.pt.2016.10.010

Smith, M.A. and Clegg, J.A. (1984) *Schistosoma mansoni*: decay of resistance induced by gamma irradiated cercariae in the mouse. *Transactions of the Royal Society of Tropical Medicine and Hygiene* 78(2), 190–192. DOI: 10.1016/0035-9203(84)90275-X

Smithers, S.R. and Terry, R.J. (1965) Acquired resistance to experimental infections of *Schistosoma mansoni* in the albino rat. *Parasitology* 55(4), 711–717. DOI: 10.1017/S0031182000086261

Smithers, S.R. and Terry, R.J. (1969) Immunity in schistosomiasis. *Annals of the New York Academy of Sciences* 160(2), 826–840. DOI: 10.1111/j.1749-6632.1969.tb15904.x

Smythies, L.E., Betts, C., Coulson, P.S., Dowling, M.A. and Wilson, R.A. (1996) Kinetics and mechanism of effector focus formation in the lungs of mice vaccinated with irradiated cercariae of *Schistosoma mansoni*. *Parasite Immunology* 18(7), 359–369. DOI: 10.1046/j.1365-3024.1996.d01-115.x

Stanisic, D.I. and Good, M.F. (2023) Malaria vaccines: progress to date. *BioDrugs* 37(6), 737–756. DOI: 10.1007/s40259-023-00623-4

Stertman, L., Palm, A.E., Zarnegar, B., Carow, B, *et al.* (2023) The Matrix-M™ adjuvant: a critical component of vaccines for the 21st century. *Human Vaccines & Immunotherapeutics* 19, 2189885. DOI: 10.1080/21645515.2023.2189885

Sturrock, R.F., Butterworth, A.E. and Houba, V. (1976) *Schistosoma mansoni* in the baboon (*Papio anubis*): parasitological responses of Kenyan baboons to different exposures of a local parasite strain. *Parasitology* 73(3), 239–252. DOI: 10.1017/s003118200004693x

Sturrock, R.F., Cottrell, B.J., Lucas, S., Reid, G.D., Seitz, H.M. *et al.* (1988) Observations on the implications of pathology induced by experimental schistosomiasis in baboons in evaluating the development of resistance to challenge infection. *Parasitology* 96(1), 37–48. DOI: 10.1017/s0031182000081646

Tallima, H., Abou El Dahab, M., Kareem, S., Dalton, J.P. and El Ridi, R. (2017a) Protection against *Schistosoma haematobium* infection in hamsters by immunization with *Schistosoma mansoni* gut-derived cysteine peptidases, SmCB1 and SmCL3. *Vaccine* 35(50), 6977–6983. DOI: 10.1016/j.vaccine.2017.10.069

Tallima, H., Dvořák, J., Kareem, S., Abou El Dahab, M., Abdel Aziz, N. *et al.* (2017b) Protective immune responses against *Schistosoma mansoni* infection by immunization with functionally active gut-derived cysteine peptidases alone and in combination with glyceraldehyde 3-phosphate dehydrogenase. *PLoS Neglected Tropical Diseases* 11(3), e0005443. DOI: 10.1371/journal.pntd.0005443

Tendler, M., Vilar, M.M., Brito, C.A., Freire, N.M., Katz, N. *et al.* (1995) Vaccination against schistosomiasis and fascioliasis with the new recombinant antigen Sm14: potential basis of a multi-valent anti-helminth vaccine? *Memórias do Instituto Oswaldo Cruz* 90(2), 255–256. DOI: 10.1590/s0074-02761995000200022

Tran, M.H., Pearson, M.S., Bethony, J.M., Smyth, D.J., Jones, M.K. *et al.* (2006) Tetraspanins on the surface of *Schistosoma mansoni* are protective antigens against schistosomiasis. *Nature Medicine* 12(7), 835–840. DOI: 10.1038/nm1430

van Diepen, A., Van Der Velden, N.S.J., Smit, C.H., Meevissen, M.H.J. and Hokke, C.H. (2012a) Parasite glycans and antibody-mediated immune responses in *Schistosoma* infection. *Parasitology* 139(9), 1219–1230. DOI: 10.1017/S0031182012000273

van Diepen, A., Smit, C.H., Van Egmond, L., Kabatereine, N.B., Pinot de Moira, A. *et al.* (2012b) Differential anti-glycan antibody responses in *Schistosoma mansoni*-infected children and adults studied by shotgun glycan microarray. *PLoS Neglected Tropical Diseases* 6(11), e1922. DOI: 10.1371/journal.pntd.0001922

van Diepen, A., Van der Plas, A.-J., Kozak, R.P., Royle, L., Dunne, D.W. *et al.* (2015) Development of a *Schistosoma mansoni* shotgun *O*-glycan microarray and application to the discovery of new antigenic schistosome glycan motifs. *International Journal for Parasitology* 45(7), 465–475. DOI: 10.1016/j.ijpara.2015.02.008

Vance, G.M., Khouri, M.I., Neto, A.P. da S., James, S., Leite, L.C.C. *et al.* (2023) Antigenic epitope targets of rhesus macaques self-curing from *Schistosoma mansoni* infection. *Frontiers in Immunology* 14, 1269336. DOI: 10.3389/fimmu.2023.1269336

Villella, J.B., Gomberg, H.J. and Gould, S.E. (1961) Immunization to *Schistosoma mansoni* in mice inoculated with radiated cercariae. *Science* 134(3485), 1073–1075. DOI: 10.1126/science.134.3485.1073

West, J.B. (2013) Fragility of pulmonary capillaries. *Journal of Applied Physiology* 115(1), 1–15. DOI: 10.1152/japplphysiol.00229.2013

Wilkins, H.A., Goll, P.H., Marshall, T.F. and Moore, P.J. (1984) Dynamics of *Schistosoma haematobium* infection in a Gambian community. III. Acquisition and loss of infection. *Transactions of the Royal Society of Tropical Medicine and Hygiene* 78(2), 227–232. DOI: 10.1016/0035-9203(84)90283-9

Wilson, R.A. and Coulson, P.S. (1998) Why don't we have a schistosomiasis vaccine? *Parasitology Today* 14(3), 97–99. DOI: 10.1016/S0169-4758(97)01198-8

Wilson, R.A. and Coulson, P.S. (1999) Strategies for a schistosome vaccine: can we manipulate the immune response effectively? *Microbes and Infection* 1(7), 535–543. DOI: 10.1016/S1286-4579(99)80093-8

Wilson, R.A. and Coulson, P.S. (2006) The development of a schistosome vaccine. In: Maule, A.G. and Marks, N.J. (eds) *Parasitic Flatworms: Molecular Biology, Biochemistry, Immunology and Physiology*. CAB International, Wallingford, UK, pp. 303–326. DOI: 10.1079/9780851990279.0303

Wilson, R.A. and Coulson, P.S. (2009) Immune effector mechanisms against schistosomiasis: looking for a chink in the parasite's armour. *Trends in Parasitology* 25(9), 423–431. DOI: 10.1016/j.pt.2009.05.011

Wilson, R.A. and Jones, M.K. (2021) Fifty years of the schistosome tegument: discoveries, controversies, and outstanding questions. *International Journal for Parasitology* 51(13–14), 1213–1232. DOI: 10.1016/j.ijpara.2021.11.002

Wilson, R.A., Langermans, J.A.M., van Dam, G.J., Vervenne, R.A., Hall, S.L. *et al.* (2008) Elimination of *Schistosoma mansoni* adult worms by rhesus macaques: basis for a therapeutic vaccine? *PLoS Neglected Tropical Diseases* 2(9), e290. DOI: 10.1371/journal.pntd.0000290

Wilson, R.A., Li, X.H. and Castro-Borges, W. (2016) Do schistosome vaccine trials in mice have an intrinsic flaw that generates spurious protection data? *Parasites & Vectors* 9(1), 89. DOI: 10.1186/s13071-016-1369-9

Wilson, R.A., Li, X.H. and Castro-Borges, W. (2017) Schistosome vaccines: problems, pitfalls and prospects. *Emerging Topics in Life Sciences* 1(6), 641–650. DOI: 10.1042/ETLS20170094

Woellner-Santos, D., Tahira, A.C., Malvezzi, J.V.M., Mesel, V., Morales-Vicente, D.A. *et al.* (2024) *Schistosoma mansoni* vaccine candidates identified by unbiased phage display screening in self-cured rhesus macaques. *NPJ Vaccines* 9(1), 5. DOI: 10.1038/s41541-023-00803-x

Yamey, G., McDade, K.K., Anderson, R.M., Bartsch, S.M., Bottazzi, M.E. *et al.* (2024) Vaccine value profile for schistosomiasis. *Vaccine* in press, 126020. DOI: 10.1016/j.vaccine.2024.05.068

Yang, Y.Y.M., Li, X.H., Brzezicka, K., Reichardt, N.-C., Wilson, R.A. *et al.* (2017) Specific anti-glycan antibodies are sustained during and after parasite clearance in *Schistosoma japonicum*-infected rhesus macaques. *PLoS Neglected Tropical Diseases* 11(2), e0005339. DOI: 10.1371/journal.pntd.0005339

Yang, Y.Y.M., Wilson, R.A., Thomas, S.R.L., Kariuki, T.M, *et al.* (2019) Micro array-assisted analysis of anti-schistosome glycan antibodies elicited by protective vaccination with irradiated cercariae. *The Journal of Infectious Diseases* 219, 1671–1680. DOI: 10.1093/infdis/jiy714

Yole, D.S., Pemberton, R., Reid, G.D.F. and Wilson, R.A. (1996a) Protective immunity to *Schistosoma mansoni* induced in the olive baboon *Papio anubis* by the irradiated cercaria vaccine. *Parasitology* 112(1), 37–46. DOI: 10.1017/S0031182000065057

Yole, D.S., Reid, G.D.F. and Wilson, R.A. (1996b) Protection against *Schistosoma mansoni* and associated immune responses induced in the vervet monkey *Cercopithecus aethiops* by the irradiated cercaria vaccine. *The American Journal of Tropical Medicine and Hygiene* 54(3), 265–270. DOI: 10.4269/ajtmh.1996.54.265

Zhang, W., Molehin, A.J., Rojo, J.U., Sudduth, J., Ganapathy, P.K. *et al.* (2018) Sm-p80-based schistosomiasis vaccine: double-blind preclinical trial in baboons demonstrates comprehensive prophylactic and parasite transmission-blocking efficacy. *Annals of the New York Academy of Sciences* 1425(1), 38–51. DOI: 10.1111/nyas.13942

Zhang, W., Le, L., Ahmad, G., Molehin, A.J., Siddiqui, A.J. *et al.* (2020) Fifteen years of Sm-p80-based vaccine trials in nonhuman primates: antibodies from vaccinated baboons confer protection *in vivo* and *in vitro* from *Schistosoma mansoni* and identification of putative correlative markers of protection. *Frontiers in Immunology* 11, 1246. DOI: 10.3389/fimmu.2020.01246

10

Reproductive System

10.1 Overview

Most trematodes are hermaphrodites so the 85–100 known members of the family Schistosomatidae, with separate sexes (dioecy/gonochorism), are anomalous in this respect. They are a monophyletic group, exclusively parasitic in endothermic birds and mammals, largely inhabiting the portal venous system. Their closest relatives, the largely hermaphroditic Spirorchiidae of turtles, are vascular system generalists inhabiting the heart and arterial system. The evolution of separate sexes has been linked to the higher metabolic rate of endotherms, with their consequent higher uptake of nutrients conveyed to the liver via the hepatic portal system providing obvious benefits from colonizing this habitat. Additionally, a filiform body shape that permits insinuation into the tiniest venules of the intestinal wall minimizes the distance an egg must travel to reach the exterior (Loker and Brant, 2006). It must be assumed that colonization of the bladder wall by *Schistosoma haematobium* is a trade-off foregoing that nutritional advantage for an easier access of eggs to exterior in the liquid medium of urine.

In this chapter we are concerned only with the genus *Schistosoma*, where it is certainly true that females are significantly more slender than their male counterparts. Within the genus there is another consideration that impacts on the reproductive system. Analysis of mitochondrial gene order has revealed that the Asian species *Schistosoma japonicum*, *Schistosoma mekongi* and *Schistosoma malayensis* are basal, while other species are derived (Webster and Littlewood, 2012). This is reflected in the morphology of the female reproductive system, especially the number of eggs in the uterus and the daily egg output per female worm, which has implications for pathogenesis. How is the generation of separate sexes controlled at the genetic level? Pioneering work on chromosomal complement showed that the female was heterogametic (ZW) while the male had a ZZ constitution (Short, 1983). Genome sequencing and assembly at the chromosome level for *Schistosoma mansoni* and *S. japonicum* has provided insights into the genetic modifications associated with the move to separate sexes. The complexity of interactions between males and females that facilitate pairing, sexual maturation of females and oviposition is being elucidated, but some puzzles such as the manner of insemination remain.

10.2 Layout of the Male System

The male reproductive system has a relatively simple layout, situated in the anterior third of the body immediately after the bifurcation of the gut at the level of the ventral sucker, lying dorsal to the start of the gynaecophoric canal (Fig. 10.1.1)

DOI: 10.1079/9781800625167.0010

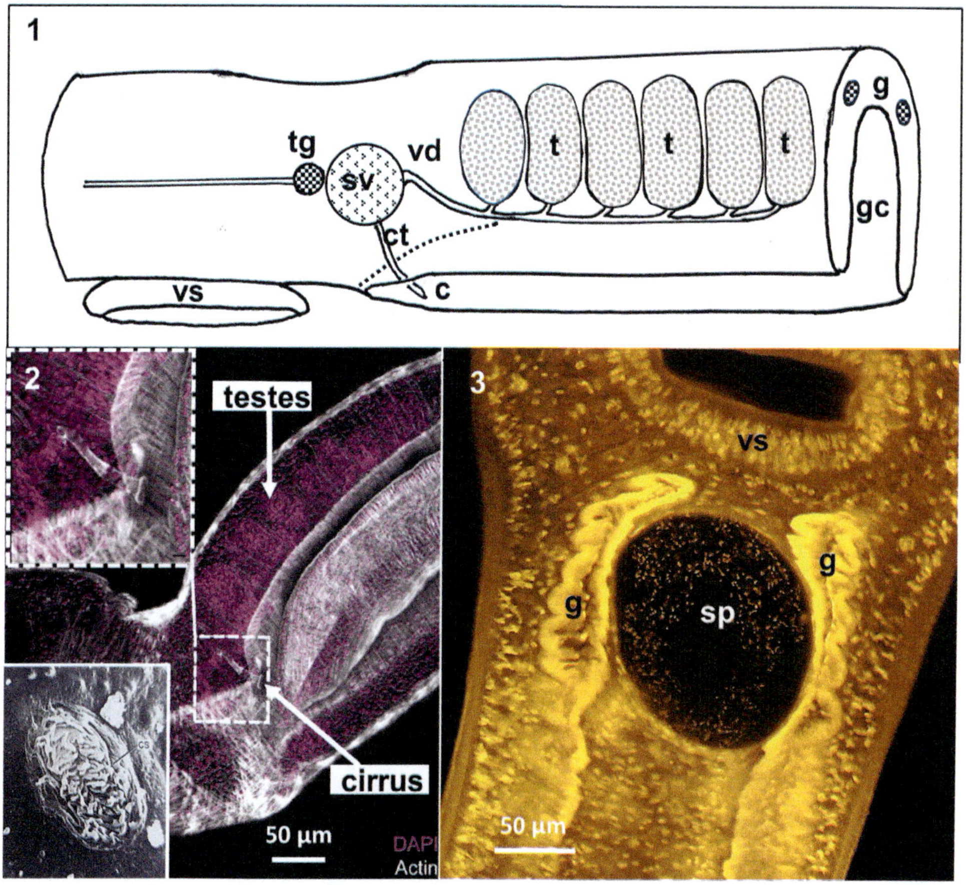

Fig. 10.1. The male reproductive system. **1**) Schematic lateral view of the layout. Approximately six testis lobes (t) lie centrally, posterior to the ventral sucker (vs) and transverse gut (tg) between two branches of the gut (g) (not shown). Spermatozoa travel along a common vas deferens (vd) and are stored in a seminal vesicle (sv) prior to exit down a cirrus tube (ct) to inseminate the female, held in the gynaecophoric canal (gc), via an eversible cirrus (c). **2**) Adult male with a unique image of an everted cirrus. The second inset is a SEM of the holdfast through which the cirrus is everted. **3**) Seminal vesicle with spermatozoa (sp) lying posterior to the ventral sucker (vs), between two branches of the gut (g). (**2** from Collins *et al.*, 2011; inset from Otubanjo, 1980.) **1** and **3**) Figures author's own. **2**) Figure used under license CC-BY-4.0; inset figure used with permission from Cambridge University Press.

(Otubanjo, 1980). In *S. mansoni* there are around six compact testes lobes lying in sequence (the precise number of lobes can vary with species), each with a short vas efferens joining a common ventral vas deferens. This leads forward to a seminal vesicle in which spermatozoa accumulate, and from which a cirrus tube emerges ventrally to terminate in an eversible cirrus for insemination of the female.

10.2.1 Testes, spermatogenesis and spermatozoa

Individual testis lobes (~40 µm × 80 µm) are surrounded by a fibrous capsule which aids in their isolation in a reasonably intact state by protease treatment of male bodies, each lobe still interconnected by the vas deferens (Hahnel *et al.*, 2013). Within the lobe there is a loose mass of cells in various stages of the cell cycle which culminates in spermatogenesis (Fig. 10.2.1). The process has been followed by *in vitro* pulse labelling of the three main human species with ^{3}H-thymidine followed by transplantation back into the portal vein of hamsters (Nollen *et al.*, 1976). In *S. japonicum* the label is incorporated into cells immediately beneath the capsule, but in *S. mansoni* and *S. haematobium* the spermatogonia are scattered throughout the tissues. This has made the mitoses and meiosis occurring during spermatogenesis impossible to follow because there are no groups of adherent cells; it is also unclear if support cells exist. By three days the label is diluted and scattered throughout each lobe, and by day 6 labelled sperm are present in the seminal vesicle. In mated females they appear in the seminal receptacle on the same day. Experiments with labelled males were proposed to follow the movement of spermatozoa in females after mating, but never published (Nollen, 1983).

The spermatozoa distributed throughout the testis lobe can be visualized by staining with antibody to acetylated tubulin which binds to microtubules (Fig. 10.2.2 and 10.2.3) (Collins *et al.*, 2011). In appearance they are ~12 μm long and relatively stubby with a large head and short tail. Viewed by transmission electron

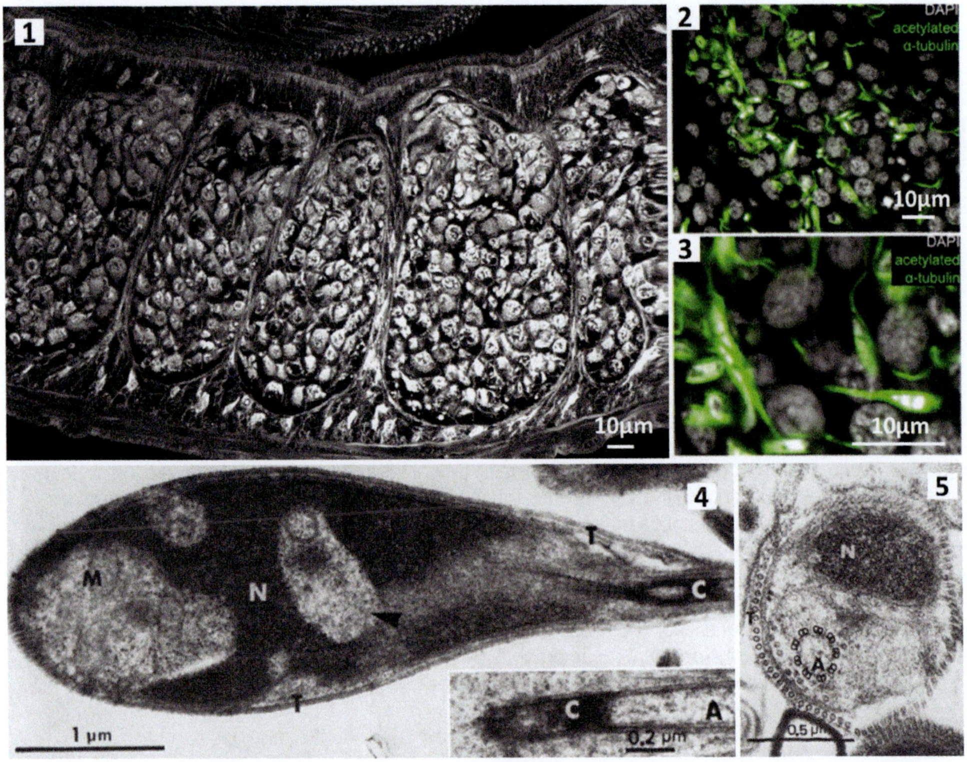

Fig. 10.2. Structure of testes and spermatozoa. **1**) Testis lobes occupy the full depth of tissue between dorsal and ventral body wall muscles. The internal structure is not organized, with dividing cells and spermatozoa fully intermingled. **2**) The spermatozoa are readily visualized by staining with anti-tubulin antibody (green) and other cells with DAPI (grey). **3**) Higher magnification reveals that the sperm tails are stumpy. **4**) Longitudinal TEM through the spermatozoan head. The anterior region where the acrosome would normally be is packed with small mitochondria (M). The nucleus (N) lies centrally, and microtubules (T) underlie the entire plasma membrane. The centriole (C) gives rise to the axoneme (A) which runs into the tail. **5**) Transverse section showing the tight ring of microtubules beneath the surface, and the axoneme (A) which lacks the central pair of microtubules. (**2** and **3** from Collins *et al.*, 2011; **4** and **5** from Kitajima *et al.*, 1976.) **1**) Figure author's own. **2** and **3**) Figures used under license CC-BY-4.0. **4** and **5**) Figures used with permission from Allen Press.

microscopy (TEM), a tight ring of longitudinal microtubules lies peripherally beneath the plasma membrane and continues around the axoneme into the tail (Fig. 10.2.4 and 10.2.5) (Kitajima *et al.*, 1976). At the anterior, instead of an acrosome normally involved in ovum penetration, there is a dense cluster of mitochondria. Coincidentally these organelles appear to be lacking in the tail, where they would normally provide the ATP for locomotion. The haploid nucleus lies in the centre of the head and the basal body is just posterior to it, with a nine doublet/zero central pair of microtubules, not the normal 9 + 2 arrangement, which continues down to the axoneme of the flagellum. To what extent this atypical spermatozoan morphology is related to dioecy, mating behaviour, insemination and fertilization remains to be elucidated. Whether the unusual mitochondria contribute to the complement in the zygote after fertilization or are destroyed by autophagy, the normal situation in animals (Al Rawi *et al.*, 2011), is also unknown.

10.2.2 Vas deferens, seminal vesicle and eversible cirrus

The vas deferens consists of a single layer of flattened epithelial cells lying of a fibrous basal lamella and forming a tube (~10 μm diameter) for conveying mature spermatozoa to the seminal vesicle (Otubanjo, 1980). Its luminal surface is lamellate, and the individual cells appear to produce granular secretory bodies. The spherical seminal vesicle (~30 μm diameter), containing dispersed spermatozoa, has a different ultrastructure. It is lined with a thin (0.25 μm) layer of modified tegument syncytium lacking inclusions, lying on an extracellular basal lamella and muscle layer, with nucleated cell bodies positioned externally. The cirrus tube connecting the seminal vesicle to the male pore is similarly lined with syncytial tegument, this time with multilaminate vesicles, and the same arrangement of circular muscles and cell bodies. By scanning electron microscopy (SEM), the evaginated cirrus was originally described as a disc-shaped and sponge-like structure (~15 μm diameter), raised above the tegument surface with the genital orifice lying at its centre (Otubanjo, 1980). However, confocal microscopy has revealed that a narrow eversible tube, the cirrus proper, can be projected from the centre of the disc (Collins *et al.*, 2011). Its function is presumably to deliver spermatozoa to an 'aperture' on the female body, and the basal disc is best considered as a holdfast to keep the female in position for insemination.

10.3 Layout of the Female System

As in the male, the gut bifurcates at the level of the ventral sucker and the bulk of the female system lies between the two branches, which unite post-ovary to pass as a single caecum to the posterior extreme. The ovary is situated about one-third of the way down the body while the vitellaria occupy the posterior two-thirds laterally alongside the caecum (Fig. 10.3.1) (Chen *et al.*, 2022). A simplified sketch of the female reproductive system, produced long before advanced microscopical techniques, captured the principal features of the layout (Fig. 10.3.2) (deWalick *et al.*, 2012). The common vitelline duct and the oviduct run forward to unite at the junction with the ootype, where egg formation occurs. Both ducts are described as being surrounded by a thin muscle layer, contractions of which could propel vitelline cells and zygotes towards the ootype (Erasmus, 1973). The enigmatic Mehlis gland also delivers its secretions to the entrance of the ootype. Formed eggs are then conveyed along the uterus to be expelled at the female pore, situated just posterior to the ventral sucker. It is notable that in unmated/virgin females the ovary and vitellaria are developmentally repressed whereas the uterus, oviduct and vitelline duct, the ootype and Mehlis' glands develop normally before mating (Erasmus, 1973). This clearly illustrates the need for a male 'factor', but only in ovary and vitellaria maturation.

10.3.1 Ovary

The ovary, like the testes, is surrounded by a fibrous capsule that allows it to be isolated reasonably intact from worm bodies by tissue digestion (Hahnel *et al.*, 2013). It is best described as an elongate tapered sausage (~200 μm long) with rounded ends, narrow at the anterior and widening to the posterior (Fig. 10.3.3). This reflects the marked increase in size of the individual oocytes from anterior to posterior as they proceed through oogenesis, but at the ultrastructural level relatively little is known about the process. However, distinct gradients of expression for the developmental genes *nanos1*, *meiob* and *bmpg* in the ovary have been demonstrated by WISH (Fig. 10.4.1) (Wendt *et al.*, 2020). Expression of the gene *bmpg* is notably lacking in virgin female worms, confirming its role in oocyte maturation. The oocytes themselves are unusual

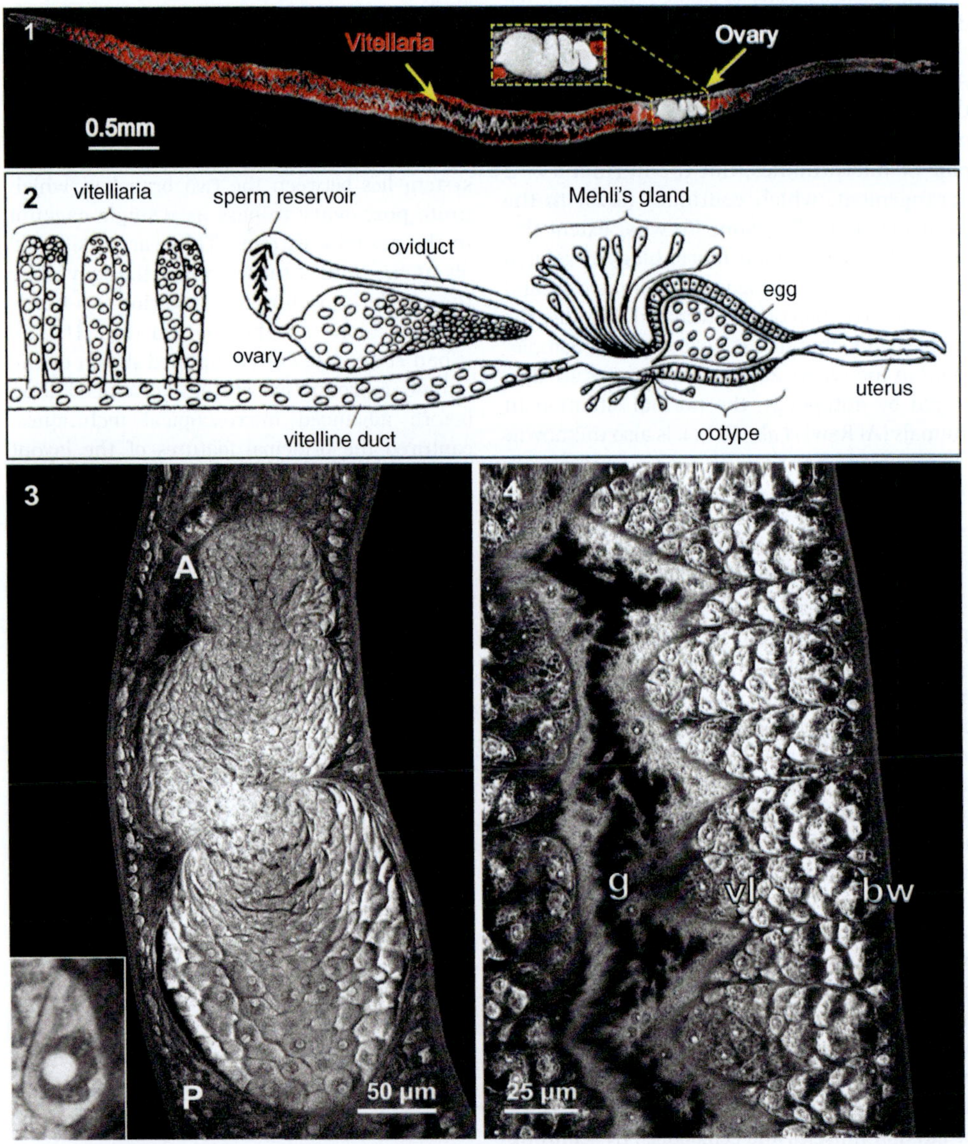

Fig. 10.3. Layout of the female reproductive system. **1**) A mature female with the ovary (white) and vitellaria (red), highlighting their respective contributions to a single egg. **2**) Sketch of the female system created from light microscope observations. **3**) Ovary showing the progression in gamete maturation from anterior (A) to posterior (P). Inset is a single mature oocyte with large nucleolus. **4**) A series of vitelline lobes (vl) filling the space between the gut (g) and body wall (bw). (**1** from Chen *et al.*, 2022; **2** from deWalick *et al.*, 2012.) **1** and **2**) Figures used with permission from Elsevier. **3** and **4**) Figures author's own.

because they lack the nutrient content required for miracidial development; this is provided by the vitellocytes in the ectolecithal egg. However, each oocyte possesses numerous cortical granules (~1 μm diameter) produced at Golgi bodies and positioned immediately beneath the plasma membrane (Fig. 10.4.2 and 10.4.3) (Erasmus, 1973). Their composition is unknown, but they are presumably released on penetration of the first spermatozoan into the oocyte to create a barrier preventing further entries. Perusal of the late female germ cell cluster (Wendt *et al.*, 2020) does not provide any obvious clues, apart from an abundant tyrosinase mRNA (Smp_013540) perhaps indicative of protein cross-linking.

10.3.2 Vitellaria and vitellogenesis

It has been assumed that both oocytes and vitellocytes arise from common mother cells in the developing liver worm (Kunz, 2001). These probably equate to germline stem cells (GSCs) identified by single-cell RNA sequencing (RNA-Seq) (Wendt *et al.*, 2020). The progeny of such stem cells undergo gametogeny in the female ovary (and in the testes in males), but also give rise to the vitelline tissues, primarily (but not exclusively) in the female. When these GSCs progeny are present in the female and will become either oocytes or vitellocytes, they clearly have a checkpoint in the cell cycle, which requires supply of the 'male factor' for its continuation. The vitelline lobules extend in closely packed formation either side of the gut all the way to the tail and each is an autonomous unit (Fig. 10.3.4). Early TEM observations revealed that they contain an admixture of cells representing a sequence of developmental stages (Fig. 10.5.1) (Erasmus and Popiel, 1980). Stage 1 cells are actively proliferating, with a large nucleus, mitochondria and ribosomes. Relatively scarce Stage 2 cells show the beginnings of protein synthetic activity with the appearance of endoplasmic reticulum. Stage 3 cells are actively synthesizing protein, with rough endoplasmic reticulum, Golgi bodies and the first aggregates of vitelline droplets. At mature Stage 4, vitelline droplets are abundant, larger than at Stage 3, with granules of more uniform size. Lipid droplets are also present, many associated with clusters of glycogen granules (Fig. 10.5.2). A method for isolating vitelline

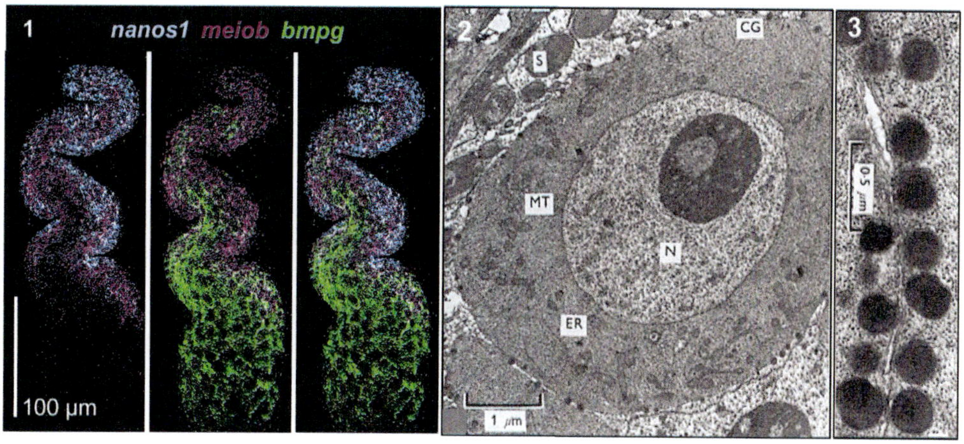

Fig. 10.4. Oogenesis. **1**) The differentiation of oocytes from oogonia as they progress down the ovary from anterior to posterior revealed by triple *in situ* hybridization. The three genes are markers for: *nanos1*, S-phase DNA synthesis (=stem cells), *meiob*, meiosis in stem cell progeny (=oocyte); *bmpg*, C-type lectin expressed in the late female germ cell cluster (=ovum). **2**) TEM of a mature ovum showing a nucleus with large nucleolus (N), endoplasmic reticulum (ER) and numerous mitochondria (M). Cortical granules (CG) are located beneath the plasma membrane. **3**) TEM showing the cortical granules beneath the surface of two adjacent ova. (**1** original image kindly provided by Professor J.J. Collins, UTSouthwestern Medical Center, Dallas, TX, USA, published by Wendt *et al.*, 2020; **2** and **3** from Erasmus, 1973.) **2** and **3**) Figures used with permission from Cambridge University Press.

cells by enzymatic digestion of female tissue was developed (Lu *et al.*, 2015). The viable cells could then be stained with vital dyes for lipids and DNA, with shell granules detected by autofluorescence (does this mean some cross-linking had occurred?) (Fig. 10.6.1). They could also be separated by flow cytometry into four populations corresponding to morphological Stages 1–4 (Fig. 10.6.2). Some characterization of gene expression was on these isolated cells was performed by RT-PCR to identify known components of the vitelline cells.

The mature vitelline cells exit each lobule via a short connection to the ventrally located vitelline duct and proceed towards the ootype. The duct itself comprises flattened epithelial cells with luminal lamellate extensions, lying on fibrous basal lamella, external to which are circular and longitudinal muscles fibres. Their contractile activity presumably provides the motive force to drive progression of the tightly packed vitelline cells (Erasmus, 1973). A novel serine/threonine (S/T)-rich protein, designated female-specific mucin (FsMucin), has been identified by cloning techniques (Menrath *et al.*, 1995) and its expression localized to the oviduct proximal to the ovary where it may serve a protective function. Note that it is also expressed in early and late vitellocyte clusters (Wendt *et al.*, 2020) so its function requires clarification.

A series of genetic markers that identify stages in vitelline cell maturation has also been identified in the clusters assembled from single-cell RNA-Seq and localized to vitelline tissues by WISH (Wendt *et al.*, 2020). For the record, these genes are *nanos1* for stem cells in S-phase, *msantd3* encoding a DNA-binding protein for S1 progeny, eggshell protein *p48* for late vitellocytes and *ataxin2* for mature vitellocytes. The mature vitelline cells have a bimodal function, containing

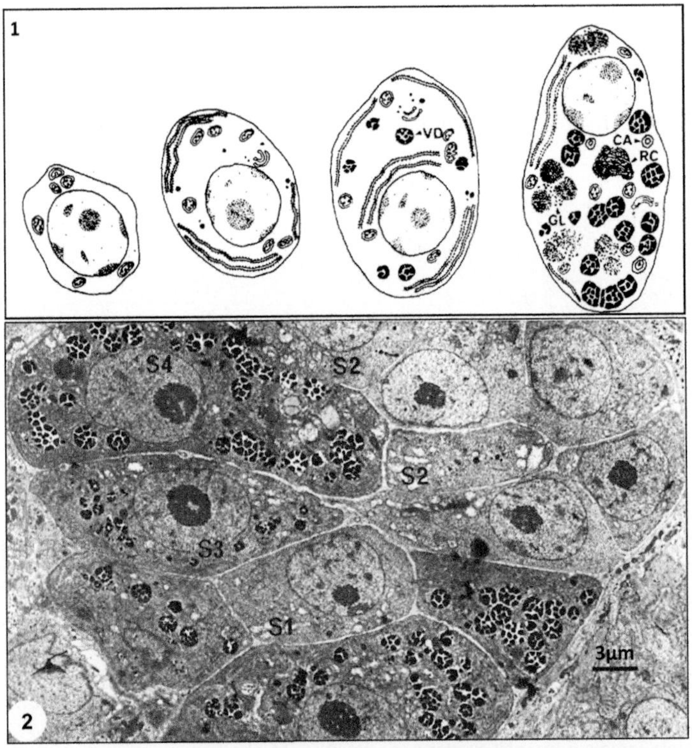

Fig. 10.5. Sequence of vitellocyte developmental stages. **1**) Morphological stages matched to gene expression stages of Wendt *et al.*, 2020. Stage 1 = S1 progeny, Stage 2 = early vitellocytes, Stage 3 = late vitellocytes, Stage 4 = mature vitellocytes. VD, vitelline droplets; CA, calcium granules; GL, glycogen; RC, ribosomal complex. **2**) TEM of the four stages of vitelline cell development: S1, S2, S3 and S4. (**1** and **2** from Erasmus and Popiel, 1980.) Figure used with permission from Elsevier.

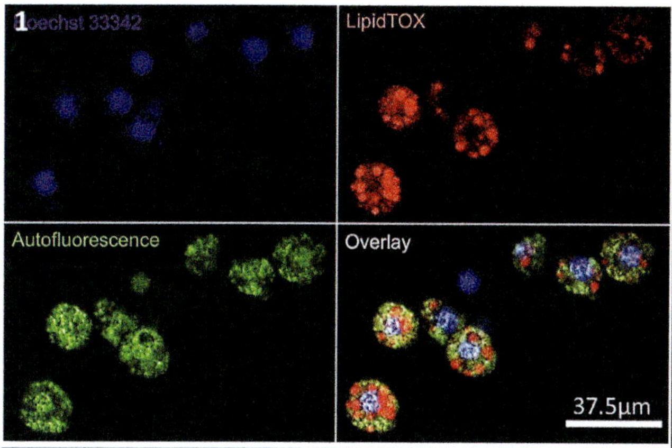

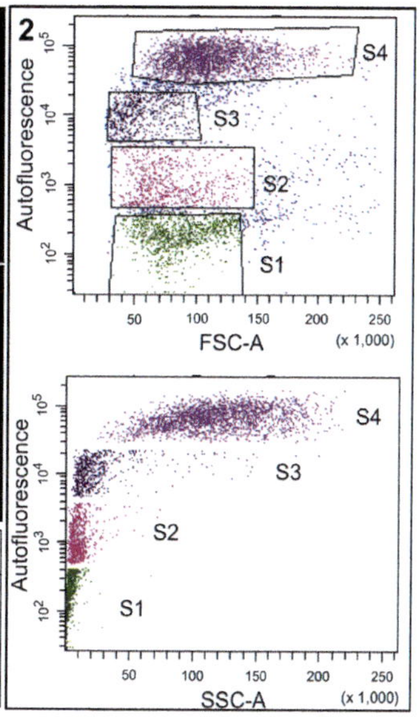

3 Smp	Identity	Smp	Identity
191910	Egg shell p19	000270 (2)	Egg shell p800
316140 (3)	Egg shell p14	050270 (2)	Tyrosinase
241610 (2)	Egg shell p48	302980	S/T rich protein

Fig. 10.6. Features of vitelline cells. **1**) Vitelline cells isolated by tissue digestion, stained for DNA (blue) and lipids (red), with shell granule autofluorescence (green). (Does this mean some cross-linking had occurred during cell isolation?). **2**) Vitelline cell populations separated by flow cytometry. **3**) A list of genes expressed in the vitelline cells found by RT-PCR of eggshell protein families and the enzyme tyrosinase. The numbers in parentheses are the copy number of those genes. The S/T-rich protein has mucin-like properties. (**1–3** from Lu *et al.*, 2015.) Figure used with permission from Elsevier.

the protein precursors required for eggshell formation in the ootype, but also those components (e.g. the lipids) that will partly nourish the developing miracidium during its development in the host tissues (see Chapter 11). The proteins that form the eggshell by a process of cross-linking (tanning) of tyrosine residues have been characterized but the role of others in shell formation is less clear. Partly this is because there are multiple gene copies, and their annotations have been updated in successive versions of the *S. mansoni* database. The key players are listed in Fig. 10.6.3.

There are three families of shell precursor proteins, p14, p19 and p48, designated on the basis of molecular weight. They are notable for the amounts of tyrosine residues (11%, 11.6% and 26%), respectively (Cogswell *et al.*, 2012), which are the initial substrate of the tyrosinase enzymes in the tanning process (see ootype in Section 10.3.3). The tyrosine residues are frequently flanked by a glycine residue, particularly on the carboxy side, which may favour their oxidation. A second group found in the eggshell, designated female-specific 800 (Fs800), contain a trematode eggshell synthesis (TES) domain, and have less tyrosine (6%); they are prominently expressed in the mature vitellocytes (Cogswell *et al.*, 2012; Wendt *et al.*, 2020) but their function is unknown. The tyrosinase enzymes are also localized to the vitelline granules with gene expression in late but not mature vitellocytes (Wendt *et al.*, 2020).

10.3.3 Mehlis gland, ootype and egg formation

The Mehlis gland is a discrete compact structure first identified in trematodes by a German doctor Karl Mehlis over 200 years ago, positioned where the oviduct and vitelline duct enter the ootype. The dense cluster of uninucleate cell bodies (Erasmus, 1973; Collins *et al.*, 2011) lies external to the muscle layers around the oviduct (Fig. 10.7.1). From these cells, individual funnel-like cytoplasmic extensions pass between the muscle fibres and through the lining epithelium to deliver their vesicular contents to the lumen (Fig. 10.7.2) (Moczon *et al.*, 1992). The cell bodies are typical

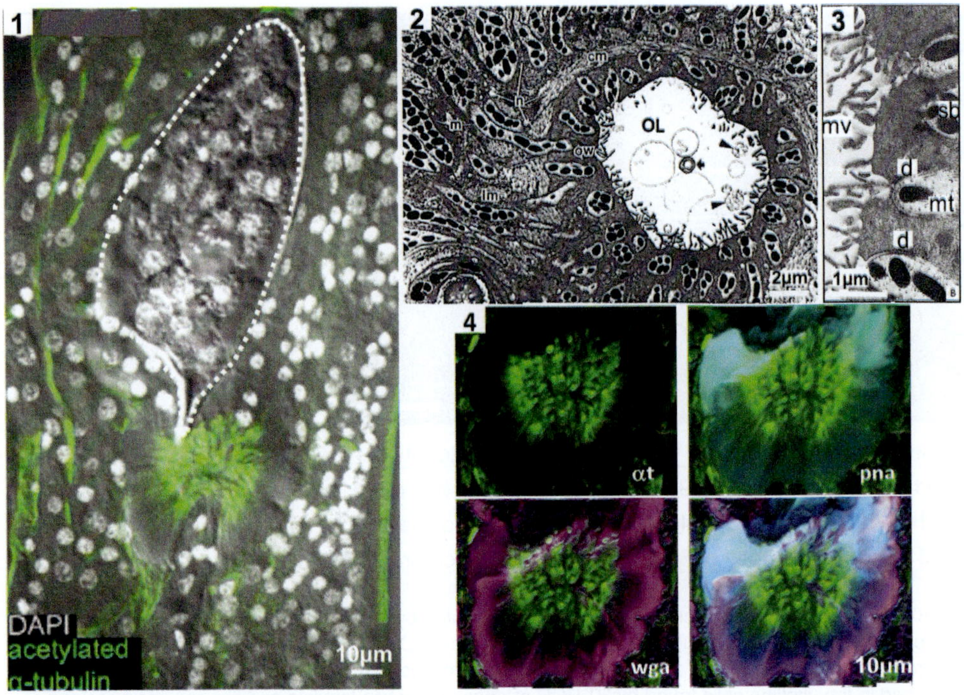

Fig. 10.7. Mehlis gland. **1**) Confocal image of a female worm stained with DAPI for nuclei and α-tubulin for microtubules. A forming egg delineates the ootype lumen with the gland lying immediately posterior (P). **2**) TEM of the proximal ootype lumen (OL) showing the position of ducts through the muscle layers (cm, lm) and epithelium. Arrows points to disintegrating vesicles. **3**) High magnification of the luminal surface showing the duct termini anchored by desmosomes (d), lined with microtubules (mt) and containing secretory bodies (sb). The luminal surface is covered with short microvilli (mv). **4**) Confocal images of the gland stained with anti-α-tubulin (αt), wheat germ agglutinin (wga), peanut agglutinin (pna) and an overlay of the three. (**1** and **4** from Collins *et al.*, 2011; **2** from Moczon *et al.*, 1992; **3** from Erasmus, 1973.) **1** and **4**) Figures used under licence CC-BY-4.0. Figures used with permission from **2**) Elsevier and **3**) Cambridge University Press.

of cells synthesizing proteins for export, with rough endoplasmic reticulum and Golgi bodies, the *trans* cisternae of which are positive for glycans. Dense ovoid membrane-bound vesicles (0.2 × 0.6 µm) are assembled close to the *trans* face, and process down the funnels towards the luminal surface. The region of the ducts carrying the vesicles through the muscle layers is lined with a cytoskeleton of microtubules which keeps the lumen patent (Fig. 10.7.3). TEM images suggest that intact vesicles are simply extruded into the gland lumen in a process not involving membrane fusion events. It is a reasonable supposition that these glycoprotein secretions play an integral role in egg formation, but we can only conjecture what that might be.

Confocal microscopy has been used to visualize regional differences between parts of the gland (Collins *et al.*, 2011). The cell bodies, but not the ducts, react with wheat germ agglutinin which targets *N*-acetylglucosamine residues (Fig. 10.7.4). There is also a weak reaction with peanut agglutinin which targets Gal-β(1–3)-GalNAc residues, strongest at the junction with the ootype (Fig. 10.7.4). The microtubules that line the gland cell ducts can also be stained with antibody to α-acetylated tubulin (Fig. 10.7.4). Single-cell RNA-Seq generated a cluster identified as the Mehlis gland (Wendt *et al.*, 2020) but inspection of the list of genes, ordered by *P* value, does not emphasize any obvious function for the potential secretions.

The ootype is a hollow chamber ~120 µm long that provides a physical template within which egg formation takes place. It is lined by a typical cuboidal epithelium, with the cells resting on an extracellular fibrous basal layer, and their luminal surfaces bearing short villi or lamellae (Fig. 10.8.1). In *S. mansoni* there is short lateral pocket at the posterior that moulds the egg spine (Fig. 10.7.1). The whole chamber is invested by outer longitudinal and inner circular muscle layers (Erasmus, 1973), which provide the motive force to propel a formed egg into the adjacent uterus. A sphincter is present at this junction to hold cells in the lumen until the egg has formed and then to allow its exit. There must be a similar tight control of oviduct and vitelline duct deliveries into the ootype lumen. For *S. mansoni* the complement is one zygote and around 30 vitelline cells and the process of shell formation takes ~5 min, equating to an output of ~300 eggs per female per day. The eggs of *S. japonicum* are smaller with fewer vitelline cells and they are produced at the rate of around 1 per minute, an output greater than 1500 per day.

The process of shell formation results from release/shedding of the vitelline granules containing the shell precursor proteins (see 10.3.2) and the tyrosinases into the ootype lumen (Fig. 10.8.2), but the cross-linking process only occurs at the luminal surface, implying a mechanism to prevent premature tanning. Chemically, the action of tyrosinase requires oxygen in a two-step mechanism on the tyrosine residues of shell proteins to convert them first to L-DOPA (l-3,4-dihydroxyphenylalanine) and then to *o*-quinone. The *o*-quinones are highly reactive compounds, which by interacting with lysine residues, cross-link neighbouring proteins to form a highly resistant matrix. This chemical reaction explains the autofluorescence of the eggshell, but it retains a degree of elasticity/flexibility, not seen in *Fasciola* eggs shells, that allows an increase in size during miracidial development (see Chapter 11). As noted above, the contribution of Mehlis gland secretions to egg formation must be vital but presently remains a mystery. Microdissection of the Mehlis gland and ootype for proteomics would be one route to explore this question (Neves *et al.*, 2023).

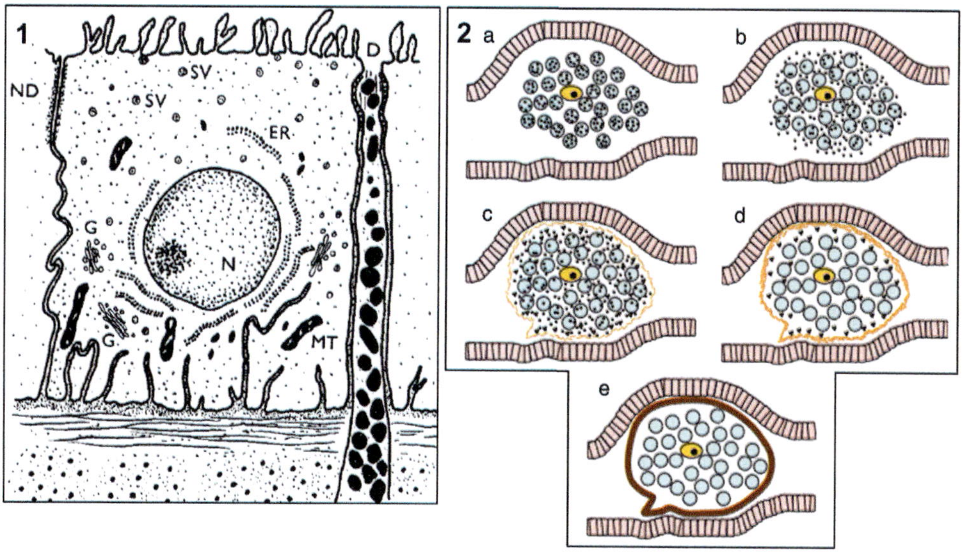

Fig. 10.8. The ootype and egg formation. **1**) Diagram of a cuboidal epithelial cell from the proximal lining of the ootype with an adjacent Mehlis gland duct (D). The cells are firmly attached to each other at the luminal border by a desmosome (ND) while the cytoplasm contains a central nucleus (N), mitochondria (MT), endoplasmic reticulum (ER) and Golgi bodies (G). A few small vesicles (SV) are present but there is little evidence for significant protein export. **2**) A diagram of the stages in eggshell formation when a single zygote (chrome) and 30 vitelline cells (blue) aggregate in the ootype lumen. Vitelline granules (dots) are released and move to the periphery, where the eggshell proteins are cross-linked by the action of tyrosinases (triangles). (**1** From Erasmus, 1973; **2** from deWalick *et al.*, 2012.) Figures used with permission from **1**) Cambridge University Press and **2**) Elsevier.

10.4 The Unsolved Question of Insemination

The way in which hermaphroditic trematodes inseminate each other or themselves is an open question. Many families of flukes possess a clearly demarcated pore on the dorsal surface that opens into a short duct, called Laurer's canal after the German anatomist Johann Friedrich Laurer who first described it in 1830. This canal delivers spermatozoa directly into the seminal receptacle, a specialized part of the proximal oviduct. In the liver fluke (*Fasciola hepatica*) this makes sense because the uterus is filled with thousands of eggs, which would present an enormous obstacle to spermatozoa delivered via the female pore on the ventral surface immediately behind the ventral sucker. The situation in the genus *Schistosoma* is unclear because no Laurer's canal has ever been described and the consensus has emerged that insemination must occur via the female pore. That might seem feasible in *S. mansoni* where there is only a single egg in the uterus at any one time but less so for species like *S. japonicum* with many eggs in the uterus. In all schistosomes the spermatozoa would still have to transit through the ootype, where egg formation is occurring. This seems rather implausible, given that the spermatozoa would be swimming against the flow of materials, but especially would become entangled with the released vitelline granules which coalesce and form the shell, using the ootype as a mould (see Section 10.3.3). They would also need to distinguish between the apertures of the oviduct and vitelline duct where they meet at the entrance to the ootype and pick the right one.

10.4.1 The seminal receptacle

The oviduct emerging from the posterior of the ovary is a tube comprising specialized epithelial cells resting on a fibrous basal lamella (Erasmus, 1973). Its luminal surface is extended into fine lamellae running longitudinally. The presence of vesicles near the luminal surface is suggestive of endo- or exo-cytotic activity (Fig. 10.9.3). Morphologically, the oviduct is divided into three distinct regions, distally towards the ootype bearing lamellae and cilia, centrally just lamellae, and proximally it is highly modified to form a seminal receptacle (Fig. 10.9.1). The spermatozoa are firmly attached head-first to the lining around the periphery of the duct of the receptacle (Fig. 10.9.2), between projecting lamellae, presumably via a specific docking mechanism (Fig. 10.9.4). A mature ovum entering the oviduct must pass the waiting spermatozoa, fertilization occurs and its cortical granules are instantly released to harden the surface and prevent further entry. The zygote then travels through the central and distal regions aided by beating of cilia, to reach the point of entry into the ootype at the junction with the vitelline duct. How the spermatozoa arrive in the seminal receptacle remains an open question.

10.4.2 Laurer's canal in bird schistosomes

The blood flukes of turtles, members of the Spirochiidae, the taxonomic sister group of the Schistosomatidae, do possess a Laurer's canal and the structure has been described in one schistosome of birds, *Trichobilharzia regenti* (Skírnisson *et al.*, 2012). As the name suggests, this schistosome is threadlike, with the anatomy of the female very extended, up to 1.9 cm long. The short Laurer's canal runs between the oviduct and the body surface and application of pressure results in spermatozoa being expelled to the exterior confirming it is a patent duct. Paradoxically, the authors consider it an ancestral feature that functions as an overspill channel, not used for insemination, because it has not been described in the more evolved schistosomes.

10.4.3 A hypothesis for insemination

A feature of self-cure in rhesus macaques is that females slowly starving to death cease to produce eggs, while the males are still active and capable of mating. As a result, some white emaciated *S. japonicum* females recovered by perfusion at week 21 had spermatozoa filling the seminal receptacle and overflowing into the oviduct in large numbers, but not as far as the ootype (Videos 10.1 and 10.2) (Li *et al.*, 2015). These spermatozoa were non-adherent, presumably because their docking sites are present only in the seminal receptacle, the proximal region adjacent to the ovary. Add to this the fact that

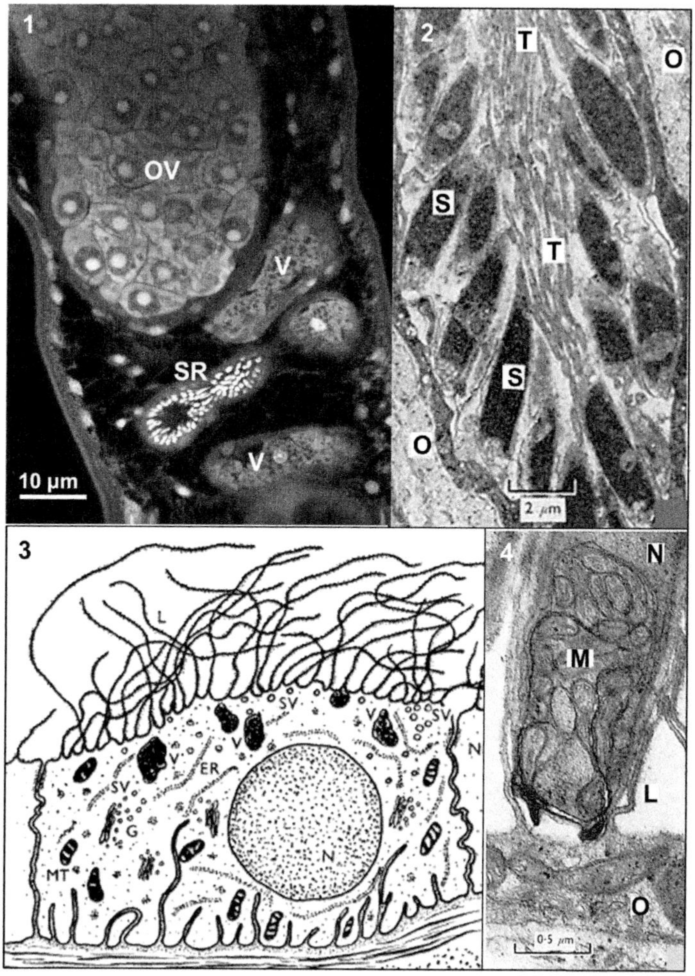

Fig. 10.9. Seminal receptacle. **1**) Confocal image showing lumen of receptacle (SR) lined with docked spermatozoa posterior to ovary (OV). V, vitelline duct. **2**) TEM of receptacle with spermatozoa (S) attached to the oviduct wall (O) and tails (T) projecting into the lumen. **3**) Diagram of an oviduct wall cell with surface lamellae (L), nucleus (N) and vesicles (V, SV) proximal to the lumen. **4**) High magnification TEM of spermatozoan head docked between lamellae (L) of the oviduct wall (O). Mitochondria (M) are prominent anterior to the nucleus (N). (**2–4** from Erasmus, 1973.) **1**) Figure author's own. **2–4**) Figures used with permission from Cambridge University Press.

the stumpy spermatozoa of *S. mansoni* have been described as 'only a little motile', so do not appear to be designed for swimming (Justine and Mattei, 1981). The conclusion must be that they are delivered very close to the seminal receptacle via a Laurer's canal. It simply has not been found but would be located on the female dorsal surface (Fig. 10.10). The situation in bird schistosomes would thus be the norm in all schistosomes, not just a residual feature.

10.5 Gender Interplay and the Male Factor

There has been a long history of speculation and experimentation in attempts to solve the question of how males regulated female maturation. Progress was only made when worm transfer techniques and adequate *in vitro* culture methods were developed (Popiel and Basch, 1984). These allowed immature females from unisexual

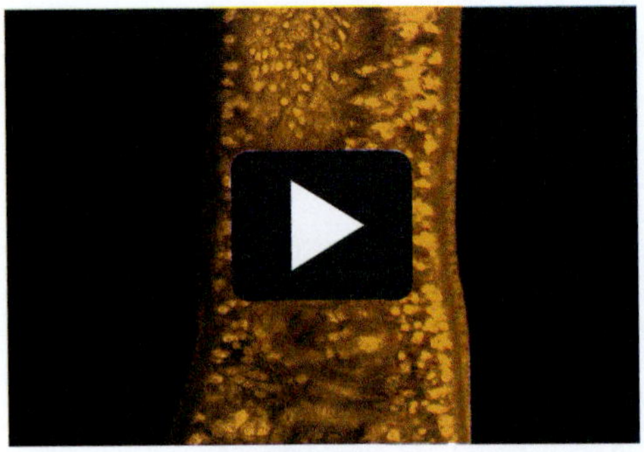

Video 10.1. An animated Z-stack of a super-impregnated *S. japonicum* female worm lying on its side. The stack progresses from one branch of the bifurcated gut to the other, passing through the ovary, oviduct and vitelline duct. The spermatozoa fill the lumen of the oviduct far beyond the seminal receptacle. The ovary at the top with large cells is clearly defective, with a vacuole where mature ova should be leaving to be fertilized. The distal oviduct (top left) is devoid of spermatozoa. Video courtesy of Mr Grant Calder, Imaging and Cytometry Laboratory, Department of Biology, University of York, York, UK.

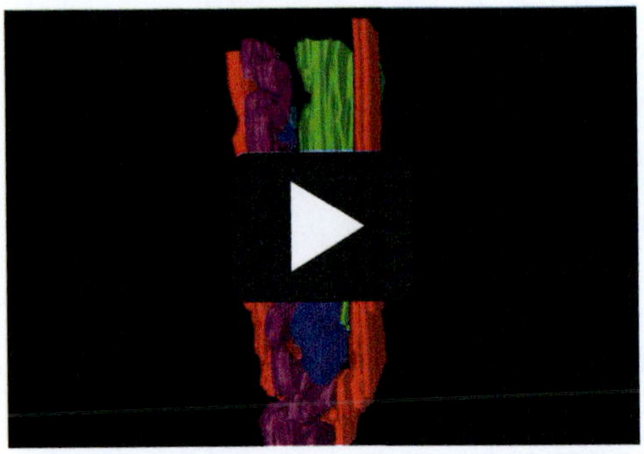

Video 10.2. A mapping of the female reproduction organs and gut from consecutive Z-stacks of a super-inseminated *S. japonicum* female worm which had ceased to produce eggs but was still held in the gynaecophoric canal of a male. Colour code: crimson red, intestinal branches; emerald green, ovary; purple, common vitelline duct; bright blue, proximal oviduct filled with excess spermatozoa; turquoise blue, distal oviduct, sperm free.

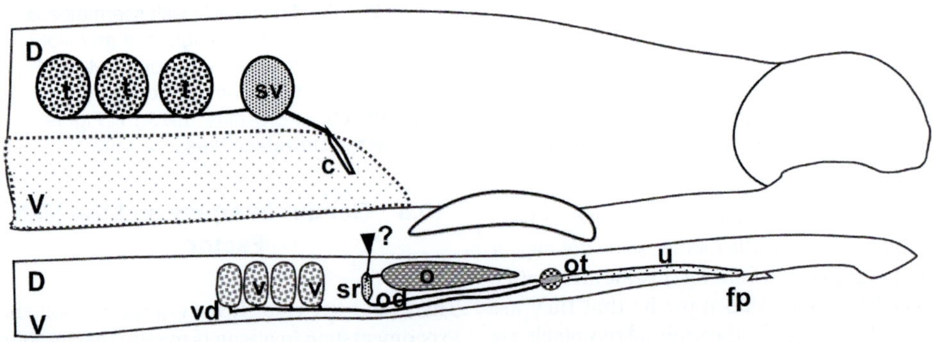

Fig. 10.10. A hypothesis for schistosome insemination. The layout of the male system with testes (t), seminal vesical (sv) and cirrus (c) is not in question. The female system comprises ovary (o), seminal receptacle (sr), vitellaria (v), oviduct (od) and vitelline duct (vd) delivering their respective cargoes to the ootype (ot) where egg formation occurs. Eggs pass down the uterus (ut) to be deposited in host tissues via the female pore (fp). Do schistosomes possess a Laurer's canal (arrow) running from a pore on the dorsal surface to the seminal receptacle? Figure author's own.

infections and mature males to be transected into body segments and kept alive by transfer back to the mesenteric veins of hamsters or cultured *in vitro* for long periods. In both situations pairing took place between intact worms of each sex and segments of the other, and between segments of both sexes. A specific staining assay (Fig. 10.11.1) was developed to assess vitelline cell development, revealing that the majority of female worms and their segments that paired showed some reproductive development. More recently the culture methods have been further improved with the formulation of ABC169 (ascorbic acid, blood cells, cholesterol and M169 medium) (Wang *et al.*, 2019). In this medium, intact unisexual females paired with small male segments show vitelline gland development limited to that portion of the worm held by the male (Fig. 10.11.1 and 10.11.2). The study also identified a factor termed vitellogenic factor 1 (VF1; Smp_248100), a nuclear receptor that is activated by pairing. Such receptors possess conserved N-terminal DNA-binding and C-terminal ligand-binding domains. The former was present in VF1 but a ligand has yet to be identified. The Smp_248100 gene is expressed within vitelline stem cells and plays a key role in vitelline stem cell differentiation, which remains to be elucidated.

Both early and recent culture experiments have concluded that worm pairing, male stimulation and the female developmental response are independent of central nervous control by the cerebral ganglia; males do not have a centralized source for the female-stimulating factor. Furthermore, vitelline gland differentiation in the female requires local stimulation through male contact, which is not propagated throughout the worm. Female development is thus dependent on stimulation from the somatic tissue of mature males rather than the reproductive system. However, the effect of pairing is not instantaneous. It takes 3–4 days after pairing *in vivo*, and 6 days *in vitro*, for mature vitelline cells to appear (Popiel and Basch, 1984). It was also apparent that uncoupling of worms and fragments very rapidly resulted in regression of female reproductive structures (see Section 10.5.2). The stimulus required for maturation must therefore be continuously applied.

10.5.1 Gonad-specific and pairing-dependant transcriptomes

There was an interval of 30 years before the observations on male stimulation of female

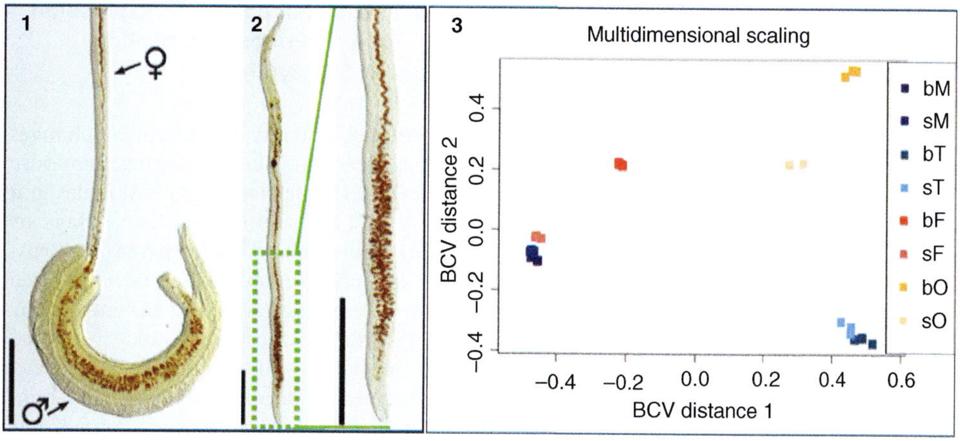

Fig. 10.11. Male–female interactions. **1**) A unisexual female cultured *in vitro* with a male segment before separation, showing vitellaria development is restricted to paired region. **2**) Female after separation from a male segment showing vitellaria development in the posterior region. Enlargement shows vitelline cells are packing the lumen of the vitelline duct anterior to the formed vitellaria. Scale bars: 500 μm.
3) Multidimensional scaling of transcriptomes from isolated ovaries and testes compared with intact males and females. b, bisex (paired); s, single sex (unpaired); M, male; F, female; T, testes; O, ovary. All replicates cluster tightly together. The isolated O and T are widely separated from each other and from the bF and bM worms. The sO is distinct from the bO. Strikingly, the sF clusters with sM and bM. BCV: biological coefficient of variation. (**1** and **2** from Wang *et al.*, 2019; **3** from Lu *et al.*, 2016.) Figures used under license CC-BY-4.0.

maturation gained any real traction at the molecular level. Then an RNA-Seq comparison of isolated ovaries and testes from paired and unpaired schistosomes provided some profound insights into the impact of pairing on maturation (Lu *et al.*, 2016). Bioinformatic analyses revealed a high congruence between replicates (Fig. 10.11.3). Isolated testes from single or mated males occurred in one cluster, as did entire single and mated male worms. This indicated only a small impact of mating on both testes and male bodies. In contrast, ovaries from single and mated females split in two separate clusters, as did entire single and mated female worms. Pairing, therefore, had a more pronounced effect on ovaries and female bodies than on testes and male bodies. Viewed at the level of gene expression, the number of genes affected by pairing was 15-fold greater in the ovaries than the testes. In the intact female bodies schistosome eggshell precursor genes p14 and p48, plus the two tyrosinases were among those most affected by pairing, reflecting maturation of the vitellaria. There was also high number of differentially expressed genes putatively involved in neural processes, including multiple neuropeptides. This is a little surprising considering the conclusions from male–female interactions that maturation is a local, not a central phenomenon (Popiel and Basch, 1984).

Compared with mated females, the transcriptome of single-sex females was remarkably similar to that of males (Fig. 10.11.3). This observation has prompted speculation on the evolution of separate sexes in schistosomes. Protandry, the development of the male gonad before that of the female, is a common form of sequential hermaphroditism that occurs in spirorchid trematodes of turtles, the most closely related sister group to schistosomes (Platt and Brooks, 1997). Alternatively, the evolution of dioecy in schistosomes may have proceeded via androdioecy, where hermaphrodites initially deposit eggs in the vascular system and then develop into larger functional males (Lu *et al.*, 2016). This implies that the origin of dioecy in schistosomes resulted from the evolution of genes suppressing female function in males and, according to physiological and molecular data, also in single females, while male functions are suppressed in mated females.

10.5.2 Identification of the *gli1* gene as a key regulator

A key developmental pathway essential for male-induced female reproductive development was finally identified using a suite of techniques based on culture of worms in ABC169 (Chen *et al.*, 2022). The first step was a comprehensive RNA interference (RNAi) screen focused on 50 components of major metazoan signalling pathways (Fig. 10.12.1). Virgin females were targeted at day 0 and then added to cultures of male worms, with RNAi continued up to day 10. The knockdown of a single gene, the transcriptional activator *gli1*, almost completely suppressed egg production. RNAi of *gli1* had no effect in female worms, but female worms mated with *gli1* RNAi male worms displayed little vitellaria development, scant ovary differentiation and were incapable of egg production post-pairing. The directionality of signalling was confirmed by *in situ* hybridization that revealed *gli1* expression in cells of the male ventral surface (Fig. 10.12.2). Note that this cannot be the whole story because the *gli1* gene is expressed widely in females and expression increases with maturation.

10.5.3 Effect of pairing on expression of a non-ribosomal peptide synthetase

In a scheme to identify *gli1*-dependent changes in gene expression following pairing, immature females were associated with RNAi males in a variety of conditions and after 3 days of cocultivation, they were prepared for RNA-Seq. The most notable difference observed was in the expression of a gene encoded by Smp_158480, induced >20-fold in paired versus unpaired control males. This gene, now annotated as (β-alanyl-bioamine) non-ribosomal peptide synthetase (Sm*nrps*), has orthologues in many invertebrate phyla. It is expressed primarily in cells along the ventral groove of males (Fig. 10.12.3) alongside 7b2, a marker for nerve cells. Its expression increases in the days after pairing and expression rapidly decreases after males are separated from females (Fig. 10.12.4). Note that a time lag of 3–4 days between mating *in vivo* and the appearance of

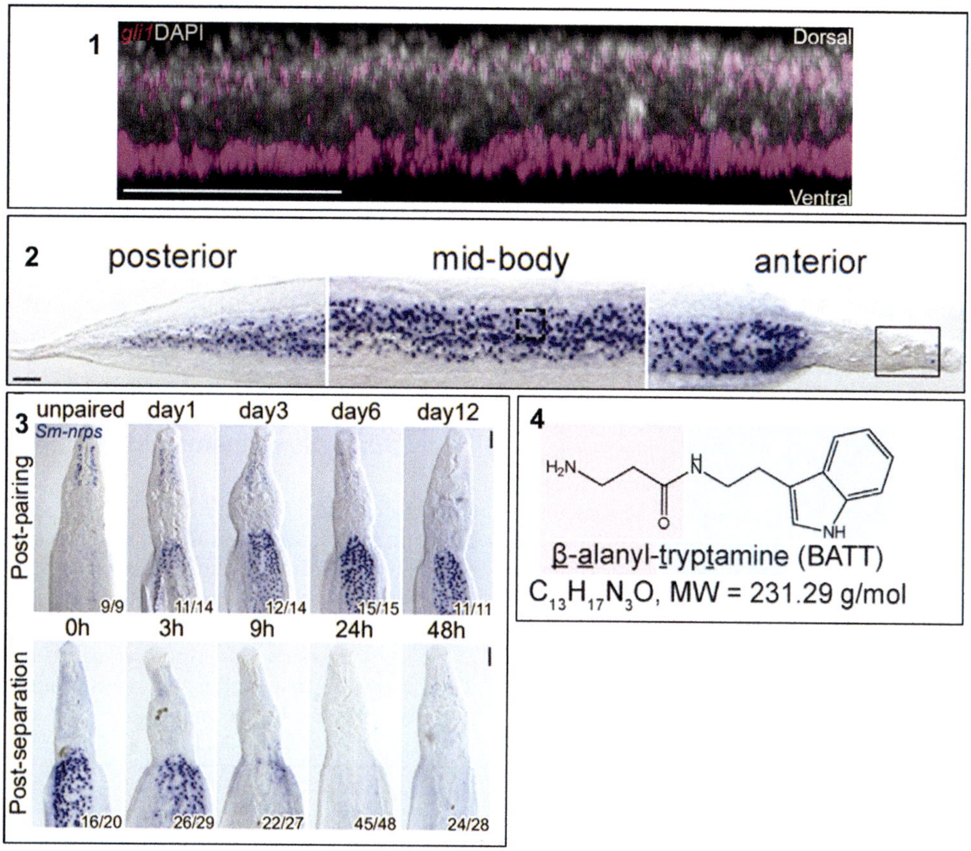

Fig. 10.12. Identification of the male pheromone. **1**) Sagittal confocal section showing expression of mRNA for the developmental gene *gli1* (magenta) enriched in the ventral part of a male worm where the male–female interaction occurs. **3**) The peptide synthase gene, Sm*nrps*, is strongly expressed (together with a neural marker *7b2*) along the male ventral groove. **4**) The Sm*nrps* gene was activated in the days following mating with a female, and equally, expression was turned off within hours of separation. **5**) Molecular formula of the pheromone β-alanyl-tryptamine synthesized by the NRPS enzyme. (From Chen *et al.*, 2022.) Figures used with permission from Elsevier.

mature vitelline cells was observed in early pairing experiments (Popiel, 1986).

It is also worth noting that the expression of Sm*nrps* (Smp_158480) had been previously identified, using a quantitative RT-PCR approach, as stably upregulated in paired versus never-paired males of *S. mansoni* (referred to as Sm*ebony*) (Haeberlein *et al.*, 2019). Separation of pairs led to a reduction in transcription while re-pairing reversed the effect completely. A second gene was also identified in this study, encoding a DOPA/tyrosine decarboxylase (Smp_135230), involved in neurotransmitter metabolism (Lu *et al.*, 2019). Further evidence for the involvement of biogenic amines in female maturation was also found by transcript analysis of *S. japonicum*, which identified the orthlogue of Sm*nrps* (Sjp_0068110) as induced in male *S. japonicum* upon coupling with a female (Wang *et al.*, 2017).

10.5.4 Identification of β-alanyl-tryptamine as a pheromone

Examination of Sm*nrps* expression in the single-cell RNA-Seq atlas of adult schistosomes (Wendt *et al.*, 2020) found that this gene was most highly expressed in a subpopulation of neurons that expressed the *7b2* neural marker. Subsequent studies also found that these positive cells express *tppp2* (Smp_097490), which encodes a tubulin polymerization protein, a marker for ciliated sensory cells. Such sensory endings are distributed throughout the gynaecophoric canal in both paired and unpaired male worms (Chen *et al.*, 2022). As noted above, the protein encoded by Sm*nrps* has homology to the *Drosophila* protein, Ebony, that conjugates β-alanine to biogenic amines. In practice, the correctly folded recombinant SmNRPS enzyme reacts with a number of monoamine neurotransmitters, confirming that it possesses β-alanyl-bioamine synthase activity. The *in vivo* product of SmNRPS was identified by isotopic labelling and liquid chromatography as β-alanyl-tryptamine (BATT) (Fig. 10.12.5). The molecule can be detected in media conditioned by males continuously paired with female worms and its production drops rapidly in the absence of those females. Synthetic BATT is sufficient to induce egg laying in virgin female parasites, which began egg production in the presence of >0.5 μM BATT as early as 4 days after initial incubation. It is presumed that BATT is synthesized in the cell bodies of the sensory nerves and potentially released from the ciliated endings, but concrete evidence has yet to be produced. Its receptor in the female worm and the associated signalling pathways are still to be elucidated. It is known that males of one schistosome species can induce the sexual development of females of another (Armstrong, 1965), suggesting that the effects of BATT are generalizable between species, but it is possible that other schistosome species use different monoamines (Chen *et al.*, 2022).

10.6 Sex Determination

Schistosome chromosomes have been assembled into seven pairs of autosomes, with sex determined by heterogametic females (ZW sex chromosomes) and homogametic males (ZZ sex chromosomes) (Fig. 10.13.1). The evolution of dioecy/gonochorism and the marked sexual dimorphisms of male and female schistosomes must be reflected in the make-up of the sex

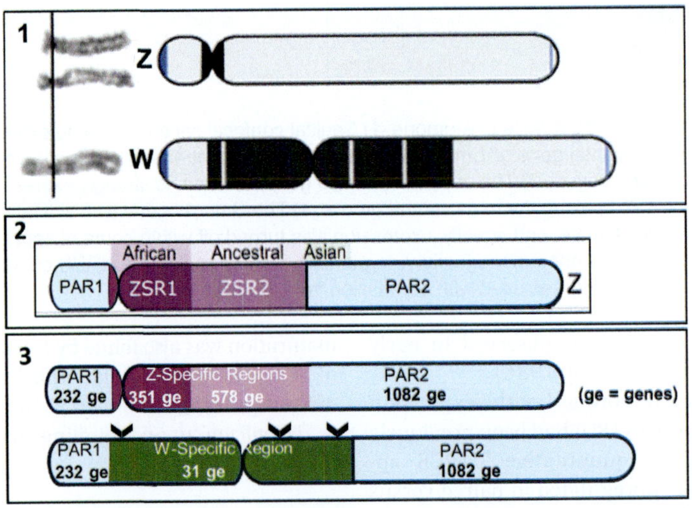

Fig. 10.13. Sex chromosomes. **1**) Male Z and the longer female W chromosomes. Euchromatic DNA, grey; constitutive heterochromatin (C-band), black; telomeric sequence, blue; subtelomeric sequence, light blue. **2**) Strata of the *S. mansoni* Z chromosome. PAR, pseudoautosomal region. African-specific stratum (dark purple) defines ZSR-1 with 50% shared coverage. Ancestral stratum contains orthologues shared between all schistosome species. Asian stratum has coverage specific to *S. japonicum*. **3**) Annotated idiograms of Z and W sex chromosomes. All but 31 genes and five pseudogenes have been lost from the WSR. Two are present as duplicate and triplicate copies. Chevrons indicate the position of three euchromatin bands. (Redrawn from Buddenborg *et al.*, 2021.) Figures used with permission from Dr Sarah Buddenborg (Wellcome Sanger Institute, Cambridge, UK).

chromosomes. However, the assembly of the Z and W chromosome sequences has lagged behind that of the autosomes due to both genetic divergence and the large amounts of highly repetitive regions.

10.6.1 Chromosome sequencing

A new chromosomal assembly that includes a full-length (88 Mb) Z chromosome has been published (Buddenborg *et al.*, 2021). It comprises a Z-specific region (ZSR), flanked by two pseudoautosomal regions (PAR) common to both sex chromosomes (Fig. 10.13.2). These >50 Mb shared PAR1 and PAR2 regions of the Z and W chromosomes contain 229 and 1071 protein-coding genes, respectively (Fig. 10.13.3). Synteny relationships of Z chromosome orthologues from four schistosome species, with the trematode *Echinostoma caproni* providing a hermaphroditic comparator, revealed three strata. ZSR1 contained genes common to African species, an Asian stratum had genes specific to *S. japonicum*, and an Ancestral stratum ZSR2 had orthologues common to all schistosomes.

Like the human Y chromosome, the *S. mansoni* W chromosome is largely heterochromatic with much of its length composed of satellite repeats. Apart from the PAR1 and PAR2 regions, there are just three small bands of euchromatin on the W-specific region (WSR) that correspond to the 932 protein-coding genes of the ZSR. Only 33 genes in these bands have clear homologous copies on the Z chromosome (termed gametologues) all within the WSR (Fig. 10.13.3). Five of the 33 are pseudogenes, indicating that degeneration of this region is continuing. In addition, repeat expansions and insertion of transposable elements have largely disrupted any co-linearity between the WSR and the ZSR. Gametologues are virtually absent in the Ancestral stratum, which is consistent with this part of the chromosome having become sexually differentiated earlier with degenerative processes thus having been under way for longer. However, among the few gametologues, one is predicted to encode the large subunit of splicing factor U2AF (Smp_019690 on Z and Smp_348790 on W). Strikingly, the sequences of these two versions are almost identical (>95%) for most of their lengths but with divergent N-terminal sequences.

Synteny with tapeworm genomes showed that one end of the *S. mansoni* Z chromosome is highly related to chromosome 3 of *Echinococcus multilocularis* and the other end is highly related to chromosome 5. In several taxa, a chromosomal fusion has underpinned the genesis of sex chromosomes, and it was speculated that a similar event occurred in the ancestral schistosome, creating a new pre-sex autosomal chromosome. This fusion event could have isolated a sex-determining locus that was advantageous to females and/or antagonistic to hermaphrodite worms. The *U2AF* gene is located in the oldest part of the ZSR, common to all African and Asian schistosomes. Its encoded protein is a component of the spliceosome located primarily within the nucleus, which removes the introns in transcribed pre-mRNA to form the mature mRNA.

An analogy has been made with *Drosophila*, where the protein encoded by the sex-lethal gene (*sxl*) uses U2AF to influence female-specific development by inhibiting certain splicing pathways when it is active in females. Potentially, the *S. mansoni* female-specific W copy of U2AF could antagonize the activity of the Z copy to inhibit the splicing of one or more genes. The *S. mansoni* sex-specific regions also contain a homologue of the U2AF small subunit, further implicating U2AF in sex determination. The failure to find a W chromosome-specific gene suggests that multiple sex-determining loci were isolated on the sex chromosomes to produce separate sexes. Thus, the W copy of U2AF could regulate other gametologues, or even genes located on the autosomes, to control the suppression of male or female function. Identifying the downstream interactions of U2AF with other genes will be a critical next step for uncovering the mechanisms involved in schistosome sex determination.

10.6.2 Evolution of sexual systems, sex chromosomes and sex-linked gene transcription

Investigating the origin of sex chromosomes and sexual dimorphism from a very broad perspective has also been tackled (Wang *et al.*, 2022). It involved a comparison of trematodes and cestodes with a range of nematode species, including the androdioecious model organism *Caenorhabditis elegans*. Among all the platyhelminth species studied, only the schistosome genome sequences exhibited the signature indicating the presence of sex chromosomes. Moreover, recombination was first suppressed between the Z and W chromosomes in the ancestor of all schistosomes, estimated to be about 21 million years ago. The study used the hermaphroditic fluke *Clonorchis sinensis* and the tapeworm *Taenia multiceps* as the comparators for synteny relationships. There was general agreement about chromosomal rearrangements, and a second candidate sex-determining gene *mag1* was located close to *U2AF* on the Ancestral (SO) region of the Z chromosome. In *C. elegans* expression of *mag1* (a homologue of *Drosophila mago nashi* involved in oogenesis) is responsible for feminization of the normally hermaphroditic germ line. The protein is part of the exon junction complex deposited on spliced mRNAs after intron removal and transported to the cytoplasm. A comparison was made of the downstream gene transcriptome patterns in testes and ovaries from the hermaphroditic platyhelminths to the ZW system in the gonochoristic *S. mansoni*. It suggested that the transition involved mostly defeminization, a lesser or similar extent of masculinization and demasculinization, and an even lower extent of feminization of gonad gene expression. Clearly, as our knowledge of schistosome genomes deepens, it should be possible to flesh out the pathways that led to separate sexes with such marked sexual dimorphism.

10.7 Summary

- The site of schistosome parasitism in the hepatic portal system, with the requirement for the egg transmission stage to escape from the host, has been the likely evolutionary pressure leading to separate sexes in the otherwise entirely hermaphroditic trematodes. The much thinner female can progress further into the mucosal tissues to deposit eggs. Assembly of Z and W chromosomes and use of synteny has revealed a large amount of heterochromatin and an enormous reduction in the number of genes present in the WSR. The precise genes involved in feminization and masculinization have yet to be determined.
- The control of female maturation upon pairing with a male is now better understood. The maturation of vitellaria is under local, not central nervous system control. A small molecule 'hormone', BATT, has been identified. It is synthesized continuously by the male ventral surface and released to stimulate localized vitelline lobule maturation.
- Movement of vitelline cells and ova in the female system must be down to body peristalsis because neither the oviduct nor vitelline ducts are ciliated nor invested with musculature. The ovary has its own coat of muscles, as do the ootype and uterus. Sphincters control the entry of eggs and vitelline cells into the ootype and exit of the formed egg from the chamber into the uterus. All this must require significant nervous control about which nothing is known.
- The Mehlis gland and its secretions are very much an unknown quantity. The products are released into the lumen at the proximal end of the ootype and we must presume are essential for shell formation.
- The motility of the stumpy spermatozoa in the male system is an open question. The 9 + 0 arrangement of axonemes in the tail, and the absence of mitochondria to provide energy, do not suggest a great ability for locomotion. The docking of each spermatozoan, head-first, on the wall of the seminal receptacle also indicates that it waits for the ovum rather than swimming to locate it.
- The prevailing opinion that the male impregnates the female via the female pore just posterior to the ventral sucker is a non-starter for good physiological reasons. Bird schistosomes possess a Laurer's canal, and the author's hypothesis is that there is an anchor point, most likely on the female dorsal surface, via which the male attaches using its holdfast. It then everts its cirrus into the transiently open canal to deposit feebly motile spermatozoa into the region of the seminal receptacle. We have just not found that canal yet.

References

Al Rawi, S., Louvet-Vallée, S., Djeddi, A., Sachse, M., Culetto, E. *et al.* (2011) Postfertilization autophagy of sperm organelles prevents paternal mitochondrial DNA transmission. *Science* 334(6059), 1144–1147. DOI: 10.1126/science.1211878

Armstrong, J.C. (1965) Mating behavior and development of *Schistosomes* in the mouse. *The Journal of Parasitology* 51, 605–616. DOI: 10.2307/3276242

Buddenborg, S.K., Tracey, A., Berger, D.J., Lu, Z., Doyle, S.R. *et al.* (2021) Assembled chromosomes of the blood fluke *Schistosoma mansoni* provide insight into the evolution of its ZW sex-determination system. *bioRxiv* 2021.08.13.456314. DOI: 10.1101/2021.08.13.456314

Chen, R., Wang, J., Gradinaru, I., Vu, H.S., Geboers, S. *et al.* (2022) A male-derived nonribosomal peptide pheromone controls female *Schistosome* development. *Cell* 185(9), 1506–1520. DOI: 10.1016/j.cell.2022.03.017

Cogswell, A.A., Kommer, V.P. and Williams, D.L. (2012) Transcriptional analysis of a unique set of genes involved in *Schistosoma mansoni* female reproductive biology. *PLoS Neglected Tropical Diseases* 6(11), e1907. DOI: 10.1371/journal.pntd.0001907

Collins, J.J., King, R.S., Cogswell, A., Williams, D.L. and Newmark, P.A. (2011) An atlas for *Schistosoma mansoni* organs and life-cycle stages using cell type-specific markers and confocal microscopy. *PLoS Neglected Tropical Diseases* 5(3), e1009. DOI: 10.1371/journal.pntd.0001009

deWalick, S., Tielens, A.G.M. and van Hellemond, J.J. (2012) *Schistosoma mansoni*: the egg, biosynthesis of the shell and interaction with the host. *Experimental Parasitology* 132(1), 7–13. DOI: 10.1016/j.exppara.2011.07.018

Erasmus, D.A. (1973) A comparative study of the reproductive system of mature, immature and 'unisexual' female *Schistosoma mansoni*. *Parasitology* 67(2), 165–183. DOI: 10.1017/s0031182000046394

Erasmus, D.A. and Popiel, I. (1980) *Schistosoma mansoni*: drug induced changes in the cell population of the vitelline gland. *Experimental Parasitology* 50(2), 171–187. DOI: 10.1016/0014-4894(80)90018-1

Haeberlein, S., Angrisano, A., Quack, T., Lu, Z., Kellershohn, J. *et al.* (2019) Identification of a new panel of reference genes to study pairing-dependent gene expression in *Schistosoma mansoni*. *International Journal for Parasitology* 49(8), 615–624. DOI: 10.1016/j.ijpara.2019.01.006

Hahnel, S., Lu, Z., Wilson, R.A., Grevelding, C.G. and Quack, T. (2013) Whole-organ isolation approach as a basis for tissue-specific analyses in *Schistosoma mansoni*. *PLoS Neglected Tropical Diseases* 7(7), e2336. DOI: 10.1371/journal.pntd.0002336

Justine, J.L. and Mattei, X. (1981) Ultrastructural study of sperm flagella *Schistosomes* (Trematoda: Digenea). *Journal of Ultrastructure Research* 76(1), 89–95. DOI: 10.1016/s0022-5320(81)80053-6

Kitajima, E.W., Paraense, W.L. and Correa, L.R. (1976) The fine structure of *Schistosoma mansoni* sperm (Trematoda: Digenea). *The Journal of Parasitology* 62(2), 215–221. DOI: 10.2307/3279270

Kunz, W. (2001) Schistosome male–female interaction: induction of germ-cell differentiation. *Trends in Parasitology* 17(5), 227–231. DOI: 10.1016/s1471-4922(01)01893-1

Li, X.-H., Xu, Y.-X., Vance, G., Wang, Y., Lv, L.B. *et al.* (2015) Evidence that rhesus macaques self-cure from a *Schistosoma japonicum* infection by disrupting worm esophageal function: a new route to an effective vaccine? *PLoS Neglected Tropical Diseases* 9(7), e0003925. DOI: 10.1371/journal.pntd.0003925

Loker, E.S. and Brant, S.V. (2006) Diversification, dioecy and dimorphism in *Schistosomes*. *Trends in Parasitology* 22(11), 521–528. DOI: 10.1016/j.pt.2006.09.001

Lu, Z., Quack, T., Hahnel, S., Gelmedin, V., Pouokam, E. *et al.* (2015) Isolation, enrichment and primary characterisation of vitelline cells from *Schistosoma mansoni* obtained by the organ isolation method. *International Journal for Parasitology* 45(9–10), 663–672. DOI: 10.1016/j.ijpara.2015.04.002

Lu, Z., Sessler, F., Holroyd, N., Hahnel, S., Quack, T. *et al.* (2016) *Schistosome* sex matters: a deep view into gonad-specific and pairing-dependent transcriptomes reveals a complex gender interplay. *Scientific Reports* 6(1), 31150. DOI: 10.1038/srep31150

Lu, Z., Spänig, S., Weth, O. and Grevelding, C.G. (2019) Males, the wrongly neglected partners of the biologically unprecedented male–female interaction of *Schistosomes*. *Frontiers in Genetics* 10, 796. DOI: 10.3389/fgene.2019.00796

Menrath, M., Michel, A. and Kunz, W. (1995) A female-specific cDNA sequence of *Schistosoma mansoni* encoding a mucin-like protein that is expressed in the epithelial cells of the reproductive duct. *Parasitology* 111(4), 477–483. DOI: 10.1017/s0031182000065987

Moczon, T., Swiderski, Z. and Huggel, H. (1992) *Schistosoma mansoni*: the chemical nature of the secretions produced by the Mehlis' gland and ootype as revealed by cytochemical studies. *International Journal for Parasitology* 22(1), 65–73. DOI: 10.1016/0020-7519(92)90081-u

Neves, L.X., Wilson, R.A., Brownridge, P., Holman, S.W., Harman, V.M. *et al.* (2023) Dissection of *Schistosome* tissues under LC-MS compatible preservative conditions for quantitative proteomics. *Rapid Communications in Mass Spectrometry* 38(Suppl. 1), e9523. DOI: 10.1002/rcm.9523

Nollen, P.M. (1983) Patterns of sexual reproduction among parasitic platyhelminths. *Parasitology* 86(4), 99–120. DOI: 10.1017/s0031182000050861

Nollen, P.M., Floyd, R.D., Kolzow, R.G. and Deter, D.L. (1976) The timing of reproductive cell development and movement in *Schistosoma mansoni*, *S. japonicum*, and *S. haematobium*, using techniques of autoradiography and transplantation. *The Journal of Parasitology* 62(2), 227–231. DOI: 10.2307/3279273

Otubanjo, O.A. (1980) *Schistosoma mansoni*: the ultrastructure of the ducts of the male reproductive system. *Parasitology* 81(3), 565–571. DOI: 10.1017/s0031182000061941

Platt, T.R. and Brooks, D.R. (1997) Evolution of the *Schistosomes* (Digenea: Schistosomatoidea): the origin of dioecy and colonization of the venous system. *The Journal of Parasitology* 83(6), 1035. DOI: 10.2307/3284358

Popiel, I. (1986) Male-stimulated female maturation in *Schistosoma*: a review. *Journal of Chemical Ecology* 12(8), 1745–1754. DOI: 10.1007/BF01022380

Popiel, I. and Basch, P.F. (1984) Reproductive development of female *Schistosoma mansoni* (Digenea: Schistosomatidae) following bisexual pairing of worms and worm segments. *The Journal of Experimental Zoology* 232(1), 141–150. DOI: 10.1002/jez.1402320117

Short, R.B. (1983) Presidential address: sex and the single *Schistosome*. *The Journal of Parasitology* 69(1), 2. DOI: 10.2307/3281269

Skírnisson, K., Kolářová, L., Horák, P., Ferté, H. and Jouet, D. (2012) Morphological features of the nasal blood fluke *Trichobilharzia regenti* (Schistosomatidae, Digenea) from naturally infected hosts. *Parasitology Research* 110(5), 1881–1892. DOI: 10.1007/s00436-011-2713-9

Wang, J., Chen, R. and Collins, J.J. (2019) Systematically improved *in vitro* culture conditions reveal new insights into the reproductive biology of the human parasite *Schistosoma mansoni*. *PLoS Biology* 17(5), e3000254. DOI: 10.1371/journal.pbio.3000254

Wang, J., Yu, Y., Shen, H., Qing, T., Zheng, Y. *et al.* (2017) Dynamic transcriptomes identify biogenic amines and insect-like hormonal regulation for mediating reproduction in *Schistosoma japonicum*. *Nature Communications* 8(1), 14693. DOI: 10.1038/ncomms14693

Wang, Y., Gasser, R.B., Charlesworth, D. and Zhou, Q. (2022) Evolution of sexual systems, sex chromosomes and sex-linked gene transcription in flatworms and roundworms. *Nature Communications* 13(1), 3239. DOI: 10.1038/s41467-022-30578-z

Webster, B.L. and Littlewood, D.T.J. (2012) Mitochondrial gene order change in *Schistosoma* (Platyhelminthes: Digenea: Schistosomatidae). *International Journal for Parasitology* 42(3), 313–321. DOI: 10.1016/j.ijpara.2012.02.001

Wendt, G., Zhao, L., Chen, R., Liu, C., O'Donoghue, A.J. *et al.* (2020) A single-cell RNA-seq atlas of *Schistosoma mansoni* identifies a key regulator of blood feeding. *Science* 369(6511), 1644–1649. DOI: 10.1126/science.abb7709

11

The Egg and its Secretions

11.1 Overview

Many parasitic helminths void their egg transmission stage via the faeces, and it is common to find different species in the same sample (Fig. 11.1). Nothing illustrates the difference between nematodes and schistosomes better than the structure of these eggs. Nematodes, in the clade Ecdysozoa, daily lay unembryonated eggs in vast numbers. These develop in the external environment, but a frequent life cycle strategy is for the resistant eggs to persist and ultimately infect the definitive host by contamination of food. The eggshell, composed of chitin, is extraordinarily resistant and the larva inside is protected by an impermeant vitelline membrane. Schistosomes, in the clade Lophotrochozoa, lay eggs in small numbers, and they undergo full development in the tissues to the infective stage before being voided from the host. These eggs are not resistant or persistent and the miracidium must hatch into fresh water to infect the molluscan host by direct penetration. Schistosome eggs have a tanned protein eggshell, beneath which a living subshell envelope develops. Its secretions are a vital component of the mechanism permitting eggs to transit from blood vessel to gut lumen. Those secretions and the contents of eggs sequestered in host tissues are also the agents of the pathology that is the hallmark of schistosomiasis.

11.2 Egg Deposition and Development

The maturation of female worms following mating with males in the intrahepatic portal veins was covered in Chapter 10, and the subsequent migration of mated pairs up the portal tract to the intestinal wall in Chapter 3. We are reliant primarily on murine studies for what is known about egg deposition, but the laboratory mouse has limitations due to its small size. The thickness of the human small intestinal wall is ~3–5 mm, that of the large intestine ~1–5 mm, depending on the degree of distension. In comparison, values for the mouse are approximately ~0.25 and ~0.5 mm, respectively. This means that there is 10 times more physical space in human/primate intestines for worm manoeuvres. Set alongside this, the length of extended *Schistosoma mansoni* males is up to 12 mm and of females is 16 mm (*Schistosoma japonicum* worms are even longer). The blood vessels associated with the small intestine, large intestine and rectum are the inferior and superior mesenteric arteries, and the portal veins. Within the intestinal wall, the main arterioles run parallel to the longitudinal axis, lying both beneath the serosa and within the submucosa, sending smaller branches into the muscle layers and the mucosa, where they give rise to capillary networks. These coalesce to form the portal venules in the same locations. Female

DOI: 10.1079/9781800625167.0011

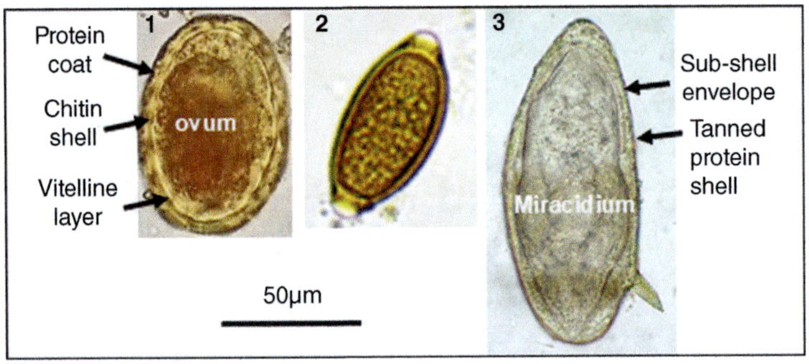

Fig. 11.1. Helminth eggs in human faeces, approximately to scale. **1**) *Ascaris lumbricoides*. **2**) *Trichuris trichiura*. **3**) *Schistosoma mansoni*. (**3** kindly provided by Mr Idzi Potters, Institute of Tropical Medicine, Antwerp, Belgium.) **1** and **2**) Figure author's own.

worms must press forward upstream of the males in these venules to deposit their eggs. Given the greater thickness of human (and primate) intestines it seems likely that they can reach deeper into the tissues than in mice, but we have no concrete *in vivo* information. In parenthesis, it is worth noting that for *Schistosoma haematobium* there is an additional migratory phase involving transit of pairs through the rectal venous plexus to the vesical veins of the bladder wall (see Chapter 3). The thickness of the human bladder wall varies between 2 and 5 mm, again depending on distension.

11.2.1 Pair migration and the site of egg deposition

In larger primate hosts, longitudinal histopathological studies have revealed that the walls of the colon are the favoured site for egg deposition. In one baboon study, ~85% of eggs were recovered by tissue digestion from the colon compared with 5% from the small intestine and 10% from the liver (Farah *et al.*, 1997). In a second study, distributions were ~65% in the large intestine, ~26% in the small intestine and ~12% for other locations (Damian *et al.*, 1976). The structure and thickness of the mucosal layer is relevant in this context. Together, the crypts and microvilli in the small intestine provide a greater barrier to egg egress compared with the crypts and flatter surface of the colon, related to the respective functions of the small and large bowel. Again, it would appear that the structure of the colon provides less of an obstacle to egg escape than does the small intestine. Within the intestinal walls of rhesus macaques with a light infection, eggs have been recorded from serosal surface locations, but especially from the submucosa which was thickened, oedematous and infiltrated with leucocytes (Cheever and Powers, 1972). The situation in primates has been contrasted with the mouse where a much larger proportion of eggs are carried downstream to lodge in the liver (Farah *et al.*, 1997). It undoubtedly reflects the inability of females to penetrate far enough into the thinner wall of the mouse intestine, due to its correspondingly smaller portal venules.

With all the above caveats in mind, one experiment using mice has provided information about the manner of egg deposition (Pellegrino and Coelho, 1978). The process was examined in animals harbouring only a single worm pair, using oogram scanning to plot the location of first-stage eggs in the whole intestine from duodenum to rectum. The tacit assumption was that these eggs represented the population deposited in the previous 24 h. In four mice the mean number was 297 first-stage eggs, very close to accepted values for daily egg production (300 per day). The pattern of deposition revealed that first-stage eggs were largely distributed along the small intestine (cf. the colon in primates), reflecting a remarkable wandering capacity of the pair (Fig. 11.2.1). They were present in clusters, confirming the observation that eggs distend the venule in a beadlike row as the female retreats depositing eggs as she goes. Then the pair withdraws and relocates to another vessel, which may be some distance away. This must require a

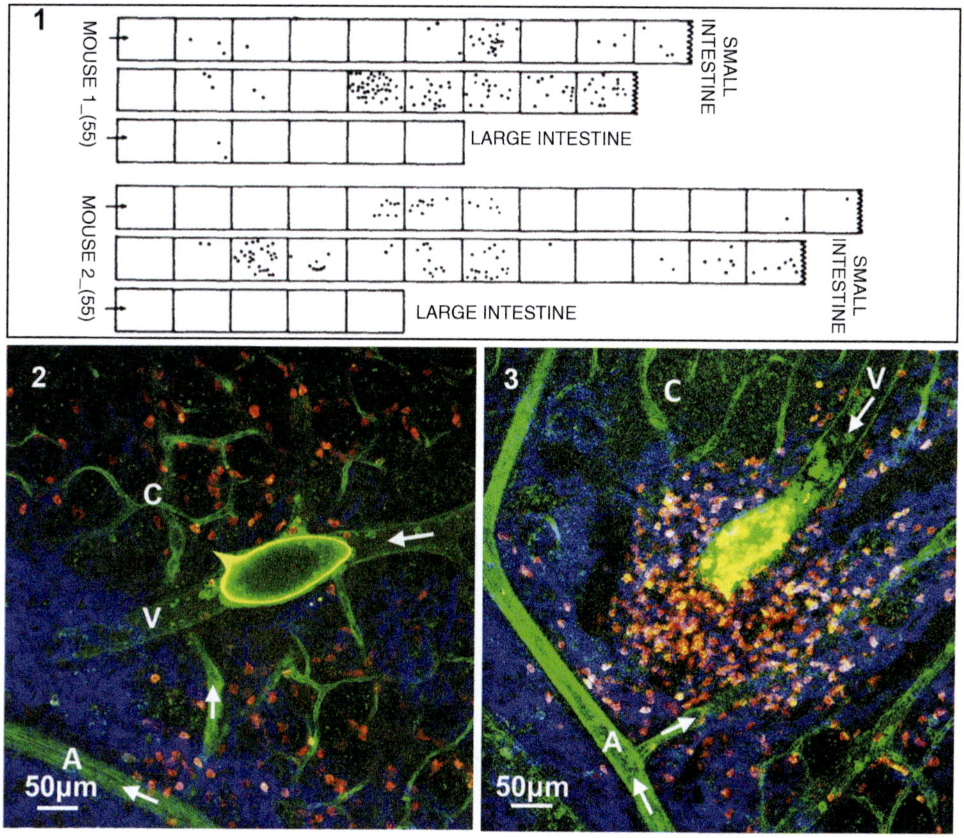

Fig. 11.2. Egg deposition in portal venules of the intestinal wall. **1**) Oograms from the intestines of two mice infected with single worm pairs showing the discontinuous, patchy distribution of first-stage eggs, primarily in the small intestine. **2** and **3**) The layout of vessels in the submucosa of the mouse small intestine viewed by multiphoton microscopy. Arteries (A), veins (V) and capillaries (C) are highlighted in green by *in vivo* staining with FITC-tomato lectin. The extracellular matrix between serosal and submucosal layers appears blue due to the second harmonic. CD4⁺ T cells have intrinsic VADs red fluorescence. The *S. mansoni* egg with backward-pointing spine displays yellow autofluorescence from phenolic groups in the tanned protein shell. **2**) An immature egg lodged in a venule attracts no attention from the randomly distributed T cells. **3**) A mature egg is surrounded by numerous T cells, apparently clustering most densely in the downstream region. Arrows indicate direction of blood flow. (**1** reproduced with permission from *The Journal of Parasitology*, KGL Publishing Services, Pellegrino and Coelho, 1978; **2** and **3** from Wilson, 2012.) Figure used with permission from Elsevier.

significant degree of neuromuscular coordination between the male and female.

Newly deposited eggs of *S. mansoni* are laid with spine pointing backward to snag into the wall of a portal venule (Fig. 11.2.2) (Wilson, 2012). At this stage they do not attract attention from CD4⁺ T cells. However, once they have matured, an inflammatory cluster of cells collects around the still intravascular egg (Fig. 11.2.3). Clearly the lack of reactivity during the tissue phase of development is a device to prevent premature expulsion of the partially developed egg (Ashton *et al.*, 2001). The marked increase in reactivity upon maturation initiates its passage into the extravascular space and then through the submucosal and mucosal layers to reach the gut lumen. The ability of mature eggs to secrete specific proteins formed the basis of a now obsolete diagnostic test for schistosomiasis in human populations, called the circumoval precipitin (COP) test, whereby characteristic deposits would form on the surface of eggs incubated with serum from infected individuals (Hillyer *et al.*, 1980).

11.2.2 Stages and timing of egg development

Schistosome eggs long resisted transmission electron microscopy (TEM) analysis because fixatives, dehydrating agents and embedding media penetrate poorly through the shell. This speaks volumes about the properties of that shell, and special cryo-techniques (Neill *et al.*, 1988) or hand-pricking with a fine entomology pin (Ashton *et al.*, 2001) were needed to allow penetration of resin, prior to sectioning. The shell itself is extremely dense, but with some spherical 50 nm lacunae, and bears a coat of microspines, ~200 μm long. There is no information about how the luminal surface of the ootype is organized to regulate the formation of these spines during eggshell tanning. In the mature egg only, these spines appear to hold in position a layer of mucus-like material potentially exuded from within the shell (Fig. 11.3.1). No direct sieve-like pores were found after eggshell pricking (Ashton *et al.*, 2001) but it was noted that

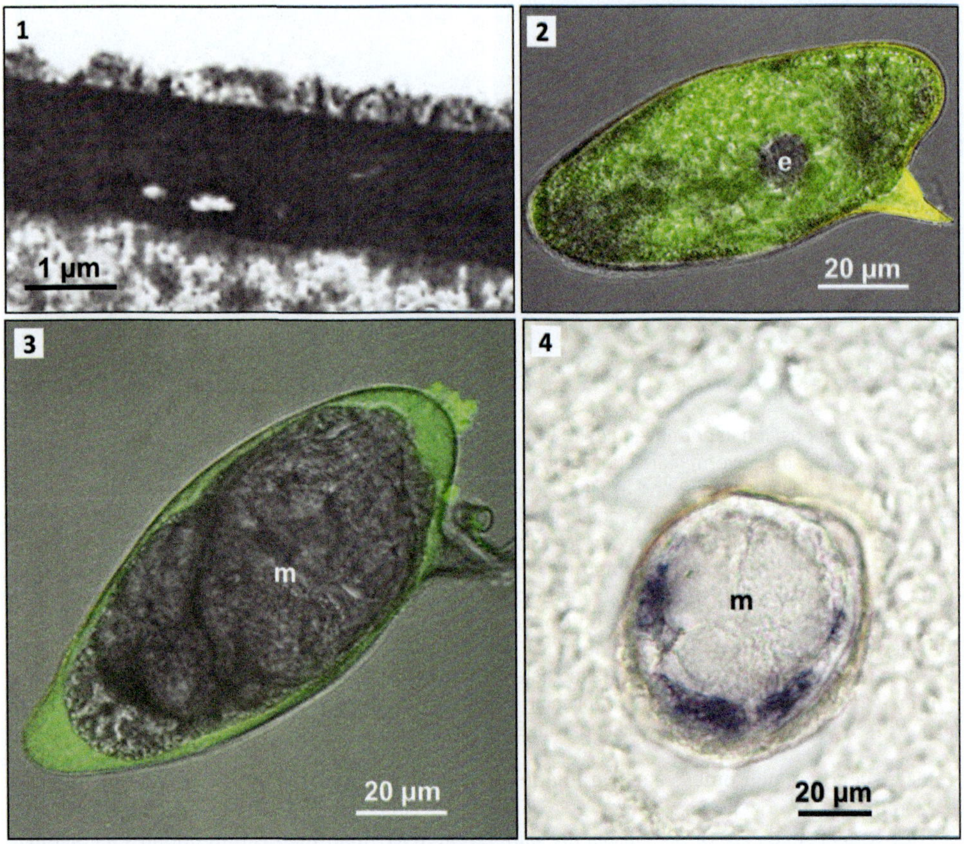

Fig. 11.3. Properties of the developing egg. **1**) The shell in a mature egg showing small vacuoles and the surface extended into short microspines, which appear to hold a layer of material *in situ*. **2**) A newly deposited egg with a tiny embryo, incubated with FITC-dextran (10 kDa). The dextran has passed through the shell and stained all the vitelline cells, but the embryo is unstained. **3**) Mature egg (scale as in **2**) given the same treatment. The dextran has entered the subshell envelope but not the internal lacuna containing the miracidium (m), which is unstained. **4**) Expression of the *meg3.2* gene encoding one of the ESPs, localized by *in situ* hybridization; the gene (blue) is active in the subshell envelope but not the miracidium. (**1** from Ashton *et al.*, 2001; **2–4** from Wilson, 2012.) **1**) Figure used with permission from Cambridge University Press. **2–4**) Figures used with permission from Elsevier.

quenching of eggs in liquid nitrogen produced minute fractures in the shell (Neill *et al.*, 1988), so it is not possible to determine whether such sieve pores exist, or are an artefact of the cryotechnique. Incubation of isolated eggs with fluorescently labelled dextran (10 kDa) reveals that the immature eggshell is completely permeable to low-molecular-weight compounds, with the entire vitelline contents but not the growing embryo being stained (Fig. 11.3.2). There is a lack of information on egg structure in both *S. japonicum* and *S. haematobium*, but observations on the former species confirm the presence of microspines on the shell surface and suggest the presence of micropores in the shell (Cao *et al.*, 1982). In view of the relevance for pathogenesis, the situation needs clarification in both species.

At the start of development in a venule, an egg comprises the zygote and around 30 intact vitelline cells. The zygote begins division to form a compact ball of embryonic cells while the vitelline cells, full of lipid droplets and other inclusions (Fig. 11.4.1), begin a controlled degradation which has not been characterized. Very early in embryonic development, a small number of cells detach and migrate peripherally to lie beneath the shell (Fig. 11.4.2) (Neill *et al.*, 1988; Ashton *et al.*, 2001). They coalesce to form a 0.5 μm thick syncytial layer, referred to as the subshell envelope, with cytoplasm that contains mitochondria, vesicles and endoplasmic reticulum, clearly a tissue preparing to synthesize proteins for export (Fig. 11.4.3) (Ashton *et al.*, 2001). At this stage the envelope excludes labelled dextran, which no longer reaches the interior, indicating its continuity (Fig. 11.3.3). Localization by *in situ* hybridization of genes putatively secreted from the mature egg revealed that they originate not in the miracidium but in the envelope (Fig. 11.3.4). This makes it crucial to distinguish between live and dead eggs in pathogenic processes.

Focusing on the envelope in the maturing egg, by the time ciliated plates appear on the miracidial surface, it is 2 μm thick and highly differentiated with an external surface extended into short, branched microvilli reminiscent of transporting epithelium (Fig. 11.4.4). The cytoplasm contains abundant rough endoplasmic reticulum, and large vacuoles of granular material. In the mature egg a new layer of heterogenous, flocculent material (1 μm thick) originating in the envelope, accumulates beneath the shell (Fig. 11.4.5). This has been referred to as Reynolds' layer (Neill *et al.*, 1988). An attempt to characterize egg development based on light microscopy, which lacks the resolution of TEM, has overcomplicated the process designating eight stages (Jurberg *et al.*, 2009). It describes the subshell envelope as the inner envelope and the secreted layer as the outer envelope, when one is a living syncytium and the other comprises secreted material; the classification will not be adopted here.

It was observed in early studies on development that there was an increase in egg size between oviposition and maturation *in vivo* (Michaels and Prata, 1968). Treating the egg as a prolate spheroid, using the dimensions provided, gives a 2.1-fold increase in volume. More recently a value of 3.24-fold was obtained (Ashton *et al.*, 2001) (compare the eggs in Fig. 11.3.2 and 11.3.3). Taking account of the different densities of undeveloped ($\rho = 1.06$) and mature eggs ($\rho = 1.09$), based on Percoll gradient isolation, an increase in mass by a factor of 3.3 times is implied during development (Ashton *et al.*, 2001). This suggests that around two-thirds of the nutrients for egg development are derived from external sources. It also explains why development of the schistosome egg during *in vitro* culture requires supplementation of the medium; unlike the *Fasciola* egg it is not self-sufficient in nutrients. The observations on increase in egg volume and mass have been reinforced by *in vitro* experiments. Immature eggs isolated *ex vivo* for short-term culture released 0.32 μg of protein per 1000 eggs, whereas mature eggs were 8 times more active, releasing 2.63 μg/1000. Nevertheless, both egg types were biosynthetically active, as confirmed by culturing eggs with ^{35}S-labelled amino acids. The immature and mature eggs incorporated roughly comparable amounts of label, but the mature eggs released 10 times as much precipitable protein. Furthermore, fractionation of the labelled protein released from mature eggs had a quite distinct composition, compared to the soluble fraction of the whole egg (Fig. 11.5.1).

11.3 Egg Secretions

11.3.1 Biochemical methods to identify egg secreted proteins

Although discrete patterns of secreted proteins could be identified by gel electrophoresis (Ashton *et al.*, 2001) there was no easy way to identify

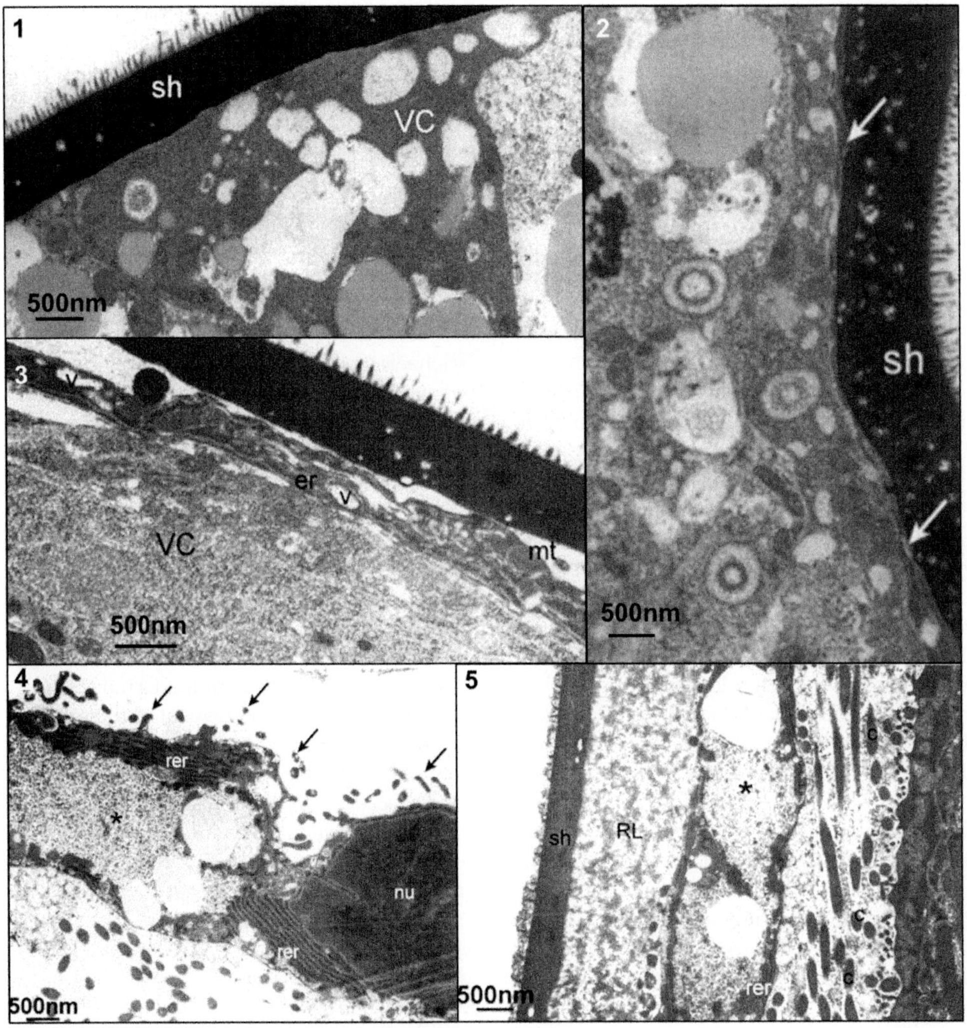

Fig. 11.4. Development of the subshell envelope. **1**) Newly laid egg with vitelline cell (VC) lying in direct contact with the shell (sh). **2**) Partially developed egg with a layer of cytoplasm (arrowed) representing the nascent envelope interposed between the shell and vitelline cell. **3**) The subshell envelope is now differentiating, with mitochondria (mt), endoplasmic reticulum (er) and vesicles (v) apparent. **4**) Fully developed subshell envelope with external surface extended into short microvilli (arrowed), nucleus (nu), extensive rough endoplasmic reticulum (rer) and large vacuoles (asterisk) full of granular material (shell absent). **5**) Mature egg. The space between the subshell envelope and the shell is now full of granular material, comprising Reynolds' layer (RL). Numerous cilia (c) are visible on the miracidium and material is also present around the shell surface microspines. (**1**–**5** from Ashton *et al.*, 2001.) Figures used with permission from Cambridge University Press.

them before the advent of proteomic techniques. Consequently, the first breakthrough came via recombinant DNA technology, and it is worth noting just how laborious this was (Schramm *et al.*, 2003). An abundant protein was isolated from total egg extract using a combination of cation exchange and *Aurelia aurantia* lectin chromatography. N-terminal sequencing of the first 20 amino acids by Edman degradation provided a tag which was used to search dbEST at GenBank to identify a corresponding nucleotide sequence for screening of an egg cDNA library.

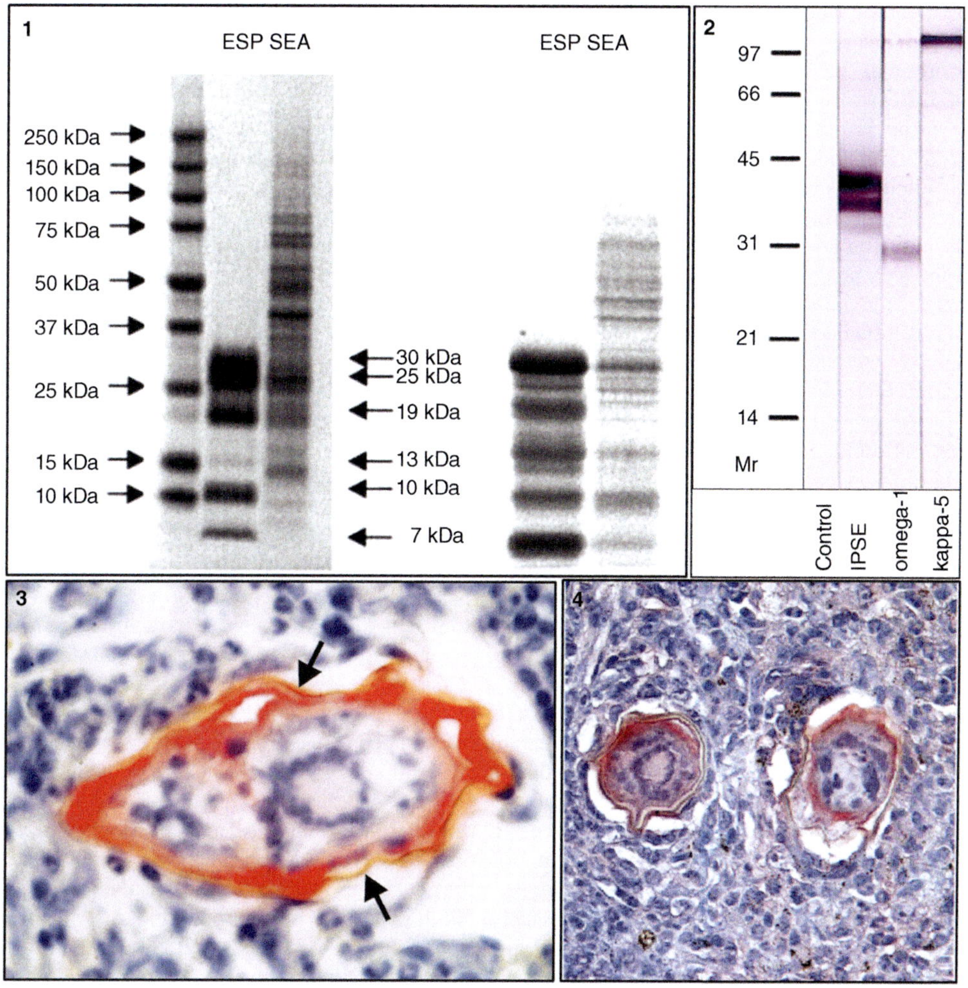

Fig. 11.5. Secretions of the subshell envelope. **1**) One-dimensional separation on SDS-PAGE gel of ESPs from mature eggs and total soluble protein extract (SEA). On the left, Coomassie staining reveals that ESP comprises a simple mixture of six bands between 7 and 30 kDa while the SEA has much greater complexity. On the right autoradiography of samples from mature eggs cultured with ^{35}S-labelled amino acids reveals a similar and intense pattern of ESP protein synthesis, compared to SEA. **2**) Western blot of egg proteins reacted with rabbit polyclonal antibodies to the three principal proteins synthesized by the envelope reveals their respective molecular weights. **3**) The localization of IPSE protein (red) to the subshell envelope of the mature egg using a specific monoclonal antibody. The arrows point to the yellow autofluorescence of the shell. **4**) Localization of kappa-5 to the subshell envelope using specific rabbit antiserum. (**1** from Ashton *et al.*, 2001; **2** and **4** from Schramm *et al.*, 2009; **3** high-resolution image kindly provided by Dr Gabrielle Schramm, Borstel, Germany, from Schramm *et al.*, 2003.) Figures used with permission from **1**) Cambridge University Press and **2–4**) Elsevier.

The full-length clone was then expressed as a recombinant protein in *E coli* for functional assays and antibody production (GenBank AY028436). The protein, given the name interleukin-4-inducing principle of *S. mansoni* eggs (IPSE), was shown to be the bioactive principal leading to the activation of human basophils and their expression of IL-4 and IL-13, that predispose the immune response towards the Th2 pole and IgE production. IPSE activated basophils by cross-linking surface membrane IgE receptors, independent of their antigen specificity. Immunocytochemistry revealed its origin in the mature egg as a product of the subshell envelope, not the miracidium (Fig. 11.5.3). Important pro-inflammatory products of human basophils include histamine, heparin, chondroitin sulphate, peroxidase, platelet activating factor and proteases. Collectively this information fits with the concept of the schistosome egg deliberately provoking an inflammatory response that aids its passage through the tissues. IPSE proved to be identical to an egg protein called alpha-1/CEF6 identified two decades earlier but not characterized at the time, and to the egg secreted protein ESP3–6 on two-dimensional gels (Schramm *et al.*, 2009). There are at least 13 virtually identical copies of *ipse* in v10 of the *S. mansoni* genome (was Smp_112110, now, e.g. Smp_335430, etc.).

In a very different approach, based on the idea that virus genomes encode chemokine binding proteins, a search of all schistosome life cycle stages was made using ^{125}I-CXCL8 and ^{125}I-CCL3 as bait in a protein binding assay (Smith *et al.*, 2005). A single complex was identified in egg secretions, which contained a 36 kDa schistosome protein. A peptide was identified by mass spectrometry and used to obtain a match on dbEST (AI820476). The encoded protein was named chemokine binding protein (SmCKBP) but the authors also noted sequence identity with IPSE. However, the two studies differed in one respect, the expression of CKBP in an insect cell system, which could affect binding and glycosylation properties. The authors concluded that schistosome eggs secrete SmCKBP to block the activity of certain chemokines both *in vitro* and *in vivo*. It is thus anti-inflammatory and a potent suppressor of inflammatory responses in acute murine inflammation models. The contradictions between the claims for pro- and anti-inflammatory properties of the same ESP have not to date been satisfactorily resolved. However, the inflammation that facilitates egg egress from the gut, also creates perforation channels that enable bacteria to enter the gut wall. These could in turn exacerbate intestinal inflammation via lipopolysaccharide–Toll-like receptor interactions on macrophages. The role of IL-4/IL-13 release from basophils would not be Th2 induction, but rather the promotion of alternatively activated anti-inflammatory macrophages, which possess wound healing and resolution phase properties (Knuhr *et al.*, 2018).

The CEF6 fraction of egg secretions contained a second protein, termed omega-1, that was subsequently cloned by the same route as IPSE (Fitzsimmons *et al.*, 2005) and shown to be a hepatotoxic T2 ribonuclease. To exert its action of breaking down intracellular RNA, omega-1 needs to enter host cells, so the question is which cells, and how does this benefit the mature egg that has released it. Its hepatotoxic properties, while bad news for the host liver cells, are only tangential to its primary role in aiding egg escape from the gut. It too is synthesized in the subshell envelope and secreted from the mature egg, with multiple copies of the gene present in v10 of the *S. mansoni* genome (was Smp_193860, now, e.g. Smp_339930). There is no information on its effect on venule endothelium, the first tissue it will encounter on release from the sequestered egg.

A third protein, given the name kappa-5 (GenBank AY903301), was characterized using a similar methodology to omega-1 (Schramm *et al.*, 2009). There are at least five copies of *kappa5* in the v10 genome (e.g. Smp_335490). When fractionated by electrophoresis it has a molecular weight of ~97 kDa, but under reducing conditions it appears as a dimer of 45 and 50 kDa, the difference being the degree of occupation of the four *N*-glycosylation sites. The protein is synthesized in the subshell envelope (Fig. 11.5.4) but the authors noted that, unlike IPSE and omega-1, kappa-5 is not secreted from eggs and only appears in ESP if some miracidia hatched during sample preparation. Envelope products separated on a non-reducing gel and reacted with specific rabbit polyclonal antibodies revealed the respective molecular weights of the native proteins (Fig. 11.5.2). One further piece of evidence came from the COP test using the same specific rabbit sera, which was strongly positive for IPSE, omega-1 and crude ESP, but negative for kappa-5, indicating its retention beneath the eggshell (Schramm *et al.*, 2009). Additionally, in contrast to IPSE and omega-1, kappa-5 transcripts were present in miracidia. We must assume that kappa-5 is too large to pass through the eggshell pores, and this would make it a principal component of Reynolds' layer, between the envelope and shell. Proteomic analysis identified the presence of albumin (60 kDa) but not IgG (160 kDa) in hatch fluid (Mathieson and Wilson,

2010), supporting this idea of differential shell permeability. This poses the question that if kappa-5 is not involved in promoting egg escape, what is its role in the mature egg? Its presence in the miracidium, as well as Reynolds' layer, suggests that it may function as a protective barrier for the miracidium against attack by inflammatory mediators generated in the tissues, or acute-phase proteins present in the circulation resulting from schistosome infection (Gonçalves-Silva *et al.*, 2022). The release of such mediators on interaction of IPSE with basophils was noted above and the recruitment of intraepithelial mucosal mast cells to the mouse gut wall following schistosome egg deposition has also been recorded (Miller *et al.*, 1994; De Jonge *et al.*, 2002). This suggests contrasting roles for mouse mast cell products, with mast cell protease-1 (β-chymase) acting on the extracellular matrix to facilitate egg migration, while the miracidium inside the egg needs protection against the released inflammatory mediators.

From experiments on human monocyte-derived dendritic cells it has been established the glycan residues on omega-1 are recognized by the surface mannose receptor (C-type lectin; CD206) (Everts *et al.*, 2012). After internalization by endocytosis, and translocation into the cytosol, omega-1 interferes with ribosomal function and protein synthesis in a way that drives Th2 polarization of the immune response. This may be important in the overall immunology, especially with respect to granuloma formation but it is unclear how it assists egg transit through the gut tissues.

11.3.2 Proteomic approaches to identify egg secretions

The first proteomic study of the *S. mansoni* egg described a secretome comprising 188 proteins, including several histones, multiple glycolytic enzymes and heat shock protein chaperones as constituents (Cass *et al.*, 2007). Although the listed constituents are indicative of cytosol and nucleoplasm, the authors used SecretomeP (https://services.healthtech.dtu.dk/service.php?SecretomeP-2.0) to justify the presence of these internal constituents, supposedly exported via a non-classical pathway. This conclusion has been questioned, particularly secreted histones and cytoskeletal proteins, raising doubts about whether the secreted fraction was contaminated with leakage products from dead eggs (DeMarco and Verjovski-Almeida, 2009). A second study, using two-dimensional electrophoretic separation, investigated the soluble proteome of undeveloped eggs, mature eggs, hatched miracidia and residual hatch fluid (Mathieson and Wilson, 2010). Additionally, the proteins released by mature eggs during culture (ESP) in unsupplemented RPMI medium were characterized. The composition of ESP was relatively simple, with the previously identified IPSE dominant (83% of the crude content), and omega-1 as the second most abundant protein; other spots appeared only faintly in the background (Fig. 11.6.1). Note that kappa-5 was not present, adding further support to its non-secretory status. Passage of ESP down an *Aleuria* lectin column to deplete IPSE and omega-1 left a more complex protein mixture in the flow-through, comprising multiple members of the micro-exon gene-encoded MEG-2 and -3 protein families (Fig. 11.6.2) (DeMarco *et al.*, 2010).

The two-dimensional electrophoretic analysis of soluble proteins in mature eggs identified SmE16 calcium-binding protein (Smp_096390) as 1.2% of the proteome, and 1.9% of the miracidium larva (Mathieson and Wilson, 2010). (This protein should not be confused with Sm16/Stathmin protein recently described in eggs; Shiels *et al.*, 2020.) Smp40 α-crystallin/HSP20 (Smp_049250, now Smp_302280) was the most abundant protein in the same two fractions (10.9% and 15.2%, respectively). As both SmE16 and Smp40 clearly reside in the miracidial body, they are most relevant to pathogenesis when released from dead eggs trapped in liver or gut tissues.

More recent proteomic analyses of putative egg secretions, including those of *S. haematobium* and *S. japonicum*, have been published and the reader is referred to a review for a detailed appraisal (Castro-Borges and Wilson, 2022). The secretome (ES fraction) of the *S. haematobium* egg was reported to contain 138 different proteins, a heterogeneous mixture that included histones, ribosomal and mitochondrial proteins as well as numerous cytosolic and cytoskeletal constituents (Sotillo *et al.*, 2019). The authors seem unaware of the complex structure of the

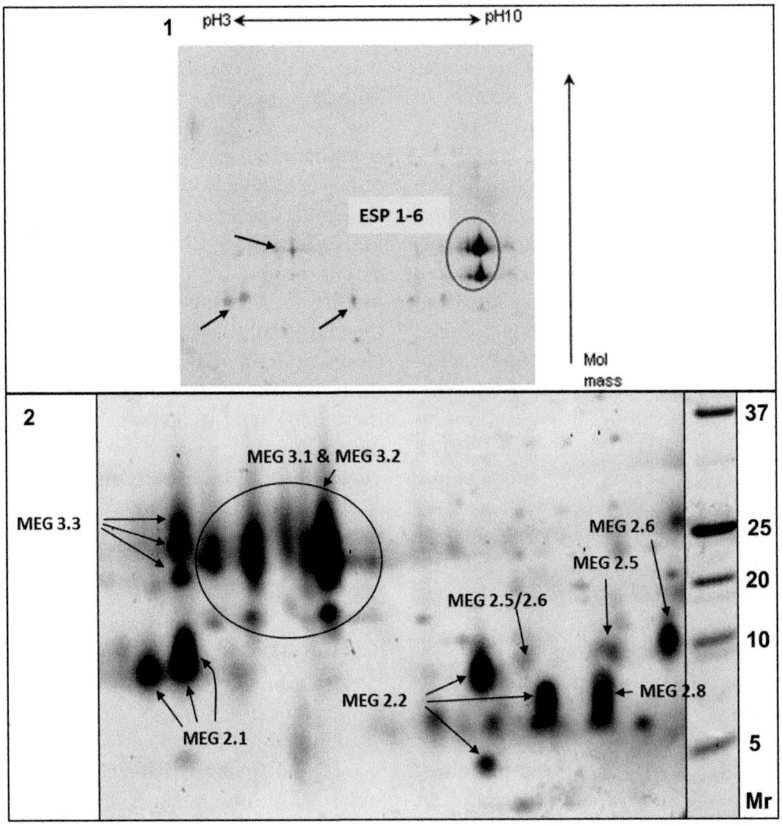

Fig. 11.6. Characterization of ESPs. Eggs were recovered from the livers of mice, infected 7 weeks previously, by trypsin digestion, washing and sieving. Mature eggs, separated by centrifugation on a Percoll gradient and cultured in RPMI medium for 3 days, were judged to be 96% viable. **1**) Two-dimensional electrophoretic separation of ESP concentrated from culture medium. ESP 1–6 was a simple mixture, predominantly IPSE with a minor component of omega-1. **2**) ESP depleted of ESP 1–6 on a lectin column comprises multiple MEG-2 and MEG-3 family proteins, most with splice variants. (**1** from Mathieson and Wilson, 2010; **2** from DeMarco *et al.*, 2010.) Figures used with permission from **1**) Elsevier and **2**) Cold Spring Harbour Laboratory Press.

mature egg, concluding that the egg secretions 'likely originate from an active secretion process by the miracidium'. However, there does not appear to be a TEM description of the mature *S. haematobium* egg that would clarify this issue. A second study involved analysis of the secretions of *S. japonicum* eggs after 3 h of culture in RPMI-1640 medium (De Marco Verissimo *et al.*, 2019). A total of 95 proteins, again a heterogenous mixture of cytosolic, cytoskeletal and nuclear origin, was uniquely identified in the ES fraction, and justified using SecretomeP to indicate a non-classical secretory pathway. The third study compared the eggs of all three main human schistosomes (Carson *et al.*, 2020), identifying a total of 266, 90 and 50 proteins within the *S. mansoni*, *S. japonicum* and *S. haematobium* putative egg secretomes, respectively. Of note, there was little in common between the 'secretomes' of the three species.

How are we to explain the large discrepancies in the claims made by the four studies that find egg secretomes with over 100 constituents, versus the positively frugal list identified in the author's laboratory? (Mathieson and Wilson, 2010). All studies used liver eggs to maximize sterility in culture, but this means a mixture of eggs in different developmental stages were present. A major distinction was that our analysis of egg secretions used only mature eggs, separated from the mixture on a Percoll gradient. In one of the studies eggs were extracted by mechanical disruption of livers, previously stored overnight at 4°C in 200 mM sodium chloride solution (in retrospect rather harsh conditions), followed by sieving (Cass *et al.*, 2007), while the other used protease (trypsin or collagenase) to digest the eggs free of tissue. Viabilities of between 80% and 96% were recorded, and this certainly allows for contamination from a few damaged/dead eggs leaking their intracellular constituents. Turning that situation on its head, it is arguable that the presence of intracellular markers in the supposed secretions is the best indicator of such damage. It would also explain the apparently random nature of constituents in the egg secretomes. Equally, the practice of using SecretomeP to justify 'non-classical' secretory pathways should ring alarm bells (DeMarco and Verjovski-Almeida, 2009).

There is one further point of contention about egg secretions. It has been suggested that *S. mansoni* eggs cultured in RPMI-1640 medium for 24 h release extracellular vesicles (51–172 nm diameter) that can be recovered from the supernatant for vaccination experiments (Mossallam *et al.*, 2021). Unfortunately, the limits to shell pore size set out in Section 11.3.1 make it very unlikely that an intact schistosome egg would be capable of secreting formed membrane vesicles. With all the above caveats, we are left with a small number of dominant proteins (IPSE, omega-1, kappa-5, MEG-2 and MEG-3 family members) that originate in the subshell envelope. The majority are secreted by the live mature egg to facilitate its escape to the gut lumen, with the shell serving as a slow-release capsule to control egress; kappa-5 appears to remain *in situ* beneath the shell performing a protective function.

There is information on the existence of *ipse*, *omega1* and *kappa5* genes in the deposited genome sequences for *S. haematobium* and *S. japonicum*, but for the most part their protein products have not been characterized, nor do they appear in the lists of supposed ESPs from the two species. The exception is H-IPSE, where the encoded protein contains both a signal peptide and a C-terminal nuclear localization sequence SKR(R/G)RKY (Pennington *et al.*, 2017), as with the *S. mansoni* IPSE. The H-IPSE sequence was shown to direct the endocytosed protein to the nucleus of urothelial cells in culture. The authors speculated that H-IPSE release by eggs deposited in the urothelium of the bladder wall may aid egg escape but were uncertain about the target cell(s). In this context, the injection of *S. haematobium* eggs into the murine bladder wall was found to have a marked suppressive effect on genes encoding claudins involved in junctional complexes between cells, and uroplakins that control bladder wall permeability (Ray *et al.*, 2012). Again, it is unclear whether this would aid egg escape to the lumen. Given the central role of schistosome eggs in pathogenesis this lack of a focus on the major egg secretions really needs to be remedied.

11.3.3 Secretions and egg escape

We are accustomed to the idea that parasites survive in the host by developing immune evasion strategies, but the schistosome egg is an exception to the rule. An active immune response to the egg is essential in mice and humans to facilitate its escape; see Schwartz and Fallon (2018) for a summary of the literature. The weight of evidence has shown that T-cell-deficient, *nu*/*nu* and *scid* mice have severely reduced levels of egg excretion, demonstrably dependent on a deficiency of Th2 cytokines or their receptors. Human patients with HIV-infection and reduced $CD4^+$ T cell counts also showed reduced faecal egg excretion. In terms of the cell biology, the live schistosome egg is deliberately secreting powerful immunoreactive proteins that recruit the host immune response to aid its escape. Immunologists have had a field day exploring the manifold interactions of the immune system with the products of live and dead schistosome eggs, especially as the agents of pathogenesis. However, seen from the viewpoint of the egg that needs to escape, these are largely academic. Put simply, what does the egg recruit from the host response to facilitate its egress, potentially from the blood vessel where it was deposited and then from the gut (or bladder) wall to the lumen?

An analogy can be drawn between the migrating lung schistosomulum and the mature egg, both located in the lumen of blood vessels, and both secreting a mixture of MEG-2 and -3 family protein isoforms. They have different goals, the lung schistosomulum to progress through the pulmonary capillary bed to reach a venule for onward migration, and the egg to burst out into the extravascular space to begin its tissue transit. The general postulate about the protein variation generated by differential splicing of MEG genes is as an immune evasion strategy (DeMarco *et al.*, 2010). Indeed, it is unclear why the schistosome needs three *meg3* and up to eight *meg2* genes encoding closely related proteins, which operate in the close confines of a blood vessel. We can only speculate about the nature of the targets of these small proteins, and to date the MEG-2 family has attracted no interest. The longest isoforms of the MEG-3 family proteins possess 16 cysteine residues that can be aligned in two groups of four pairs, each separated by three amino acids (Wilson, 2012). It is tempting to conclude that the mature protein is a dimer capable of cross-linking surface receptors on the vascular endothelium to achieve a biological effect. It is also possible that the secreted MEGs could be translocated across the vascular endothelium in coated pits to affect the extracellular matrix. It seems clear that the release of these proteins from egg and migrating schistosomulum in the close confines of a blood vessel is intimately linked to their respective goals, but the nature of the interactions remains to be elucidated.

Although proteolytic activity, at 14 and 31 kDa, was detected in casein-substrate gels of fractionated egg secretions (Ashton *et al.*, 2001) no obvious proteases have been identified by proteomic analysis of egg secretions. Indeed, it is more likely that the egg makes use of the enzymatic activity of granuloma cells, especially macrophages in its tissue transit.

T cells are the source of the cytokines that instruct the effector functions of other immune response cells. While immature eggs lodged in portal venules of C57BL/6 mice fail to attract $CD4^+$ T cells (Fig. 11.2.2), once such eggs mature and begin to secrete their complement of proteins from the subshell envelope there is a marked and intense accumulation in the immediate vicinity (Fig. 11.2.3) (Wilson, 2012). Such an aggregation might qualify for the epithet of a proto-granuloma. Histopathological studies have shown that ileal and colonic granulomas around eggs in mice are smaller and contain a much larger proportion of macrophages than hepatic granulomas (Weinstock and Boros, 1983). A low level of collagen and fibronectin in ileal and colonic compared to hepatic granulomas has also been noted (Grimaud *et al.*, 1987), indicating an altogether looser focus of cells around an intestinal egg. The preponderance of Th2 type cells in the mouse intestine resulting from IL-4/IL-13 production leads to the generation of alternatively activated (M2) macrophages, involved in resolution of inflammation. It is possible that a balance between the expression of matrix metalloproteases (MMPs), tissue inhibitors of metalloproteases (TIMPs) in M2 macrophages, acting on collagen isoforms regulates fibrosis in the intestine (Singh *et al.*, 2006) allowing eggs to progress towards the lumen.

The capabilities of IPSE and omega-1, the major egg secretions, need to be integrated into this scheme. In addition to chemokine binding capacity, and interaction with IgE on basophils (and potentially on mucosal mast cells), IPSE also has a nuclear localization signal near the C-terminus giving it the capability to enter cells and translocate to the nucleus (Kaur *et al.*, 2011). What effect this has on the host cells surrounding an egg in transit remains to be established. Omega-1 also has the ability to enter host cells, via C-lectin-type mannose receptors. Its hepatotoxicity via T2 ribonuclease activity was established (Fitzsimmons *et al.*, 2005), but its role in egg escape is less clear. Again, we must assume that it has a deleterious effect on the host response cells that are attracted to the egg in transit. There is one additional factor that may be relevant to egg escape, namely intestinal peristalsis, where repeated waves of smooth muscle contraction and relaxation will deform interstitial spaces in the submucosa and mucosa through which an egg is moving.

A series of experiments with schistosome eggs in a very unusual model of inflammation established to investigate tuberculoid granulomas has provided novel information on the immunological properties of immature versus mature eggs (Takaki *et al.*, 2021). A major problem in following egg transit through the gut wall is that it relies on single timepoint histologic studies of human clinical samples and animal models – hamsters, mice and monkeys. The optical transparency of the zebrafish (*Danio rerio*) hindbrain ventricle has permitted description of the early events of tuberculous granuloma formation in real time using non-invasive, high-resolution, serial intravital microscopy. In this model, *in vitro*-laid immature and mature eggs were implanted into the hindbrain ventricle. The mature eggs induced macrophage recruitment, including granuloma formation, whereas the immature eggs did not. Moreover, the eggshell itself proved to be immunologically inert. The observations confirm that the immature egg is essentially invisible to the host, even as a foreign body, until it reaches maturity and the subshell envelope begins to secrete proteins.

11.4 Host Responses to Eggs

The mature egg deposited in the gut or bladder wall is the vehicle by which the schistosome exits its host to continue the cycle. The least damage with which this is achieved the better for both host and parasite. However, while most infections in humans are subclinical or debilitating, some can in the long term be life threatening. It is worth considering how serious clinical conditions can arise, as a result of responses to eggs.

11.4.1 Granulomas and pipe-stem fibrosis

A potential outcome of prolonged schistosomiasis mansoni or schistosomiasis japonica is the development of pipe-stem fibrosis in the liver, followed by portal hypertension, porta-systemic anastomoses and resulting downstream sequela such as pulmonary hypertension. Porta-caval shunting occurs in chronically infected mice, but in a period of 12–20 weeks, and as a result of fibrous granuloma formation around eggs embolized in hepatic portal distributaries of the liver (McHugh *et al.*, 1987). This is not the aetiology of pipe-stem fibrosis in humans, which appears after a long period of exposure. Its origin is poorly understood and the only animal model to provide pointers to its cause is the baboon given repeated exposures (Farah *et al.*, 2000). Periportal fibroblast infiltration and extracellular matrix deposition (fibrosis), angiogenesis and bile duct hyperplasia were observed in some animals (Fig. 11.7). The extent of fibrosis correlated with production of the cytokines transforming growth factor-β and IL-4 by T lymphocytes primed by egg antigens. To what extent are the secretions of the subshell envelope responsible for driving this process?

11.4.2 Severe bladder wall pathology

The human bladder is a remarkably plastic organ, which accommodates large distensions and contractions of its wall during normal excretory function. The most important regions for

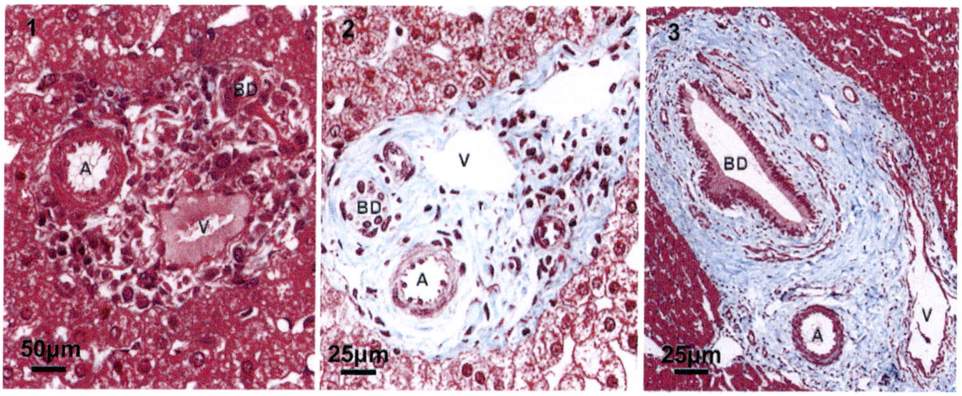

Fig. 11.7. Histopathology of periportal fibrosis in schistosome-infected baboons. **1**) Without fibrosis but a significant mononuclear cell infiltrate. **2**) With periportal fibrosis. **3**) Periportal hyperplasia and angiogenesis. A, artery; V, vein; and BD, bile duct, which constitute the characteristic triad of the portal tract. Collagen deposits are stained blue with Masson's Trichrome (From Farah *et al.*, 2000, reproduced with the permission of Dr Thomas Kariuki, Science for Africa Foundation, Nairobi, Kenya).

schistosomes are the lamina propria connective tissue layer, and its overlying transitional epithelium, the urothelium (Fig. 11.8.1) (Birder and Kullmann, 2018). In normal bladder the lamina propria appears as a loose fibrous network well supplied with arterioles and venules, while the

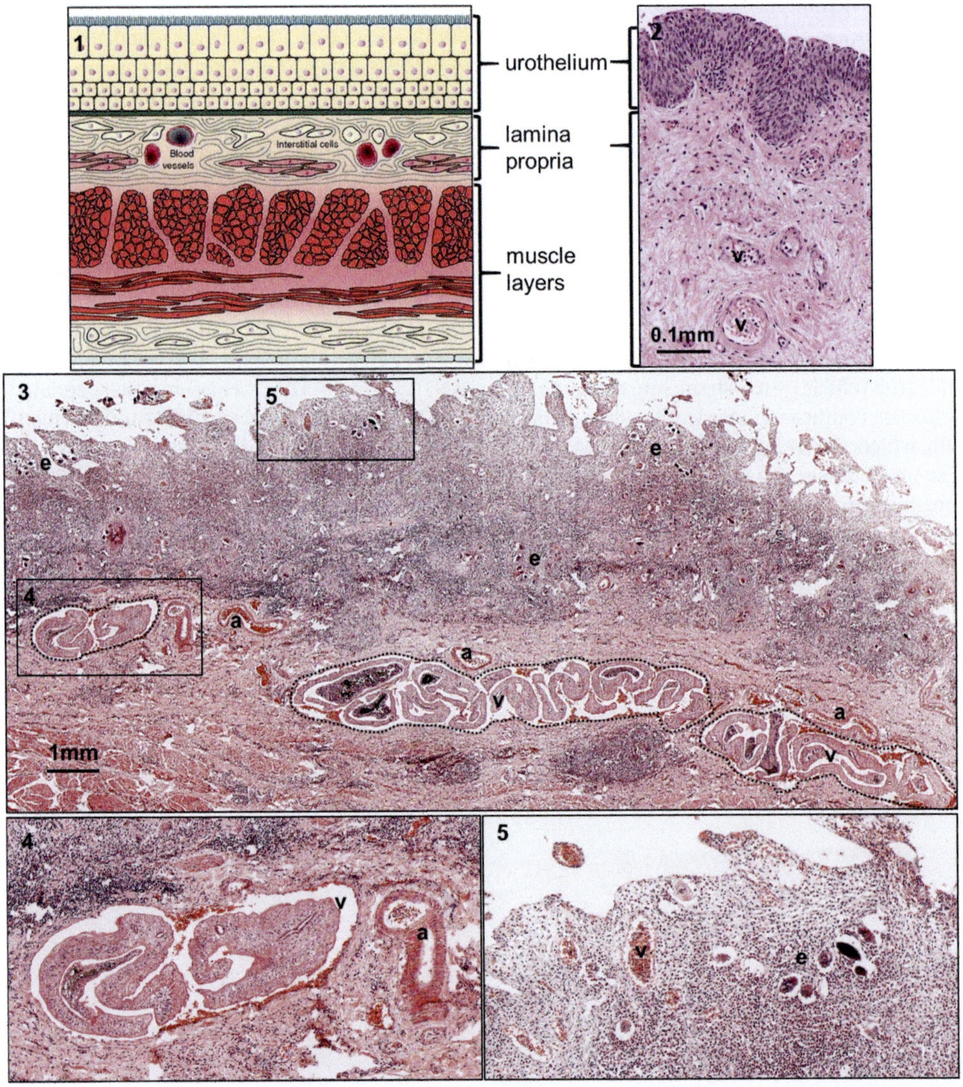

Fig. 11.8. Histopathology of the human bladder wall after *S. haematobium* infection. **1**) Diagram of the normal wall with muscle layers, plus overlying lamina propria and urothelium. **2**) Histology of the lamina propria, a largely fibrous extracellular matrix and the overlying urothelial transitional epithelium. **3**) Low magnification of bladder wall pathology with nests of adult schistosomes (circled) located in lamina propria venules. There is enormous hyperplasia of the urothelium with loss of organized structure and massive leucocytic infiltration. **4**) Higher magnification of worms in a venule of the lamina propria, showing cellular infiltrates, especially dense in the overlying urothelial layer. **5**) The outer edge of the urothelial layer revealing neovascularization, and numbers of eggs, some with defined contents. e, eggs; v, venule; a, arteriole. (**1** from Birder and Kullman, 2018; **2** from Sardana R. and Parwani, A. Histology. PathologyOutlines.com (https://www.pathologyoutlines.com/topic/bladderhistology.html); **3–5** courtesy of Professor Bobbi Pritt, The Mayo Clinic, Rochester, WI, USA.) **1**) Figure used under license CC-BY-4.0.

urothelium is a deep layer of cells which differentiate towards the surface, culminating in an impermeable surface barrier (Fig. 11.8.2). Our knowledge of the impact of schistosomiasis haematobia on the human bladder derives largely from classical histopathology studies on organs at autopsy (Von Lichtenberg *et al.*, 1971) or after surgical removal, often because of squamous cell carcinoma (Cheever *et al.*, 1975; Cheever, 1985). The adult worm pairs are recorded as 'nesting' in a small area of the bladder wall in clusters (Fig. 11.8.3 and 11.8.4), which in turn leads to localized egg deposition and focal lesions. Our knowledge of disease progression in the bladder wall and ureters derives from histopathological observations on a small number of chimpanzees, performed >50 years ago (Sadun *et al.*, 1970). The lesions progress from bulky (polypoid) inflammatory masses to fibrous patches, finally ending up as 'sandy patches'. Many deposited eggs become calcified, contributing to the persistence of the lesions. The urothelium is thickened, losing its organized structure, and showing massive leucocytic infiltrations. Eggs must now cross a much wider and disorganized barrier. New blood vessels form in this layer, which may aid egg deposition (Fig. 11.8.5). The lack of a suitable animal model means that the role of both adult worm and mature egg products in the generation of bladder pathology is poorly understood. The way in which *S. haematobium* infection causes bladder cancer is also still an open question. Does it result from prolonged production of egg secretions that are putatively carcinogenic or from damage to the urothelial permeability barrier that allows ingress of concentrated toxic compounds, or pathogenic microbes, from the urine?

11.4.3 Adult worms and eggs in the wrong place

On occasion adult worms and their eggs can end up in the wrong location. This is evident when porta-caval anastomoses in humans and animal models breach the integrity of the portal tract allowing both stages to escape downstream to the lungs, with ensuing damage to that organ. There are hundreds of case reports in the literature of ectopic schistosomes and their eggs in the brain or spinal cord region, but no explanation of how they developed there. It is probably the strongest argument for not trialling the radiation-attenuated cercarial vaccine (see Chapter 9) in human populations. The other and increasingly appreciated occurrence is in schistosomiasis haematobia where eggs are found in parts of the female genital tract, especially the cervix, fallopian tubes and vagina, potentially because of anastomoses between blood vessels of the pelvic organs (Kjetland *et al.*, 2012). The 'sandy patch' lesions are present on mucosal surfaces and may persist in adult humans, where the eggs become calcified long after praziquantel treatment has removed the adult worms. These lesions are also associated with increased susceptibility to sexually transmitted diseases. The reasons why *S. haematobium* eggs should spill over from the bladder wall to pelvic organs are unclear but provide another argument for the detailed appraisal of their structure and secretions.

11.5 Summary

- The ectolecithal schistosome egg has unusual properties that set it apart, even from other trematode eggs. It is deposited in a subsurface venule of the intestine or bladder. The zygote then develops into the miracidium over about 5–6 days *in situ*, acquiring two-thirds of its nutrients from the host. Consequently, the egg actually increases in size, during which time a syncytial subshell envelope develops.
- The maturation of this envelope and the start of secretion is the trigger for escape from the blood vessel. Host inflammatory cells are recruited to its vicinity, aiding its passage through mucosal tissues and exit to the exterior. This is a remarkable employment of what would normally be considered host-protective, to the schistosome's advantage. The detailed role of host cells in egg expulsion remains sketchy, especially with respect to tissue 'solubilization'.
- The properties of the tanned protein eggshell determine what can enter or escape from the living egg. Evidence points to an upper limit for proteins of around 60 kDa, certainly not large enough to permit the release of preformed membrane vesicles.

- Labelling studies, combined with proteomic analysis of cultured egg secretions, indicate that only a very discrete cohort of proteins is released from the mature living egg, not the hundreds of internal components advocated in some publications. IPSE and omega-1 glycoproteins are the major constituents, together with minor MEG-2 and MEG-3 family members. These MEGs were also released by intravascular lung schistosomula, suggesting a role in egg escape from the blood vessel. IPSE and omega-1 potentially alter the gene expression patters of host leucocytes.
- A third major protein synthesized by the subshell envelope, the kappa-5 dimer, appears too large to pass through the shell but accumulates beneath it as Reynolds' layer. Its function may be protection of the enclosed miracidium from the ingress of host leucocyte toxins. The identity of such toxins is an important outstanding question.
- Host responses to egg secretions and the products released from dead eggs/miracidia are central to the generation of fibrotic pathology in the liver or bladder wall. The conditions are slow to develop, have a massive impact on tissue function, and are largely irreversible when the infection is terminated by chemotherapy. The persistence of these lesions in the liver or urogenital organs is one of the strongest arguments for the development of a prophylactic vaccine.

References

Ashton, P.D., Harrop, R., Shah, B. and Wilson, R.A. (2001) The *Schistosome* egg: development and secretions. *Parasitology* 122(3), 329–338. DOI: 10.1017/S0031182001007351

Birder, L.A. and Kullmann, F.A. (2018) Role of neurogenic inflammation in local communication in the visceral mucosa. *Seminars in Immunopathology* 40(3), 261–279. DOI: 10.1007/s00281-018-0674-0

Cao, H.M., Wang, Y.F. and Long, S. (1982) A study of ultrastructure of egg shell of *Schistosoma japonicum*. I. Transmission electron microscopic observation of *S. japonicum* egg. *Annales de Parasitologie Humaine et Comparée* 57(4), 345–352. DOI: 10.1051/parasite/1982574345

Carson, J.P., Robinson, M.W., Hsieh, M.H., Cody, J., Le, L. *et al.* (2020) A comparative proteomics analysis of the egg secretions of three major *Schistosome* species. *Molecular and Biochemical Parasitology* 240, 111322. DOI: 10.1016/j.molbiopara.2020.111322

Cass, C.L., Johnson, J.R., Califf, L.L., Xu, T., Hernandez, H.J. *et al.* (2007) Proteomic analysis of *Schistosoma mansoni* egg secretions. *Molecular and Biochemical Parasitology* 155(2), 84–93. DOI: 10.1016/j.molbiopara.2007.06.002

Castro-Borges, W. and Wilson, R.A. (2022) *Schistosome* proteomics: updates and clinical implications. *Expert Review of Proteomics* 19(4–6), 247–261. DOI: 10.1080/14789450.2022.2142565

Cheever, A.W. (1985) *Schistosoma haematobium*: the pathology of experimental infection. *Experimental Parasitology* 59(2), 131–138. DOI: 10.1016/0014-4894(85)90065-7

Cheever, A.W. and Powers, K.G. (1972) *Schistosoma mansoni* infection in rhesus monkeys: comparison of the course of heavy and light infections. *Bulletin of the World Health Organization* 46, 301–309. DOI: 10.665/263445

Cheever, A.W., Torky, A.H. and Shirbiney, M. (1975) The relation of worm burden to passage of *Schistosoma haematobium* eggs in the urine of infected patients. *The American Journal of Tropical Medicine and Hygiene* 24(2), 284–288. DOI: 10.4269/ajtmh.1975.24.284

Damian, R.T., Greene, N.D., Meyer, K.F. and Cheever, A.W. (1976) *Schistosoma mansoni* in baboons. III. The course and characteristics of infection, with additional observations on immunity. *The American Journal of Tropical Medicine and Hygiene* 25, 299–306. DOI: 10.4269/ajtmh.1976.25.299

De Jonge, F., Van Nassauw, L., Van Meir, F., Miller, H.R.P., Van Marck, E. *et al.* (2002) Temporal distribution of distinct mast cell phenotypes during intestinal schistosomiasis in mice. *Parasite Immunology* 24(5), 225–231. DOI: 10.1046/j.1365-3024.2002.00457.x

De Marco Verissimo, C., Potriquet, J., You, H., McManus, D.P., Mulvenna, J. *et al.* (2019) Qualitative and quantitative proteomic analyses of *Schistosoma japonicum* eggs and egg-derived secretory-excretory proteins. *Parasites & Vectors* 12(1), 173. DOI: 10.1186/s13071-019-3403-1

DeMarco, R. and Verjovski-Almeida, S. (2009) *Schistosomes* – proteomics studies for potential novel vaccines and drug targets. *Drug Discovery Today* 14(9–10), 472–478. DOI: 10.1016/j.drudis.2009.01.011

DeMarco, R., Mathieson, W., Manuel, S.J., Dillon, G.P., Curwen, R.S. *et al.* (2010) Protein variation in blood-dwelling *Schistosome* worms generated by differential splicing of micro-exon gene transcripts. *Genome Research* 20(8), 1112–1121. DOI: 10.1101/gr.100099.109

Everts, B., Hussaarts, L., Driessen, N.N., Meevissen, M.H.J., Schramm, G. *et al.* (2012) *Schistosome*-derived omega-1 drives Th2 polarization by suppressing protein synthesis following internalization by the mannose receptor. *Journal of Experimental Medicine* 209(10), 1753–1767. DOI: 10.1084/jem.20111381

Farah, I.O., Nyindo, M., Suleman, M.A., Nyaundi, J., Kariuki, T.M. *et al.* (1997) *Schistosoma mansoni*: development and modulation of the granuloma after single or multiple exposures in the baboon (*Papio cynocephalus anubis*). *Experimental Parasitology* 86(2), 93–101. DOI: 10.1006/expr.1997.4152

Farah, I.O., Mola, P.W., Kariuki, T.M., Nyindo, M., Blanton, R.E. *et al.* (2000) Repeated exposure induces periportal fibrosis in *Schistosoma mansoni*-infected baboons: role of TGF-β and IL-4. *The Journal of Immunology* 164(10), 5337–5343. DOI: 10.4049/jimmunol.164.10.5337

Fitzsimmons, C.M., Schramm, G., Jones, F.M., Chalmers, I.W., Hoffmann, K.F. *et al.* (2005) Molecular characterization of omega-1: a hepatotoxic ribonuclease from *Schistosoma mansoni* eggs. *Molecular and Biochemical Parasitology* 144(1), 123–127. DOI: 10.1016/j.molbiopara.2005.08.003

Gonçalves-Silva, G., Vieira, L.G.M. dos S., Cosenza-Contreras, M., Souza, A.F.P., Costa, D.C. *et al.* (2022) Profiling the serum proteome during *Schistosoma mansoni* infection in the BALB/c mice: a focus on the altered lipid metabolism as a key modulator of host-parasite interactions. *Frontiers in Immunology* 13, 955049. DOI: 10.3389/fimmu.2022.955049

Grimaud, J.A., Boros, D.L., Takiya, C., Mathew, R.C. and Emonard, H. (1987) Collagen isotypes, laminin, and fibronectin in granulomas of the liver and intestines of *Schistosoma mansoni*-infected mice. *The American Society of Tropical Medicine and Hygiene* 37(2), 335–344. DOI: 10.4269/ajtmh.1987.37.335

Hillyer, G.V., Ramzy, R.M.R., El Alamy, M.A. and Cline, B.L. (1980) Immunodiagnosis of infection with *Schistosoma haematobium* and *S. mansoni* in man. *The American Journal of Tropical Medicine and Hygiene* 29(6), 1254–1257. DOI: 10.4269/ajtmh.1980.29.1254

Jurberg, A.D., Gonçalves, T., Costa, T.A., de Mattos, A.C.A., Pascarelli, B.M. *et al.* (2009) The embryonic development of *Schistosoma mansoni* eggs: proposal for a new staging system. *Development Genes and Evolution* 219(5), 219–234. DOI: 10.1007/s00427-009-0285-9

Kaur, I., Schramm, G., Everts, B., Scholzen, T., Kindle, K.B. *et al.* (2011) Interleukin-4-inducing principle from *Schistosoma mansoni* eggs contains a functional C-terminal nuclear localization signal necessary for nuclear translocation in mammalian cells but not for its uptake. *Infection and Immunity* 79(4), 1779–1788. DOI: 10.1128/IAI.01048-10

Kjetland, E.F., Leutscher, P.D.C. and Ndhlovu, P.D. (2012) A review of female genital schistosomiasis. *Trends in Parasitology* 28(2), 58–65. DOI: 10.1016/j.pt.2011.10.008

Knuhr, K., Langhans, K., Nyenhuis, S., Viertmann, K., Kildemoes, A.M.O. *et al.* (2018) *Schistosoma mansoni* egg-released IPSE/alpha-1 dampens inflammatory cytokine responses via basophil interleukin (IL)-4 and IL-13. *Frontiers in Immunology* 9, 2293. DOI: 10.3389/fimmu.2018.02293

Mathieson, W. and Wilson, R.A. (2010) A comparative proteomic study of the undeveloped and developed *Schistosoma mansoni* egg and its contents: the miracidium, hatch fluid and secretions. *International Journal for Parasitology* 40(5), 617–628. DOI: 10.1016/j.ijpara.2009.10.014

McHugh, S.M., Coulson, P.S. and Wilson, R.A. (1987) The relationship between pathology and resistance to reinfection with *Schistosoma mansoni* in mice: a causal mechanism of resistance in chronic infections. *Parasitology* 94(1), 81–91. DOI: 10.1017/S0031182000053476

Michaels, R.M. and Prata, A. (1968) Evolution and characteristics of *Schistosoma mansoni* eggs laid *in vitro*. *The Journal of Parasitology* 54(5), 921–930. DOI: 10.2307/3277120

Miller, H.R.P., Newlands, G.F.J., McKellar, A., Inglis, L., Coulson, P.S. *et al.* (1994) Hepatic recruitment of mast cells occurs in rats but not mice infected with *Schistosoma mansoni*. *Parasite Immunology* 16(3), 145–155. DOI: 10.1111/j.1365-3024.1994.tb00334.x

Mossallam, S.F., Abou-El-Naga, I.F., Abdel Bary, A., Elmorsy, E.A. and Diab, R.G. (2021) *Schistosoma mansoni* egg-derived extracellular vesicles: a promising vaccine candidate against murine schistosomiasis. *PLoS Neglected Tropical Diseases* 15(10), e0009866. DOI: 10.1371/journal.pntd.0009866

Neill, P.J.G., Smith, J.H., Doughty, B.L. and Kemp, M. (1988) The ultrastructure of the *Schistosoma mansoni* egg. *The American Journal of Tropical Medicine and Hygiene* 39(1), 52–65. DOI: 10.4269/ajtmh.1988.39.52

Pellegrino, J. and Coelho, P.M.Z. (1978) *Schistosoma mansoni*: wandering capacity of a worm couple. *The Journal of Parasitology* 64(1), 181. DOI: 10.2307/3279647

Pennington, L.F., Alouffi, A., Mbanefo, E.C., Ray, D., Heery, D.M. *et al.* (2017) H-IPSE is a pathogen-secreted host nucleus-infiltrating protein (Infiltrin) expressed exclusively by the *Schistosoma haematobium* egg stage. *Infection and Immunity* 85(12). DOI: 10.1128/IAI.00301-17

Ray, D., Nelson, T.A., Fu, C.-L., Patel, S., Gong, D.N. *et al.* (2012) Transcriptional profiling of the bladder in urogenital schistosomiasis reveals pathways of inflammatory fibrosis and urothelial compromise. *PLoS Neglected Tropical Diseases* 6(11), e1912. DOI: 10.1371/journal.pntd.0001912

Sadun, E.H., Von Lichtenberg, F., Cheever, A.W., Erickson, D.G. and Hickman, R.L. (1970) Experimental infection with *Schistosoma haematobium* in chimpanzees. *The American Journal of Tropical Medicine and Hygiene* 19(3), 427–458. DOI: 10.4269/ajtmh.1970.19.427

Schramm, G., Falcone, F.H., Gronow, A., Haisch, K., Mamat, U. *et al.* (2003) Molecular characterization of an interleukin-4-inducing factor from *Schistosoma mansoni* eggs. *Journal of Biological Chemistry* 278(20), 18384–18392. DOI: 10.1074/jbc.M300497200

Schramm, G., Hamilton, J.V., Balog, C.I.A., Wuhrer, M., Gronow, A. *et al.* (2009) Molecular characterisation of kappa-5, a major antigenic glycoprotein from *Schistosoma mansoni* eggs. *Molecular and Biochemical Parasitology* 166(1), 4–14. DOI: 10.1016/j.molbiopara.2009.02.003

Schwartz, C. and Fallon, P.G. (2018) *Schistosoma* 'eggs-iting' the host: granuloma formation and egg excretion. *Frontiers in Immunology* 9, 2492. DOI: 10.3389/fimmu.2018.02492

Shiels, J., Cwiklinski, K., Alvarado, R., Thivierge, K., Cotton, S. *et al.* (2020) *Schistosoma mansoni* immunomodulatory molecule Sm16/SPO-1/SmSLP is a member of the trematode-specific helminth defence molecules (HDMs). *PLoS Neglected Tropical Diseases* 14(7), e0008470. DOI: 10.1371/journal.pntd.0008470

Singh, K.P., Gerard, H.C., Hudson, A.P. and Boros, D.L. (2006) Differential expression of collagen, MMP, TIMP and fibrogenic-cytokine genes in the granulomatous colon of *Schistosoma mansoni*-infected mice. *Annals of Tropical Medicine & Parasitology* 100(7), 611–620. DOI: 10.1179/136485906X118530

Smith, P., Fallon, R.E., Mangan, N.E., Walsh, C.M., Saraiva, M. *et al.* (2005) *Schistosoma mansoni* secretes a chemokine binding protein with antiinflammatory activity. *The Journal of Experimental Medicine* 202(10), 1319–1325. DOI: 10.1084/jem.20050955

Sotillo, J., Pearson, M.S., Becker, L., Mekonnen, G.G., Amoah, A.S. *et al.* (2019) In-depth proteomic characterization of *Schistosoma haematobium*: towards the development of new tools for elimination. *PLoS Neglected Tropical Diseases* 13(5), e0007362. DOI: 10.1371/journal.pntd.0007362

Takaki, K.K., Rinaldi, G., Berriman, M., Pagán, A.J. and Ramakrishnan, L. (2021) *Schistosoma mansoni* eggs modulate the timing of granuloma formation to promote transmission. *Cell Host & Microbe* 29(1), 58–67. DOI: 10.1016/j.chom.2020.10.002

Von Lichtenberg, F., Edington, G.M., Nwabuebo, I., Taylor, J.R. and Smith, J.H. (1971) Pathologic effects of *Schistomiasis* in Ibadan, Western State of Nigeria. II. Pathogenesis of lesions of the bladder and ureters. *The American Journal of Tropical Medicine and Hygiene* 20(2), 244–254. DOI: 10.4269/ajtmh.1971.20.244

Weinstock, J.V. and Boros, D.L. (1983) Organ-dependent differences in composition and function observed in hepatic and intestinal granulomas isolated from mice with *Schistosomiasis mansoni*. *The Journal of Immunology* 130(1), 418–422. DOI: 10.4049/jimmunol.130.1.418

Wilson, R.A. (2012) Virulence factors of *Schistosomes*. *Microbes and Infection* 14(15), 1442–1450. DOI: 10.1016/j.micinf.2012.09.001

12

Diagnostics: Can the Deficit be Fixed?

12.1 Overview

The landscape of schistosomiasis control has changed dramatically over the last 50 years, especially since the introduction of praziquantel as a potent anti-schistosomal agent by Bayer AG (Gonnert and Andrews, 1977) and its adoption by the World Health Organization (WHO) as the principal treatment for human infections. Mass drug administration programmes have reduced the frequency of severe cases and overall morbidity, but transmission continues in most endemic countries, with few successful eradication programmes. This is where a shortfall in diagnosis comes to the fore. A range of diagnostic techniques has been developed and form the subject matter of this chapter. However, while their sensitivity is adequate for individuals with medium or high worm burdens, they struggle to detect low levels of infection. Indeed, it is easy to miss infections completely in a disease that has a prolonged time course and no outward symptoms.

In recent years, the sensitivity of diagnosis has increased and so has the realization that there are more low-level infections, which translates to a higher overall prevalence (Colley *et al.*, 2017). This has significant implications for national control and eradication programmes. The most obvious starting point for detection of a current infection is to look for eggs in urine or faeces, depending on species. The other major avenue is to detect parasite products in the blood or urine, which worms must release in their interaction with the host. In this context, the use of a urine sample for diagnosis is non-invasive so highly desirable but requires that blood analytes must be small enough to cross the kidney filtration barrier. A different angle is provided by detection of antibodies to schistosomes in blood or other body fluids, popular but with serious limitations. There are two criteria against which progress can be measured. The first is to evaluate how far towards the goal of single worm pair detection we have travelled. The second is to assess how user-friendly diagnostic techniques have become. Are they suitable for 'point-of-care' (POC) diagnosis in surveys of human populations for the prevalence of schistosome infection?

12.2 Eggs

12.2.1 Eggs and haemoglobin in urine

Theoretically the diagnosis of *Schistosoma haematobium* infections ought to be very straightforward. The adult pairs live in the blood vessels of the bladder wall, where eggs are deposited in the lamina propria between the detrusor muscles and the stratified urothelium. After a period of

DOI: 10.1079/9781800625167.0012

development, the mature egg then crosses these layers to reach the bladder lumen for expulsion in the urine. Unfortunately, there is no animal model that replicates this, and human tissue samples are usually taken from cases of advanced infection or bladder carcinoma, so our knowledge is therefore largely conjectural. However, one fact is clear, the escape of eggs is accompanied by release of blood via the exit tunnel so must involve significant tissue disruption. This has made detection of haematuria one of the most frequently used and recommended test for *S. haematobium* infection, albeit using an indirect correlate. This can be achieved in almost any setting using a cheap commercially available dipstick (e.g. Hemastix) that can detect as little as 1.5 μg of haemoglobin in 10 ml of urine (Savioli *et al.*, 1990). Taking 30 pg of haemoglobin as the content of one erythrocyte, that is equivalent to a mere 50,000 erythrocytes.

The complementary approach is to concentrate a volume of urine, e.g. through a filter disc with a pore size of 20 μm. The disc can then be stained and the eggs counted under a dissector by a trained microscopist. Egg counts of 0–50 eggs/10 ml urine have been taken as indicators of a light to medium infection. This brings us to another problem with detection of *S. haematobium* infections. Unlike the situation for *Schistosoma mansoni* or *Schistosoma japonicum*, it is difficult to define infection intensity. We must rely on material from patients scheduled for cystectomy due to carcinoma or exstrophy of the bladder, where the number of eggs passed in the urine was assessed preoperatively (Cheever *et al.*, 1975). There is an additional problem of locating worms by tissue dissection. With those caveats, a linear regression of the number of embryonated eggs passed in the urine against worm pairs gave a daily estimate of 432 embryonated eggs per pair. This would place *S. haematobium* as somewhere between *S. mansoni* and *S. japonicum* in its fecundity. More than half of tissue eggs were found in the bladder wall or tumour. The fraction of eggs that escape is uncertain and currently the thinking to explain the pathogenic sequelae is that majority become inadvertently sequestered in tissues rather than passed into the urinary tract (Donnelly *et al.*, 2024). Where the methods of detection have been compared, yet another factor has emerged, namely the daily variability of egg excretion (Savioli *et al.*, 1990). In a survey over 6 consecutive days, monitoring of daily egg counts in individuals revealed extreme fluctuation from negative to heavily infected (>50 eggs/10 ml of urine). At the population level, the prevalence of heavy infection in those <20 years of age was higher based on egg counts compared to gross haematuria, while for adults >25 years, haematuria predicted a higher prevalence. As with other aspects of *S. haematobium* infection, this situation underlines the scarcity of reliable data.

A different approach not relying on the visual identification of eggs for diagnosis has been to detect their associated DNA in urine samples. This was made feasible by the discovery of a repeated DraI sequence, consisting of tandemly arranged 121 bp repeats, originally suggested as a tag to detect the presence of cercariae in fresh water (Hamburger *et al.*, 2001). The repeats comprise ~15% of the *S. haematobium* genome. Using RT-PCR it proved possible to detect as little as 10 fg of DNA or a single cercaria, but the analogous repeat sequence from *S. mansoni* was not amplified. The detection of DraI repeats was subsequently developed as a diagnostic test for schistosomiasis haematobia in urine samples. It has been trialled in comparison with haematuria reagent strips and urine filtration for eggs, detecting more than twice as many positive urine samples (Keller *et al.*, 2020). The internal transcribed spacer-2 sequence from *S. haematobium* ribosomes has been used as another target for RT-PCR on 0.2 ml of patient urine (Obeng *et al.*, 2008). It was found to be 100% positive in high-intensity and 87% positive in low intensity infections (<50 eggs/10 ml urine). However, while quantitative PCR may be able to assess more accurately the prevalence and incidence of *S. haematobium* infections than classical parasitological methods, it is not a rapid diagnostic test. It requires a well-equipped laboratory, experienced technicians and a considerable amount of time, particularly for DNA extraction. It seems better suited to a clinical environment where individual diagnosis is important, and where migrants, travellers and tourists may present with very light infections.

With these limitations in mind, attempts have been made to find DNA detection methods that are both sensitive and adaptable to a POC setting. These include loop-mediated isothermal amplification and recombinase polymerase amplification (RPA). Both are single-tube systems performed at constant temperature, so dispensing with the need for a thermal cycler. At present, the RPA method seems to be the front runner, operating best at temperatures of 37–42°C, and more slowly at room temperature. It has already been used to diagnose several other pathogens at POC (Archer *et al.*, 2020) and shown to be capable of detecting 10 copies of synthetic DraI DNA, or one *S. haematobium* egg spiked in a urine sample. Current efforts are directed towards making the RPA assay suitable for use in endemic settings (Donnelly *et al.*, 2024; Mesquita *et al.*, 2025). See also https://www.cor-ntd.org/research-outcomes/studies/molecular-isothermal-diagnostics-schistosomiasis-mids.

12.2.2 Eggs in faeces

The number of eggs laid per female *S. japonicum* or *S. mansoni* worm presents a surprising limitation for the simple approach of diagnosis by faecal sampling as there is no equivalent to urine concentration (Ogongo *et al.*, 2018). The reported values are in the region of 2000 and 300 per day, respectively, with <100% excreted in the faeces. Human faecal output in a low-income setting has been estimated as 250 g per day (Rose *et al.*, 2015). This translates to a maximum of 8 eggs per gram of faeces for *S. japonicum* and 1.2 per gram for *S. mansoni*.

The standard approach for decades to measure intestinal schistosomiasis has been the Kato-Katz (KK) faecal smear. This standardized method requires a template with a hole 6 mm diameter and 1.5 mm deep, which is filled level with ~50 mg of stool sample. The template is then removed and replaced with a strip of cellophane, with glycerol/malachite green stain added, and gently compressed. The strip is then examined under a microscope to count the eggs. In the most favourable circumstances, using the estimates above, the theoretical number of worm pairs needed to provide one egg in 50 mg, i.e. 20 eggs per gram, is 17 for *S. mansoni* or 2.5 for *S. japonicum*. In practice, the odds are worse than this. For example, loose stools are difficult to read and *S. japonicum* eggs are much smaller.

In fact, it is possible to perform a direct calibration of the KK smear using data from primate experiments, where the surrogate technique for worm number (eggs per gram of faeces) was determined before the animals were perfused to estimate actual worm burden (Fig. 12.1) (Wilson *et al.*, 2006). The regression of eggs on worm burden was based on data from 37 baboons, which had burdens ranging between 25 and 555 worms, after a 600 cercarial challenge. A total of nine KK smears were made when egg

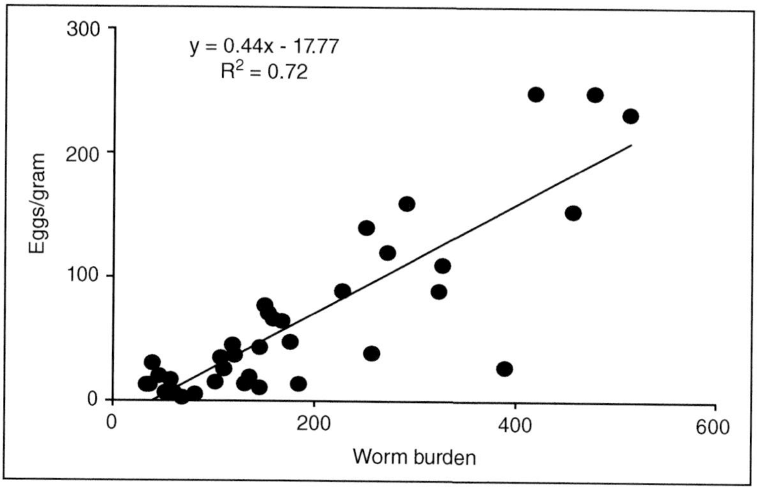

Fig. 12.1. Calibration of the faecal smear technique. The detection limit for the KK smear in baboons infected with *S. mansoni.* Worm burdens were determined by portal perfusion at 10 weeks. Values are means of triplicate smears performed at weeks 8, 9 and 10 after cercarial exposure = a total of nine smears. (From Wilson *et al.*, 2006.) Figure used with permission from Elsevier.

output reached a steady state, three each at weeks 8, 9 and 10 post-infection. The intercept on the *x*-axis gives a value of 40 worms which, adjusted for the observed 1.5:1 male:female sex ratio, equates to 16 worm pairs. (A similar calibration for *S. japonicum* is not available.) Can anything be done to improve the sensitivity of faecal egg detection?

Flotation techniques have been used to enrich helminth parasite eggs in faeces. They work well with *Ascaris* and *Trichuris* when a larger faecal sample is comminuted using zinc sulphate or sucrose solutions of high specific gravity (1.18–1.25). The eggs are protected by their impermeant vitelline membrane and float off the debris for easy counting. This approach, referred to as FLOTAC, has been tried with *S. mansoni* using 5 g of faeces, 100 times the amount for a KK smear (Glinz *et al.*, 2010). The technique detected a higher prevalence of infection than the KK smear on the same samples, but a lower intensity, suggesting that many eggs were not recovered by flotation; this was confirmed by the images of eggs displayed, which were seriously deformed, with fluids sucked out.

In primate experiments a different flotation approach was developed to solve the problem of reading KK smears from animals with diarrhoea, while preserving the integrity of *S. mansoni* eggs (Eberl *et al.*, 2002). This involved layering 0.25 g of faeces over a 60% Percoll gradient, with a slightly higher density than eggs, and negligible osmolarity. The debris and particulates float off and the eggs are pelleted for counting on a slide. The method was 10–20 times more effective than a KK smear. Moreover, when used with human faecal samples in Egypt, it detected not just *S. mansoni* eggs but also those from other pathogenic helminths, including *Ascaris lumbricoides*, *Trichuris trichiura*, *Enterobius vermicularis*, *Hymenolepis nana* and *Fasciola hepatica*. Unfortunately, the method requires laboratory equipment and an expensive reagent so is only suited to laboratory studies.

A third enrichment method for eggs, based on the physical their properties, has been named Helmintex (Fagundes Teixeira *et al.*, 2007). It has a starting sample of 30 g faeces, processed through a series of sieves to exclude debris but permit egg passage, and claims to detect 1.3 eggs per gram of faeces, with a sensitivity of 100%, far outperforming the KK smear. The eggs in the sample were reacted with a variety of lectins and concentrated using paramagnetic beads – these are essential as latex beads cannot substitute. The way the beads bind to eggs has been explored, with a rather hazy conclusion that it is more likely to be related to surface charge-based electrostatic interactions between eggs and magnetic iron oxide rather than through a direct magnetic interaction (Candido *et al.*, 2015). A second study demonstrated that eggshells contained iron in measurable amounts, detectable in the lacunae, most likely as an iron–phosphate complex (Karl *et al.*, 2013). However, the eggs did not move in a magnetic field, so the binding of microspheres was unlikely to be magnetic in origin. Spontaneous binding of microspheres to *S. japonicum* eggs occurred to a greater degree than to *S. mansoni* eggs, and this was attributed to a filamentous coat detected by scanning electron microscopy (SEM). Given that fresh eggs are likely to be coated in secreted IPSE and omega-1 proteins (see Chapter 11), the possibility of improving the efficiency of binding by coating microspheres with specific antibodies to those proteins ought to be investigated.

12.2.3 DNA in faeces

The detection of *S. mansoni* egg DNA in faeces has a long history, based on the 121 tandem repeat sequence (Hamburger *et al.*, 1991), using RT-PCR as the amplification method (Pontes *et al.*, 2002). It was capable of detecting 1 fg of DNA in as few as 2.4 eggs per gram of faeces, 10 times more sensitive than the KK smear. It has proved to have some clear advantages in regions of low endemicity, where individuals may have low parasite loads but are still capable of transmitting infection to snails (Magalhães *et al.*, 2020). In this cross-sectional study of a community in Brazil, using RT-PCR on the tandem repeat, it performed better at identifying cases with low (<100 eggs per gram) or very low (<12 eggs per gram) parasite loads than either a consolidated reference standard (KK smear, saline gradient, Helmintex) or a POC circulating cathodic antigen test (POC-CCA). The DNA was recovered using a QIAamp DNA Stool Mini Kit and it is not clear if steps were taken to lyse any eggs, e.g. by sonication, before extraction.

The same RT-PCR approach with *S. japonicum* infections used an abundant tandemly repeated genomic DNA sequence of 101 base pairs, designated SjTR1 (Halili *et al.*, 2021). The assay could detect a single egg spiked into a 1 g faecal sample and out-performed the traditional KK smear, especially at low infection intensity. One downside was that the assay also detected the closely related *Schistosoma mekongi*. However, these two Asian species barely overlap in their geographical range, so RT-PCR may provide a method for confirming the occurrence of *S. mekongi* in human populations. It is also notable that human stool samples were processed using a FastPrep Spin Kit for soil microorganisms that lyses samples to recover the DNA, an important step where tough eggshells are involved.

12.3 Circulating Antigens

Eggs are the principal output from paired female worms, deposited in the blood vessels of intestinal or bladder tissues. For an *S. mansoni* female laying 300 eggs per day, this has been estimated as ~1 μg of protein (excluding shell) (Castro-Borges and Wilson, 2022). Male testes appear to mature without the need for mating but there is no information about whether such unmated males release spermatozoa into the bloodstream. (This would be easily testable in animals or humans with a single-sex infection.) The adult worms, resident in blood vessels, also release specific macromolecules into the bloodstream as part of their normal biological activities, and these are the other potential source material for diagnosis of a current infection (see Chapter 8). The protein output per worm pair has been estimated as 75 ng per day, predominantly alimentary tract vomitus. Those figures give some idea of the scale of the task for a diagnostic, given that the products will be dispersed through 3.5 l of plasma in an adult human. Of course, death of worms contributes much larger quantities of protein (41 μg for a male, 19 μg for a female) but such occurrences are sporadic except after chemotherapy. The release of proteins from eggs trapped in tissues superficially looks a better source of worm products, but it seems unlikely that they reach the bloodstream from within the fibrous granuloma capsule. For reasons that may reside in their molecular properties, the emphasis has been on detection of the polysaccharide circulating antigens from the worm gut.

12.3.1 Gut-derived circulating cathodic antigen and circulating anodic antigen

A circulating antigen migrating towards the anode was first detected by immunoelectrophoresis in the serum of mice and hamsters with massive worm infections (Berggren and Weller, 1967). Subsequently, this antigen was shown to be soluble in 15% trichloroacetic acid (TCA) so likely to be polysaccharide, with a molecular weight >100 kDa (Nash *et al.*, 1974). A rabbit polyclonal antibody raised against this antigen was used to demonstrate its origin in the worm gastrodermis (Fig. 12.2.1) (Nash, 1974). Working independently, researchers in Leiden, The Netherlands, demonstrated two circulating polysaccharide antigens in the serum of heavily infected hamsters (Deelder *et al.*, 1976). The first later proved to be identical to the high-molecular-weight anodic antigen, the second had a molecular weight <30,000 and migrated towards the cathode. This second was also detectable in urine, presumably due to its lower molecular weight, and the two were given the epithets circulating anodic antigen (CAA) and circulating cathodic antigen (CCA), which are current today.

These were exciting times for diagnostic techniques, with the description of monoclonal antibodies in 1976 (Köhler and Milstein, 1976) and the popularization of the ELISA technique (Voller *et al.*, 1979). In the ensuing years attempts were made to use both monoclonal and polyclonal antibodies, raised against CAA and CCA, as diagnostic tools in radio- or enzyme-linked immunoassays to detect schistosome infections (e.g. Feldmeier *et al.*, 1986). The group in Leiden developed a panel of monoclonal antibodies from which an IgG1 against CAA was selected (Deelder *et al.*, 1989). It was used both as the capture antibody immobilized on ELISA plates and as the detection antibody, directly labelled with alkaline phosphatase, to diagnose *S. mansoni* infections in a group of patients in Zaire. The study relied on and highlighted the fact that CAA contains multiple identical epitopes (see below). At this early stage, it was believed to detect CAA down to a level of 1 ng/ml, based on the assumed

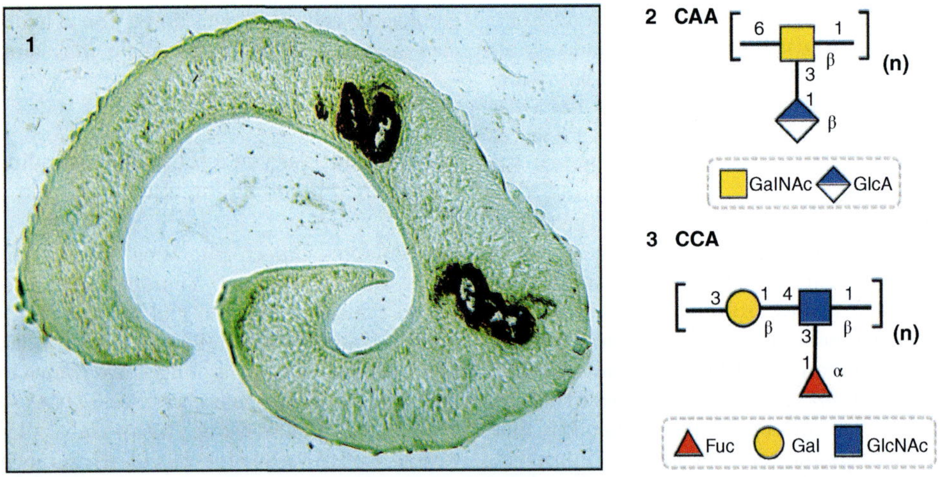

Fig. 12.2. Circulating polysaccharide antigens. **1**) Localization of circulating antigen in a section of adult male gut epithelium using the original rabbit polyclonal antibody, detected using peroxidase-labelled secondary antibody. **2**) Diagram of the repeating unit in CAA, with the formula [–6(GlcAβ1–3)GalNAcβ1–]$_n$. **3**) Diagram of the repeating unit in CCA, with the formula [–3Galβ1–4(Fucα1–3)GlcNAcβ1–]$_n$. GalNAc, *N*-acetylgalactosamine; GlcA, glucuronic acid; Fuc, fucose; Gal, galactose; GlcNAc, *N*-acetylglucosamine. (**2** and **3** and the text describing their properties in Section 12.3.1 were kindly provided by Professor C.H. Hokke, Leiden University Medical Centre, Leiden, The Netherlands; the antibody in **1** was a gift from Dr T. Nash, NIH, Bethesda, MD, USA.)

10% CAA content of the TCA precipitate of adult worm antigen. Subsequent work showed that the precipitate contained much less CAA so limits of detection were ~30 pg/ml. The ELISA assay could detect infection in human patients shedding 7 eggs per gram of faeces, measured by triplicate KK smears.

A variant of the ELISA technique using monoclonal antibodies was also developed for the detection of CCA, with an IgG3 for capture and a biotinylated IgM for detection. Reactivity was then measured using enzyme-labelled streptavidin (de Jonge *et al.*, 1990). The assay was believed at the time to have a dynamic range between 1 and 62.5 ng/ml of a crude preparation containing 20% CCA, later found to be 3%. It was able to detect *S. mansoni* infections in both serum and urine samples from infected patients. The two ELISAs were subsequently used to evaluate schistosomiasis infections using sera and urine from a cohort of Egyptian patients and uninfected controls (Van Lieshout *et al.*, 1992). The assays were performed on TCA-treated supernatants, used at a 1:4 dilution, apart from for urine CAA, which was concentrated 5-fold. This probably reflects the relative molecular sizes of the two antigens, which affects their ability to cross the glomerular filtration barrier, but the strong negative charge of CAA may also be an important factor. The study also identified the higher intrinsic background of the CCA assay, using samples from the controls. Nevertheless, combinations of the assays achieved a sensitivity of 97–98% for detection of schistosome infection.

The chemical structures of the antigenic epitopes exhibited by CAA (Bergwerff *et al.*, 1994) and CCA (van Dam *et al.*, 1994) have been analysed at the Leiden University Medical Centre using a range of glycomic approaches to arrive at consensus sequences (Fig. 12.2). For both CCA and CAA the key to understanding is that they are polysaccharides, perhaps attached to a core lipid or peptide. The structure of the CAA epitope comprises units of [–6(GlcAβ1–3) GalNAcβ1–]$_n$ (Fig. 12.2.2). As far as is known, this repeating CAA structure is unique to schistosomes, accounting for the exquisite specificity of the assay. The specific antigenic epitope is formed by a number of the repeats, and anion-exchange chromatography indicates that there may be more than 30 glucuronic acid residues in a typical

CAA molecule (Bergwerff *et al.*, 1994). By mass spectrometry it is very difficult to define CAA due to the variable chain lengths and the high negative charge. Indeed, separation on SDS-PAGE gels probed by Western blotting detects a smear ranging from 50 to >500 kDa, but this simply reflects the atypical behaviour of polysaccharides in electrophoretic separations. Thus, CAA may be pure polysaccharide or could comprise between 20 and 100 chains attached to a core peptide. As well as multiple epitope binding sites on one CAA molecule, it is also likely that the chains take on a conformational structure when they elongate, potentially due to the acidic groups repelling each other.

The situation with the CCA epitope is even more complex. The specific monoclonal antibody binds to a linear polymer of the trisaccharide [–3Galβ1–4(Fucα1–3)GlcNAcβ1–]$_n$ similar but not identical to Lewis X (LeX) (Fig. 12.2.3). There was an estimated average of 25 of these repeating units per CCA chain (van Dam *et al.*, 1994). CCA may contain an *O*-glycan core linked via Ser/Thr to a protein backbone, but this has yet to be identified, primarily because mucin-like clustered *O*-glycan domains are difficult to analyse. The assay detecting CCA has a higher intrinsic host background, since neither the LeX structure nor the repeating LeX are unique to schistosomes but occur, in addition to sialyl-LeX, on human cells and some human bacterial pathogens such as *Helicobacter pylori*.

The CAA and CCA assays have been used in numerous studies of populations in endemic areas, and research has been directed to improving their sensitivity to the point where they are capable of detecting single worm pair infections. As human mass drug administration programmes have progressed the overall intensity of infections has declined, and the limits of detection become more crucial. The location of the worms in the portal tract or the bladder wall/ureters means that direct estimation of their numbers is not feasible. For *S. mansoni* infection in baboons, where worm burdens have been determined by portal perfusion, a calibration of CAA and CCA ELISA has been possible (Fig. 12.3) (Wilson *et al.*, 2006). The threshold for detection for CAA, based on linear regression, is 24 worms. Adjusted for the observed 1.5:1 male:female ratio this

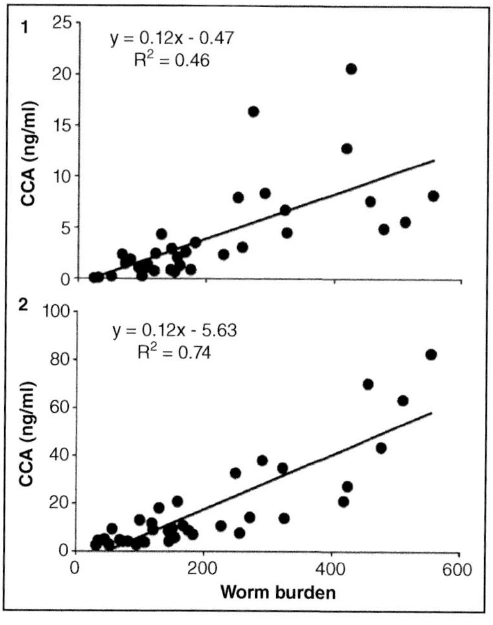

Fig. 12.3. Calibration of the circulating antigen assays. **1**) The detection limits of ELISA for CAA, based on serum levels at weeks 6, 8 and 10 in baboons infected with *S. mansoni*. **2**) The detection limits of ELISA for CCA, based on serum levels at weeks 8 and 10. Worm burdens were determined by portal perfusion of baboons at 10 weeks. (From Wilson *et al.*, 2006.) Figure used with permission from Elsevier.

equates to 16 worm pairs. For CCA, the comparable values are 47 worms equating to 19 worm pairs. It is noticeable that the amounts of CCA detected by the ELISA are ~4 times the amounts of CAA detected in the same samples by the comparable ELISA. Nevertheless, CAA provides the best surrogate assay for worm burden.

The detection of CCA in patient urine and the ease of obtaining urine samples led to the development of a lateral flow (LF) assay applicable as a POC diagnostic tool (van Dam *et al.*, 2004). As a result of the COVID-19 pandemic readers will be familiar with the principle and a range of formats have been developed. In the initial assay, monoclonal antibody conjugated to carbon particles was mixed with test urine sample to create immune complexes. A nitrocellulose strip on a vinyl backing provided the matrix through which the analytes flow. A transverse line of anti-CCA monoclonal antibody was immobilized on the strip to capture any immune complexes present. A second line of anti-mouse antibody that detected the excess carbon-labelled monoclonal acted as a positive control. The test had a higher positivity for *S. mansoni* infections than duplicate KK smears and semi-quantitative scoring of the strips was feasible. It also had a high specificity and the prepared strips were stable for at least 3 months at room temperature. The CCA test has been widely used and is currently commercially available (https://www.rapid-diagnostics.com). In the standard cassette format drops of urine can be applied to the test well and the reaction read later. However, consistency and the problem of a high background threshold has limited its applicability in areas of low endemicity (Graeff-Teixeira *et al.*, 2021). At the time of writing (January 2025), Mondial Diagnostics in The Netherlands is working with international partners on an updated version of the POC-CCA test using recombinant antibodies. The aim is an improved reliability of the test with an associated higher specificity and sensitivity. See https://www.landcent.nl/schistosomiasis.

The CAA test has also undergone a period of development since its inception, not least because of it very high specificity. The CAA ELISA format was converted to a LF assay, using ultrasensitive fluorescent up-converting phosphor (UCP) reporter particles to detect CAA in serum, with the intensity of reaction determined on a portable reader (van Dam *et al.*, 2013). Serum and urine samples were pretreated with TCA to remove interfering proteins and dissociate immune complexes prior to assay. The UCP-LF assay format could detect CAA concentrations <30 pg/ml and had the added value of a dry assay design (Corstjens *et al.*, 2014). In a further improvement a larger 0.5 ml sample was concentrated in a centrifugal filter with a 10 kDa cutoff 25-fold to ~20 μl. With this format, the detection of <1.0 pg/ml is possible and the assay can be calibrated using serial dilutions of TCA extracts from adult worms. Applied to baboon serum samples with known egg counts and worm burdens, it provided a better resolution at low worm burdens than the standard CAA ELISA. Using higher urine sample concentration devices (4, 15 and 40 ml) the threshold for detection was reduced even further and the UCP-LF assay was able to detect very low-level infections in baboons as early as 3 weeks after cercarial exposure (Corstjens *et al.*, 2020). This assay, now termed the UCAA2000 signifying U for urine and 2000 for the microlitres analysed, has been applied to human samples originating in South America, Africa and Asia in locations where transmission was believed to be low or interrupted. Prevalence levels were found to be dramatically higher for *S. mansoni*, *S. japonicum*, *S. mekongi* and *S. haematobium*, compared to those based on egg microscopy of urine or stools (Fig. 12.4). This is a telling illustration of the diagnostic deficit that has to be overcome before the goal of schistosomiasis eradication can be reached.

A recent comparison of the UCP-LF assay (without concentration) for the detection of *S. mansoni* and *S. haematobium* infections in stored serum and urine samples has revealed important features of the two circulating antigens (Fig. 12.4) (Hoekstra *et al.*, 2024). CCA levels were significantly higher in *S. mansoni*- than *S. haematobium*-infected individuals, with the greatest differences in the urine. However, CAA concentrations were higher in serum than in urine, irrespective of species, providing more evidence for the disparities in molecular weights or the effect of negative charge. Given the much lower threshold for detection of CAA in the UCP-LF assay, efforts are being made to develop it as a fingerprick blood test for rapid diagnosis of all schistosome species (https://www.eliminateschisto.org/sites/gsa/files/content/attachments/2020-10-12/PR_Schisto-collab_12Oct20_FINAL.pdf).

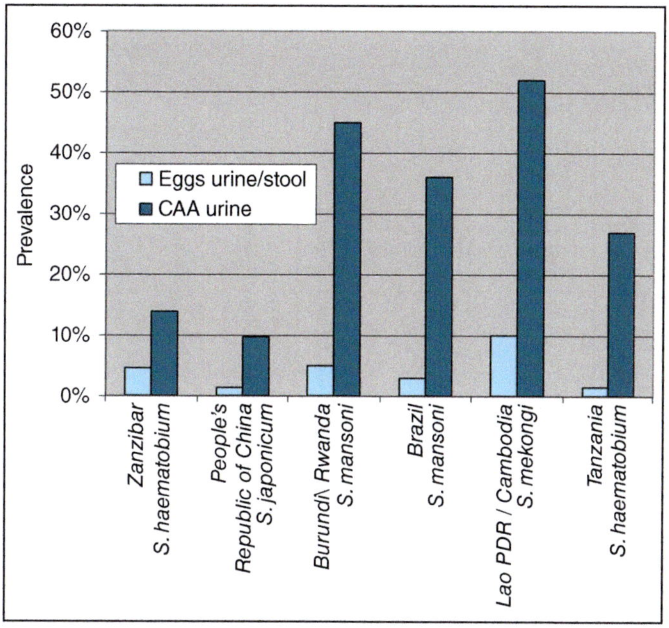

Fig. 12.4. The greater sensitivity of the CAA test across four schistosome species on three continents. A comparison of the prevalence of infection detected by schistosome eggs in urine (*S. haematobium*) or stool samples (*S. mansoni*, *S. japonicum* and *S. mekongi*) with that determined by CAA in urine using the UCAA2000 assay. The plot is © Dr Govert van Dam, Leiden University Medical Centre, Leiden, The Netherlands, reproduced with his kind permission.

12.3.2 Other worm products

The advantages of the circulating polysaccharide antigens include multiple repeating epitopes on a single molecule, the separation of the polysaccharide moieties from interfering proteins using TCA treatment and their stability in long-term storage. It is possible that schistosome eggs secrete antigens with similar properties but to date none has been identified. Some products of the subshell envelope, like IPSE and omega-1, are glycoproteins but it is very unlikely that the decorating glycan residues would be amenable to enrichment by TCA treatment. Omega-1 has enzymatic activity which might provide a means of signal amplification if present in serum (or urine). There is a range of oesophageal secreted proteins that are low molecular weight so should easily pass through the glomerular filtration barrier into Bowman's space, with potential for concentration in the kidney tubules before entry into the urine. Furthermore, peptide array screening indicates that many of these oesophageal gland proteins are immunologically unreactive, which would facilitate their persistence in the bloodstream. To date there do not appear to have been any direct proteomic analyses of urine from schistosome-infected humans that might reveal their presence.

The enzymes secreted by the gastrodermis and released into the bloodstream alongside CCA and CAA are another potential source of diagnostic molecules but little is known about their persistence in the circulation. However, one gut-derived enzyme has been tested for diagnostic potential (González *et al.*, 2016). Polyclonal rabbit antibodies were raised against a highly purified preparation of cathepsin B1.1 (Smp_103610; Sm31) and used as the capture agent on ELISA plates to bind the enzyme in positive or negative patient sera. Enzymatic activity was then assessed by addition of a chromogenic substrate and the colour read on a plate reader. It proved to be as accurate as the KK smear in identifying infected individuals. Whether this enzyme capture approach has the potential to rival circulating polysaccharides remains to be explored – it certainly provides a signal amplification step that could be the key.

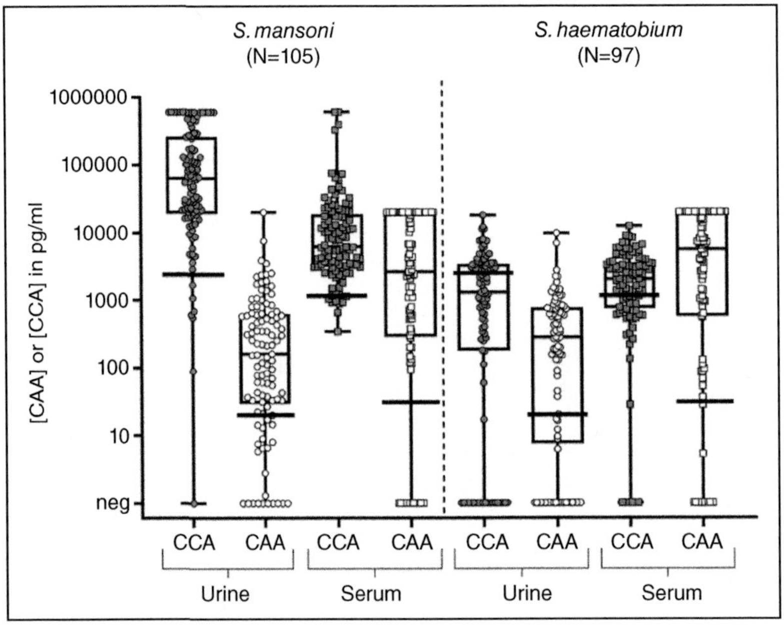

Fig. 12.5. A comparison of the efficacy of CAA and CCA. Box-and-whisker plot of circulating antigen concentrations in humans infected with *S. mansoni* or *S. haematobium.* The boxes delimit the 25th to 75th percentiles of CCA or CAA concentrations in urine (circles) and serum (squares) (note ln *y*-axis scale). The central line in each box denotes the median antigen concentration. For *S. mansoni*, the median values for CCA are 10-fold higher in urine than serum, for *S. haematobium* they are much closer. For CAA, the median serum values are >10-fold higher than those in urine. The whiskers mark the minimum and maximum antigen concentrations, and the horizontal thick lines are cutoffs above which a value is considered positive. They are a dramatic illustration of the sensitivity of CAA over CCA. The values for CCA are 2460 pg/ml for urine and 1140 pg/ml for serum. The values for CAA are 20 pg/ml for urine and 30 pg/ml for serum. (With permission from Hoekstra *et al.*, 2024.)

12.4 Anti-schistosome Antibodies

The serological diagnosis of schistosomiasis has a long history going back at least to the 1960s. Irrespective of the techniques and antigens used, the approach had serious shortcomings, not least the persistence of specific antibodies in the circulation long after the infection had terminated, either naturally or after chemotherapy. Serological diagnosis is most applicable for previously unexposed travellers returning from endemic areas, but least useful for assessing infection status in endemic populations. Nevertheless, the detection of schistosome infection via antibodies in the circulation has had its advocates and both a wide variety of antigen sources and a range of vehicles have been used to visualize the reaction. The reader is referred to a comprehensive review of the literature covering the six schistosome species infecting humans (Hinz *et al.*, 2017). The list of antigen sources includes: homogenates of cercariae, adult worms and eggs; secretions from cercariae and schistosomula; individual recombinant proteins; cryosections of adult worms; and keyhole limpet haemocyanin for its shared glycans. Techniques for detecting antibody in serum include: ELISA, indirect immunofluorescence on sections, indirect haemagglutination, immunoblotting and circumoval precipitation. The Global Schistosomiasis Alliance website lists the commercially available diagnostic tests (https://www.eliminateschisto.org/resources/diagnostics-collection).

These numerous commercial products available for detection of antibody in serum are a testament to the reality of schistosome diagnosis in a clinical setting, especially in non-endemic countries. The case of Scotland with a population of around 5.5 million, where schistosomiasis is the most frequently reported parasitic disease in travellers, well illustrates this point (Alexander *et al.*, 2018). At the central parasite diagnostic reference laboratory from 2001 to 2015, 8163 travellers were tested for schistosome IgG by ELISA using soluble egg antigen. A total of 25% was found to be seropositive, and focusing on a subset of eight African countries, 435/1284 individuals coming from Malawi (25%) and 112/279 from Uganda (40%) tested positive.

The success of mass drug administration programmes in reducing the overall prevalence of schistosomiasis to low levels has recently given the question of serological testing more prominence, especially in view of the WHO's stated aim to eliminate schistosomiasis as a public health problem. This is critical in countries like Brazil, where prevalence has been driven to low levels by public health measures, but elimination has not been achieved because the thresholds of detection mean that low-level, frequently subclinical infections are not identified. An immunoproteomic analysis of soluble egg extract identified Smp40 (α-crystallin/HSP20; see Chapter 11.3.2) as a major egg immunogen, detected by sera from both acute and chronically infected human patients (Silva-Moraes *et al.*, 2019). A recombinant version of this major egg antigen, used to coat ELISA plates, performed better than KK smears in identifying individuals with extremely low levels of infection. It was also not cross-reactive with sera from individuals infected with three soil-transmitted helminths. This may be the kind of test that needs to be incorporated into the final stages of eradication programmes, to identify cryptic infections.

In the same vein, a serological assay has been developed for CAA (Kildemoes *et al.*, 2025). In a microarray-based evaluation of a panel of representative schistosome antigens, CAA emerged as the best-performing target with overall high sensitivity (IgM ≥100% and IgG ≥97%) and specificity (IgM ≥93% and IgG ≥97%) for serological detection of primary schistosomiasis infections. This underlined the superior specificity of anti-CAA antibodies as primary infection markers, and it is anticipated that they will be pan-schistosome species specific, as CAA is excreted by several schistosome species. In contrast to CCA, anti-CAA IgG responses are much stronger, and the isotype switch from IgM manifests with an infection dose-dependent timing. Individuals exposed to 30 cercariae elicit anti-CAA IgG responses earlier and with higher titres compared to those exposed to only 10 parasites. The authors suggest that anti-CAA antibody detection can be a powerful surveillance tool in near- and post-elimination settings. Specifically, antibody detection tools fit into the WHO's Target Product Profile for diagnostics to determine when transmission has been interrupted and when to conduct post-mass drug administration surveillance. Ideally, a rapid diagnostic fingerprick anti-CAA test format would be developed, based on detection of IgG, as this shows the highest specificity. In turn the CAA target would need to be produced and validated, preferably by a chemical, enzyme-assisted or biotechnological methods; synthesis of complex glycan structures is not a trivial task.

12.5 Summary

- Historically, the detection of blood in the urine was an initial indicator of *S. haematobium* infection, still in use as a POC test.
- As an appreciation of the cryptic morbidity associated with schistosome infection increased over the last 60 years, parasitological methods to detect schistosome eggs in urine or faeces became the mainstay for direct diagnosis.
- Following the widespread use of safe and effective praziquantel chemotherapy around 1980, the intensity of infection has reduced, revealing the limitations of the parasitological methods for detection – the diagnostic deficit.
- Over the same period the sensitivity of tests to detect antigens released into the bloodstream by adult worms has increased, focusing in on the polysaccharides in gut vomitus. The unique specificity of the CAA epitope as a pan-schistosome marker and its detection in urine makes it a serious candidate for a POC test to detect infections in low intensity transmission foci.
- For *S. haematobium*, the amplification of the repeat DraI DNA sequence in urine, using isothermal amplification, has provided an alternative route to a POC diagnostic that can detect a single egg.

- For intestinal schistosomiasis, the holy grail of an ability to detect a single worm pair in an infected human has yet to be reached, even after concentration of serum or urine. There is a possibility that a mature egg product or a different gut antigen might exist, but the multi-epitope structure of the gut polysaccharides may simply make them the best candidates.
- Does detection of anti-schistosome antibodies for detection of ongoing versus previous infections have a role to play in confirming eradication? Finding an antigen target which elicited a strong detectable antibody response to a few worms, which then declined to background in the absence of worms, is a tall order.

References

Alexander, C.L., Cottom, L., Smith, K., Perrow, K., Coyne, M. *et al.* (2018) Schistosomiasis in Scottish travellers: public health importance of laboratory testing and the need for enhanced surveillance. *Journal of Public Health* 40(1), 138–145. DOI: 10.1093/pubmed/fdx024

Archer, J., Barksby, R., Pennance, T., Rostron, P., Bakar, F. *et al.* (2020) Analytical and clinical assessment of a portable, isothermal recombinase polymerase amplification (RPA) assay for the molecular diagnosis of urogenital schistosomiasis. *Molecules* 25(18), 4175. DOI: 10.3390/molecules25184175

Berggren, W.L. and Weller, T.H. (1967) Immunoelectrophoretic demonstration of specific circulating antigen in animals infected with *Schistosoma mansoni*. *The American Journal of Tropical Medicine and Hygiene* 16(5), 606–612. DOI: 10.4269/ajtmh.1967.16.606

Bergwerff, A.A., van Dam, G.J., Rotmans, J.P., Deelder, A.M., Kamerling, J.P. *et al.* (1994) The immunologically reactive part of immunopurified circulating anodic antigen from *Schistosoma mansoni* is a threonine-linked polysaccharide consisting of →6)-(β-D-GlcpA-(1→3))-β-D-GalpNAc-(1→ repeating units. *The Journal of Biological Chemistry* 269(50), 31510–31517.

Candido, R.R.F., Favero, V., Duke, M., Karl, S., Gutiérrez, L. *et al.* (2015) The affinity of magnetic microspheres for *Schistosoma* eggs. *International Journal for Parasitology* 45(1), 43–50. DOI: 10.1016/j.ijpara.2014.08.011

Castro-Borges, W. and Wilson, R.A. (2022) *Schistosome* proteomics: updates and clinical implications. *Expert Review of Proteomics* 19(4–6), 247–261. DOI: 10.1080/14789450.2022.2142565

Cheever, A.W., Torky, A.H. and Shirbiney, M. (1975) The relation of worm burden to passage of *Schistosoma haematobium* eggs in the urine of infected patients. *The American Journal of Tropical Medicine and Hygiene* 24(2), 284–288. DOI: 10.4269/ajtmh.1975.24.284

Colley, D.G., Andros, T.S. and Campbell, C.H., Jr (2017) Schistosomiasis is more prevalent than previously thought: what does it mean for public health goals, policies, strategies, guidelines and intervention programs? *Infectious Diseases of Poverty* 6(1), 63. DOI: 10.1186/s40249-017-0275-5

Corstjens, P.L.A.M., De Dood, C.J., Kornelis, D., Fat, E.M.T.K., Wilson, R.A. *et al.* (2014) Tools for diagnosis, monitoring and screening of *Schistosoma* infections utilizing lateral-flow based assays and upconverting phosphor labels. *Parasitology* 141(14), 1841–1855. DOI: 10.1017/S0031182014000626

Corstjens, P.L.A.M., de Dood, C.J., Knopp, S., Clements, M.N., Ortu, G. *et al.* (2020) Circulating anodic antigen (CAA): a highly sensitive diagnostic biomarker to detect active *Schistosoma* infections-improvement and use during SCORE. *The American Journal of Tropical Medicine and Hygiene* 103(1_Suppl.), 50–57. DOI: 10.4269/ajtmh.19-0819

de Jonge, N., Kremsner, P.G., Krijger, F.W., Schommer, G., Fillié, Y.E. *et al.* (1990) Detection of the *Schistosome* circulating cathodic antigen by enzyme immunoassay using biotinylated monoclonal antibodies. *Transactions of the Royal Society of Tropical Medicine and Hygiene* 84(6), 815–818. DOI: 10.1016/0035-9203(90)90094-u

Deelder, A.M., Klappe, H.T., van den Aardweg, G.J. and van Meerbeke, E.H. (1976) *Schistosoma mansoni*: demonstration of two circulating antigens in infected hamsters. *Experimental Parasitology* 40(2), 189–197. DOI: 10.1016/0014-4894(76)90081-3

Deelder, A.M., De Jonge, N., Boerman, O.C., Fillié, Y.E., Hilberath, G.W. *et al.* (1989) Sensitive determination of circulating anodic antigen in *Schistosoma mansoni* infected individuals by an enzyme-linked immunosorbent assay using monoclonal antibodies. *The American Journal of Tropical Medicine and Hygiene* 40(3), 268–272. DOI: 10.4269/ajtmh.1989.40.268

Donnelly, O., Mesquita, S., Archer, J., Ali, S.M., Bartonicek, Z. *et al.* (2024) Refining the *Schistosoma haematobium* recombinase polymerase amplification (Sh-RPA) assay: moving towards point-of-care use in endemic settings. *Parasites & Vectors* 17(1), 321. DOI: 10.1186/s13071-024-06380-9

Eberl, M., al-Sherbiny, M., Hagan, P., Ljubojevic, S., Thomas, A.W. *et al.* (2002) A novel and sensitive method to monitor helminth infections by faecal sampling. *Acta Tropica* 83(2), 183–187. DOI: 10.1016/s0001-706x(02)00089-x

Fagundes Teixeira, C., Neuhauss, E., Ben, R., Romanzini, J. and Graeff-Teixeira, C. (2007) Detection of *Schistosoma mansoni* eggs in feces through their interaction with paramagnetic beads in a magnetic field. *PLoS Neglected Tropical Diseases* 1(2), e73. DOI: 10.1371/journal.pntd.0000073

Feldmeier, H., Nogueira-Queiroz, J.A., Peixoto-Queiroz, M.A. and Doehring, E. (1986) Detection and quantification of circulating antigen in schistosomiasis by monoclonal antibody. II. The quantification of circulating antigens in human schistosomiasis mansoni and haematobium: relationship to intensity of infection and disease status. *Clinical and Experimental Immunology* 65, 232–243.

Glinz, D., Silué, K.D., Knopp, S., Lohourignon, L.K., Yao, K.P. *et al.* (2010) Comparing diagnostic accuracy of Kato-Katz, Koga agar plate, ether-concentration, and FLOTAC for *Schistosoma mansoni* and soil-transmitted helminths. *PLoS Neglected Tropical Diseases* 4(7), e754. DOI: 10.1371/journal.pntd.0000754

Gonnert, R. and Andrews, P. (1977) Praziquantel, a new broad-spectrum antischistosomal agent. *Zeitschrift für Parasitenkunde* 52(2), 129–150. DOI: 10.1007/BF00389899

González, A.Y., Sulbarán, G.S., Ballen, D.E. and Cesari, I.M. (2016) Immunocapture of circulating *Schistosoma mansoni* cathepsin B antigen (Sm31) by anti-Sm31 polyclonal antibodies. *Parasitology International* 65(3), 191–195. DOI: 10.1016/j.parint.2015.12.008

Graeff-Teixeira, C., Favero, V., Pascoal, V.F., de Souza, R.P., Rigo, F. de V. *et al.* (2021) Low specificity of point-of-care circulating cathodic antigen (POCCCA) diagnostic test in a non-endemic area for schistosomiasis mansoni in Brazil. *Acta Tropica* 217, 105863. DOI: 10.1016/j.actatropica.2021.105863

Halili, S., Grant, J.R., Pilotte, N., Gordon, C.A. and Williams, S.A. (2021) Development of a novel real-time polymerase chain reaction assay for the sensitive detection of *Schistosoma japonicum* in human stool. *PLoS Neglected Tropical Diseases* 15(10), e0009877. DOI: 10.1371/journal.pntd.0009877

Hamburger, J., Turetski, T., Kapeller, I. and Deresiewicz, R. (1991) Highly repeated short DNA sequences in the genome of *Schistosoma mansoni* recognized by a species-specific probe. *Molecular and Biochemical Parasitology* 44(1), 73–80. DOI: 10.1016/0166-6851(91)90222-R

Hamburger, J., He, N., Abbasi, I., Ramzy, R.M., Jourdane, J. *et al.* (2001) Polymerase chain reaction assay based on a highly repeated sequence of *Schistosoma haematobium*: a potential tool for monitoring schistosome-infested water. *The American Journal of Tropical Medicine and Hygiene* 65(6), 907–911. DOI: 10.4269/ajtmh.2001.65.907

Hinz, R., Schwarz, N.G., Hahn, A. and Frickmann, H. (2017) Serological approaches for the diagnosis of schistosomiasis – a review. *Molecular and Cellular Probes* 31, 2–21. DOI: 10.1016/j.mcp.2016.12.003

Hoekstra, P.T., de Dood, C.J., Abdoel, T., Hilt, S., van Diepen, A. *et al.* (2024) Detecting two *Schistosoma* circulating antigens – CCA and CAA – in urine and serum to improve diagnosis of human schistosomiasis. *Frontiers in Parasitology* 3, 1460331. DOI: 10.3389/fpara.2024.1460331

Karl, S., Gutiérrez, L., Lucyk-Maurer, R., Kerr, R., Candido, R.R.F. *et al.* (2013) The iron distribution and magnetic properties of *Schistosome* eggshells: implications for improved diagnostics. *PLoS Neglected Tropical Diseases* 7(5), e2219. DOI: 10.1371/journal.pntd.0002219

Keller, D., Rothen, J., Dangy, J.P., Saner, C., Daubenberger, C. *et al.* (2020) Performance of a real-time PCR approach for diagnosing *Schistosoma haematobium* infections of different intensity in urine samples from Zanzibar. *Infectious Diseases of Poverty* 9(1), 128. DOI: 10.1186/s40249-020-00726-y

Kildemoes, A.O., Veldhuizen, T., Hilt, S.T., van Lieshout, L., Supali, T. *et al.* (2025) Identification of a circulating carbohydrate antigen as a highly specific and sensitive target for schistosomiasis serology. *Journal of Clinical Microbiology* 63(2), e0100824. DOI: 10.1128/jcm.01008-24

Köhler, G. and Milstein, C. (1976) Derivation of specific antibody-producing tissue culture and tumor lines by cell fusion. *European Journal of Immunology* 6(7), 511–519. DOI: 10.1002/eji.1830060713

Magalhães, F. do C., Resende, S.D., Senra, C., Graeff-Teixeira, C., Enk, M.J. *et al.* (2020) Accuracy of real-time polymerase chain reaction to detect *Schistosoma mansoni*-infected individuals from an endemic area with low parasite loads. *Parasitology* 147(10), 1140–1148. DOI: 10.1017/S003118202000089X

Mesquita, S.G., Donnelly, O., Archer, J., Lugli, E.B. and Webster, B. (2025) Advances in the recombinase polymerase amplification platform for urogenital schistosomiasis diagnosis (ShDraI-RPA) towards implementation at the point-of-care. *Scientific Reports* 15(1), 13590. DOI: 10.1038/s41598-025-95887-x

Nash, T.E. (1974) Localization of the circulating antigen within the gut of *Schistosoma mansoni*. *The American Journal of Tropical Medicine and Hygiene* 23(6), 1085–1087. DOI: 10.4269/ajtmh.1974.23.1085

Nash, T.E., Prescott, B. and Neva, F.A. (1974) The characteristics of a circulating antigen in schistosomiasis. *Journal of Immunology* 112(4), 1500–1507. DOI: 10.4049/jimmunol.112.4.1500

Obeng, B.B., Aryeetey, Y.A., de Dood, C.J., Amoah, A.S., Larbi, I.A. *et al.* (2008) Application of a circulating-cathodic-antigen (CCA) strip test and real-time PCR, in comparison with microscopy, for the detection of *Schistosoma haematobium* in urine samples from Ghana. *Annals of Tropical Medicine and Parasitology* 102(7), 625–633. DOI: 10.1179/136485908X337490

Ogongo, P., Kariuki, T.M. and Wilson, R.A. (2018) Diagnosis of schistosomiasis mansoni: an evaluation of existing methods and research towards single worm pair detection. *Parasitology* 145(11), 1355–1366. DOI: 10.1017/S0031182018000240

Pontes, L.A., Dias-Neto, E. and Rabello, A. (2002) Detection by polymerase chain reaction of *Schistosoma mansoni* DNA in human serum and feces. *The American Journal of Tropical Medicine and Hygiene* 66(2), 157–162. DOI: 10.4269/ajtmh.2002.66.157

Rose, C., Parker, A., Jefferson, B. and Cartmell, E. (2015) The characterization of feces and urine: a review of the literature to inform advanced treatment technology. *Critical Reviews in Environmental Science and Technology* 45(17), 1827–1879. DOI: 10.1080/10643389.2014.1000761

Savioli, L., Hatz, C., Dixon, H., Kisumku, U.M. and Mott, K.E. (1990) Control of morbidity due to *Schistosoma haematobium* on Pemba Island: egg excretion and hematuria as indicators of infection. *The American Journal of Tropical Medicine and Hygiene* 43(3), 289–295. DOI: 10.4269/ajtmh.1990.43.289

Silva-Moraes, V., Shollenberger, L.M., Castro-Borges, W., Rabello, A.L.T., Harn, D.A. *et al.* (2019) Serological proteomic screening and evaluation of a recombinant egg antigen for the diagnosis of low-intensity *Schistosoma mansoni* infections in endemic area in Brazil. *PLoS Neglected Tropical Diseases* 13(3), e0006974. DOI: 10.1371/journal.pntd.0006974

van Dam, G.J., Bergwerff, A.A., Thomas-Oates, J.E., Rotmans, J.P., Kamerling, J.P. *et al.* (1994) The immunologically reactive *O*-linked polysaccharide chains derived from circulating cathodic antigen isolated from the human blood fluke *Schistosoma mansoni* have Lewis x as repeating unit. *European Journal of Biochemistry* 225(1), 467–482. DOI: 10.1111/j.1432-1033.1994.00467.x

van Dam, G.J, Wichers, J.H., Ferreira, T.M.F., Ghati, D., van Amerongen, A. *et al.* (2004) Diagnosis of schistosomiasis by reagent strip test for detection of circulating cathodic antigen. *Journal of Clinical Microbiology* 42(12), 5458–5461. DOI: 10.1128/JCM.42.12.5458-5461.2004

van Dam, G.J., de Dood, C.J., Lewis, M., Deelder, A.M., van Lieshout, L. *et al.* (2013) A robust dry reagent lateral flow assay for diagnosis of active schistosomiasis by detection of *Schistosoma* circulating anodic antigen. *Experimental Parasitology* 135(2), 274–282. DOI: 10.1016/j.exppara.2013.06.017

Van Lieshout, L., De Jonge, N., el Masry, N.A., Mansour, M.M., Krijger, F.W. *et al.* (1992) Improved diagnostic performance of the circulating antigen assay in human schistosomiasis by parallel testing for circulating anodic and cathodic antigens in serum and urine. *The American Journal of Tropical Medicine and Hygiene* 47(4), 463–469. DOI: 10.4269/ajtmh.1992.47.463

Voller, A., Bidwell, D.E. and Bartlett, A. (1979) *The Enzyme Linked Immunosorbent Assay (ELISA): A Guide with Abstracts of Microplate Applications*. Dynatech Laboratories, Alexandria, VA.

Wilson, R.A., van Dam, G.J., Kariuki, T.M., Farah, I.O., Deelder, A.M. *et al.* (2006) The detection limits for estimates of infection intensity in *Schistosomiasis mansoni* established by a study in non-human primates. *International Journal for Parasitology* 36(12), 1241–1244. DOI: 10.1016/j.ijpara.2006.07.002

Index

Note: Page numbers in **bold** type refer to **figures**; page numbers in *italic* type refer to *tables*

Printed and bound by CPI Group (UK) Ltd, Croydon, CR0 4YY
13/09/2026
14961117-0004